AF747010

Communicating about Risks and Safe Use of Medicines

Priya Bahri
Editor

Communicating about Risks and Safe Use of Medicines

Real Life and Applied Research

Adis

Editor
Priya Bahri
European Medicines Agency (EMA)
Amsterdam, Noord-Holland
The Netherlands

ISBN 978-981-15-3012-8 ISBN 978-981-15-3013-5 (eBook)
https://doi.org/10.1007/978-981-15-3013-5

© Springer Nature Singapore Pte Ltd. 2020
This work is subject to copyright. All rights are reserved by the Publisher, whether the whole or part of the material is concerned, specifically the rights of translation, reprinting, reuse of illustrations, recitation, broadcasting, reproduction on microfilms or in any other physical way, and transmission or information storage and retrieval, electronic adaptation, computer software, or by similar or dissimilar methodology now known or hereafter developed.
The use of general descriptive names, registered names, trademarks, service marks, etc. in this publication does not imply, even in the absence of a specific statement, that such names are exempt from the relevant protective laws and regulations and therefore free for general use.
The publisher, the authors, and the editors are safe to assume that the advice and information in this book are believed to be true and accurate at the date of publication. Neither the publisher nor the authors or the editors give a warranty, expressed or implied, with respect to the material contained herein or for any errors or omissions that may have been made. The publisher remains neutral with regard to jurisdictional claims in published maps and institutional affiliations.

Adis is a brand of Springer

This Adis imprint is published by the registered company Springer Nature Singapore Pte Ltd.
The registered company address is: 152 Beach Road, #21-01/04 Gateway East, Singapore 189721, Singapore

Foreword

Communicating about Risks and Safe Use of Medicines: Real Life and Applied Research offers an encompassing vision for fulfilling the duty to inform that accompanies all use of medicines. It begins with case studies that demonstrate the complexity of such communications and serve as an antidote to simplistic, box-checking approaches. By featuring cases from around the world, it shows the universality of these decisions and the value of the international community of collaborators that it seeks to empower. It also shows the richness of the social and cultural context that must be addressed when tailoring communications to any setting. These chapters are good reading on their own, even for spectators.

Having shown that responsible communication is complicated, the book then shows that it is not impossibly so. It offers chapters summarizing the research on essential ingredients for successful communication in accessible form. A theme common to these chapters is the need for evidence. Professionals who know the research will have better intuitions about identifying the information that people want and need, designing and delivering it, and creating trusted, respectful relations with those who depend on them. However, those are still but intuitions, which need to be evaluated empirically with people who depend on them.

These chapters on the science are bracketed by ones describing the ethical and legal constraints that circumscribe the place of communications about medicines in society. They lead to a concluding chapter on patients' role in shaping communications to serve their interests. The ethical and legal chapters show the importance of such active participation. The scientific chapters show its feasibility. Together, they dispel any sense, or claim, that decisions about medicines should be left to professionals because laypeople cannot handle them. The science creates opportunities to understand and aid people in situations where their behavior may seem refractory without it.

This book also sets out a challenge: How to mobilize all the forms of expertise needed to fulfill the duty to inform. Even the best summary of a field cannot afford competence in it. However, it can provide the common language needed for collaboration among experts and practitioners. By facilitating an intellectually and culturally diverse community of individuals committed to this mission,

Communicating about Risks and Safe Use of Medicines may also facilitate convincing governments, firms, and healthcare systems to provide the resources for that community to do its work.

Pittsburgh, PA, USA
May 2019

Baruch Fischhoff

Preface: Guide to Readers

Dear Reader,

There are many ways to read and use this book. You may read it from the beginning to the end to follow its logical built-up or start with any chapter that catches your interest. Each chapter is self-standing and understandable in its own right. The chapters are cross-referenced and held together not only by a common vision for patient-centred care, but the methods presented in Chaps. 6–15 of Part II on the various scientific disciplines are all seen as belonging to a multidisciplinary approach to research.

A framework in which multiple disciplines can come together to collaborate and complement each other for getting a fuller understanding of medicinal product risk communication and the causality of communication and outcomes is set out in Chap. 1. A visualisation of this multilayered research framework for establishing humanities and epidemiology of medicinal product risk communication is provided in Fig. 1.1. Typologies of communication events and outcomes are added in Tables 1.1 and 1.2 to lay the groundwork for collaborative research across disciplines. Chap. 1 also explains the overall terminology used in the book and touches upon some terminological discrepancies, which exist between disciplines, research governance systems, and jurisdictions regarding the regulation of medicines.

The scientific disciplines included have been selected for being highly relevant at the present time to progress this research field. However, the contributions and potential of other disciplines of the medical humanities, social sciences, neurosciences, and health services research need to be explored in the future. As the chapters have been written for researchers from different disciplines as well as for readers with a general interest in the topic, attention has been given to explaining terms and concepts in a way that is accessible without having prior knowledge in the given discipline. Please forgive the authors and me as editor that despite all efforts there may still be parts of the book where easy accessibility has not been achieved, although this is ironic for a book aiming at improving communication, I admit.

Part I contains Chaps. 2–5 on major real-life communication experiences with hormonal contraceptives, COX-2 inhibitors, isotretinoin, and pandemic influenza vaccines. These chapters reflect more deeply on some of the key experiences introduced in Chap. 1. Anybody who wants to start reading the book with a taste of what the complexity and challenges feel like for those in charge of medicines safety and communication should pick one of these chapters first before reading about the methods in Part II, where one can see how particular methods can generate the evidence for overcoming the challenges and improving communication. Understanding the historical experiences is important for current and future communication practitioners, policy-makers, and researchers, as these have influenced current communication practices and policies, and the lessons learnt should not be forgotten in the future.

While this book aims at being comprehensive, it is at the same time far from complete. I have collected many more examples, research articles, and evaluation frameworks that I could possibly review and incorporate, as communication, in simple words, is life, and the aspects to consider seem indefinite. In fact, all authors had to select a focus and could not address all aspects of their discipline. Any omission of aspects and existing work that could have been discussed and referenced should therefore not be understood as a deliberate exclusion from the book. Rather, we need to accept this as a human limitation to understanding or synthesising everything at a given moment in time. In order to provide an overview of the current evidence as well as gaps in evidence and evidence-generating methods, Table 1.3 has extracted the relevant review articles. Being more inclusive and at the same time filtering out less relevant items, to keep the reading of the content and its application in studies manageable, will be another task for developing medicinal product risk communication research in the future.

Please accept that this book will not answer all the questions you may have about medicinal product risk communication research as it is not a textbook or research guide on any of the methods presented. It rather intends to introduce you to methods you might not yet have heard about, or have only a vague awareness, or are familiar with in a different context. It will guide you to resources to consult, should a method appear useful for your research endeavour. Actually, the book might leave you with even more questions, and if so, I hope they will not be questions of confusion, but questions born of curiosity and motivation to understand more and develop your research interests.

If you are among those who deal with the communication challenges in your profession, please do not take any critique you may find in this book as blame. Instead, we are coming together as researchers to understand each other's contributions and improve things together, as ultimately, we all remain learners.

If you are a patient, healthcare professional, communication practitioner, or journalist, I am most delighted that you want to read this book, which might seem to be addressed only to formal researchers. It is definitely not! This book is about patient-centred care, and those interacting with patients and those caring for them, or people in general—as we all can be patients tomorrow—have major knowledge about communication and what works and feels good, and what does not, which should be collected and analysed. Of course, the patients themselves have information interests and needs as well as communication expectations, which they may consider be fulfilled or not. Chaps. 1 and 16 therefore close the research circuit by discussing how patients can involve themselves in research for planning and evaluating communication events.

As you will see, most examples come from high-income regions of the world, and even for those regions, countries with research published in languages other than English will be underrepresented. There is generally less medicinal product risk communication research available in middle- and low-income countries, but effort has been made for this book to find and reference examples from these countries too. It has also to be stressed that less published research does not mean that there are no good communication practices in these countries; the contrary may be the case. Public health campaigns, traditional communication channels embedded in contemporary culture, and local creative measures using modern technology can be highly effective, as has been learnt through conferences and personal encounters. It is my hope that this book will support collaborative research across regions and mutual learning on best communication practices.

Finally, the most exciting way to read this book might be to go to the index at the end, find a key word you do not know or are surprised about, and see to which chapter and aspects it brings you. This is the way I often enjoyed reading books during most of my student years, and I still do so. In digital times where we use search functions for documents on our computers, an index might be forgotten as a useful tool. Considerable time has been invested in this index to allow you to quickly find concepts and methods that you are most familiar with as your entry point, or examples from your world region or class of medicines you are interested in. As the authors come from different disciplines and countries, they are used to different terms, and while some terms have been harmonised across the book, most had to stay with the term known in their disciplines. Therefore, the index refers readers between key words, which sometimes are synonyms, but more often are related concepts, and the degrees of their distinctiveness, overlap, or identical meaning remain open for the time being. Reading across chapters along related concepts is another way the book may support multidisciplinary research collaborations. Hopefully, in the future, we will come to consensus on terms for greater clarity.

Each chapter has been complemented with an abstract at the beginning, which summarises the scope of the chapter, and bullet-pointed conclusions at the end, which are supposed to serve quick repetition of the key contents after reading the chapter, and also as a reminder, should you want to refresh your memory of the chapter later on.

May you find your own way of reading this book as you enjoy it best and gain the most for your interests and for our joint progress in the field.

Amsterdam, Netherlands   Priya Bahri
December 2019

Editor's Acknowledgements

This book has been a special journey of research and exchange between many colleagues and friends.

It began with Nitin Joshi, chief editor of the journal *Drug Safety* at Springer Nature, approaching me with the suggestion to edit a book on medicines risk communication, and I convey my thanks to him, as well as to Bert Leufkens and Brian Taylor for their immediate encouragement and support throughout. Specifically, thanks go to Bert for his idea to name the research framework I have developed in my chapter "multilayered", and to Alex Dodoo, University of Ghana, for stressing the need to establish with this book medicinal product risk communication practice and research as a self-standing discipline. I thank Patrick Waller, specialist in pharmacovigilance and pharmacoepidemiology, Kornelia Grein, scientific-regulatory specialist, and Andrew Brown, specialist in health systems strengthening, for their most helpful advice; Marion Schaefer, Humboldt University of Berlin, and Jamie Wilkinson, at the time at the Pharmaceutical Group of the European Union (PGEU), for reflecting with me on the role of the pharmacist in communication research; Jeffrey Aronson, University of Oxford, for increasing my awareness of language aspects relevant to pharmacovigilance; and Lorna Woods, University of Essex, for enhancing my understanding on legal aspects of social media research. Thanks are also conveyed to the Springer Nature team, in particular to Palani Murugesan, Rajesh Gopalakrishnan, Jo Grant, and previously Cam Wright, as well as my graphic designer Angelika Keck for bringing the book out in its beautiful printed and online formats.

Looking back to the time long before this book was foreseeable, I want to express my thanks to Bruce Hugman, Uppsala Monitoring Centre, and Benjamin Lozare, Johns Hopkins University, and his colleagues for their teaching on health communication and firm belief and experience that communication can bring positive change; as well as to Ragnar Löfstedt, King's College London, and Frédéric Bouder, now University of Stavanger, and their colleagues for the enriching conferences and discussions on risk communication—all that I learnt from them prepared me for undertaking this book. Thanks are also due to Mira Harrison-Woolrych, as we co-edited the *Drug Safety* special theme edition on risk communication in 2012, and to all its authors, who jointly provided a comprehensive picture of the still current challenges of medicinal product risk communication—this theme edition has been the starting point for the book. Thanks also go to my colleagues at the US Food and

Drug Administration, who hosted me for a fellowship in 2012—they gave me valuable insights into risk communication from the perspectives of their multiple departments. And I do not want to forget late Giampaolo Velo, University of Verona, who as a pharmacologist was so visionary about communication that he convened regular international expert meetings at the Ettore Majorana Foundation and Centre for Scientific Culture in Erice, resulting in the fundamental *Erice Declaration on Effective Communications in Pharmacovigilance* of 1997 and further statements during the following 20 years—I am glad that he involved me in 2009 and let me find my special community.

Moreover, I feel amazed and grateful for having had the opportunity to work with and learn from so many colleagues at the European Medicines Agency (EMA) and the whole regulatory network of the European Union across its member states as well as all those I met through collaborations with the World Health Organization (WHO) and the Council for International Organizations of Medical Sciences (CIOMS)—it has always been our common goal to inform patients, healthcare professionals, and the general public on the risks and safe use of medicines, including vaccines, as best as possible, and our shared work and discussions over many years on the challenges, solutions found in the different settings and open questions have been an immense experience.

I am, of course, most grateful to all authors who embraced the vision of this book without hesitation and had the enthusiasm to be part of it and work so diligently, applying their expertise to this still rather new field of medicinal product risk communication research and sometimes even conducting original research for their chapters. I enjoyed very much working together and discovering something wonderful in each of them—some I have known for a long time, and some I crossed ways with, as destiny had it, while I was developing the concept, structure, and contents of the book. It has been important to me that in the early days of conceptualisation Baruch Fischhoff reassured me that a book that brings together methods across sciences is needed for progress, and his foreword is a special honour for the book, as is the afterword from Nilima Kshirsagar, endorsing its global relevance and applicability.

Last but not least I thank my parents, family, friends, fellow dancers, and also the people with whom I could only share a shortest moment in time, as life is the greatest teacher on communicating and loving.

The journey of this book shall not end with its publication, but the book is meant to serve as a platform where anybody who is passionate about supporting and empowering people when using medicines and wants to do or contribute to research in this field can hopefully find know-how and inspiration to move on in collaboration with scientists from other disciplines. I look forward to continuing the journey together and progressing medicinal product risk communication research.

Contents in Chapters

Part II: Tackling the Challenges: Methods for Medicinal Product Risk Communication Research

Contents

About the Authors

Priya Bahri holds degrees in pharmacy and epidemiology, focused her PhD at Humboldt University of Berlin on healthcare quality management, and is trained in strategic communication and global health diplomacy. She worked in pharmacies and for projects of health insurance physicians' associations and the German international development agency before joining the European Medicines Agency (EMA) in 1996 and specialising in pharmacovigilance. She is active for the Utrecht WHO Collaborating Centre for Pharmaceutical Policy and Regulation and also in learned societies, including as fellow of the International Society of Pharmacovigilance.

Michael A. Cacciatore has a research focus on science topics and the framing of risks in traditional and social media. His work analyses how science and risk information is presented to audiences and how audiences make sense of that information based on their values. The research has been published in *Public Understanding of Science*, *Science Communication*, *New Media & Society and Risk Analysis*, among others. He is assistant professor at the Grady College of Journalism and Mass Communication, University of Georgia, United States.

Ineke Crijns graduated from the Medical School of the University of Nijmegen, Netherlands, and worked as a physician and was in leading positions for pharmaceutical companies. Since 2000, she has been a (senior) assessor at the Dutch Medicines Evaluation Board, and from 2001 to 2009 she was the (alternate) Dutch member of the Pharmacovigilance Working Party at the European Medicines Agency (EMA). In her PhD, she investigated the pregnancy prevention programme for isotretinoin, and she is a known expert on medicines in pregnancy.

Nabarun Dasgupta is an epidemiologist who studies the use and adverse effects of medicines, with a focus on controlled substances. He has worked with WHO, non-profit organisations, health departments, and pharmaceutical industry. He was co-founder of surveillance and harm prevention systems in the United States, including the RADARS System, Project Lazarus, and Epidemico, which developed the reporting app MedWatcher and MedWatcher Social for making use of social media data. He now is adjunct professor of epidemiology at the Eshelman School of Pharmacy, University of North Carolina.

Nicola Diviani holds a PhD in communication sciences from the Università della Svizzera italiana and conducted research on health communication at the Harvard School of Public Health, United States, and at the Amsterdam School of Communication Research, Netherlands. Currently, he is postdoctoral researcher and lecturer at the University of Lucerne, Switzerland, Department of Health Sciences and Medicine and at Swiss Paraplegic Research, Person-Centered Health Care and Health Communication Group.

Maddalena Fiordelli is researcher and lecturer at the Faculty of Communication Sciences at the Università della Svizzera italiana, where she obtained her PhD in 2009. During her PhD, she was visiting scholar at the University of Amsterdam, Netherlands. Her research interests include eHealth, mHealth, participatory research, and social isolation. She collaborates with the Faculty of BioMedicine and Swiss Paraplegic Research. Since 2019, she is the treasurer of EACH, the International Association for Communication in Healthcare.

Baruch Fischhoff holds degrees in mathematics and psychology from the United States and Israel and now is the Howard Heinz University professor at the Institute for Politics and Strategy and Department of Engineering and Public Policy at Carnegie Mellon University, Pittsburgh. He is a member of the US National Academy of Sciences and the US National Academy of Medicine, and a fellow of several societies. He was founding chair of the US Food and Drug Administration Risk Communication Advisory Committee.

Jörg Fuchs is a professional advocating for user-friendly information for medicines, readability and usability tests and related research across the field of regulatory affairs. Having completed pharmacy studies at Greifswald University, Germany, in 1996, he immediately applied himself to research for improving and testing patient information leaflets. This work led to a PhD at Humboldt University of Berlin. Since 2005, his research has been continued at the Department of Drug Regulatory Affairs at the University of Bonn and activities at PAINT-Consult.

Kerr Grieve is a research fellow at the Medicines Monitoring Unit (MEMO) at Ninewells Hospital and Medical School, belonging to the University of Dundee, Scotland, United Kingdom. He is a hospital physician who is training in clinical neurology, and his research interests lie in the interaction between observational research and clinical trial design. He is also interested in regulation of medicines and post-authorisation safety surveillance.

François Houÿez is director of Treatment Information and Access at the European Organisation for Rare Diseases (Eurordis). He has been working in patient advocacy since the early 1990s, first in HIV/AIDS and since 2003 in rare diseases. His European and international expertise includes community advisory boards, cross-border care, compassionate use, shortages and repurposing of medicines, as well as regulatory and health technology assessment activities, in particular marketing authorisation, pharmacovigilance, pricing, and reimbursement.

Emilie Karafillakis is a research fellow with the global Vaccine Confidence Project at the London School of Hygiene & Tropical Medicine, United Kingdom. Her work focuses on understanding determinants of vaccine hesitancy and levels of confidence in vaccination in parents, adolescents, pregnant women, and healthcare workers, in particular in Europe. Her research interests include human papillomavirus vaccination, the role of social media in spreading concerns, and communication strategies.

Nilima A. Kshirsagar holds a medical postgraduate degree, a doctorate, and fellowships of learned societies in India, the United Kingdom, and the United States. She has over 40 years of experience and received national and international awards. She is the National Chair of Clinical Pharmacology of the Indian Council of Medical Research, member of the WHO Advisory Committee on Safety of Medicinal Products, the Scientific Advisory Committee of the Drugs for Neglected Diseases initiative (DNDi), and further chairs and contributes to several national and international committees.

Heidi Larson is professor of anthropology, risk and decision science at the London School of Hygiene & Tropical Medicine, United Kingdom, clinical professor at the Department of Health Metrics Sciences, University of Washington, United States, and director of the global Vaccine Confidence Project. Her research focuses on social and political factors affecting acceptance of health interventions. She previously headed Global Immunisation Communication at UNICEF, and she has served in advisory groups for the European Union, US Food and Drug Administration and WHO.

Teresa Leonardo Alves studied pharmaceutical sciences in Porto, Portugal, and holds an MPH from the Netherlands Institute of Health Sciences as well as a PhD in pharmaceutical policy from Utrecht University, Netherlands. Teresa has more than 15 years of experience in the coordination and public relations of not-for-profit organisations in project management, communications, and evidence-based policy advocacy. From 2012 to 2017, she was international policy advisor for the medical bulletin *Prescrire* in Paris, France.

Hubert G. Leufkens is trained in pharmaceutical sciences and epidemiology. His research aims at gaining deep insight on why and how medicines are developed, regulated, and used in clinical practice. After his positions as professor of pharmacoepidemiology and chair of the Dutch Medicines Evaluation Board, he is now professor of pharmaceutical policy and regulatory science as well as scientific director of the Utrecht WHO Collaborating Centre for Pharmaceutical Policy and Regulation, Netherlands. He has been active at several European Union and international platforms.

Thomas M. MacDonald is professor of clinical pharmacology and pharmacoepidemiology and honorary consultant physician at the University of Dundee, Scotland, United Kingdom. He is also the director of its Medicines Monitoring Unit (MEMO) and Hypertension Research Centre, and member of the European Network of Centres for Pharmacoepidemiology and Pharmacovigilance (ENCePP). He has been principal investigator of large, multi-national safety studies, and his research focus includes hypertension, cardiovascular disorders, and safety of medicines, especially of non-steroidal anti-inflammatory drugs.

Barbara Mintzes is a senior lecturer in the Faculty of Pharmacy and Charles Perkins Centre at the University of Sydney, Australia, and Affiliate Associate Professor at the School of Population and Public Health, University of British Columbia, Canada. A key focus of her research is on effects of promotion of medicines, including direct-to-consumer advertising, on medicine use. She has worked for many years with consumer and women's health groups.

Mathias Møllebæk is a PhD fellow at the Copenhagen Centre for Regulatory Science at the University of Copenhagen, Denmark. His research examines the effectiveness of regulatory medicines risk communication using qualitative methodologies and rhetorical theory. He holds an MA in rhetoric from the University of Copenhagen and has been a visiting graduate student at the University of Texas at Austin, United States. He has previously worked as a public relations and communication consultant in public and private sectors.

S. Anne Moorhead is lecturer and director of courses in health communication at the School of Communication at Ulster University, Northern Ireland, United Kingdom. She has an MA in psychology, an MSc in nutrition and dietetics, and a PhD in biomedical sciences and is an accredited healthcare communicator. She is senior fellow of the UK Higher Education Academy and member in research and ethics committees. She is board member and section editor for the *Journal of Medical Internet Research*.

Elaine H. Morrato was associate dean and professor at the Colorado School of Public Health, United States, before being appointed founding dean of the Parkinson School of Health Sciences and Public Health at Loyola University Chicago in 2020. Her research focuses on accelerating the translation of medical innovation and drug warnings into clinical practice. She has advised the US Food and Drug Administration on issues of risk communication and management. Her commercialisation experience as a product development manager in a pharmaceutical company informs her research and practice.

Sérgio Nishioka is a physician and infectious disease specialist with a PhD in epidemiology. He worked as a lecturer at the Universidade Federal de Uberlandia, Brazil, at Anvisa, the Brazilian medicines regulatory authority—first responsible for the registration of new medicines and clinical trial authorisation and later for post-marketing surveillance—and at WHO for vaccine prequalification. In 2015, he became coordinator at the Department of Communicable Disease Surveillance at the Ministry of Health, and now is a consultant.

Glen J. Nowak has his research focus on health communication, social marketing, and infectious disease prevention. He is the author or co-author of 40 peer-reviewed journal articles, including articles in *Social Marketing Quarterly*, *Journal of Health Communication*, and *Vaccine*. He spent 14 years with the US Centers for Disease Control and Prevention, including 6 years as the media relations director. He is now professor at the Grady College of Journalism and Mass Communication, University of Georgia, United States, and director of the College's new Center for Health and Risk Communication.

Carrie Pierce pioneers artificial intelligence-powered capabilities and novel data sources for pharmacovigilance. Previously at Booz Allen Hamilton, United States, she oversaw the development of data collection, data processing, and crowdsourcing tools for product safety surveillance and risk communication. She worked with pharmaceutical companies and regulatory authorities on applying pharmacovigilance standards to social media data and served as an expert for academia and other organisations in the United States and Europe. She holds a BA from New York University and a dual MBA and MPH from Boston University.

Amy Rogers is a physician trained as a general practitioner (GP) and now working in safety and effectiveness research with the Medicines Monitoring Unit (MEMO) at Ninewells Hospital and Medical School, belonging to the University of Dundee, Scotland, United Kingdom. Her special interests include novel methodologies in comparative effectiveness research and the integration of such research into evidence-based healthcare. As a GP, she has experienced the challenges of effective risk communication in facilitating shared decision-making with diverse patient populations.

Sara Rubinelli holds a degree in classics and philosophy from the Catholic University of Milan, Italy, and a PhD from the University of Leeds, United Kingdom, in the areas of argumentation theory, persuasion, and rhetoric. She is associate professor in health sciences at the Department of Health Sciences and Medicine of the University of Lucerne, Switzerland, and leads the Person-Centered Healthcare Group at Swiss Paraplegic Research. Currently, she is president of EACH, the International Association for Communication in Healthcare.

Meredith Y. Smith is a behavioural and health services scientist with over 15 years of pharmaceutical industry experience. Now as director of risk management at Alexion, she builds systems and capacities for risk management tracking, digital risk minimisation measures, structured benefit-risk assessment and patient-centred approaches. She has been an invited member of expert panels at the US Food and Drug Administration and international working groups, including CIOMS and IMI-PREFER. She also holds an adjunct professor position at the School of Pharmacy, University of Southern California.

Burkhard Sträter is an honorary professor at Bonn University, Germany, where he leads the Drug Regulatory Affairs degree programme. His career started in 1977 as a judge at the regional and administrative courts in Berlin, and after heading the legal service at the German health agency, he established his own law firm. He advises the German parliament and task forces. In 2002, he was named by the Global Counsel among the Top 10 Life Science Lawyers of the World and received the PMI Pharmaceutical Law Award.

Brian J. Taylor is professor of social work at Ulster University, Northern Ireland, United Kingdom, and leads its Research Cluster on Decision, Assessment, Risk and Evidence Studies. Previously, he spent 25 years as practitioner and manager in health and social care. His first degree was in physics and his PhD in epidemiology. He cooperates with the Harding Centre for Risk Literacy, Berlin, Germany, and the Cochrane Collaboration, Oxford, and is fellow of the UK Academy of Social Sciences.

Ghislaine van Thiel is associate professor at the Department of Public Health, Healthcare Innovation and Evaluation and Medical Humanities which is part of the Julius Center for Health Sciences and Primary Care at the University Medical Center (UMC) Utrecht, Netherlands. She studied health sciences and has specialised in ethics of medicines and technology development, end-of-life decisions, and clinical trials. She is member of the Dutch Health Council and chairs the Medical Research Ethics Committee Utrecht. She teaches ethics at the medical school.

Carly Winokur is a public health professional at Carrum Health, Customer Success, Account Management and Implementation, United States. Previously, she was a health analyst for Booz Allen Hamilton's digital health surveillance services team and for Epidemico, and a health policy analyst at Israel's Ministry of Health and the US Centers for Disease Control and Prevention's Laboratory of Infectious Diseases and Malaria. She has an MPH in health policy and management from Emory University, 2011, and a BS in International Relations and Communication Studies from the University of Miami, 2009.

A Multilayered Research Framework for Humanities and Epidemiology of Medicinal Product Risk Communication

1

Priya Bahri

Abstract

Modern medicines are among the most successful health interventions, and as such are part of our daily lives and conversations. However, they do not come without risks, and safe use advice from healthcare professionals, conversations between friends and debates in the media are some of the many forms communication about risks with medicines can take. With a view to improving communication for the benefit of patients and society as a whole, this chapter discusses how to approach communication about medicine risks with curiosity and compassion for communication as a vital human behaviour and with consideration for the social spheres where such communication actually happens. Reflecting on past and current safety challenges with medicines, the chapter proposes a multilayered research framework that combines different data types and methods from various scientific disciplines to gain a wider and deeper understanding of the complexity of communication as well as the causal relationships, risk and success factors and pathways towards outcomes. This research approach advocates for the active participation of patients, healthcare professionals and journalists in research and mutual learning. It should generate evidence relevant for communicators in high- and low-income countries alike and prepare the ground for establishing a self-standing inclusive discipline of humanities and epidemiology of medicinal product risk communication.

P. Bahri (✉)
European Medicines Agency (EMA), Amsterdam, The Netherlands
e-mail: comm-research@priyabahri.de

© Springer Nature Singapore Pte Ltd. 2020

P. Bahri (ed.), *Communicating about Risks and Safe Use of Medicines*,
https://doi.org/10.1007/978-981-15-3013-5_1

1.1 The Triad of Medicines, Risks and Communication

Medicines, risks and communication—how to approach this triad as a researcher, or anybody interested in such research, is the question this chapter discusses with suggestions for ways forward. It aims to do so by viewing communication as the vital behaviour of human beings and combining a range of data types and methods from different scientific disciplines to obtain a wider and deeper understanding. Without understanding what influences the use of medicines and which role risks and risk communication in the different medical and societal contexts play, one can do very little for improving communication outcomes—not for patients with their individual needs nor for societies as a whole. Communication means interacting with each other, exchanging information and creating relationships. New information enters and settles in us through a process of perception. How we process new input and form knowledge and beliefs as well as which emotions drive our motivations define how we shape mental models and attitudes and how we behave (Morgan et al. 2002; Slovic 2010). As good health is among the basic human needs and desires, and as medicines are among the most successful health interventions that can prolong and improve life, but do not come without risks, communication about risks with medicines nowadays is manifold and omnipresent. Hence, medicinal product risk communication is a highly important and exciting research field of relevance for global health.

1.1.1 Developing a Humane Perspective

A full understanding of communication as human behaviour is a huge scientific undertaking as much as a personal life journey. In this section of the chapter, short reflections on selected aspects are offered for taking a humane perspective on medicinal product risk communication as a starting point.

Appreciating Complex Dialogues

In the past, information about medicines was mainly provided to patients by their healthcare professionals in an instructive or educational manner. Those providing the information also decided what, when and how to communicate. This corresponded to what is called a one-way, or unidirectional, information flow (Rimon 2007).

Before a medicine can be used in healthcare, it requires a license or marketing authorisation. This is issued by authorities regulating medicines, which—important to note—do not oversee healthcare, public health polices, such as recommendations for immunisation, or pricing of medicines. For those in regulatory bodies, the paradigm is to value medicines for their health benefits, try to prevent harm, and view information as an enabler for safe and effective use. This communication model has originally been, and largely still is, likewise unidirectional, with an information flow about risk assessments and advice on the appropriate use of medicines from regulatory bodies to patients, healthcare professionals and the wider public. Nowadays this happens not only via printed information but also via the regulatory bodies' websites, which can in principle be accessed by everybody.

The package leaflet might be the first information patients see when they obtain a medicine new to them. Package leaflets are approved by the regulatory body as part of medicinal products. The pharmaceutical company that holds the marketing authorisation and is hence responsible for the product is also responsible for developing and disseminating this and other officially required information materials. In addition, companies are allowed to issue advertising materials, but inappropriate advertising should be prevented. Some countries have legal restrictions, mandatory compliance with the approved product information and regulatory oversight in place, or impose self-regulation. The approved product information is usually also reflected in official, healthcare setting-specific or academic reference materials, such as pharmacopoeias, medicine formularies and pharmacological textbooks.

While this unidirectional communication model still prevails, the aims and ideals of communication in healthcare have changed tremendously (Hugman 2009). Patients search more and more independently for information through their communities and the internet and expect a two-way flow of information. Through such a dialogue they wish not only to receive information in comprehensive and understandable manner and possibly ask their healthcare professionals for details, but to express their views and contribute information too. Thereby, they may want to explore and clarify their own therapeutic expectations, risk tolerance and preferences. This input from patients is essential for shared decision-making between the physician and the patient on which treatment is right for this patient as an individual. It is crucial that patients have access to information upon their own initiative as well as that they are actively informed, in particular by their healthcare professionals. Further, patients should have the opportunity to report, to their healthcare professionals and the authorities, their experiences of side effects, i.e. suspected adverse reactions. The therefore relevant concept of health literacy describes people's knowledge, skills and motivation to access and apply health information, to take health-beneficial decisions and to effectively use and participate in healthcare (Squiers et al. 2012).

The roles of the different healthcare professionals, e.g. physicians, nurses, community health workers and pharmacists, in communicating about medicines are multiple. As receivers of new information, they continuously update their professional knowledge, and as information senders, they discuss information with their patients. At the same time, they may also contribute data to the overall evidence through leading or participating in research or through reporting to the authorities adverse reactions they may suspect in a patient.

The two-way communication model manifests not only in the interpersonal dialogue in healthcare. Communities and societies expect a public dialogue too. Patient and healthcare professional groups can provide collated information about their experiences and preferences regarding the risks they are willing to take for possible treatment benefits to public bodies through citizen participation mechanisms. For example, regulatory bodies may welcome patients and healthcare professionals to public hearings, advisory meetings or written consultations, and take their input into account for decision-making on regulatory action for a medicine. Such participation should not only be an option for those in high-income countries with strong regulatory and health systems as well as infrastructure. The Ebola crisis of 2014 has most dramatically shown that the involvement of communities in West African countries is equally demanded and feasible in low resource settings, in this case for preventing further virus spread and developing an effective vaccine (World Health Organization (WHO) 2016a, 2014–2017). A multi-stakeholder dialogue requires mechanisms for voicing information, mutual listening and reaching agreement on what needs to be done for achieving best outcomes.

However, communication about medicines happens not only between patients, communities, healthcare professionals, manufacturers and regulators. Many more parties are involved, such as academic researchers, health policy makers and politicians, health insurance and technology assessment bodies, and of course journalists, bloggers and those active in the social media. All these stakeholders provide different types of communication and raise questions about medicines from different perspectives and for various purposes and objectives. In addition, each party may be heterogeneous, consisting of subgroups or individuals who express different, potentially opposing views, and a subgroup may even become a separate opinion leader. This makes communication complex with many interactions between and within stakeholder groups.

In particular the impact of the change in communication stipulated by the digital revolution and its internet-based communication channels, 24-h news channels and social media with far and fast reach around the globe cannot be overestimated, and is challenging to predict and optimise. Respect should be paid to those who had foreseen issues, such as Marshall McLuhan had in the 1960s about the intertwined relationship of the media, the messages and mobile technology, and the influence of this intertwined relationship on the perception of messages, as we experience it today (McLuhan 1964).

On the whole this means that a massive change is happening with increasing complexity of constant, simultaneous and multi-stakeholder dialogues and growing importance of the patients' voice.

Acknowledging Cognitive Processes of Perception and Trust-Building

It further contributes to the complexity that communication about medicines happens in a world of augmenting technicalisation, described by some social scientists since the 1980s as "risk society" and "post-trust society". The concept of risk society refers to societies viewing new technical choices primarily in terms of benefit-risk trade-offs and trying to deal with probabilities of harm and uncertainties (Beck 1986; Giddens 1998). In parallel, societies may experience some erosion of their trust towards industry providing new technologies, like medicines, and the authorities regulating them. This erosion of trust has been explained, partially at least, by developments in politics overall and the internet with its 24-h news channels and social media allowing everybody to disseminate news and opinions quickly, as well as by regulatory shortcomings in various domains causing public outrage (Löfstedt 2005). The related phenomenon of public debates leading to heightened perceptions of risks in terms of their likelihood and severity has been named by Roger Kasperson and colleagues the "social amplification of risk" (Kasperson et al. 1988). Fast dissemination of misinformation like rumours and so-called fake news, nowadays also through mobile technology and internet-based media, may contribute to amplification of risk perceptions (Vosoughi et al. 2018). Fake news has been defined as fabricated messages that mimic news media content in form but not in organisational process or intent, in particular in terms of editorial norms and ensuring the accuracy and credibility of information (Lazer et al. 2018).

Risk perceptions and information needs are interrelated, and they differ among and between patients and healthcare professionals (Bongard et al. 2002). The underlying beliefs and values of those bearing a risk are rational in their own right and often more complex than those of experts (Frewer 1999). Experts should also be aware that their own perceptions depend on the current scientific paradigms. Prominent examples are the lack of awareness in the 1950/60s that medicines can pass the placenta and expose the foetus (see Sect. 1.2.1) and the news of 2008 that the genome of a person is not static but changes over lifetime due to ageing and environmental factors (Johns Hopkins Medical Institutions (JHMI) 2008). Researching risk perceptions of the various stakeholders and the psychology of risk is therefore crucial for understanding debates and interactions, in order to create constructive dialogues and improve risk communication outcomes.

Dialogues and mutual beneficial outcomes are however not possible if the communicating parties do not trust each other (Renn and Levine 1991). Generally, trust refers to the firm belief in the reliability, truth or ability of someone or something (Oxford Dictionary 2017). In relation to risk communication, trust has been defined as the generalised expectancy that a message received is true and reliable and that the communicator demonstrates competence and honesty by conveying accurate, objective and complete information (Renn and Levine 1991). Trust in the physician-patient relationship has been defined as the belief or confidence that the physician will provide reliable information and will act in the patient's interests (Thom et al. 1999). With regard to medicines specifically, two components of trust have been identified: (1) the willingness to assume a position of vulnerability in relation to the provision of healthcare and medicines and (2) the reliance on the competence of companies, authorities and healthcare professionals to fulfil their responsibilities (Hernandez et al. 2014). From a human relationship perspective, trust is the willingness to open oneself to risk by engaging in relationships with others (Grunig, and National Academies of Sciences, Engineering, and Medicine 2015).

Lately, scientists have felt the need to engage in trust-building with the general public regarding the value of evidence (Rosenbaum 2017). On the other hand, if scientists themselves ignore factual data demonstrating trust from societies in science and society's wish for evidence-based decisions in politics, scientists may lose credibility and nourish a self-fulfilling prophecy (Spiewak 2017). Some sociologists have called science the last resort for good policy-making (Maasen and Weingart 2006). Also, the majority of patients, e.g. in European countries and the United States (US), trust their healthcare professionals. Despite searching the internet, they expect and seek information from their physicians, in particular in the case of chronic or serious diseases (Ahlqvist-Radstad et al. 2016; Blendon et al. 2014; Higgins et al. 2011; Jacobs et al. 2017), and the majority prevent and treat diseases with medicinal products. These findings seem to contradict the description of post-trust societies, but future research might find more details about parallel phenomena, maybe depending on differences in the involved actors and their roles in given systems. Trust and more broadly political climate develop over time within given cultures, but can also change suddenly. Therefore, the monitoring and analysis of sentiments in different population segments and how they affect behaviours is important for understanding risk communication.

Fostering Compassion and Curiosity

Since good health is a basic human need and aspiration, and medicines are among the most successful health interventions, they have become part of daily life. As such, medicines are as essential as water, food, housing and education, and have been recognised at global level as a life-saving commodity everybody should have access to (United Nations (UN) Commission on Life-Saving Commodities 2012). Likewise, communication about medicines is omnipresent in daily life, whether in healthcare, among family and friends or in the news and social media.

Even fiction media allocate major roles to medicines. For example, the Australian novel "Addition" depicts a woman with an obsessive-compulsive disorder. As the medication causes her weight gain, perceived loss of self and decreased interest in her partner, she decides to stop the medicine and accept the disorder as part of her life (Jordan 2008). The US thriller movie "Side Effects" tells the story of a woman claiming not to be guilty of murdering her husband, as she was under the influence of an antidepressant making her sleep-walk (Soderbergh and Burns 2013). This big box office hit as well as "Addition" as a bestseller in many countries may well have raised general awareness about medicines used for mental disorders and impacted on patients' attitudes and therapeutic choices. On the other hand, fiction may only mirror concerns about medicines already widely prevalent. Other famous movies take a more semi-documentary approach, incorporating details from actual events in a fictional story. The multiple award-winning movie "Wit", for example, has its audience witnessing the severe adverse reactions of chemotherapy (Wikipedia 2018a). "120 BPM" won likewise many awards in 2017/18 and touched people with its story about the French activists fighting for treatments against infection with the human immunodeficiency virus (HIV) (Wikipedia 2018b). Fiction media are an opportunity to disseminate important health information. As an example, the television series "Tsha Tsha", highly popular in South Africa, was an entertaining story around a dance community and successfully encouraged young people to test for HIV and obtain medication (Govender 2013).

Medicines have also been portrayed in the arts, such as in installations—very famous is "Pharmacy" by Damien Hirst (Hirst 1992)—as well as in staged choreographies, all animating viewers to reflect about what role medicines play in their own lives. The piece "Side Effects" by the dance group Dante or Die with support from the Royal Pharmaceutical Society and the Wellcome Trust in the United Kingdom (UK) offered a performance of manifestations of adverse effects of medicines in the body and mind. The dancers confronted the audience with the explicit question: "What is in your medicine cabinet?" (Dante or Die 2011). The arts collaboration Pharmacopoeia concludes an article about their installation "Cradle to Grave" in the British Museum with the following thoughts: "In the end we are asked to consider the deeply complex relationship we have with prescription drugs. They are both wonderful and dangerous. They allow us to live longer, they allow us to suffer less, but they may also offer false promises of happiness and health and immortality that they cannot possibly deliver. In this they are more like the spirits and gods of other cultures than we care to believe" (Freeman et al. 2010).

Given the health relevance of medicines, the omnipresence of communication about medicines as well the complexity of message flows, it seems timely to conduct research in wider and deeper ways than has been done so far. As discussed later in this chapter with a range of examples, communicating about risks with medicines is difficult for many reasons, and it is not easy to achieve informed therapeutic choices and safe use behaviours. When a behaviour change does occur, evidence is often limited with regard to what the main driver was and how to sustain positive changes. Medicines use and communication both depend on the given healthcare setting and overall environment, the medical culture and general views upon health and life of individuals and communities.

Communication about medicines also raises questions of ethics and tact, about what is appropriate to say and ask, and how. Communication with patients is considered ethical when it promotes patient autonomy and assures high quality and equitable healthcare (Jarosch and Allhoff 2006). Wrong words can discriminate, victimise or stigmatise patients; questions can be indiscreetly private and personal; and thoughtless public statements can be judgemental and disrespectful in relation to priorities and choices of individuals.

In order to gain a wider and deeper understanding, we therefore could, rather than looking at medicines, risks and communication only from the perspective of the medicine as a product to regulate and use appropriately, approach this triad from the angle of communication as the fundamental process of life. It is one of the very human desires that we want to relate to others, understand them, trust them, express ourselves and engage in exchange. As individuals, we engage first of all with our close contacts, family and friends, join wider communities where we live and work, and through belonging to our village, city or country have further duties, rights and options to influence what affects us locally or goes beyond. All of these exchanges impact on our emotions, mental models, attitudes and behaviours. A framework for understanding the interactive effects of personal and social factors that determine our behaviour as individuals and communities can be found in the social-ecological model (SEM). This model distinguishes between the personal sphere of an individual and the social spheres surrounding any individual. It depicts that individuals together form private circles of family and friends, communities at the places where they live, work or meet for common interests, and all together form society (Storey and Figueroa 2012; United Nations Children's Fund (UNICEF) 2017). A model of communication for studying a specific medicine and safety concern in a specific social-ecological environment will describe actors, flows of communication content as well as structures of power and influence across the personal, private, community and society spheres.

Considering the above, we, as researchers or being interested in such research, can approach communication about risks of medicines with humanity, i.e. with compassion and curiosity: compassion for patients and everybody involved and challenged by having to deal with disease, medicines and risks; and curiosity for how we seek understanding of the world and interact with each other within social spheres, how this relates to our perceptions and choices in life as well as our longings and goals, and how this impacts on our behaviours and health, and last but not least the use of medicines. It is the vision of this book that a research framework approaching the triad from this humane perspective could generate more complete evidence for improving medicinal product risk communication for the benefit of individual patients and societies as a whole.

1.1.2 Fundamental Terms and a Typology of Medicinal Product Risk Communication

Differences in terminology of concepts and methods exist between scientific disciplines, in particular those of the natural, medical and social sciences, and even between domains of the medical-pharmaceutical field, such as clinical trials, pharmacovigilance (see Sect. 1.2.1) and systems for patient safety in healthcare. Terms may be identical but have different meanings, or be similar but not refer to the same, or be different but describe common concepts. Also, the relationships between terms may differ between disciplines and domains, creating different distinctions, inclusions and overlaps. For a multidisciplinary research field such as medicinal product risk communication, researchers need to be aware of terminological discrepancies and always clarify what is subject to their research and which terms they apply with which meanings.

While this chapter does not have the aim nor the authority to harmonise terminology across disciplines, this section clarifies in which sense terms are used in this book, focussing on the fundamental terms relevant to its scope of medicinal product risk communication research. Meanings of terms from the communication sciences have been sourced from an authoritative textbook (Littlejohn et al. 2016). Many clarifications for medicines-related terms are provided with a general pharmaceutical expertise. Specific terms for the regulation and surveillance of medicines have been incorporated too with their references. Those internationally agreed have been preferred, but when not available, those from the European Union (EU) have been applied, in particular from its guidelines on good pharmacovigilance practices (EU-GVP) (European Medicines Agency (EMA), Heads of Medicines Agencies 2012–2019), given that the EU-GVP is a frequent reference in many jurisdictions outside the EU too. The chapters in part II of this book introduce further terminology relevant to the respective disciplines they present.

In order to clarify which kind of communication may be subject to medicinal product risk communication research, a tabulated overview of major communication types is provided at the end of this section.

Researcher

Researchers, for the purpose of this book, are not only those conducting formal studies, reviews of the scientific literature and other research projects. The term is meant to include those who, in whatever setting, seek to collect or analyse information for understanding, planning or evaluating communication. The term "research" itself is applied in this book accordingly.

Patients

Patients, for the purpose of this book, are not only those individuals with a medical condition against which a medicine is used or considered to be used, but the term includes healthy individuals, or consumers, who use or consider using a medicinal product for diagnostics, disease prevention or the modification of physiological functions or who may have a future need to use medicines, i.e. in practice any individual. For the ease of reading, the term "patient" furthermore includes, unless clearly distinguished, parents, family members, friends or others who care for a patient or speak and may take decisions on behalf of a patient in their personal, not professional capacity. It also includes, likewise for the ease of reading and unless clearly distinguished, patient advocates, who speak for patients and their interests.

Medicines

Medicines, or medicinal products, are defined by their properties for treating or preventing disease, restoring, correcting or modifying physiological functions or making a medical diagnosis (European Union 2004a; Uppsala Monitoring Centre (UMC) 2018). We value medicines most for curing disease or easing symptoms and improving quality of life when one falls sick. Vaccines are the major example for medicinal products successfully preventing diseases of infectious origin, and hormonal contraceptives for products modifying a physiological function not related to a disease. The active substance of a medicinal product can have different origins, i.e. chemical (naturally occurring or synthesised), biological (from a living human or animal organism, or its products) or vegetable (from a micro-organism or plant) (European Union 2004b).

A medicine becomes available through a product development process and a marketing authorisation, also called license. It is developed by a sponsor, usually a pharmaceutical company. The marketing authorisation is issued by the regulatory body based on their thorough assessment of data on quality, safety and efficacy obtained from pharmaceutical tests and clinical trials during the development process. The authorisation is issued when the data assessment comes to the conclusion that the product is beneficial and its risks are acceptable in relation to the benefit (i.e. a positive risk-benefit balance). Once a product has been authorised, the company becomes marketing authorisation holder and is also the manufacturer, unless the marketing authorisation is sold to another company or the manufacturing is outsourced. For the ease of reading, the terms "manufacturer" and "pharmaceutical company" are used in this book as the more colloquial terms for marketing authorisation holder. Once a product has been authorised for use in healthcare, it is legally mandatory for the pharmaceutical company and the regulatory authority to conduct continued product-related safety surveillance and risk minimisation, i.e. pharmacovigilance (see Sect. 1.2.1). Medicines are available to patients upon medical prescription-only (POM) or without prescription (e.g. "over-the-counter" (OTC), "pharmacy-only", general sale), depending on the legal status of the product.

Part of the authorised medicinal product is the product information; that is the way the product is labelled on its outer packaging, the package leaflet for patients (also called patient information leaflet) and the summary of product characteristics for healthcare professionals (also called "the label"). Additional information materials may be required as part of the authorisation to mitigate specific risks.

Depending on the jurisdiction, there may be products on the market with reference to their traditional use as a remedy and these may not undergo the same rigorous regulatory procedures described above. As they may be referred to as medicines too, at least in common language, and may require advice for safe use on their own or in combination with (other) medicines, or impact on risk perception of (other) medicines (e.g. "Traditional is safer and preferable"), it is appropriate to address them through medicinal product risk communication research too.

Medicines are also called pharmaceutical products or drugs, sometimes excluding vaccines. The term "drug" is sometimes used in the meaning of the active substance in a medicinal product, as opposed to the whole product. As the term "drug" is also used to describe illicit drugs of abuse, this book prefers the terms "medicine" and "medicinal product", and applies these two interchangeably.

Risks

Risks with medicines can arise from the active substance they contain, as any substance will have multiple effects on the body—positive ones we expect to benefit from, and sometimes also negative ones we want to avoid. A substance can remedy one body function but may harm another, healthy body part of the patient. This is commonly called side effect. Harm can occasionally also be due to an excipient the medicine contains, i.e. an added substance that brings the active substance into a pharmaceutical form, like a tablet, liquid or patch, that can actually be administered by or to a patient or makes the active substance travel to the interior body part where it is needed. Residues from substances used in the manufacturing process may be present, after cleaning processes, only in very small trace amounts if at all, and usually do not constitute a risk, but effects on allergic patients may still be possible.

Individual patients have different susceptibilities to experience negative effects from the ingredients, e.g. due to genetic factors (which may be more prevalent in a specific ethnic group) or addtional diseases a patient may have, or due to physiological conditions related to biological sex or age and development. However, risk factors are not always known or detectable, and hence, harm may be unpredictable or unpreventable.

Overall, serious risks caused by the ingredients of a medicine are rare, as only those medicinal products are allowed on the market by the regulatory authority for which the available data on quality and safety do not show the frequent occurrence of serious harm. Occasionally though a certain level of harm is accepted for medicines used to save patients from serious diseases such as cancer.

Another, more frequent cause of harm is using a medicine knowingly, in error or with a lack of understanding in a way that is not appropriate in terms of the authorised product information or standards of good medical care. This concerns, for example, use in a medical condition the medicine is not intended for or even officially contraindicated, i.e. "forbidden", use of the wrong dose or route of intake, wrong use of an administration device or inappropriate use together with interacting other medicines, food or beverages. Also, there may be intentional misuse or abuse of a medicine, in particular where psychotropic effects are involved.

A further type of risk results from contamination. For example, valsartan-containing products that following a manufacturing change were contaminated with N-nitrosodimethylamine (NDMA), a substance classified as a probable human carcinogen (i.e. a substance that could cause cancer), have been a major communication challenge for regulators and healthcare professionals worldwide (European Medicines Agency (EMA) 2018a; United States Food and Drug Administration (US FDA) 2018a) (however, the cancer risk has been assessed as low) (European

Medicines Agency (EMA) 2018b). Furthermore, the potential of contamination with infectious agents, such as viruses and prions, is a risk to avoid through high-quality manufacturing and surveillance for blood- and plasma-derived products, other biological products or so-called advanced therapy products based on genes, cells or tissues. In general terms, harm can be caused by products that have an accidental quality defect, or are substandard, i.e. do not meet the legally demanded quality requirements, or are deliberately falsified. Substandard or falsified products can enter the market of any country in the world, and are sometimes sold through unlicensed internet sellers. Especially in countries with low resources for regulatory oversight, consumer protection and enforcement action, the sale of such products may be frequent. Falsified products, also known as "fakes", may contain undeclared toxic ingredients or therapeutically ineffective ingredients. Such products, including those sold as antimalarials, are a significant problem in Africa and Asia (Lancet Respiratory Medicine (eds) 2018).

Lack of efficacy of a medicinal product, whatever the cause, is part of the risk concept, because it may cause harm, in particular in the cases of treatment of a life-threatening condition, vaccination or contraception.

In some instances, inappropriate use may not only harm the patient, but can have severe negative impact on the entire potential patient population. For example, the inappropriate prescribing of antibiotics can make infectious agents resistant to the active substance and lead to lack of therapeutic efficacy of this medicinal product, a phenomenon called antimicrobial resistance (AMR).

Beyond patient harm, there may be specific risks for other individuals. Most importantly medicines taken during pregnancy can possibly damage the unborn child (i.e. teratogenicity) (however, there are medical conditions that require medication for treating or protecting the pregnant woman and/or the child). Furthermore, there can be harm due to accidental exposure, e.g. children mistaking medicines for sweets, or following diversion of prescribed medicines to others in good will to help or against money, or for healthcare professionals and carers when handling a medicine (i.e. occupational exposure to a medicinal product), or to those involved in its manufacturing. Contamination of the environment may result from negligent manufacturing processes, from elimination from the body when using the medicine, or from disposal of unused highly potent medicines, such as medicines against cancer.

There is a conceptual difference between harm and risk, but the term "risk" is often used to cover both concepts, as the terms "risk-benefit balance" and "benefit-risk trade-offs" show. Based on the evidence of harm that has occurred, probabilities of future harm, i.e. risks, are established. Apart from probabilities in the statistical-mathematical sense or calculated frequencies, risk in colloquial language relates more generally to the possibility, or potential, or uncertainty that something negative, however small or big its extent and probability, may happen. In this book the two terms "risk" and "harm" are used interchangeably, as, for example, a discussion with a patient about harm experienced with a medicine and measures how to reduce the risk of future harm can overall be referred to as risk communication.

Two officially defined terms describe events related to harm or the potential for harm with medicines:

- *Adverse reaction*: Concretely, harm with a medicine in an individual manifests as a so-called adverse reaction (also referred to as adverse effect and undesirable effect), which has been internationally defined as a response to a medicinal product that is noxious (i.e. harmful or unpleasant) and unintended (ICH Secretariat 2003). As the causal relationship of harm that has occurred in an individual and the medicine is often, at least initially, unknown, the term "suspected adverse reaction" is used to describe this uncertainty. Depending on the context, the term "adverse reaction" is usually used as an umbrella term that includes suspected adverse reactions (ICH Secretariat 2003). Adverse reactions may arise from use of a product in accordance with the terms of the marketing authorisation (also termed "on-label"), or outside these terms, or from occupational exposure of healthcare professionals. Use outside the terms of marketing authorisation includes overdose, intentional abuse and misuse, unintended medication errors and off-label use, i.e. situations where a product is intentionally used for a medical purpose not in accordance with the terms of the marketing authorisation. Notably, in the cases of abuse (i.e. persistent or sporadic, intentional excessive use that is accompanied by harmful physical or psychological effects) and misuse (including in the case of misuse with a criminal intent) harmful effects can be intended by the user, but these effects still fall under adverse reactions (despite the definition characterising adverse reactions as unintended), because in principle it is against the intent of a medicinal product to cause such harm. Adverse reactions may also arise from a product having a quality defect, being substandard or falsified. Lack of efficacy of some medicinal products like those used in a life-threatening condition, vaccines or contraceptives are considered adverse reactions too for the purpose of pharmacovigilance (European Medicines Agency (EMA), Heads of Medicines Agencies 2012–2019; 2013).

  The term "adverse reaction" is applied in two ways: first, it may describe the harm that has been experienced in a specific individual and been attributed to or be suspected to be causally associated with the medicine, i.e. a case of an adverse reaction; second, it may describe the potential for harm as a characteristic of a medicine with higher or lesser certainty based on the available evidence, including that from reported cases. Adverse reactions have a number of aspects, such as what actually occurs in the body (i.e. mode of pharmacological-toxic action and severity), the proportion of individuals who are affected (i.e. frequency), how serious the outcomes can be (i.e. seriousness) and which factors might make the harm more severe or more likely to occur (i.e. risk factors).

  In common language, the term "side effect" describes adverse reactions, although side effect in its strict sense refers to the additional, mostly undesirable, pharmacological effect of the active substance itself, and not to the broader concept of adverse reaction. This book prefers the term "adverse reaction" but occasionally uses the term "side effect" interchangeably.
- *Medication error*: A medication error has been defined by various organisations in different ways, but may generally be understood as an unintended failure in the treatment process with a medicine that leads to, or has the potential to lead to, harm in the patient (European Medicines Agency (EMA) 2015). Medication errors relating to prescribing, dispensing, storing, preparation and administration

of a medicine are common preventable causes. Medication errors specifically in relation to vaccines have been termed immunisation errors. These comprise errors in the storage and handling of the vaccine product (which may impair its quality and hence efficacy or safety, e.g. if a cold chain is interrupted), in prescribing/applying (i.e. not in accordance with the marketing authorisation or immunisation recommendations) or in the administration to the person to be vaccinated (Council for International Organizations of Medical Sciences (CIOMS), World Health Organization (WHO) 2012).

The term "medication error" is applied in two ways: first, it may relate to a situation where harm has occurred (this is classifiable as a case of adverse reaction (European Medicines Agency (EMA) 2015)); second, it may relate to a situation with the potential for harm, i.e. where no harm has occurred, e.g. because the error was not so severe or managed before harm occurred, or because the error was discovered in the course of the process and corrected before its completion.

Before a risk is confirmed and then termed in the regulatory context "identified risk", considerations take place whether a medicine may carry risks. These originate from theoretical reflections, such as on the molecular structure of the active substance, toxicological studies, experience with similar medicines or from inconclusive data for the given medicine (due to, e.g. limitations, weakness or inconsistency of the data and study results). Where considerations provide some basis for a suspicion, but without confirmation of a causal association, issues are termed "potential risks" (ICH Secretariat 2010). Often first reports of suspected adverse reactions from patients or healthcare professionals signal a potential risk. Another data source may be a pharmacoepidemiological study in relevant patient populations. During the course of data gathering and risk assessment, situations of variable strength of available evidence may be encountered, and while potential risk and identified risk are two distinct concepts (however on a continuum of increasing evidence), the term "risk" in this book covers, unless clearly distinguished, both concepts.

Dealing with both potential and identified risks entails scientific uncertainties on the evidence continuum. These uncertainties may concern the diagnosis whether a given medicinal product has actually caused the harm seen in a specific patient or the assessment of the data from all sources on whether a given medicinal product can cause a certain adverse reaction, the data on the frequency of the reaction and the factors increasing the likelihood of a reaction, and the data on the potential for medication errors in day-to-day healthcare. Further, every study has a degree of some uncertainty around its findings, arising from limited study power, the statistical assumptions or residual confounding. It may hence be recognised that more data need to be collected to check for safety, in particular in sub-populations (also termed "missing information" (ICH Secretariat 2013)). Unless clearly distinguished, the term "risk" in this book includes the various aspects of scientific uncertainty.

People might also have broader concerns with using medicines. Some religious or moral grounds or health beliefs are not compatible with using a certain medicine, such as "A natural infection leads to stronger immunity than vaccination" in some parents (McKee and Bohannon 2016), or "My body should be strong and not become dependent on medicines" in some young people (Atkins et al. 2010). Or there might be doubts over the integrity of an expert consensus or over financial and political interests. For example, vaccination against human papillomavirus (HPV) had to be stopped in two Indian states, as initial high vaccine acceptance turned into mistrust over questions regarding appropriateness of funding, healthcare for women and health equity overall (Larson et al. 2010). Even rumours can be a risk. A school-based deworming programme in Ghana, as one example, had to be stopped for public outrage about rumours of adverse reactions. These were possibly triggered by the fact that a child had been taken to hospital following an accident outside the school building. Rapid official investigations and public communication was successful in restoring trust and order (Dodoo et al. 2007). Concerns in the public domain may however persist even when risks have long been ruled out, as discussed later in this chapter with the example of the measles-mumps-rubella (MMR) vaccines (see Sect. 1.2.2). Likewise, healthcare professionals may have doubts and not follow official advice. For example, a number of countries around the world have reported that many healthcare professionals opt out of getting vaccinated against seasonal influenza, as they believe it is not effective, not safe or not needed (Abalkhail et al. 2017; Cheung et al. 2017; Elias et al. 2017; Fernández-Villa et al. 2017; Habib et al. 2017; Hagemeister et al. 2018; Ko et al. 2017; Looijmans-van den Akker et al. 2009; Maridor et al. 2017; Marshall et al. 2017; Mustafa et al. 2017; Rabensteiner et al. 2018; Riedel 2017). Although there may not be any risk with a medicinal product involved, those voicing concerns see possible links. This can lead to not using a medicinal product when actually beneficial or may otherwise constitute risks to health and require communication.

Therefore, this book takes the view that any concern that people may have about medicines falls under the scope of medicinal product risk communication. For the purpose of the book and the ease of reading, concerns, whether or not related to potential or identified risks or scientific uncertainties, are included, unless clearly distinguished, in the term "risk". As no medicine, even under the most optimised circumstances, comes without risks or concerns, communication is necessary. However, insufficient or poor communication can have negative health outcomes and thus become in itself a risk to patient and public health, and can even lead to crisis situations (see Sect. 1.2).

Communication

Communication in the general language may refer to the content, the tools, the process, the underlying structures or the achievement of communication, and as a starting point for this book should be thought of in this wide meaning. Communication scientists themselves find the term "communication" not easy to define, but agree that it is a process and recommend developing a specific model which maps and best describes the involved parties, underlying systems and specific processes for any given communication situation. These models describe the senders and receivers of messages as well as the message flows between them. Modelling helps to gain clarity about the communication processes and underpins the scope and focus of communication research projects (Littlejohn et al. 2016).

The content of communication is often referred to as messages or information. The latter is an equally difficult term to define. In usual language, information describes facts provided or learned about something or someone (Oxford Dictionary 2017) and is related to knowledge and data (Merriam-Webster Dictionary 2017). It has also been defined as a collection of words, numbers, dates, images, sounds, etc. put into context to give them meaning (BBC 2017). In the communication sciences, information is a concept independent from meaning. There, it refers to the quantification of signals, or sensory input, that are perceived as new for making an uncertain situation more certain and hence providing an answer and guiding a choice (Littlejohn et al. 2016). However as discussed in this chapter, not all information about medicines will provide more or complete certainty. This is due to the nature of their risks and the evidence at hand. Further, the complexity of medicinal product risk communication and the variability of the quality of information content and presentation as well as the phenomena of rumours and fake news make the perception of information from multiple sources for knowledge formation challenging for individuals. This chapter intends to mainly use the term "information" in relation to evidence or experiences, and the term "messages" as an umbrella term for different kinds of communication content, whether true or not.

When developing a model for communication about medicines, different levels of communication need to be considered (Littlejohn et al. 2016):

- *Interpersonal level*: Most important from the perspective of patients is the personal communication with their physician, the pharmacist and other healthcare professionals. More generally other one-to-one exchanges with close contacts, such as family members and friends, is usually essential for every individual. Interpersonal communication also happens between individual healthcare professionals or health policy makers as colleagues.
- *Intra-group/organisation level*: Patients and cares may engage in communication within groups, like self-help groups, patient organisations and social media groups, and healthcare professionals may communicate within their healthcare teams or professional organisations, such as self-regulatory bodies or learned societies. Exchanges among medicinal product assessors and regulators in scientific committees for making decisions on medicines can be seen as happening at intra-group level too.
- *Inter-group/organisation level*: Furthermore, there is communication about medicines between groups or organisations, such as between pharmaceutical companies, regulatory bodies and/or other bodies, like between a public body and a patient organisation.
- *Mass level*: Messages that are disseminated in the public domain or are accessible by everybody constitute communication at mass level. Debates about medicines happen in the news and social media, research is published in the scientific media, and many organisations publish information for patients or healthcare professionals.

These four levels are proposed as an initial structure to consider when developing a communication model to underpin research into medicinal product risk communication. In real life, levels may overlap or not be clearly distinguishable. For example, groups may constitute a formal organisation, like a registered learned society or patient organisation, but could also be more personal in character. Social media exchanges may only be accessible to a closed community, or be publicly available and then be classified as mass level communication. While articles in scientific journals target a specialist community, they can be accessed by everybody. On the other hand, information that may be available in the public domain might only be known about and accessed by a very limited number of people. Hence, a communication model for a specific research project will have to describe who is involved and what precisely is happening at the relevant levels in the real-world situation of the studied communication event.

As already mentioned with reference to the social-ecological model (SEM), communication also occurs in different social spheres, i.e. the

- *Private sphere*;
- *Community sphere*; and
- *Society sphere* (see Sect. 1.1);

and a communicative interaction may occur in more than one spheres at the same time. For example, the communication between a patient and a healthcare professional at interpersonal level happens in the private sphere, but some of the information will be shared within the healthcare setting as a community sphere, and further the interpersonal communication contributes to (and is influenced by) the given medical and general culture as well as the healthcare system and overall infrastructure of society as the wider spheres. Also, an interpersonal exchange between two medical opinion leaders can happen in the private sphere or the community sphere at a conference. Inter-organisation exchange may also ultimately become available for everybody through transparency provisions. This illustrates that levels and spheres of communication describe different dimensions of communication events, albeit related, in particular for public communication events. News media stories and debates in parliaments, for example, happen in the society sphere and at mass communication level.

A Note on Communicating Risks in the Context of Benefits of Medicines
While this book is dedicated to risk communication, it should not be forgotten that patients and healthcare professionals expect from communication about medicines to also cover their benefits and the benefit-risk trade-offs. Indeed, risks are assessed and communicated in the light of the expected benefits and the context of the risk-benefit balance. Where heightened perceptions of risk lead to not using a medicine in a patient for whom the benefit-risk expectations are positive, the patient may get deprived from an actually needed benefit. Therefore, studying the relationship between benefits and risks with regard to communication is part of medicinal product risk communication research. However, practice and research of benefit communication as such requires a different expertise. Information about benefits refers to another kind of evidence base and different study designs for generating the evidence. It is also subject to different perceptions, and its communication has specific objectives and faces its own challenges. These relate to efficacy endpoints, effectiveness in real life, non-responders and the relevance of benefit to individual patients. In the case of infections and vaccines the dynamics of disease spread, herd immunity and health at population level are additional complex items of benefit information. Further challenges lie in presenting benefit information in a way that

does not result in unrealistic expectations in those using medicines, or inappropriate overuse, or in unhealthy behaviours as a consequence of feeling protected from disease by the medicine. Benefit communication can hence be seen as a separate research field, yielding findings that should be brought together with the findings from medicinal product risk communication research, in order to ultimately improve information about medicines comprehensively.

Medicinal Product Risk Communication
To date there is no worldwide agreed definition, but for this book, medicinal product risk communication comprises the structures, processes and outcomes of information exchanges about risks and any concerns people may have with medicines, about the measures to support safe use and minimise risks and about risk governance overall in private, community and society spheres.

A Typology of Medicinal Product Risk Communication
In order to clarify the range of communication events which may be subject to research into medicinal product risk communication, an overview of major communication types with examples has been compiled from experience in the area of medicines information and regulation in Table 1.1. The communication types have been linked to the major senders of messages who engage in speaking, listening and discussing about medicines. Some types are formal and planned, e.g. the product information and campaigns to encourage the safe use of medicines, and as such these may be referred to as communication interventions. Regional specifics or legal differences may apply to the examples given in the table and have to be checked for a given research project. The overview also covers documents that are not actively communicated, or "pushed", to audiences but are available on the internet and may serve as a public information source, e.g. risk assessment reports from regulatory bodies. Pharmaceutical companies may be legally obliged to regularly access and act upon these assessment reports. In addition, such official assessment reports fulfil transparency obligations and accountability of public bodies towards citizens. The different communication types can be oral, written or make use of other tools, such as audio or video clips and digital tools, as well as be disseminated through multiple channels, such as personal interactions, conferences and news, social or scientific media. They may present the information in words, numbers and/or pictures. The different communication types could be further related to the different social spheres and communication levels (see Sect. 1.1). Other communication types may exist, but the typology in Table 1.1 already shows how omnipresent information about medicines risks is and to how many different senders, contents and objectives of communication patients and healthcare professionals are exposed to. What this means for their risk perceptions and therapeutic choices is only one of many important research questions. How to disseminate certain safe use advice widely and consistently is another challenging question, as the Table makes obvious too. The important work in information sharing of patient organisations is included in the last row, not because it is least important, but to close the Table—like this chapter (see Sect. 1.4.1) and the series of chapters (see Chap. 16)—with the increasingly active role patients take in communication processes and research.

Table 1.1 Types of medicinal product risk communication events

Senders	Communication event type
Patients, parents, carers, physicians, nurses, pharmacists, other healthcare professionals, family planning advisors, teratogenicity counsellors	*Interaction between patient or carer and healthcare professional*: e.g. healthcare professional's oral instructions and explanations; information and questions from patient/parents/carer; discussion between patient/parents/carer and healthcare professional/family planning advisor/teratogenicity counsellor; medication monitoring; pharmaceutical care; patient-tailored written/printed information supporting the instructions or decision-making
Patients, parents, carers, traditional healers, alternative or complementary health practitioners	*Interaction between patient and healer or practitioner*: e.g. traditional healer/alternative/complementary health practitioner not prescribing the medicinal product but giving information or an opinion about it
Patients, parents, carers, family members, friends, neighbours, community members	*Interaction between patient and close contact or community face-to-face*: e.g. patient/parents/carer receiving information, news or advice from family member/friend/neighbour/community member face-to-face; patient parents/carer engaging in personal or face-to-face group discussion with close contacts
Patients, parents, carers, family members, friends, social media community members	*Interaction among patients in the internet*: e.g. patient/parents/carer receiving or sharing information, news, advice from/with family member/friend/social media community member; patient parents/carer engaging in discussion with close contacts personally/a defined social media group/the wider social media audience/chatrooms; posting messages in words or pictures; following messages from close contacts/celebrities/opinion leaders; information seeking via social media
Religious leaders, members of a religious community, ethicists, philosophers, followers of a philosophy, world view or belief	*Expression of health-related opinions or beliefs by community or world view leaders*: e.g. expression of concerns about medicinal products or on their safety or other impact originating from religious, philosophical or moral world views and health beliefs orally or in writing in various media
Physicians, dentists, nurses, pharmacists, pharmacy technicians, medical assistants, other healthcare professionals	*Interaction among healthcare professionals*: e.g. general or patient-related exchanges among healthcare professionals in ambulatory, hospital or other healthcare settings, nursing homes or regional pharmacovigilance centres; informal discussions on a medicinal product at interpersonal level, within healthcare settings, professional organisations, social media communities or at conferences
Healthcare professional organisations	*Information about a medicinal product from a healthcare professional organisation*: e.g. safety information in newsletters for members; statements/advice to the public for the safe use of a medicinal product; comments on public debates or official decisions about safety concerns and risks with a medicinal product; materials for continuing professional education; risk information for patients
Patients, parents, carers, family members, friends, healthcare professionals, scientists	*Information seeking on websites*: e.g. searches using web browsers, scientific literature databases, specific websites of organisations, news media outlets, scientific journals

Table 1.1 (continued)

Senders	Communication event type
Physicians, dentists, nurses, pharmacists, coroners, patients parents, carers, family members, friends, lawyers	*Submission of a case report by the original reporter*: e.g. submission of a suspected adverse reaction in a patient to the regional/national pharmacovigilance reporting system/ pharmaceutical company; submission of a medication error or patient incident to the regional/national patient safety reporting system
Academia, pharmaceutical companies, contract research organisation	*Material for the conduct of a study*: e.g. investigator's brochure for physicians conducting clinical trials; informed consent forms for patients participating in clinical trials; risk information in protocols of clinical trials or post-authorisation safety studies submitted to ethical committees for approval
Regulatory bodies, pharmaceutical companies	*Interaction between regulatory body and pharmaceutical company*: e.g. requests from a regulatory body for data submission in relation to a safety concern, risk or risk minimisation; exchange in writing or at oral explanations; announcements of and responses to public hearing; responses to public consultations on guidelines and policies
Pharmaceutical companies	*Submission of data by a pharmaceutical company to a regulatory body*: e.g. submission of case reports of suspected adverse reactions to the national pharmacovigilance reporting system; legally required submission of clinical trial data, pre-clinical toxicology data, post-authorisation safety study findings, risk management plans (RMPs) (European Medicines Agency (EMA), Heads of Medicines Agencies 2012–2019)/ risk evaluation and mitigation strategies (REMS) (United States Food and Drug Administration (US FDA) 2018b), periodic safety update reports (PSURs) (ICH Secretariat 2013), signals of a new potentially causal association or new aspects between a medicinal product and an adverse event (CIOMS) 2010), urgent new safety information/emerging safety issue (European Medicines Agency (EMA), Heads of Medicines Agencies 2012–2019), data in support of changing the terms of marketing authorisation and product information, other data concerning potential risks under investigation to the regulatory body; submission of data to a public body as legally required or as responses to consultations
Regulatory bodies, pharmaceutical companies	*Statutory product information (PI)* (authorised by the regulatory body): e.g. summary of product characteristics/ label; package/patient information leaflet; labelling of container, blister or other packaging (Council for International Organizations of Medical Sciences (CIOMS) 1999; 2014); boxed warnings as part of the PI; audio and video clips of PI
Pharmaceutical companies, regulatory bodies	*Direct healthcare professional communication (DHPC)*: e.g. communication intervention by which important information is delivered directly to individual healthcare professionals to inform them of the need to take certain actions or adapt their practices in relation to a medicinal product (Council for International Organizations of Medical Sciences (CIOMS) 2014), often as a printed letter delivered by postal service

(continued)

Table 1.1 (continued)

Senders	Communication event type
Pharmaceutical companies	*Material for additional risk minimisation measures (aRMM)* (required and approved by the regulatory body): e.g. educational and training materials for patients/healthcare professionals; medication guides; counselling tools (e.g. patient card); materials for patients/healthcare professionals supporting restricted access programmes, controlled distribution systems or pregnancy prevention programmes; certificates allowing a certain healthcare professional to prescribe or dispense the medicinal product; registry enrolment forms; patient-provider agreements, information acknowledgement forms, patient monitoring forms, informed consent forms (Council for International Organizations of Medical Sciences (CIOMS) 2014)
Pharmaceutical companies, healthcare professionals	*Interaction between company representative and healthcare professional for early post-marketing phase vigilance (EPPV) or all-case surveillance (ACS)* (required by the regulatory body at the Ministry of Health, Labour and Welfare in Japan): for EPPV: information on appropriate use of a medicinal product in given healthcare setting through visit of medical representative 2 weeks prior to first use and follow-up visits and correspondence during first 6 months after product delivery to ensure the information has been understood by healthcare professionals and requesting appropriate use and reporting of adverse reactions (Ministry of Health, Labour and Welfare (MHLW) 2006); for ACS: information on prescribing a new medicinal product and collecting information on its use and outcomes in those healthcare settings allowed to prescribe the new medicinal product until a certain exposure and safety reassurance or adjustment of risk minimisation measures has been reached (Ministry of Health, Labour and Welfare (MHLW) 2009)
Pharmaceutical companies, healthcare professionals	*Interaction between company representative and healthcare professional*: e.g. visits of company representatives to physicians/pharmacies/hospitals for presenting a new medicinal product; information from healthcare professional on experience with medicinal product and suspected adverse reaction in a patient
Regulatory bodies, national pharmacovigilance centres	*Information on the website of the regulatory body or national pharmacovigilance centre about the assessment and the authorisation process of a medicinal product*: e.g. public assessment reports; marketing authorisation/licensing information; information about risk management plans (RMPs)/risk evaluation and mitigation strategies (REMS); statutory product information; information on additional risk minimisation materials; overviews on signals/potential risks under investigation; agenda and minutes of regulatory meetings for risk assessment; announcements about new risks, reassurance on safety or safe use advice, product or batch suspensions or withdrawals; publication on the website of the regulatory body of direct healthcare professional communications (DHPCs) that have been disseminated by a pharmaceutical company as required by the regulatory body or disseminated by the regulatory body itself; summaries of any such information in language generally understandable to the public

Table 1.1 (continued)

Senders	Communication event type
Regulatory bodies, national pharmacovigilance centres, patient organisations, healthcare professional organisations, citizens	*Interaction between regulatory body or national pharmacovigilance centres and patients, healthcare professionals and citizens*: e.g. information motivating and providing for reporting of adverse reaction cases; announcement of and responses to public consultations on product-, policy- or guideline-related matters; submission of data to a public body as responses to specific questions posed to the public; announcements of and responses to public hearings; meetings of the regulatory body with patients/ healthcare professionals/members of the general public; individual responses to patients/healthcare professionals/ academic researchers/members of the general public; news bulletins about medicinal products; educative materials using multiple media targeted at children and adolescents
Regulatory bodies, national pharmacovigilance centres	*Interaction between regulatory body or national pharmacovigilance centres and the media*: e.g. media releases about new risks, reassurance on safety or safe use advice disseminated to media outlets and published on the website of the regulatory body; social media messages with short warnings and safety messages; media conferences; individual responses to journalists on the phone or via e-mail
Regulatory bodies	*Regulatory guideline or policy for risk management and governance*: e.g. guidelines on pharmacovigilance conduct and processes for the regulatory body and pharmaceutical companies, including those applicable in public health emergencies; code of conduct for employees and experts of the regulatory body; policy for the management of conflict of interests of employees and experts of the regulatory body; written procedures or quality manual for pharmacovigilance, product quality or safety incidents, crisis management and communication; policies for interactions with other public bodies (of same or other jurisdiction)/patient organisations/ healthcare professional organisations/academia/international organisations/public-private consortia; summaries of any such information in language generally understandable to the public
Regional and national public health bodies, World Health Organization, other international organisations	*Official health information or announcement*: e.g. health protection campaigns using multiple media and tools; vaccination recommendations; information and advice on diseases, treatment options, medicinal products, vaccination, contraception, teratogenicity for the general public and healthcare professionals on website or in print; announcements and advice on medicinal product use and reporting of adverse events in public health emergencies; educative materials using multiple media targeted at children and adolescents

(continued)

Table 1.1 (continued)

Senders	Communication event type
Health technology assessment bodies	*Health technology assessment (HTA) report*: e.g. assessment reports of benefit, effectiveness, benefit-risk trade-offs and cost-effectiveness of a treatment with a medicinal product
Reimbursement committees, health insurance bodies	*Information on reimbursement policies for medicinal products*: e.g. reimbursement guidelines
Healthcare professional organisations	*Information about a medicinal product from a healthcare professional organisation*: e.g. safety information in newsletters for members; statements/advice to the public for the safe use of a medicinal product; comments on public debates or official decisions about safety concerns and risks with a medicinal product; materials for continuing professional education; risk information for patients
World Health Organization, other international organisations, donors, non-governmental organisations	*Recommendation for medicinal products used in a global development initiative*: e.g. WHO Model List of Essential Medicines; manuals for healthcare workers on medicinal products used in low resource settings; information for medicinal product procurement and supply chain managers; information or protocols for safe use of medicinal products in public health programmes; information about reporting of adverse reactions occurring in public health programmes
Governments, ministries of health	*Legislation and official policies*: e.g. legislation; policies; announcements of public consultations on legislative initiatives
Politicians, parliaments, governments, political parties, patient organisations, healthcare professional organisations, associations of pharmaceutical companies, health insurance bodies, civil society associations, activist groups, citizens	*Debate within and with political institutions*: e.g. parliament enquiries and hearings; opinions, comments or proposals of individual politicians/political parties debated within political institutions or public forums; responses from stakeholders to public consultations on legislation or health or risk governance policies; petitions, enquiries and signature collections for initiatives in the political or public domain; citizen petitions to parliament
Regulatory bodies, national or regional pharmacovigilance centres, poison centres, public health bodies, health technology assessment bodies, monitoring sites and centres for illicit drug use, parliaments, governments, ministries of health, official auditors, ombudsman, World Health Organization, other international organisations	*Interaction between public bodies*: e.g. interaction between public bodies at inter-organisation level about a medicinal product risk, safe use advice or risk governance policies and procedures; interaction regarding official recommendations for immunisation or other public health measures
Pharmacopoeia commissions	*Pharmacopoeia*: e.g. risk characterisation of active substances and warnings in monographs of pharmacopoeias
Healthcare settings	*Formulary*: e.g. healthcare setting-specific list of medicinal products and agreed safe use advice, taking into account risks and need for risk management for selection of the medicinal products for the list

Table 1.1 (continued)

Senders	Communication event type
Healthcare professional organisations, health technology assessment bodies, World Health Organization	*Treatment guidance:* e.g. clinical/treatment guidelines; advice on prescribing medicinal products appropriately; advice on using medicinal products in at-risk populations; decision aids for selecting the appropriate medicinal product given certain patient characteristics; classification in first, second and last line medication; advice for monitoring signs of adverse reactions in patients or the implementation of other risk minimisation measures tailored for different healthcare settings
Healthcare professional organisations	*Material for quality management of healthcare*: e.g. training for continued accreditation/practice license; quality of care management groups among practicing healthcare professionals; academic detailing (Soumerai and Avron 1990)
Health information technology providers	*Medicinal product compendium and prescribing or dispensing software*: e.g. risk information for physicians/pharmacists supporting the safe prescribing/dispensing of medicinal products and implementing risk minimisation measures in printed, downloaded or online compendia; information and pop-up alerts in prescribing/dispensing software
School teachers, school book editors, public health bodies	*Teaching in schools*: e.g. information about medicinal products and their safe use in school books and other teaching materials; opinions of teachers about medicinal products and risks
University lecturers, teachers in vocational schools or technical colleges	*Teaching of healthcare professional students or trainees*: materials used at technical colleges, universities and vocational schools for students/trainees in healthcare professions; opinions of lecturers/teachers about medicinal products and risks
Pharmaceutical companies	*Advertisement*: e.g. adverts in print news media, magazines, radio, television, posters, scientific journals, healthcare professional newsletters, websites or digital push media
Courts	*Publication of court case judgement*: e.g. published judgements in relation to harm with a medicinal product; summaries thereof for the media
Journalists, health journalists, popular science writers, scientists, healthcare professionals, bloggers, readers	*News in the general media or reader's comment*: e.g. articles about new information, current debates or interviews with affected persons/experts in print, online newspapers or magazines; news broadcasted by radio or television; articles in internet media outlets; news messages disseminated via social media; news feeds; printed or online comments on articles from readers; messages and debates in social media
Scientists, healthcare professionals, public health bodies, regulatory bodies, national pharmacovigilance centres, health technology assessment bodies	*Scientific publication*: e.g. articles in scientific journals, oral presentations, posters and panel discussions at scientific conferences; pharmacological textbooks
Scientists, healthcare professionals, popular science writers, health journalists, journalists	*Popular health book or magazine article*: e.g. popular science books; medical books for patients; articles in popular science/ health/ pharmacy magazines/internet media outlets written for the general public; infographics; booklets/articles/comics for children and adolescents

(continued)

Table 1.1 (continued)

Senders	Communication event type
Film makers, scientists, healthcare professionals, popular science writers, health journalists, journalists, patients	*Non-fiction or semi-documentary movie or video*: e.g. popular science or medical documentaries for television or internet about diseases, treatment options or patient experiences; educational video comics and games; real life based movies or documentaries of patients with certain diseases and their medication
Fiction writers	*Fiction*: e.g. novels, youth novels, hospital romance stories, movies, television series featuring patients and their medicines, reflecting on the effects of medicinal products or involving misuse or criminal use of medicinal products; entertainment education making use of movies, videos, comics
Artists, patients	*Art work:* e.g. paintings, installations, choreographies from or about patients and their medicines
Patient and consumer organisations, self-help groups, parent organisations, carer organisations, civil society associations, activist groups	*Information from patient organisation*: e.g. information on medicinal products for members and wider public or discussions of the organisation's community on websites, in writing, in newsletters, at meetings, conferences or via social media; articles in news media or magazines; surveys and contributions to research projects relating to risks with medicinal products and communication about medicines

1.2 Challenges and Outcomes of Communicating About Risks with Medicines in Real Life

The relevance of a wider and deeper scope of communication research in relation to medicines and risks becomes obvious when reviewing cases of communication challenges and their outcomes with medicines in real life. A number of cases are described in this and other chapters for highlighting important aspects and deriving an overview of communication outcome types.

1.2.1 Considering Past Challenges and the Development of Medicinal Product Risk Communication as a Scientific Dedication

Three cases have been pivotal to the development of medicinal product risk communication as a scientific dedication, namely the "VTE pill scare", the "Vioxx story" and the thalidomide re-authorisation. An excursion further back in time reminds us of what is referred to as the thalidomide disaster and summarises the establishment of pharmacovigilance for preventing harm with medicines.

The "VTE Pill Scare" of 1995

The most remembered communication crisis with medicines was the "VTE pill scare" of 1995 in the United Kingdom (UK), which concerned combined hormonal contraceptives (CHCs) containing an oestrogen and a progestogen. This crisis began with a study from the World Health Organization (WHO) and two further studies, all finding evidence of increased risks for blood clotting, or venous thromboembolism (VTE), for CHCs with certain progestogen compounds compared to other CHCs. Although the risk in absolute numbers was very small, there were plenty of news media reports and the regulatory authority had difficulties in effectively conveying reassuring messages. While the authority provided estimates of absolute and relative risks, the risk expression in relative terms as "doubled" spread more widely in the news. It has become collective memory that in consequence women got concerned and stopped their CHC, resulting in unwanted pregnancies and pregnancy terminations (Waller and Harrison-Woolrych 2017). Chapter 2 revisits the case in more detail and discusses the strength of evidence for considering this a public scare.

Realisation of the Importance of Risk Communication in the 1990s

The most important lesson learnt from these communication events was that poor communication of safety warnings can result in serious harm, and this may not only be physical, but also impact on the emotions and relationships of those affected.

It was also learnt that medicines risk communication needs to be fostered as a special skill, applying appropriate tools and best practices. It was recognised that the expression as relative risk can be misleading and that risk must be expressed carefully in a way that the actual risk and its perception match. It also became clear that whoever leads the public debate in the news media influences individual decisions (Waller and Harrison-Woolrych 2017). Therefore, an international meeting in collaboration with the WHO was convened in 1997 and resulted in the Erice Declaration, agreed by participants from 34 countries as the first global statement of principles for information, communication and education in relation to medicines (Erice Declaration 1997). These are still fundamental today and were complemented with follow-up statements in 2009 (Velo 2010), 2017 (Erice 2017) and 2019.

Whilst those responsible for safety of medicines had become sensitive for the importance and challenges of communication, further communication crises with medicines were, unfortunately, not prevented, as the case presented next shows.

The "Vioxx Story" of 2004

In 2004, one of the biggest product withdrawals in pharmaceutical history happened. The then popular new painkiller and non-steroidal anti-inflammatory substance rofecoxib, marketed globally as Vioxx®, was withdrawn from the market because of cardiovascular risks, deadly in some patients. As the pharmaceutical company withdrew the product abruptly, regulators in many countries of the world were challenged to react quickly with public statements, while the withdrawal hit the news media headlines and left patients and healthcare professionals anxious. Chap. 3 on COX-2 inhibitors discusses the Vioxx withdrawal in more detail.

Realisation of the Need of Communication for Proactive Risk Management and Trust-Building in the 2000s

Evidence of an increased risk of myocardial infarction with rofecoxib had been available before for some time, but these data had not been properly interpreted and communicated until data accumulating over time provided more clarity. Regulators were criticised for not having acted earlier, and the reputation of the pharmaceutical industry was damaged (Raine et al. 2011). Although international initiatives introducing risk management planning into safety regulation of medicines had already started (Tsintis and La Mache 2004), the "Vioxx story" pushed further into this direction of proactivity in data collection and risk minimisation as a new paradigm of pharmacovigilance (Raine et al. 2011). Interventions intended to prevent or reduce the occurrence of adverse reactions associated with the exposure to a medicine, or to reduce their severity or impact on the patient should adverse reactions occur were called, in the EU, risk minimisation measures (RMM) (European Medicines Agency (EMA), Heads of Medicines Agencies 2017), or, with a similar definition in the US, risk evaluation and mitigation strategies (REMS) (United States Food and Drug Administration (US FDA) 2018b). Activities may consist of routine risk minimisation measures (i.e. the summary of product characteristics, the package leaflet, the labelling of the packaging, the pack size, the legal status of the product and its formulation) or additional risk minimisation measures, such as educational materials and controlled access. Communication is always key to such measures and their implementation in healthcare.

The "Vioxx story" also caught the attention of social scientists and got them interested in medicinal product risk communication. Proposals arose for re-building public trust based on a continuous exchange and evaluation of accumulating data between manufactures, regulators, academic researches, patient groups, healthcare professionals and the general public (Löfstedt 2007).

The Thalidomide Re-Authorisation in the 2000s

In the EU, risk management planning found a first major application in the marketing authorisation for the active substance thalidomide in 2008. To understand the significance of this regulatory decision for risk communication, one needs to look further back in time:

- *The thalidomide disaster of 1961*:

  Thalidomide was developed and first marketed in Germany in 1956 as Contergan®, then used as a sleeping pill and thought to also ease morning sickness and vomiting in pregnant women. Unfortunately, thalidomide turned out to be a very potent teratogenic, i.e. a substance that harms the unborn child when a pregnant woman takes the medicine. By 1961, 10,000 babies were affected worldwide, tragically famous for born with deformed, incomplete or missing arms or legs. Only 5,000 children survived childhood. The product was withdrawn from the market on 2 December 1961 (Brynner and Stephens 2001). With the medical knowledge we have today, one might wonder how this could happen. At the time however, the medical teaching was that the placenta protects the unborn baby from toxic substances, ignoring previous findings of teratogenicity of viruses and alcohol (Daly 1998).
- *Establishment of pharmacovigilance and regulatory standards in 1968*:

  In response to what was called the thalidomide disaster, the WHO established in 1968 the Programme for International Drug Monitoring for the worldwide collection of suspected adverse reaction cases from member countries and early detection of signals of potential new risks (Venulet and Helling-Borda 2010).

This marks the establishment of systematic safety surveillance of medicines, or pharmacovigilance. Furthermore, strong national regulation of medicines with clinical trials for testing efficacy and safety prior to marketing authorisation, continuous pharmacovigilance of authorised medicines used in healthcare and a precautionary approach to using medicines in pregnancy became the standard to strive for (Waller and Harrison-Woolrych 2017). The judgements of the thalidomide court cases formed the legal foundation for responsibilities and liability and clarified ethical aspects. These principles are still valid today for how to deal correctly with safety concerns, unfolding evidence and risk communication, as discussed in Chap. 15 on legal frameworks. Pharmacovigilance is now defined as the science and activities relating to the detection, assessment, understanding and prevention of adverse effects or any other medicine-related problems (World Health Organization (WHO) 2002). While pharmacovigilance is well established in high-income countries with strong regulatory systems, in many countries of the world regulation and pharmacovigilance are still absent, weak or developing. Global efforts are made to overcome these shortcomings in patient and public health protection (Olsson et al. 2015).

Forty years after the thalidomide disaster, this substance had an unexpected comeback, as research demonstrated beneficial properties for some serious medical conditions, including the treatment of multiple myeloma, a specific kind of cancer. In the 2000s new marketing authorisations for thalidomide were issued.

Emergence of Communication for Societal Deliberation

However, the trauma and taboo of the thalidomide disaster had to be overcome before the re-authorisation. Surviving thalidomide victims had become adults, managing severe challenges every day of their lives and confronted with new suffering due to joint inflammation from the overuse of arms, legs and spine to compensate for missing limbs. Their "Never again!" stood against the "Give us a chance!" of those with hopes to be cured from cancer. Communication efforts were therefore vital to install a dialogue between thalidomide victims and cancer patients, so that regulatory bodies could act accountably based on the consensus of the affected populations.

From a risk governance perspective, such a situation is called ambiguity. Ambiguity arises when differences exist in the values of individuals or stakeholders in relation to a risk-related event. Resolving ambiguities requires a deliberation process, i.e. participatory involvement of stakeholders. This aims at openly discussing competing values and arguments and resolving conflicts through finding overarching common values and solutions that do not compromise the different expectations of stakeholders (Renn 2015).

For the EU, the European Medicines Agency (EMA) convened, on 30 May 2007, a meeting of representatives of thalidomide victim organisations and multiple myeloma patient organisations to comment on the proposed risk management plan (RMP). The meeting was successful in achieving mutual understanding and acceptance of a strict pregnancy prevention programme (PPP) and enabled the re-authorisation of thalidomide throughout the EU in 2008. Although the EMA had worked before with patient organisations regarding other medicinal products, such a multi-stakeholder meeting for deliberation was new for the EMA at the time. Nowadays the EMA solicits and considers input from patient and healthcare professional representatives more systematically.

The EU RMP for thalidomide is a legal requirement and includes a contraindication during pregnancy, effective contraception for female and male patients, distribution control with pregnancy testing, advice against breast-feeding, return of unused capsules to the pharmacy, restrictions to blood donation as well as patient counselling and a confirmation by the patient of understanding the risk and conditions of use. This is supported by educational materials for healthcare professionals (European Medicines Agency (EMA) 2008). A similar approach has been taken in the US with a risk evaluation and mitigation strategy (REMS), which likewise includes information materials and agreement forms for healthcare professionals and patients (United States Food and Drug Administration (US FDA) 2017a).

1.2.2 Current Challenges and a Typology of Medicinal Product Risk Communication Outcomes

The communication challenges discussed above (see Sect. 1.2.1) are not entirely historical:

- Thalidomide is now authorised in many countries, not only against multiple myeloma, but also against complications of leprosy, an infectious disease that is still highly endemic in some pockets of the world (World Health Organization (WHO) 2017a). However, complete pregnancy prevention during thalidomide exposure is difficult to achieve globally; e.g. in Brazil, millions of thalidomide tablets are distributed each year and birth defects have been reported. Poor health education and the common sharing of medicines in low resource settings lead to exposure of pregnant women. To prevent this, the WHO considers better medicines regulation and continuous communication key factors (World Health Organization (WHO) 2014).
- Differential VTE risks between CHCs were subject to new assessments by the regulators in the EU in 2001 and 2013 (European Medicines Agency (EMA) 2013). In 2018, the WHO and the US supported an updated systematic review and meta-analysis of the evidence (Dragoman et al. 2018). New research on drospirenone as a newer progestogen was published in 2017 (Larivée et al. 2017a, b). Other research from a couple of European countries and Japan in 2017 focused on identifying women at risk for VTE and improving prescribing (Dulicek et al. 2018; Hugon-Rodin et al. 2017a, b; Kobayashi et al. 2017; McDaid et al. 2017). The American Society for Reproductive Medicines published a new clinical guideline on CHCs and the risk of VTE, likewise in 2017 (Practice Committee of the American Society for Reproductive Medicine 2017).

Overall, adverse reactions to medicines are a major cause of hospital admission and contribute to substantial morbidity in patients and pressure on healthcare systems. A number of studies quantify this, and for the global scope of this book the following study comparing high- and low-income countries is of particular interest:

The prevalence of adverse reaction-related hospitalisation and mortality was found similar in the developed (6.3%, of which fatal: 1.7% (median)) and developing (5.5%, of which fatal: 1.8% (median)) worlds. Also, the main medication classes implicated were largely the same, in particular antithrombotics, non-steroidal anti-inflammatory drugs (NSAIDs) in combination with cardiovascular medicines, anti-diabetics, antineoplastics, immunosuppressants and anti-infectives. The latter were more commonly concerned in developing countries, given their higher rates for infections. Most adverse reaction-related hospitalisations were preventable (72% (median) in developed countries, 60% (median) in developing countries) (Angamo et al. 2016). This indicates the need and opportunity for communication and other measures to improve the use of medicines and reduce risks.

Hence, current challenges in medicinal product risk communication are plentiful. Some medicines that have hit the news headlines or are of global relevance have been selected here with the aim to exemplify further aspects and types of immediate and far-reaching outcomes of communication on risks with medicines. The selected examples are isotretinoin, vaccines, anti-infectives, antidepressants and opioids. Although experiences in the EU have been the starting point, the global scope of the book has been taken into account. Some of the cases are studied in more detail in part II of the book, as indicated by cross-references.

Isotretinoin

Isotretinoin is another highly potent teratogenic substance requiring a pregnancy prevention programme (PPP). While the multiple myeloma patients using thalidomide are usually older, isotretinoin is used by a younger population of highly fertile age. It is effective against otherwise untreatable acne, a skin condition that may severely impact on appearance and self-esteem. There are ongoing concerns worldwide that the PPPs for isotretinoin are not entirely successful, and this is an example for the need of audience analyses. An in-depth understanding of how to reach and motivate young women using their preferred new communication technologies is required. However, getting in contact with patients for exploring why communication has not worked and what needs to be improved can be difficult, in particular if a woman has experienced an unplanned pregnancy (Sundseth H, President of the European Institute of Women's Health. Personal communication with the author. 5 September 2017).

Teratogenicity is not the only issue to be communicated for isotretinoin. Sadly, cases of suicide have been reported in patients using this medicine. This is an example for communication in situations of scientific uncertainty. While the evidence for a causal relationship between isotretinoin and suicidal behaviour to date is inconclusive, precautionary warnings are in place in the package leaflet. But these do not, and of course cannot, address the human dimension of the issue, which pose a challenge to those in personal contact with parents of a young person who has died by suicide. The suicide cases have become subject to debate in the media and some parliaments, a yet different type of communication in the public domain. This illustrates that in real life scientific, personal and political questions may not be separate, and research on communication should illuminate interactions and their implications for communication strategies. Chap. 4 expands on the case of isotretinoin.

Vaccines

Vaccines are an even more prominent example of the interface between the personal, the communal and the political. For the last 200 years vaccines have been, besides sanitation, the most successful health intervention—the worldwide eradication of the monstrous smallpox disease in 1979 is a special achievement to remember. Thanks to the high general acceptance of vaccines, immunisation has drastically reduced many serious, often fatal infectious diseases and saves millions of lives worldwide every year (Andre et al. 2008). As with any new technology though, there has always been scepticism and refusal by some individuals or groups (Schwartz 2012). This phenomenon of refusing or delaying vaccination is nowadays referred to as vaccine hesitancy (MacDonald and SAGE Working Group of Vaccine Hesitancy 2015). The dynamics of vaccine hesitancy over the last 20 years have been allocated to a number of reasons, such as the success of vaccines that makes it difficult to recognise the severity of the prevented diseases and the benefit from vaccination, the accelerated introduction of additional vaccines into public health programmes, high-profile global immunisation initiatives, and—most relevant to note for this book—"tectonic shifts in the production and consumption of information" due to the worldwide use of the internet and social media (Hickler 2015). Among the many reasons people give for their vaccine hesitancy, concerns about vaccine safety are one of the drivers (Jarret et al. 2015).

Communicating about safety and risks of vaccines is therefore very important for supporting informed choices and safe use, and the range of themes to address through communication may be wide. For example, a global online news media monitoring study for human papillomavirus (HPV) vaccines revealed that themes of interest to the public range from safety and validity of data analysis to broader questions about the integrity of risk governance, e.g. where data originate from, how safety systems are organised and overseen, and how biased decision-making is prevented (Bahri et al. 2017). Due to the importance of vaccines for health protection, considerable research into medicinal product risk communication concerns vaccines and underpins communication guidance (Council for International Organizations of Medical Sciences (CIOMS) 2018). Different vaccines are seen differently by the public and yield specific communication requirements (Karafillakis et al. 2017). Many examples could therefore be discussed in this book; the case of MMR vaccines has been selected for this chapter, while H1N1 pandemic influenza vaccines (European Medicines Agency (EMA) 2011) are discussed in Chap. 5.

Measles, Mumps and Rubella Vaccines

The "MMR story" illustrates prominently how untrue information can lead to negative health outcomes. While it goes back to past events, it is very much a current issue. In 1998, major news media reported about the then hypothesised causal link of autism with combination vaccines against measles, mumps and rubella (MMR). This had emerged from a UK study published in a scientific journal. The hypothesis was accompanied in the news by inaccurate information on the target diseases and their prevention, while omitting other research findings not supporting the hypothesis (Goldacre 2009). It was difficult for public bodies to get balancing messages through, and the public debate in the media became politically fuelled by the privacy of the UK prime minister over the vaccination status of his son. The consequence was rapid erosion of parents' and healthcare professionals' trust in the safety of MMR vaccines, and the vaccine coverage in the UK fell to a national average of <80% (Salisbury and Council for International Organizations of Medical Sciences (CIOMS) 2018). Vaccination rates decreased in a number of other countries around the globe too (Speers and Lewis 2004). In 2010, the research was retracted by the journal due to several elements being incorrect and some claims regarding the study conduct proven to be false (Lancet (eds) 2010), but the harmful impact has been irreversible. While the MMR vaccination rate in England has recovered to above 90% (National Health Service (NHS) 2016–2017) thanks to investigational journalism and communication combined with trust-building initiatives of the government (Salisbury and Council for International Organizations of Medical Sciences (CIOMS) 2018), the untrue information stays present in the internet and mind of many people until today (Venkatraman et al. 2015). Hence some parents do not bring their children for vaccination, and measles outbreaks with fatal cases in those not or incompletely vaccinated continue to emerge in various countries (European Centre for Disease Prevention and Control (ECDC) 2017; United States Centers of Disease Control (US CDC) 2019). Among these victims are children who could have been vaccinated as well as those who cannot be vaccinated for medical reasons and need to rely on what is called "herd immunity", i.e. on others being vaccinated and not infecting them. This is an example for how individual decisions may affect others. Several reviews have concluded against a causal association between the vaccine and autism (United States Centers of Disease Control (US CDC) 2019; Demicheli et al. 2012; World Health Organization (WHO) 2017b). Today, 15 deaths an hour due to measles still occur worldwide, but the good news is that vaccination resulted in a 79% global drop in measles deaths worldwide between 2000 and 2015 (World Health Organization (WHO) 2017c).

The "MMR story" has provoked a lot of considerations by those engaged in public health and led journalists to self-critically reflect upon their responsibilities and the need to carefully check, judge and present the strength of all available evidence. It has also led to calls upon scientists to speak up more in the public domain (Speers and Lewis 2004; Illman 2013). A paediatrician and father of an autistic child has recently done so in his book "Vaccines Did Not Cause Rachel's Autism" (Hotez 2018).

Anti-infectives

Given the high global burden of disease due to infections (GBD 2016 Disease and Injury Incidence and Prevalence Collaborators 2017), not only vaccines but also anti-infectives are an important class of medicines. Anti-infectives can cure or even prevent infections, and like vaccines save lives every day. Their inappropriate use though can make an anti-infective ineffective against the infectious agent. This so-called antimicrobial resistance (AMR) has become a major global health threat. 480,000 people are affected by multi-drug resistant tuberculosis each year, and AMR has also started to complicate the fights against HIV and malaria. AMR concerns an ever-increasing range of infections and is present in every country (World Health Organization (WHO) 2016b). Regional and national plans have been developed to address AMR, as well as the WHO Global Action Plan, which includes communication, training and education as one of its five objectives (World Health Organization (WHO) 2015).

Medicinal product risk communication can support these plans through messages about AMR risks and correct indication, dosing and management of adverse reactions of anti-infectives. In particular, communication should prevent patients who suspect experiencing an adverse reaction or have another concern from stopping anti-infectives prematurely without medical advice (as this may—not necessarily though—promote AMR). Exploring, together with the patient, risk factors for adverse reactions prior to prescribing can help selecting the most appropriate anti-infective and prevent stopping. Advice on preventing lack of efficacy can also be an anti-AMR measure, as illustrated by rilpivirine. This anti-HIV medicine must be taken with food for achieving plasma levels that are high enough for therapeutic effects and AMR prevention. The regulatory authorities in the EU monitored the implementation of this instruction in the product information through requiring a study to measure physicians' awareness and adherence to informing the patients accordingly (Grainger D, Lead Investigator 2017).

Antidepressants

Next to infectious diseases, a considerable proportion of the global burden of disease falls to mental and substance abuse disorders. These are the largest contributors to disability in young people (GBD 2016 Disease and Injury Incidence and Prevalence Collaborators 2017). Promoting mental health and tackling substance abuse have therefore become integral to the United Nations Sustainable Development Agenda. With psychosocial care and medication most patients could be treated and lead normal lives again, even in resource-limited countries (World Health Organization (WHO) 2017d).

One mental disorder of major relevance is depression. More than 300 million people worldwide suffer from depression, making it a leading cause of disability in all age groups. Suicide is the second most common cause of death in 15- to 19-years old girls (World Health Organization (WHO) 2017e). Antidepressant medicines have been used in adolescents and young adults, either with a marketing authorisation specifically for this age group or as off-label use. In 2004, clinical trials showed however an increase of suicidal thoughts and behaviours in adolescents using antidepressants (4% versus 2% with placebo). As a consequence, the US Food Drug Administration (US FDA) required, and kept up-to-date since, a boxed warning in the labels of antidepressants (United States Food and Drug Administration (US FDA) 2018c). Similar warnings were introduced in the EU for specific types of antidepressants, i.e. selective serotonin reuptake inhibitors (SSRIs) and serotonin-norepinephrine reuptake inhibitors (SNRIs) (European Medicines Agency (EMA) 2005), as well as in Australia, where they soon led to intended changes in use (Dean et al. 2007).

The warning was however immediately controversial among healthcare professionals, as they feared that young people with mental disorders would in future go untreated. This exemplifies the challenging task of risk communication to advise on risks and at the same time not to discourage treatment in the case of medical need. Ten years later, in 2014, it was claimed in the US that the warning has done more harm than good, given downward trends in diagnosing depression and prescribing antidepressants for young people and upward trends in self-poisoning with psychotropic substances (interpreted as a proxy for suicidal attempt). Even prescribing in adults had declined and been attributed to the warning as a so-called spill-over effect. It was suggested that the news media debate over the warning had provoked patients to not report signs of depression or to reject treatment (Friedman 2014). Similar unintended effects were seen in Canada (Katz et al. 2008). An opposing view claimed inaccuracies and illogical interpretation of the available US data and the possible influence of changes in advertising on prescribing trends, concluding that the warning did not have negative impacts (Stone 2014). A researcher of one of the studies finding reductions in antidepressant prescribing and simultaneous "small but meaningful" increases in suicide attempts (Lu et al. 2014) explained in the news media: "This is an extraordinarily difficult public health problem, and if we don't get it right, it can backfire in serious ways…. These drugs can save lives. The media concentrated more on the relatively small risk than on the significant upside" (Soumerai 2014). In any case, the most important goal lies in detecting and treating emerging suicidal ideas and behaviours in any patient as early as possible (Friedman 2014).

Opioids

Substance abuse is a medical condition classified as a mental disorder too. Currently, opioid dependency with overdoses and deaths is seen in North America to an extent that it is now called the opioid epidemic. Opioids include illicit substances as well as prescription medicines, such as morphine, oxycodone, hydrocodone, fentanyl, tramadol, codeine and methadone. Originally most of these medicines were restricted, for use only against pain of advanced cancer or major surgery. For the last 20 years however, they have increasingly been prescribed for chronic non-cancer pain, such as backache, headaches and fibromyalgia. Between 1999 and 2015, more than 183,000 persons died from overdoses in the US, and in Canada 2,000 persons died from opioids in 2015 alone. Some analyses suggest that a similar trend of prescription overdoses is under way in Europe. There were 208 tramadol overdose deaths in the UK in 2015 (Anderson 2017). Latest data show problematic continuing increase of opioid use in the US, Canada, UK, Sweden, Norway and Ireland (Organisation for Economic Co-operation and Development (OECD) 2019). For Europe overall, the use of prescribed opioids is increasing, but at a much slower rate than in the US, and fatal incidents have so far been rare. The risk of an opioid epidemic in Europe is considered low at present but vigilance and prevention are needed (van Amsterdam and van den Brink 2015). The US opioid epidemic is seen as a warning for Europe, and also for Australia (Douglas and Holpuch 2017).

In North America multiple measures have been taken that healthcare professionals reduce opioid use and discuss risks of addiction with patients prior to prescribing (Anderson 2017). Also, media coverage raises wide public awareness of this health issue that has evolved into a political issue in the US (Blendon and Benson 2018;

Lancet (eds) 2017; McGreal 2017; Mass 2017). Although communication is only one measure among others, over 80% of the US population believe that public education programmes could be somewhat (40%) to very (44%) effective in remedying the problem (Blendon and Benson 2018). As part of the "Turn The Tide Rx" campaign, the US government sent letters and a pocket card with treatment guidance to healthcare professionals and provided further educational resources and platforms for exchange of experience between healthcare professionals (Murthy 2016). Measuring the effectiveness of this risk communication will be an important area of research.

In contrast to the situation in North America and other high-income countries, around 80% of patients worldwide have no access to adequate pain management, mainly because of strict narcotic policies or high prices. Access to pain management is however a fundamental patient right, as inadequate management of pain has serious physical, mental and societal implications (Lancet (eds) 2017).

A Typology of Medicinal Product Risk Communication Outcomes

Communicating about risks with medicines may result in intended or unintended, positive or negative and predictable or unpredictable outcomes. Outcomes manifest in full or partial achievements, increases, decreases, or other changes as well as in unchanged or newly emerging phenomena.

An intended outcome usually relates to a pre-defined communication objective in terms of what to achieve or to prevent happening. Unintended outcomes can be negative, for example if patients inappropriately stop a treatment out of concern raised by new information without consulting their healthcare professional, or positive, when, for example, advice for patients to carefully check dosing for a particular medicine creates a general awareness to always check the package leaflet for any new medicine one may use (i.e. a positive spill-over effect). An outcome of incomplete, not-understandable or otherwise ineffective communication that leaves gaps in what people want or need to know may be a so-called information vacuum in the public domain. This can result in subsequent outcomes, like rumours, misinformation and mistrust (Pang 2013).

Currently, plenty of different categorisations for outcomes are used in research. This constitutes a major obstacle for evidence consolidation and systematic reviews (see Sect. 1.3.1). Therefore, a typology of outcomes is proposed here to support formulating research objectives (see Sect. 1.3.2) and systematising findings. This may serve as a starting point for the multidisciplinary research community to agree upon common outcome categories and measurements for comparisons of findings over time, or between places, medicinal products, safety concerns, communication types or audiences. The typology in Table 1.2 has been created by deriving possible outcomes of medicinal product risk communication from the above case examples of communication challenges and grouping them into ten categories. This has been complemented by adding further outcomes studied in the research presented in Table 1.3 (see Sect. 1.3.1).

The ten categories of communication outcome types are presented in an order aligned along an idealised pathway of information flow and impact; e.g. receipt of safe use advice—increase in knowledge—motivation and intent to change behaviour—new safe use behaviour—positive health outcome through avoiding harm from the medicine. In reality information flows and pathways of impact are more complex (see Sect. 1.1), and a communication event may not only have subsequent but also different simultaneous and interacting outcomes, and any may differ by sub-populations and change over time. The first outcome of a communication event however is always the receipt of information, in particular when targeting and reaching population groups with information have been planned as part of the objectives. However, the reach of unplanned communication events or rumours can likewise be categorised under exposure to information. Then, new information may impact on one's immediate emotions and sentiments (i.e. the more enduring emotional state (Encyclopedia of Sociology 2001)) as well as one's attitudes. In line with an initial broad definition by Gordon Allport in 1935, an attitude is the mental and neural state of readiness that influences an individual's response to an object or situation (Allport 1935). Attitudes have later been described as determined by emotional, motivational, cognitive and evaluative processes (Schwarz and Bohner 2001). While trust is part of the attitude concept, it has been included in a separate category together with engagement and satisfaction. Another overlap between categories can be seen in the fact that, for example, engaging and researching are also behaviours; however, they have both been considered distinct enough to have their own categories. While ultimately the long-term health impact of using medicines is of central interest, the above case examples show that communication failures may lead to outcomes that may go far beyond the medicinal product risk to be addressed originally, such as loss of trust in science, public outrage against the government, or new legislation, policies, services and campaigns for solving problems. The typology has been developed further to cover the outcomes of stakeholder engagement, two-way communication and the information flows from, for example, patients to healthcare professionals, or patients and healthcare professionals to governments. Understanding the connections between outcomes, whether immediate and/or far-reaching, is what research with a wider and deeper scope is interested in. New research activities may also be an outcome of communication events where need for evidence-based improvements has been identified.

The outcome types in Table 1.2 are not examples of direct measurements or parameters for what cannot be directly measured. Rather, these are outcome types for which a range of measurements—quantitative ones and quality degrees—can be applied. Tools for measurement are necessary, and it requires careful consideration to define the right ways and units to characterise and measure outcomes, also with a view to evaluate underlying structural components and the processes leading to these outcomes. Likewise, indicators of needs for improvement require to be defined carefully. Where communication events have been planned with an objective, the measurement has to correspond to the objective. If, for example, the communication objective has been defined as following advice for safe medicines use or informed therapeutic decision-making, these behaviours have to be studied as outcomes. The health impact is appropriate to study as a subsequent outcome. If in future researchers can standardise how to measure outcomes, findings will become truly comparable. The research methods for studying communication outcomes are discussed in part II of the book (Table 1.2.)

Table 1.2 Types of medicinal product risk communication outcomes

Category of outcome types		Outcome types, e.g.
1	Exposure to messages	Receipt of/reading of/listening to messages by target population, addressee or interacting parties
		Re-dissemination of messages, possibly with alteration (e.g. different emphasis or framing) through news, scientific, social or other media or interactions at various communication levels and social spheres
2	Debate	Debate about safety concern, message content or integrity of risk governance in news, scientific or social media, parliaments, other political institutions or public forums or bodies or communities, including patient, parent and healthcare professional communities
		Information vacuum/unaddressed questions/uncertainty/ambiguity/misinformation in the public domain or communities, including patient, parents or healthcare professional communities and journalists
		Public/media outrage
		Activities of an individual, patient organisation, healthcare professional organisation, citizen group, other community, public body or political institution in news or social media or political forums, including petitions
3	Risk knowledge and risk minimisation skills	Knowledge of healthcare professionals, patients, parents, journalists, the public, public bodies, pharmaceutical companies and researchers on benefits, risks, safe and appropriate use and risk minimisation measures
		Knowledge of public, public bodies, pharmaceutical companies, researchers and healthcare professionals on medicines use practices and risk minimisation measures implementation status and needs in healthcare
		Communication skills of public bodies, healthcare professional organisations, healthcare professionals and others informing and counselling about risks, risk minimisation measures, safe use and available choices
		Skills of healthcare professionals, patients or parents for safe use and for implementing and adhering to risk minimisation measures
4	Attitudes	Risk awareness/risk aversion/risk acceptance/perceived risk magnitude and severity by experts in public bodies and pharmaceutical companies, healthcare professionals, patients, parents or the public with in/adequate matching to evidence and uncertainties
		Fear/negative feelings/confidence/self-efficacy (perceived ability)/motivation/intent/engagement/positive feelings of healthcare professionals or patients to use the medicinal product safely
		Fear/negative feelings/confidence/self-efficacy (perceived ability)/motivation/intent/engagement/positive feelings of healthcare professionals to effectively inform patients about risks and safe use
		Fear/negative feelings/confidence/motivation/intent/engagement/positive feelings of patients to consult healthcare professional in relation to disease and medicinal products
		Fear/negative feelings/confidence/motivation/intent/engagement/positive feelings of regulatory or other public bodies or journalists to effectively inform about risks and safe use

Table 1.2 (continued)

Category of outcome types		Outcome types, e.g.
5	Behaviours	Seeking, reading or otherwise accessing data or information by patients, parents, healthcare professionals, health policy makers and experts in public bodies and pharmaceutical companies
		Using healthcare services by patients or parents
		Listening by healthcare professionals, public bodies or others responsible for safety of medicines to experiences with medicines use, risk minimisation measures, information needs, interests and expectations of patients, parents, healthcare professionals or the public
		Providing accurate, complete and understandable information on benefits, risks, safe and appropriate use
		Informed decision-making by healthcare professionals, patients, parents, healthcare settings, regulatory bodies, health policy makers, health technology assessment bodies or health insurance systems about using the medicinal product
		Appropriate and safe prescribing/handling/dispensing/ administration of the medicinal product, including adhering to risk management/risk minimisation measures (e.g. contraindication, patient monitoring advice, pregnancy prevention programme) by healthcare professionals or patients, including the delivery of risk minimisation measures by healthcare professionals to patients
		Stopping the medicinal product appropriately and safely by healthcare professionals or patients
		Starting/switching to another treatment with a more/less favourable risk-benefit balance
		Changing medicines use not targeted by a risk communication beyond replacing the targeted medicinal product (i.e. spill-over to another indication, population or medicinal product)
		Using/not using the medicinal product when needed (adherence to treatment or vaccination schedule)
		Diagnosing diseases and recording of indications in health records
		Off-label use of the medicinal product
		Medication error
		Misuse or abuse of the medicinal product by healthcare professionals, patients or others
		Submission of a suspected adverse reaction by a healthcare professional, patient or parents to the pharmacovigilance reporting system
		Initiating/conducting/participating in monitoring activities and studies to identify and characterise risks or the effectiveness of risk minimisation measures

(continued)

Table 1.2 (continued)

Category of outcome types		Outcome types, e.g.
6	Health, quality of life and other benefits	Harm (e.g. morbidity, hospitalisation, mortality, reduced quality of life) in patient due to adverse reactions (including suicidal behaviour)/ medication errors/misuse/abuse of the medicinal product
		Harm in child/miscarriage after use of the medicinal product by mother or father before/during pregnancy
		Harm in child or carer after accidential exposure/in healthcare professional after occupational exposure to the medicinal product
		Burden of disease prevented/treated/untreated/not prevented and related quality of life/lives gained/lost in patients or populations
		Gain/loss of benefits/resources of using/not using/using inappropriately a medicinal product beyond health outcomes, e.g. patient autonomy, relationships, planned or unplanned pregnancies, economic power of individuals and societies
7	Trust, engagement and satisfaction	Trust/satisfaction of healthcare professionals, patients, parents or the public in product safety, pharmacovigilance systems, risk governance, related decision-making and outcomes in terms of product availability and risk management and science overall, including changes in political climate
		Engagement of healthcare professionals, patients or the public and regulatory or other public bodies for information exchange, risk governance, deliberation or decision-making regarding medicines or their use, including public hearings and policies
		Collaboration of healthcare professionals, patients and public bodies and satisfaction regarding their engagement, e.g. communication planning, drafting messages and policy-making
		Satisfaction of patients with communication and delivery of risk minimisation measures in healthcare and shared therapeutic decision-making and confidence in appropriateness and value-choice congruence of decisions made or decisional conflict
8	Risk governance, management and communication systems	Establishment/strengthening of legislation/policy/regulatory guidelines/ transparency provisions/communication systems and processes/capacity/ communication guidance and strategies/engagement mechanisms/ treatment guidance/formularies/risk minimisation measures for safety, safe use and risk communication for the medicinal product
		Successful/not successful multi-stakeholder deliberation and agreement to risk minimisation
		Transparency and other policies for demonstrating credibility of risk governance, e.g. transparency of data, research methods, underlying assumptions and assessments or policies for managing conflict of interests
		Establishment and operations of information services and other communication systems (e.g. medical information services, medicines hotlines, teratogenicity counselling, science media centres, quality assured websites, media offices)
		Risk communication training
		Code of conducts for science and health journalists
		Information campaigns on general medicines safe use principles for children in school or the public
9	Legal and other official procedures	Investigations of appropriate conduct of communication, litigation and taking legal action because of inappropriate or missing risk communication

Table 1.2 (continued)

Category of outcome types		Outcome types, e.g.
10	Research	Research for understanding, planning and evaluating medicinal product risk communication to foster improvements in communication
		Research for providing evidence on questions relevant to the safe and effective use of the medicinal product in healthcare or on concerns expressed by patients or healthcare professionals, and for characterising, quantifying and contextualising the risk

1.3 Multilayered Medicinal Product Risk Communication Research

The need to generate more and better evidence on medicinal product risk communication has been recognised by the global pharmacovigilance community (Bahri et al. 2015; Bahri and Harrison-Woolrych 2012), in particular regarding the impact on patients (Cox and Butt 2012). This section of the chapter provides an overview of the research that has evaluated interventions relevant to medicinal product risk communication. In order to progress the research field, this section proposes a multilayered research framework.

1.3.1 Building Upon Existing Research

Much of the available risk communication research has been reviewed and summarised in the US FDA publication "Communicating Risks and Benefits: an Evidence-Based User's Guide" (Fischhoff et al. 2011). There it is also stated that "Risk communications are all around us, but rarely evaluated" (Downs 2011). From this guide one could derive a standard against which to evaluate communication.

An overview of findings from research worldwide that has evaluated interventions relevant to medicinal product risk communication is presented in Table 1.3, together with the identified needs for further research and methods development. This overview covers the systematic reviews from the Cochrane Library (Cochrane Collaboration 2018)—as a major global resource on health interventions—and the reviews (Trevena et al. 2004; West et al. 2013; Dusetzina et al. 2012) included in the report "Health Product Risk Communication: Is the Message Getting Through?" from the international Expert Panel on the Effectiveness of Health Product Risk Communication of the Council of Canadian Academies—as the latest compilation of evidence (Council of Canadian Academies 2015). This has been supplemented with results (Hallgreen et al. 2016) from the EU project "Pharmacoepidemiological Research on Outcomes of Therapeutics by a European Consortium (PROTECT)" (European Medicines Agency 2009–2017), reviews from the EU regulatory network (Mazzaglia et al. 2018; Goedecke et al. 2018), reviews from others presented at EMA forums (Way et al. 2017; Piening et al. 2012), and two other relevant review articles (DeFrank et al. 2019; Briesacher et al. 2013).

The following becomes apparent from Table 1.3: The reviews identified by above strategy investigate communication interventions in the healthcare and regulatory contexts, but not exchanges between patients, media coverage or political debates. Most research is only about a few classes of medicines, including vaccines, and mainly from high-income countries. The reviewed studies often measure only a few outcomes identified in single data sources and hardly come to conclusions regarding causal relationships between communication and outcomes or the impact of other concurrent information flows. Behavioural and health outcomes are studied to a lesser extent, and a range of methodological limitations remain to be overcome.

The expert panel of the Council of Canadian Academies summarises the current state of evidence as follows: "There are few publicly available and publicly conducted evaluations of established health product risk communication tools in any jurisdiction. Regulators have either not evaluated their effectiveness or used the results of external evaluations, and in any case not made results public or easily accessible. This gap could have implications for the quality of risk communication. The majority of the evaluations identified for ongoing communication focused primarily on indicators of understandability (e.g. readability) and user surveys, expert analysis, and public consultations. Those identified for incident(s)-based communication examined effectiveness in terms of use and impact after implementation and completion of the communication. These studies most often used medical or pharmacy claims (e.g. prescribing rates) as indicators" (Council of Canadian Academies 2015).

Linking health outcomes to certain communication events with sufficient scientific certainty of causal relationship has so far been difficult. For example, observational data on the warnings about antidepressants and changes in diagnosis and treatment of depression (see Sect. 1.3.1) could only show trends of correlation, but not establish a causal link between the warning and changes in clinical practice (Friedman 2014). In general, it has been discussed that the absence of a strong response of a target population to a communication intervention in terms of the intended safe use behaviour may indicate either ineffectiveness of the communication or that there were already good risk awareness and positive behavioural trends in place. On the other hand, the presence of a strong response may indicate either communication effectiveness or unnecessary overcompensation on the part of patients or healthcare professionals (Vicusi 1994). Hence, any outcome has to be interpreted in relation to the situation prior to the communication event. Studying the pre- and post-situations and taking into account simultaneous, subsequent and interacting information flows and influencing factors can only be achieved through combining multiple data sources and analytical methods from different disciplines.

Some research projects have already gone into this direction. Prominently, a US pilot project combined methods from pharmacoepidemiology and the social sciences to study two drug safety communication documents (DSCs) from the US FDA, issued in 2013 for zolpidem. This sedative and sleeping aid carries a risk of next-morning impairment, and the DSCs were about this risk and the lower recommended initial dose for women. An information flow model was developed and the effects at various stages of the flows were assessed by different methods against the situation before the DSCs. The methods included an analysis of prescribing and health outcomes, interviews of patients and physicians, a patient survey as well as quantitative and qualitative reviews of news and social media stories. The project intended to test this new combination of methods for increasing understanding and optimising regulatory communications (Kesselheim et al. 2015). The news media analysis showed that only the first DSC generated high-profile news coverage, and that at least, but still only half of the news media stories reported the DSC messages correctly (Woloshin et al. 2017). Likewise, the social media analysis found substantial but short-lived uptake by Twitter, Facebook, Google and Wikipedia only for the first DSC. By contrast, the second DSC did not result in additional posts or searches (Sinha et al. 2018). The interviews of patients and physicians revealed that during their conversations side effects were discussed, but almost no patient reported that their physician had made them aware of the messages of the DSCs (Kesselheim et al. 2017). Each analysis yielded specific and complimentary conclusions, i.e. that ways for user-friendly and timely dissemination should be explored (Kesselheim et al. 2017), that it is important to find ways ensuring translation of DSC content in news media messages (Woloshin et al. 2017), and that the US FDA could contribute content to websites like Wikipedia and employ social media strategies for disseminating DSCs (Sinha et al. 2018). This "multimodal analysis" provided a multi-perspective picture of the impact of the US FDA's risk communication about zolpidem (Kesselheim et al. 2019) (Table 1.3).

Table 1.3 Reviews evaluating interventions that involve medicinal product risk communication

Objective of the review and intervention types	Studies reviewed and outcome categories	Summary of most relevant findings of the review	Gaps and needs identified by the review
Research evaluating written information about benefits and risks of medicines for patients (Nicolson et al. 2009)			
To assess the effects of information for patients about benefits and risks of prescribed and over-the-counter medicines *Interventions*: different written printed or online information	5 randomised clinical trials (in any language) *Outcomes*: (1) knowledge, attitude and behaviour; (2) health	– The trials were not clearly reported and of poor quality – Because the trials measured different outcomes in different ways, their individual results could not be combined – Written information compared to no information improved knowledge, and was not harmful in any case	Use of stronger methods and consistent, validated outcome measures; evaluation of internet-based information
Research evaluating multi-media education about medicines for patients (Ciciriello et al. 2013)			
To assess the effects of multi-media patient education interventions about prescribed and over-the-counter medications in people of all ages, including children and carers *Interventions*: delivery of information using at least two formats, i.e. text, still graphics or photographs, animation and video and/or audio	24 randomised controlled trials and quasi-randomised controlled trials (worldwide) *Outcomes*: (1) knowledge/skills; (2) compliance/adherence; (3) use, misuse/dependence; (4) health outcomes/adverse reactions; (5) quality of life; (6) self-efficacy; (7) perception, satisfaction and attitude; (8) patient use of education; (9) health service use; (10) adverse effects of education	– Studies had a high risk of bias or did not report sufficient information to judge on risk of bias – Review findings were based on very low to moderate quality of evidence – Multi-media education was more effective at improving knowledge than usual care or no education and increased the effectiveness of co-interventions, but was not more effective than control multi-media interventions – Multi-media education was more effective at skill acquisition than usual care, no education or written education, and equally effective as education by a healthcare professional – There was no difference between multi-media education and usual care or no education for compliance with medication – Interpretation whether results were of clinical importance was not possible	Evaluation of multi-media educational interventions with details about the interventions and comparators; evaluation framework with core set of outcomes; consistent, reliable and validated outcome measures
Research evaluating communication with patients about evidence (Trevena et al. 2004)			
To assess the effectiveness of communication tools and formats for probabilistic information to increase patient understanding and strategies for eliciting patient preferences *Interventions*: tailored printed information; decision aids; consultation summaries or instructions; training in a patient-centred approach ± risk communication; video; interactive computer aids; leaflets; question prompts; various formats of probabilistic information	10 systematic reviews of randomised clinical trials and 30 randomised clinical trials (in English) *Outcomes*: patient-oriented: (1) understanding; (2) knowledge; (3) comprehension; (4) satisfaction with decision; (5) adherence to decision; (6) anxiety; (7); decisional conflict; (8) involvement in decision-making	– Most formats, e.g. verbal, written, video, provider-delivered, computer-based, increased patients' understanding, but are more likely to be effective if structured, tailored and/or interactive – Probabilistic information is best understood as natural frequencies in relevant groups of people, rather than words or probabilities effect measures, e.g. relative risk reduction – Illustrations, e.g. cartoons, vertical bar charts, appear to aid understanding – Values clarification exercises may be better than standard utility techniques for eliciting preferences in individual decision-making – Pooling outcomes was not possible, as the trials were from a wide variety of clinical settings using a range of clinical problems and outcome measures – Generalising findings was difficult, but was based on the consistency of the direction of effects	Research on effectiveness of communication tools and formats; access for healthcare professionals and patients to effective communication tools in practice

Research evaluating framing of health messages (Akl et al. 2011a)			
To evaluate effects of different framings of health information *Interventions*: messages with same information but different attribute (positive vs negative) and goal (gain vs loss) framing	35 studies with randomised controlled trial, quasi-randomised controlled trial or cross-over design (in any language) *Outcomes*: (1) understanding; (2) perception of effectiveness; (3) persuasiveness; (4) behaviour of consumers	– Review findings were based on small or moderate effect sizes and very low to moderate quality of evidence – Messages were understood better when framed negatively – Although positively framed messages may have led to more positive perception of effectiveness, there was little or no difference in persuasiveness and behaviour – Loss messages led to a more positive perception of effectiveness for screening messages and may have been more persuasive for treatment messages – Different goal framing showed little or no difference in behaviour, and no study assessed understanding	Research on unexplained heterogeneity between studies and effects under specific conditions
Research evaluating statistical formats of risk communication in healthcare (Akl et al. 2011b)			
To evaluate the effects of alternative statistical presentations *Interventions*: different formats expressing same risks or risk reductions	35 studies with randomised and non-randomised controlled parallel cross-over design (in any language) *Outcomes*: (1) understanding; (2) perception; (3) persuasiveness; (4) behaviour of healthcare professionals, policy makers and consumers	– Studies related to diagnostic or screening tests – The overall quality of evidence was moderate because of the use of surrogate outcomes and/or heterogeneity – Natural frequencies were better understood than percentages – Compared with absolute risk reduction, relative risk reduction had little or no difference in understanding but was perceived to be larger and more persuasive – Numbers-needed-to-treat was less well understood – Overall there were no differences in findings between healthcare professionals and consumers – None of the studies involved policy makers – None of the comparisons assessed behaviour	Research into potential of relative risk reduction for helping people make decisions consistent with their values; improved study quality; use or randomised designs; effects in real life under specific conditions; use of validated outcome measures; behavioural outcomes; global research
Research evaluating quantitative risk and benefit information in product information and advertisement of medicines (West et al. 2013)			
To determine if the presentation of quantitative risk and benefit information in influences patients' and healthcare professionals' information processing and behaviours *Interventions*: product information; advertisement	52 studies with quasi-experimental, randomised controlled, cross-sectional, focus group or other explicit design (in English) *Outcomes*: (1) information preferences; (2) knowledge and comprehension; (3) perceived risks and benefits; (4) behavioural intention and behaviour	– The existing body of evidence is limited – While the majority of studies involved a carefully defined intervention, addressed statistical power and employed a randomised design, some suffered from comparator constraints or problematic order effects – Outcomes mainly addressed were information preferences, knowledge, understanding or risk perceptions – Numerical information appears to improve understanding of risks and benefits relative to non-numerical presentation, and presenting both numerical and non-numerical information may be best practice – No single specific format or graphical approach emerged as consistently superior	Systematic and well designed and controlled studies in populations who are the actual information users; testing of multiple format types at once and comprehensive comparisons; research into numeracy and health literacy as moderating factors

(continued)

Table 1.3 (continued)

Objective of the review and intervention types	Studies reviewed and outcome categories	Summary of most relevant findings of the review	Gaps and needs identified by the review
Research evaluating visual representation of the results of benefit–risk assessments of medicinal products (Hallgreen et al. 2016)			
To identify and appraise visual displays used for medical risk and benefit–risk communication *Interventions*: different visual displays	55 articles (in English) and 14 additional sources for visuals from websites and reports *Outcomes*: none (evaluation against criteria: (1) intended audience; (2) intended message; (3) knowledge required to understand the visual; (4) unintentional messages that may be derived from the visual and missing information that may be needed to understand the visual)	– 65 examples of visual formats were identified and classified into 14 visual types – There is not one single visual format that is consistently superior to others – Most of the drawbacks found in the visual formats could be considered general to visual communication, although some appear more relevant to specific formats and should be considered when creating visuals for different audiences depending on the exact message to be communicated – The compatibility between a visual and its target audience is very important to consider when creating visuals	Research into visual formats for addressing different types of benefit-risk analysis information
Research evaluating interventions to improve safe and effective medicines use by patients (Ryan et al. 2014)			
To assess interventions for improving safe and effective medicines use by patients *Interventions*: information/education; facilitation of communication/ decision-making; acquiring competencies; support for behaviour change; support for disease management and coping; minimisation of risks; quality of care improvements; consumer system participation	75 systematic reviews (in English; identified studies from low- and high-income countries) *Outcomes*: (1) consumer-oriented, e.g. knowledge, involvement, adverse events; (2) provider-oriented, e.g. knowledge, communication with patient; (3) health service-oriented, e.g. hospital admission	– The quality of the reviews varied and available evidence did not show the full picture – Medicines self-monitoring and self-management appeared effective to improve medicines use and health outcomes; however, some participants were unable to complete what the interventions required, suggesting they might not be suitable for everyone – Many different pathways through which the use of medicines by patients could be improved seemed possible, and simple interventions might be as effective as complex strategies – No single intervention assessed was effective to improve all outcomes across all diseases, medicinal products, patient populations or settings	Evaluation of interventions with limited or inconsistent evidence; specific populations, e.g. children, young people, carers, patients with multiple diseases

Research evaluating communication interventions about childhood vaccination (Saeterdal et al. 2014)			
To assess the effects of interventions aimed at communities to inform and/or educate people about vaccination in children 6 years and younger *Interventions*: meetings or different media, e.g. brochures, pamphlets, poster, fact sheets, videos, slide shows, web-based programmes, online communities, audio recordings, billboards, newspaper, television, radio	2 cluster-randomised trials (in English; identified studies from India and Pakistan) *Outcomes*: (1) knowledge; (2) child immunisation status; (3) unintended adverse effects; (4) attitudes; (5) involvement in decision-making; (6) confidence in the decision made; (7) resource use or cost	– Only two studies were identified and the main intervention consisted in community meetings – There was low certainty evidence that the interventions improved knowledge about vaccines or diseases and changed attitudes in favour of vaccination among parents – The interventions probably increased the number of children who are vaccinated	Assessment of knowledge of those in vaccine service delivery, confidence in vaccination decision, costs, unintended harm; transferability depending on baselines and settings; evaluation of large-scale and electronic media interventions; comparisons of community versus individual interventions
Research evaluating face-to-face communication interventions about early childhood vaccination (Kaufman et al. 2013)			
To assess the effects of face-to-face interventions for parents regarding early childhood vaccination *Interventions*: single and multiple face-to-face session strategies for informing or educating parents	6 randomised clinical trials and one cluster-randomised clinical trial (in any language; identified studies from low- or middle-income and high-income countries) *Outcomes*: (1) parental knowledge; (2) immunisation uptake; (3) intention to vaccinate child; (4) parent experience of intervention: (5) adverse effects; (6) costs	– Data could not be pooled due to heterogeneity or skewness – The studies had methodological weaknesses and provided limited evidence of low to very low quality – The review suggests that face-to-face interventions to inform or educate parents about childhood vaccination have little to no impact on immunisation status, or knowledge or understanding of vaccination – There is insufficient evidence to comment on other outcomes	Measuring both knowledge and immunisation status for understanding pathways of effects; effectiveness of single and combined interventions; comparative and controlled studies, including those between face-to-face interventions targeting individuals and groups; other barriers to immunisation; broader concept of informed choice; outcomes of intention forming, experience of communication interventions, possible adverse effects; cost-effectiveness; low literacy populations

(continued)

Table 1.3 (continued)

Objective of the review and intervention types	Studies reviewed and outcome categories	Summary of most relevant findings of the review	Gaps and needs identified by the review
Research evaluating benefit-risk communication tools for medicines used by regulatory bodies to inform patients (Way et al. 2017)			
To review studies on benefit-risk communication tools for use by patients *Interventions*: modes of benefit-risk information that are or could be available to regulatory bodies (including websites but excluding other electronic and social media tools)	Helicopter view of studies published in scientific journals *Outcomes*: (1) sharing information; (2) changing beliefs; (3) changing behaviours	– Only few studies have examined the effects of public access (transparency) to adverse event databases, the effectiveness of tools for changing beliefs, the value of infographics or the application of the mental models approach – A systematic analysis of studies on sharing clinical trial data is not available, and no studies have been done on standardised benefit-risk information frameworks – Sharing clinical trial data, adverse event databases and signals of potentially new risks may have unwanted effects, e.g. confusion of patients, heightened risk perception and discontinuation of medication – Package leaflets and other written information remains often unread, or is confusing/incomprehensible, inconsistent, incomplete and not user-friendly – Drug facts boxes with summary benefit-risk information have been successfully tested with audiences – Warnings that are tailored to audiences and well disseminated can be effective	Studies on behaviour change tools; studies on the promising mental models approach; application and studies on 'traffic light' labelling
Research evaluating the impact of medicines risk communication required by regulatory authorities (Piening et al. 2012)			
To review studies assessing the impact of risk communication *Interventions*: advisories; boxed warnings; DHPCs	50 randomised trials and quasi-experiments with interrupted time series and controlled or uncontrolled before-after design (worldwide; identified studies mainly from EU and US) *Outcomes*: (1) intended; (2) unintended	– The studies covered only a few medicines; mainly contraceptives, SSRIs, cisapride – The majority of studies assessed intended behavioural outcomes by measuring overall volume of medicinal product use – Study designs and statistical analyses were often inadequate, and none of the studies could rule out confounding – Risk communication had some impact on healthcare practice, but no firm conclusions on effect size could be drawn due to above deficiencies and inconsistency in outcome measures	Appropriate study designs and statistical analyses; impact of concomitant media coverage; impact of subsequent or concomitant risk communication; broader range of medicinal products

Research evaluating the impact of medicines risk communication required by the US FDA (Dusetzina et al. 2012)			
To review studies assessing the impact of risk communication *Interventions*: changes to the product information; boxed warnings; advisories; DHPCs	49 studies analysing empirical data (US) *Outcomes*: (1) use of the medicine; (2) use of a substitute medicine; (3) spill-over effects; (4) diagnoses, testing and non-medicines use; (5) health behaviours and outcomes; (6) patient or physician knowledge, attitudes or beliefs	– The studies covered 16 medicines or medicine classes, one third antidepressants – Most studies used claims data, others survey, medical record, prescribing audit, focus group or vital statistics data – Outcomes mostly related to medicine use – Little knowledge was gained about the impact on patient-healthcare professional communication – Populations were small or selected, and only a few studies reported on minimising non-response and socially-desirable-response biases – Few studies adjusted for influential scientific reports, media coverage, litigation or adverts – Methodological shortcomings were frequent – Risk information can have varied intended and unpredictable impact, but the complexity of the phenomenon limited further conclusions	Identifying factors that are associated with rapid and sustained intended impact; unintended impact; variations of communication across groups of physicians or other communities
Research evaluating unintended effects about safety issues with medicines (DeFrank et al. 2019)			
To review studies reporting probable unintended effects of communicating on safety issues with medicines *Interventions*: statements released by governmental bodies; direct-to-consumer advertisements; news media reports	450 abstracts resulting in 26 identified studies (23 US, 1 Canada, 1 Netherlands, 1 UK), 50% quasi-experimental, such as interrupted time-series, 2 patients surveys, 2 healthcare professional surveys, 2 media content analysis, 1 randomised controlled trial, 1 physician focus group *Outcomes*: (1) decreased use/discontinuation; (2) substitution with other medicines/alternative treatment; (3) spill-over effects; (4) shifts in diagnosis; (5) changes in clinical practice; (6) other changes in health behaviours/clinical outcomes	– 50% of the studies used administrative or health insurer claims data to examine changes in prescription medicines usage or dispensing – 14 studies concerned antidepressants and identified unintended effects of the US FDA communications and related unbalanced media coverage on antidepressant use and psychotropic drug poisoning in youth and spill-over effects to adult population – Other topics included communication about use of antidepressants in pregnancy and neonatal risks and rosiglitazone and cardiovascular risks – There are potential unintended effects from communicating about medicines safety, most commonly reported decreased use/discontinuation (21 studies); substitution/alternative (6 studies); spill-over effects (5 studies); changes in knowledge, attitudes or beliefs (4 studies), shifts in diagnosis (4 studies), changes in clinical practice (4 studies), and other changes in health behaviours/clinical outcomes (4 studies) – Evidence is limited by its inability to infer causality and challenges in defining unintended effects	Evaluation of methodological rigour and control of confounding for inference of causation between communication and outcomes; use of multiple research methods to identify for whom and under what conditions unintended effects occur, for guiding best communication practices

(continued)

Table 1.3 (continued)

Objective of the review and intervention types	Studies reviewed and outcome categories	Summary of most relevant findings of the review	Gaps and needs identified by the review
Research evaluating risk minimisation measures for medicines required by the EMA (Mazzaglia et al. 2018)			
To review studies measuring the effectiveness of risk minimisation measures for cardiovascular, endocrinology and metabolic medicines *Interventions*: routine risk minimisation measures, i.e. product information, pack size, legal status of the medicinal product; additional risk minimisation measures, e.g. education materials	59 observational studies submitted to EMA, mostly non-experimental designs, 8 quasi-experimental designs *Outcomes*: (1) knowledge; (2) behaviour; (3) safety (correlating the implementation of the risk minimisation measure with reduced incidence or reduced severity of adverse reactions); (4) more than one of the above	– The review was restricted to cardiovascular, endocrinology and metabolic medicines – Half of the studies evaluated clinical behaviour, a quarter knowledge, one safety outcomes, one multiple endpoints without safety outcomes and a quarter multiple endpoints with safety outcomes – Electronic healthcare databases were mostly used to assess the impact of routine risk minimisation measures, whereas questionnaires were mostly used to assess additional risk minimisation measures – Studies measuring any single endpoint were considered to possibly have limitations, e.g. in predicting success, providing timely results and feasibility	Process and methodological improvements; evaluation of implementation in early phase; safety outcome evaluation; integrated measurement of different elements of a set of risk minimisation; support to rapid adjustment of risk minimisation strategies
Research evaluating the impact of regulatory safety interventions for medicines (Goedecke et al. 2018)			
To provide an overview of the analytical methods for impact research on safety interventions *Interventions*: DHPCs; product information updates; boxed warnings; regulatory safety communications; additional risk minimisation measures, e.g. medication guide, PPP, controlled distribution; product suspension/ withdrawal; others, e.g. change in legal status of the medicine, pack-size restriction	229 studies with an empirical analysis evaluating impact (in English; worldwide, identified studies mainly from EU and US), two thirds of studies applied before-after time series, 16% before-after cross-sectional designs, 6 cohort studies, 1 randomised controlled trial *Outcomes*: (1) medicines utilisation; (2) knowledge and/or behaviour of patients or healthcare professionals; (3) health, e.g. reduction of disease, adverse reaction incidence, suicide rates, pregnancy related outcomes, changes in laboratory values as surrogate measure for health improvements	– Over a third of studies were on antidepressants or analgesics (paracetamol), otherwise mainly on thiazolidinediones, antipsychotics and retinoids, and further on hormonal contraceptives, non-steroidal anti-inflammatory drugs, cisapride, etc. – Main data sources were claims and electronic health record databases, and others were questionnaires, medical charts, vital statistics, registries of disease or poisoning, active medicines safety surveillance systems, patient safety incident reporting systems and electronic prescribing systems – Half of the studies evaluated medicines use patterns, a third health outcomes and 18% knowledge/behaviour – Two thirds of the studies evaluating health outcomes reported a positive impact, a third no or negligible effects and 7% were inconclusive – The effects of regulatory safety interventions remained largely unquantified and unintended consequences were rarely evaluated	Robust methods and systematic dissemination of findings; definition of population health outcome measures for intended and unintended consequences of regulatory decisions; research into whether changes in medicines use translate into health benefits

Research evaluating the impact of regulatory safety interventions taken for medicines by the US FDA (Briesacher et al. 2013)			
To conduct a literature synthesis on methods evaluating impacts of regulatory actions and to identify best practices *Interventions*: changes to product information; boxed warnings; advisories; DHPCs; product withdrawals	18 quasi-experimental studies (US) *Outcomes*: (1) use of targeted medicinal product; (2) use of substitute product or services; (3) laboratory monitoring; (4) adverse event; (5) use of product in contraindicated condition	– Almost half of the studies were on antidepressants, others on antipsychotics, antidiabetics, cisapride, etc. – Interrupted time-series was the preferred design, using data mainly from proprietary or public administrative databases – Half of the studies evaluated boxed warnings – Only half of the studies assessed changes in the use of substitute products or services, and only 11% examined patient health outcomes – Among studies meeting minimal criteria of rigour, half found no impact or weak/modest impact of regulatory actions, and a third detected unintended consequences – Rigorous evaluations of the impact of regulatory actions were limited and infrequent	Methods with stronger internal validity
Research evaluating interventions for promoting shared decision-making behaviours by healthcare professionals (Légaré et al. 2014)			
To assess communication interventions for promoting shared decision-making behaviours by healthcare professionals *Interventions*: printed educational materials; educational meetings; audit and feedback; reminders; outreach visits; patient-mediated interventions	38 randomised clinical trials and 1 non-randomised controlled trial (in English or French; identified studies from Australia, Europe, New Zealand, North America) *Outcomes*: (1) patient-reported outcomes using scales, e.g. perceived level of control in decision-making, assumed role during the consultation; (2) observer-based outcomes using scales	– No standardised instrument for assessing the adoption of shared decision-making behaviours by healthcare professionals was available – While no precise intervention was clearly recommendable over another, the review suggested that any intervention is better than none, and those targeting both the patient and the healthcare professional might be more promising than those targeting only either the patient or the healthcare professional – Due to the heterogeneity of interventions and outcomes assessed, the low quality of the studies and risks of bias, no robust conclusion could be drawn regarding the effectiveness of interventions – Lack of studies addressing interprofessional approaches was a major limitation to understanding the implementation of shared decision-making	Research quality and power; simultaneous study of healthcare professionals and patients to account for interaction, reciprocity and interdependence; interprofessional approaches; assessment of same intervention type across multiple studies and jurisdictions; low-income countries

(continued)

Table 1.3 (continued)

Objective of the review and intervention types	Studies reviewed and outcome categories	Summary of most relevant findings of the review	Gaps and needs identified by the review
Research evaluating decision aids for patients (Stacey et al. 2014)			
To assess the effects of decision aids in people facing treatment or screening decisions *Interventions*: those to help making specific and deliberated choices among options including status quo by making the decision explicit through information on options and outcomes and implicit methods to clarify values; the aid may also include information on the disease, costs, tailored outcome probabilities, explicit values clarification, information on others' opinions, personalised recommendation, guidance or coaching	105 randomised controlled trials (identified studies from Australia, China, Europe, North America) *Outcomes*: (1) knowledge; (2) accurate risk perception; (3) value-choice congruence; (4) decisional conflict; (5) patient-physician communication; (6) participation in decision-making; (7) proportion undecided; (8) satisfaction; (9) choice; (10) adherence; (11) health status and quality of life; (12) emotions; (13) costs; (14) consultation length; (15) litigation	– Review findings were based on low to high quality of evidence – People exposed to decision aids felt more knowledgeable and clearer about their values and probably had a more active role in decision-making and more accurate risk perceptions – Knowledge and accurate risk perceptions improved when decision aids were used in the consultation or its preparation – Decision aids reduced the proportion of undecided participants and appeared to have a positive effect on patient-physician communication – Those exposed were equally or more satisfied with their decision – Decision aids increased conservative choices for surgery-related decisions and new medications for diabetes; for other testing and screening choices there were mostly no differences between decision aids and usual care – The median effect of decision aids on length of consultation was 2.6 min longer – The costs of the decision aid group were lower to similar to usual care – There were no adverse effects on health outcomes	Use with lower literacy populations; use in consultations; format issues and web-based delivery; research about effects on adherence; potential negative influence on patient-physician relationship and communication; measures of preference-linked quality of life outcomes, adverse event and impact on litigation; cost-effectiveness; global research; reasons for heterogeneity of results
Research evaluating interventions for strengthening trust of patients in physicians (Rolfe et al. 2014)			
To assess the effects of interventions intended to improve patients' trust in physicians *Interventions*: those to improve patients' trust in their physicians aiming at e.g. communication skills and expression of empathy, demonstration of physician's honesty, confidentiality, demonstration of physician's competence, professionalism, continuity of care, access to care and availability of physician, demonstration of care beyond expectation	10 randomised clinical trials (identified studies from US) *Outcomes*: (1) patient trust; (2) health behaviours; (3) health status, quality of life, self-esteem; (4) use of resources, e.g. prescriptions; (5) patient's/carer's satisfaction; (6) patient's perception of physician's communication; (7) patient's perception of physician's humanistic attributes; (8) physician's perceptions of patient trust; (9) patient's perceptions of physician's trustworthiness; (10) adverse outcomes for physicians, patients/carers	– There was considerable heterogeneity among the studies in terms of aims, format and content of the interventions and measures of trust – The review was constrained by the lack of consistency between trust measurements, timeframes and populations – The studies gave conflicting results – Trials showing a small but statistically significant increase in trust included a trial of physician disclosure of financial incentives, choice of physician based on concordance between patient and physician beliefs and communication training – Evidence to conclude that any intervention may increase or decrease trust in physicians is insufficient	Trials to explore the impact of physicians' training or use of a patient-centred or decision-sharing approach on patients' trust; global research

Research evaluating interventions for involving consumers in healthcare decisions at population level (Nilsen et al. 2006)			
To assess the effects of different methods of consumer involvement at population level in developing healthcare policy and research, clinical practice guidelines and patient information material *Interventions*: methods of involvement differentiated by degree of involvement, forum for communication (e.g. one-to-one interviews, focus groups, citizens' juries, town meetings, committee meetings, working groups), involvement in decision-making, recruitment, training and support	6 randomised controlled trials (identified studies from Europe and North America) *Outcomes*: (1) participation or response rates; (2) views elicited; (3) influence on decisions, healthcare outcomes or resource utilisation; (4) consumers' or professionals' satisfaction with process or products; (5) impact on the participating consumers; (6) costs	– The review was based on evidence of very low to moderate evidence – Involving consumers in the development of information material resulted in material more relevant and understandable to patients and capable of improving their knowledge without affecting their anxiety – Informed consent documents developed with consumer input may have little if any impact on understanding – Telephone discussions and face-to-face group meetings engaged consumers better than mailed surveys for setting community health priorities and resulted in different priorities – The effects of involving consumers in developing healthcare policy and research, clinical practice guidelines and patient information material remain largely unevaluated	High-quality evidence from trials evaluating the desirable and adverse effects of different involvement methods and relationship between consumers and professionals

1.3.2 A Concept Map for Multilayered Research

Looking at medicinal product risk communication from the broader humane perspective and considering its multitude, omnipresence, complexity and potential for various immediate and far-reaching outcomes (see Sects. 1.1 and 1.2), wider and deeper research is necessary if we want to obtain a more complete picture of what is happening and improve communication outcomes for the benefit of patients. This should build on existing research (see Sect. 1.3.1), encourage researchers from all relevant disciplines to work together and go beyond what has been achieved to date. A framework is warranted that facilitates multidisciplinary collaboration, so that the different disciplines can develop a common understanding of terms and concepts, combine their approaches, data sources and methods and provide complimentary and synergistic results. In addition, it should provide for participation of those who should benefit from communication, foremost patients and healthcare professionals. Such framework for research into medicinal product risk communication and establishing causal relationships, risk and success factors and pathways towards outcomes is proposed in this section. It has been named multilayered, because pre- and post-situations and simultaneous, subsequent as well as interacting communication events in various social spheres and at multiple communication levels have to be studied, taking into account influencing factors. More concretely, this should achieve understanding of what is happening in the personal, healthcare and other social spheres, who are the involved parties, which information content flows when and where, and how personal and public attitudes are shaped within structures of influence and power. This framework is presented in Figure 1.1 in the form of a concept map. It integrates established concepts, i.e. the social-ecological model (SEM) (see Sect. 1.1.1) as well as benefit-risk and quality management with the typologies of medicinal product risk communication events (see Table 1.1) and their potential outcomes (see Table 1.2) developed in this chapter. Most importantly it is suitable for further incorporating healthcare concepts underpinning the humane perspective, namely patient-centred care and shared therapeutic decision-making, and strategic approaches to risk communication and implementation of risk minimisation.

Setting Research Intents and Objectives

The framework is meant to specifically support enlightening causal relationships, risk and success factors and pathways of communication towards outcomes. This should create understanding of how multiple communications may have synergistic or counteracting positive or negative effects on the outcomes for individuals and society, and what are the risk and success factors for certain outcomes. Where health outcomes are not as desired, studies need to be undertaken to determine where the problem lies—maybe in the process of disseminating information or the interaction between parties, in the presence of counteracting communication events, or in the failure of achieving shared knowledge or motivation. While from the viewpoint of the pharmaceutical and health sciences, the purpose of medicinal product risk communication and related research is to enable informed, safe and effective use of medicines and to contribute to patient and public health, other research questions arise when adding the viewpoint of the social and communication sciences. These questions may refer to conceptualisation, modelling, determining statistical correlations and causal relationships of communication outcomes with the characteristics of the involved individuals and groups, the news and social media and the overall societal context. Hence, such broader research could be called contextualising. Specific research objectives may be to identify and analyse those initiating communication, being targeted as audiences and interacting with each other. This may study their roles, cognitive processes, knowledge, risk perceptions, attitudes, behaviours including medicines use and information seeking, information needs and communication preferences as well as their relationships, mutual trust and expectations towards each other. This may have to be even further segmented by subgroups. Such stakeholder mapping and analysis may become part of a communication model that should be specific for a given medicinal product, safety concern and the overall situation. The model should also include the levels and social spheres where the communication happens for the main parties as senders and receivers of information as well as the directions and reach of information flows and attitude-shaping debates. Other specific research objectives may cover analysing communication content and themes, patterns of information flows by timing and locations, statistical correlations and causal relationships between communication events and intended and unintended outcomes. In general, the research may collect and use data to create new understandings, concepts, theories and hypotheses, which may be inductive, or test the validity or applicability of a hypothesis in a deductive way (Taylor et al. 2015). Table 1.4 categorises possible research objectives into five types of intents of medicinal product risk communication research. Overall, objectives should be set for generating understanding and evidence for improving communication and ultimately health outcomes.

Research for Quality Management of Communication

Improvements of communication can happen in three areas: in the structural area through improved communication systems with their policies, resources, expertise, capacity and efficiency; in the area of the communication process itself; and in achieving outcomes for individual patients, populations and society. The distinction of these three areas in the domain of health can be traced back to the structure-process-outcome model for assessing quality of healthcare pioneered by Avedis Donabedian in the 1960s (Donabedian 1966, 1988). When thinking of research in terms of quality management, such research should investigate the relationships between quality of the structures, the processes and the outcomes. The results serve as evidence for taking action to improve communication, in line with a quality improvement cycle (Deming 1982). Although a good structure is likely to run good processes that should result in good outcomes, the reality is more complex with plenty of parties, factors and simultaneous communication events impacting on the investigated structures, processes and outcomes. Identifying these impacts and their interferences is relevant for research that feeds into progressing communication quality.

Communication for Benefit-Risk Management of Medicinal Products

Communication is essential for risk management of medicinal products. Since the introduction of the risk management cycle as a proactive approach to pharmacovigilance in the 2000s (see Sect. 1.2.1), this has conceptually evolved into an iterative process of benefit-risk management with additional input from patients and healthcare professionals that aims at ensuring that the risk-benefit balance of a medicine in use remains positive. This is known as the benefit-risk assessment,

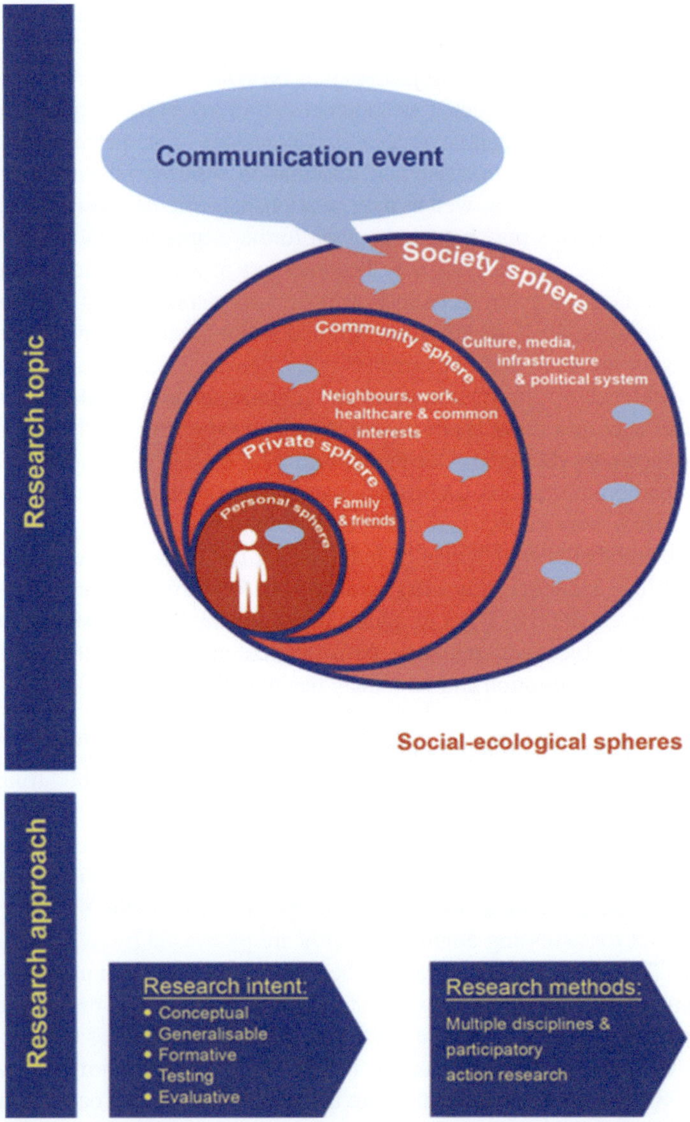

Fig. 1.1 Concept map of a multilayered research framework for medicinal product risk communication

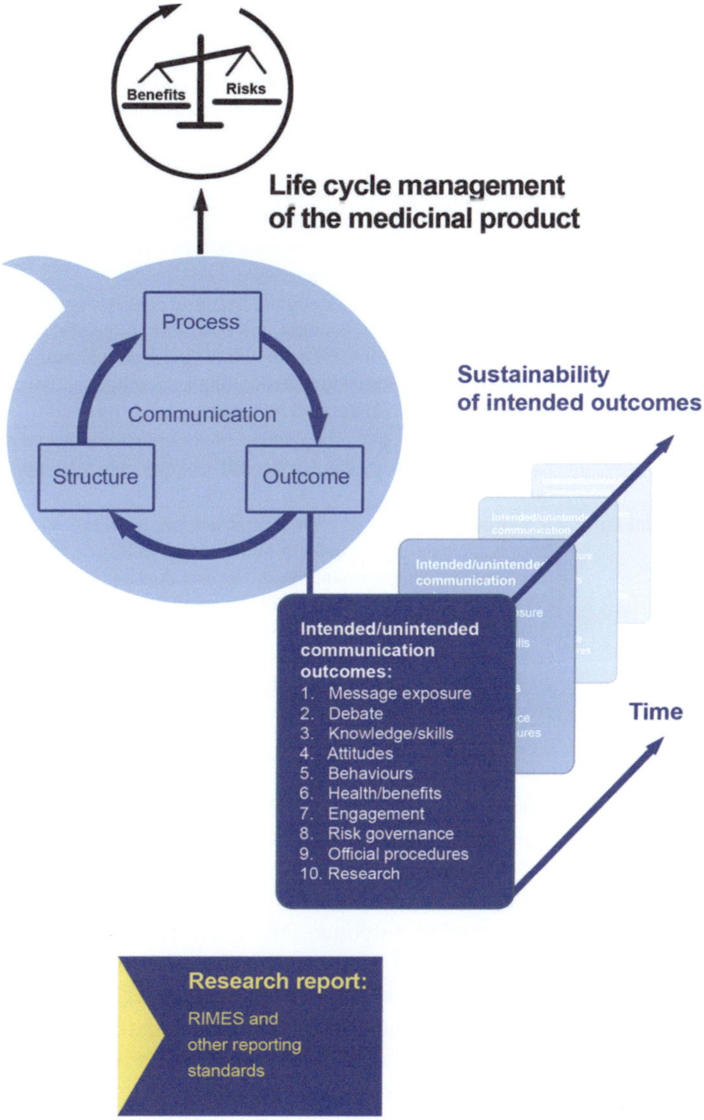

Fig. 1.1 (continued)

communication and evaluation (BRACE) cycle (Radawski et al. 2015). Within this cycle, soliciting input from patients and healthcare professionals or studying their medicines-related knowledge, attitudes, behaviours, needs and expectations can be seen as the listening part of the communication process. This is supposed to inform decisions on the best conditions of use for the medicinal product and product-related action, as well as the planning and post-event evaluation of related communication. Moreover, patient and healthcare professional input can add data to the risk assessment, or inform what a risk assessment should cover in order to address concerns

Table 1.4 Types of intents of medicinal product risk communication research

Type of research intent		Research objectives, e.g.
1	Conceptual intent	Developing or studying applicability of concepts and models in relation to phenomena relevant to medicinal product risk communication
2	Intent for generating basic and generally applicable understanding	Generating understanding of medicinal product risk communication, involved parties and audiences, applicable media and technologies, relevant phenomena and overall social, political, legal, healthcare or other contexts, with a view to establish causal relationships, risk and success factors and pathways towards outcomes
3	Formative intent	Audience mapping and analysis, situation analysis and other formative studies for planning and designing a specific communication intervention, developing a specific communication plan, strategy or policy, or establishing a specific communication system, usually with defined communication objectives
4	Testing intent	Testing of prototypes of a planned communication intervention or of its specific components or of generic components relevant to common interventions
5	Evaluative intent	Real-time monitoring or evaluating structures, processes and outcomes of (a) specific ongoing or past communication event(s), or, in the case of a planned communication intervention, of its development, implementation, effectiveness or sustainability with regard to the pre-defined communication objectives, or of the capacity and efficiency of a specific communication policy and system, including comparative evaluations of events, policies and systems, with a view to establish causal relationships, risk and success factors and pathways towards outcomes

and practical information needs of patients and healthcare professionals. The pharmacovigilance and communication processes should therefore be integrated not only for risk minimisation but also for risk assessment. Focussing specifically on evaluations of risk minimisation measures and other regulatory interventions with regard to intended and unintended outcomes, the cycle for measuring pharmacovigilance impact developed by the EU regulatory network involves regulatory bodies, pharmaceutical companies, patients and healthcare professionals, and acknowledges the need to involve healthcare systems too (European Medicines Agency (EMA) and Pharmacovigilance Risk Assessment Committee (PRAC) 2017). Both these cycles require medicinal product risk communication research for considerable parts of their evaluations. The case for establishing communication groups with risk management specialists for the coordination, effectiveness assessment and adjustments of risk communication strategies and research on communication tools has been made specifically for pharmaceutical companies too (Edwards and Chakraborty 2012).

Research for a Strategic Approach to Communication and Implementation of Risk Minimisation

For pursuing pre-defined objectives in terms of concrete outcomes, a strategic approach to communication has been applied successfully in health promotion, such as for reducing smoking or increasing safe sex behaviours, and is a major global development tool (O'Sullivan et al. 2003). It can likewise be applied to the communication of health risks (Fischhoff et al. 2011; Minister of Health, Canada 2006) and has been proposed for pharmacovigilance with the aim to achieve safe and effective use of medicines (Bahri 2010). The strategic approach fosters two-way communication and is participatory in terms of mapping and collaborating with stakeholders, and audiences in particular, in all its following steps:

1. Analysing the situation and audiences;
2. Designing and planning the event strategically for pre-defined objectives;
3. Developing and testing the various communication written materials or other events;
4. Implementing and monitoring the event; and
5. Conducting post-event evaluation against the objectives and re-planning (Health Communication Partnership (HCP) 2003).

The approach combines project, quality and change management with social marketing and participation models. Social marketing is the use of marketing principles and techniques to persuade a target audience to voluntarily change behaviour for the benefit of individuals or groups (Kotler et al. 2002). From project management, the approach has borrowed the principle of "SMART" objectives (*note*: slight differences exist in the literature in deciphering the acronym), according to which objectives should be:

- *S*pecific in terms of the behaviours called for in defined groups;
- *M*easurable for the purpose of communication evaluation;
- *A*ppropriate to remedy the given problem;
- *R*ealistic, i.e. achievable taking into account the present environment, cultures, systems and potential for change; and
- *T*ime-bound, i.e. having a realistically set point in time by which the communication intervention should be successfully completed in accordance with patient and public health needs (Williams 2007).

Most important for success is the agreement of stakeholders on the objectives and strategy.

For more than a decade now, some regulatory authorities have been using communication plans to agree communication interventions for risk minimisation with manufacturers, as in Canada and the EU (European Medicines Agency (EMA) and Heads of Medicines Agencies 2017; Health Canada 2015), or have developed full strategic risk communication frameworks, for example, in Canada and the US (Fischhoff et al. 2011; Minister of Health, Canada 2006). A strategic approach has also been suggested for communicating results from vaccine benefit-risk investigations of public-private collaborations (Larson et al. 2017) and has underpinned guidance for vaccine safety communications systems developed by the Council for International Organizations of Medical Sciences (CIOMS) for global application, in particular by the WHO Global Vaccine Safety Initiative (GVSI) (Council for International Organizations of Medical Sciences (CIOMS) 2018; Bahri et al. 2019). To apply the strategic approach in practice, its first steps should include reviewing the various options for risk minimisation and communication (Minister of Health, Canada 2006) in terms of how one could interact with and target which parties, using which messages and which communication tools and timings. Such option analysis may be based on existing or especially generated evidence and analyse the pros and cons of each option, with a view to whether the possible risk minimisation measures can actually be successfully implemented through communication and if unintended negative outcomes can be avoided. Hence, this analysis may benefit from insights from the dissemination and implementation science.

Combining Research Methods from Multiple Disciplines

Some best practice guides covering medicinal product risk communication include recommendations for research methods. For example, the Canadian "Strategic Risk Communication Framework" advises on the practical application of methods for stakeholder and situation analyses when planning a communication intervention, for testing communication materials and for evaluating their effectiveness (Minister of Health, Canada 2006). The US FDA guide "Communicating Risks and Benefits" (Fischhoff et al. 2011) gives an introduction into methods for formative research as well as evaluation of processes and outcomes (Downs 2011). The EU good pharmacovigilance practices (EU-GVP) contain some guidance, such as for surveys measuring the effectiveness of risk minimisation measures and their communication components (European Medicines Agency (EMA), Heads of Medicines Agencies 2017), and refer to further guidance on surveys, randomised controlled trials and drug utilisation studies contained in the "ENCePP Guide on Methodological Standards in Pharmacoepidemiology" from the European Network of Centres for Pharmacoepidemiology and Pharmacovigilance (ENCePP) (European Network of Centres for Pharmacoepidemiology and Pharmacovigilance (ENCePP) 2018).

Methodological shortcomings with evaluating the effectiveness of pharmaceutical risk management currently persist in the appropriateness of data collection, lack of comparators and benchmarks and difficulties in interpreting observations (Banerjee et al. 2014), similar to methodological shortcomings present in medicinal risk communication research (see Table 1.3). The expert panel of the Council of Canadian Academies specifies that "there is also no universal way to evaluate a communication tool. Different evaluation methods may be applied in different ways to address various situations, needs, motivations, and goals" (Council of Canadian Academies 2015).

So far various scientific disciplines have engaged in medicinal product risk communication research to different extents and often without linking with each other for complementation. Collaboration of pharmacovigilance experts, pharmacoepidemiologists, biostatisticians, medicinal product specialists, social and behavioural scientists, psychologists, decision scientists, risk management experts, engineers, communication and social marketing specialists, healthcare professionals and patient preference experts has however already been recommended for pharmaceutical risk communication and management (Fischhoff et al. 2011; Radawski et al. 2015; Bahri 2010). For that purpose, multidisciplinary research can be viewed as triangulation. This term from the social sciences refers to an approach that facilitates cross-validation of results through analysing data from more than two sources through different instruments, hence decreasing bias, increasing multi-perspective interpretations and deepening and widening understanding. It can also produce conceptual innovation. Overall, triangulation has been described as an attempt to explain more fully the richness and complexity of human behaviours (Better Evaluation 2018).

It is the principal aspiration of this book to present, in part II, the major methods from the disciplines most useful for medicinal product risk communication research and prepare researchers for multidisciplinary collaborations. Part II starts with Chap. 6 on ethical frameworks, as understanding whether a communication event is humane and in accordance with the societal consent on ethical aspects is fundamental. Chap. 7 on the cognitive and behavioural sciences covers research into risk perception and psychology, health literacy, therapeutic decision-making and health-related behaviours in situations perceived, or not, as risky. Chap. 8 on the social sciences explains in detail their qualitative and quantitative methods as well as underpinning theories that are relevant to other chapters too. Research into the public discourse on risks and political influences as topics of social science research are discussed in Chap. 9 on rhetoric and science and technology studies. Research methods of the media science, as a social science sub-discipline, have their own Chap. 10. While much of this chapter is not only applicable to traditional news media but also to the social media, Chap. 11 provides especially for using the social media as a source and tool for research and addresses required methods such as natural language processing. This has an addendum on legal aspects of such research, mainly on personal data protection, which may also be applicable to other data sources. Chap. 12 introduces principles and methods from design science to foster a scientifically structured approach to preparing, testing and evaluating communication interventions with a view to usability und utility for safe use of medicines. As a still rather novel approach, Chap. 13 on dissemination and implementation science looks at studying the dissemination and adoption of new information, its implementation and behaviour changes in healthcare, as well as other outcomes. Changes in medicine use following safety warnings and other communication events and their impact on patient health can be studied by pharmacoepidemiology, as discussed in Chap. 14. Part II ends with Chap. 15 on legal frameworks for assessing whether communication interventions adhere to legal requirements. This chapter reflects in particular on the historical development of the duty to warn and liability from an EU perspective (for a US perspective see Kesselheim 2012). This chapter on legal frameworks closes the circle started with the first chapter of part II on ethical frameworks, as legal requirements should be based on ethics for enforcing corresponding rights and duties and solving conflicts accordingly. All chapters provide references for more information and advice about the presented methods. Examples of studies applying the methods can be found in these methods chapters, as well as here in this chapter and those in part I.

Reporting Results from Medicinal Product Risk Communication Research

For research results to be useful to those in charge of communication interventions and their underlying systems, it is important to report the evidence, its strength, limitations and meaning clearly and in a transparent manner. For this purpose, research reports can follow the "Reporting Recommendations Intended for Pharmaceutical Risk Minimization Evaluation Studies" (RIMES Statement), which has been developed specifically for multidisciplinary research that often includes studying risk communication interventions (Smith et al. 2018). This checklist can support ensuring the quality of reporting study results as well as support assessing the quality of the studies and the strength of evidence they deliver. As it promotes a standardised way of reporting and assessing, its use should facilitate the efficient review of research for developing or correcting communication interventions. Many of the reporting items are also applicable to study reports concerning communication events that have not been planned as risk minimisation measures. For specific methods applied in a communication research project, more suited reporting standards may be available, and some of them are presented in the respective chapters in part II of this book.

1.4 Connecting with Patients, Healthcare and Society for Strengthened Research and Improved Communication

A multilayered approach to medicinal product risk communication research has been developed in this chapter to generate the evidence base for improving communication outcomes for patients and societies overall (see Sect. 1.3.2). As many parties are active in talking about medicines in private, healthcare and other social spheres, the question arises if and how research should observe and involve senders as well as receives of information and how active those, who have traditionally been seen as the passive receivers of medical and scientific information, should become in communication research. This section of the chapter discusses that establishing more active roles of patients, healthcare professionals as well as journalists in research might be timely. Moreover, this section suggests that medicinal product risk communication research should be established as a self-standing discipline.

1.4.1 Introducing Participatory Action Research

Studies for understanding medicinal product risk communication rely on the willingness, availability, openness, honesty and accuracy of patients, healthcare professionals and others to provide information in, e.g. surveys, interviews and focus groups, or patient health records and documents on healthcare processes. As regards internet-based studies, people using the internet consent explicitly or implicitly to the collection of their search data or content of what they say in the internet, and especially the social media, for purposes like market research, sentiment analysis or detection of emerging diseases. Research in its broad sense is also done by regulatory and public health bodies through involving stakeholders in the planning and evaluation of their communication events. Patient and healthcare professional representatives get, for example, involved in reviewing draft safe use advice for specifically important or sensitive safety concerns with medicines, questions & answers documents on general regulatory topics or materials for health or vaccination campaigns or through the rating of websites/-pages and surveys after high-profile communication interventions. Depending on the jurisdiction, pharmaceutical companies are legally obliged to test package leaflets in consumers or conduct studies that approach patients and healthcare professionals for evaluating the effectiveness of risk minimisation measures. The increasing involvement of patients in regulatory activities goes hand in hand with the strengthening of patient-centredness of care, shared therapeutic decision-making and the replacement of the original unidirectional communication in healthcare *to* patients with a two-way model of patient and citizen participation in decisions relevant to individuals or society. This also happens at a time when many people become "produsers"—this term has been coined for users of the internet, as they do not only *use* the internet for seeking information, but also *produce* information in terms of internet content (Bruns 2009), while data about how they use the internet and where and what they search for are produced too. Still, this current involvement of patients and others in research seems rather passive, as it might be initiated by, e.g. academia or governments, or not even be subject to a conscious consent of people when research is internet-based or makes secondary use of anonym health service data. Relatively few are actively involved in medicinal product risk communication research.

However, those who use medicines or information about medicines, as patients or professionally in healthcare, are also those who know most about what kind of information is most important to them, how they like the information to be delivered and whether it has helped them in using medicines wisely. Therefore, patients and healthcare professionals can and should take a more active role in generating real world data and evidence relevant to medicinal product risk communication. The same applies to journalists, as they know their audiences and how to cater for them. These parties may find their own ways into research, or a mechanism for collaborative research could assist.

Participatory Action Research

A promising mechanism lies in the participatory action research (PAR) approach to enquiry, developed by Kurt Lewin and already in use since the 1940s. It involves researchers and study participants for working together as partners, to become aware and understand a problematic situation and to solve it. PAR recognises the need for the persons being studied to actually participate in all phases of any research that affects them. It focuses on social change that promotes equality and democracy in a cycle of research, action and reflection. It uses a range of methods, both qualitative and quantitative, and is well-established in global development (Institute of Development Studies, United Kingdom 2019; Vollman et al. 2004).

Patients as Researchers

When applying this approach to medicinal product risk communication research, patients would not be passive but active audiences, not only be subject to research observations but be active contributors and collaborators, maybe even, in the fundamental sense of the term (see Sect. 1.1.2), be researchers themselves. When they come together in patient organisations, they can proactively gather data on their information needs and preferences, define research questions, initiate research projects and contribute to research policies. For example, for the public hearing at the EMA for the assessment of teratogenic risks and risk minimisation measures for valproate in 2017, patient organisations conducted surveys among their members about their risk knowledge and experiences with communication in healthcare, which were useful for the EMA decision-making on regulatory action (European Medicines Agency (EMA) 2018c). The last Chap. 16 of this book is dedicated to the patient voice and discusses further how patients could become best active in research.

Suggesting patients as researchers corresponds to the concepts of patient-centred care and shared therapeutic decision-making, which underpin the humane perspective of medicinal product risk communication and research. Making information available fully and in a timely manner so that patients and their family can make informed decisions has been laid down as one principle of patient-centred healthcare. Various definitions exist, but the recent Catalyst initiative of the New England Journal of Medicine defines it as care where the individual's health needs and desired outcomes are the driving force behind all healthcare decisions and quality measurements. Patients are therefore seen in partnership with their healthcare professionals and treated not only from a clinical perspective, but also from an emotional, mental, spiritual, social and financial perspective (New England Journal of Medicine (NEJM) Catalyst 2017). As healthcare is a complex system with multiple parties involved and potential for ethical conflicts between parties, a call for "collaborative care" has been made (Aronson 2016).

Healthcare Professionals as Researchers

Healthcare professionals who are directly involved in patient care may already be active in communication research, depending on their professional roles. In particular pharmacists practicing in hospital or community/retail pharmacies may engage in formal academic research about their own, patients' and other healthcare professionals' knowledge, attitude and practices regarding medicines. This is part of the area of clinical pharmacy, and such research is published, for example, in the International Journal of Clinical Pharmacy (JWF 1997). The International Pharmaceutical Federation (FIP) has issued a framework for developing medicines information strategies, applicable and tailored to the needs of physicians, nurses and pharmacists when caring for and empowering patients, and this includes research through consultations, interviews and surveys (International Pharmaceutical Federation (FIP) 2017a). The majority of healthcare professionals however have jobs in patient care that do not include options for communication research.

Unfortunately, this leaves a wealth of knowledge of healthcare professionals unused, i.e. knowledge on the understanding, missing awareness, concerns and questions their patients have about medicines. There should be mechanisms for healthcare professionals to systematically collect and analyse this. Furthermore, data from self-reflective professional practice could be collected, e.g. on the concerns and questions healthcare professionals themselves have, and how and whether they find answers to their questions, on their role, effectiveness and training needs with regard to communicating with patients, and on how they participate in pharmacovigilance through reporting of adverse reactions suspected in a patient and in risk management. They could also take the initiative to provide systematic feedback as to whether a communication intervention has reached them and the advice could be implemented usefully in practice. Even more proactively, they could provide information on whether specific risk minimisation and communication options are implementable in healthcare processes and patient routines.

For example, the Pharmaceutical Group of European Union (PGEU) have proposed communication tools that could become part of an existing healthcare process, such as a patient card with warnings that can be handed over to the patient as a discrete trigger for a conversation about a certain risk during dispensing. This was adopted by the EU regulators as a workable solution for teratogenic products like valproate (European Medicines Agency (EMA) 2018c; Pharmaceutical Group of European Union (PGEU) 2017).

Journalists as Researchers

The use of health interventions is influenced by news media stories (Grilli et al. 2002), and journalists have quite some power to change the use of medicines. The negative impact of news stories in the cases of combined hormonal contraceptives and MMR vaccines exemplify this (see Sect. 1.2.1). The need to increase the standards of journalism through knowledge on fright factors and the self-awareness that "journalists can be seduced by aspects of risk"—"often at the expense of caution and balance"—has been stated by David Ropeik, a leading representative of the profession (Ropeik 2002). On the other hand, journalists in general avoid disease mongering (Schwitzer 2008) and claim their intent to disseminate correct information and ask critical questions for good reasons (Dana Centre (host) 2006). Especially so-called watchdog journalism contributes to democracy by increasing transparency about what is going on in society and identifying wrongdoings (Waisbord 2019). In the area of health, being fast in covering complex health news adequately is however challenging for journalists, and there is high pressure to simplify and catch attention (Goldacre 2009; Schwitzer 2008; Waller et al. 2005). Part of their profession though, if time allows, is to research topics and the interests of their audiences, and therefore journalists follow news and social media debates. Gary Schwitzer, one of the few who have experience as a health journalist as well as a media researcher, has expressed his belief that journalists have a responsibility to investigate and report on citizens' needs for understanding healthcare (Schwitzer et al. 2005).

Therefore, the suggestion emerges that journalists could become engaged in a mutual learning exercise between experts, i.e. journalists who understand audiences and how to catch their attention, scientists who study medicines and risk management, and regulatory decision-makers. Together, they could improve communication that supports patients and citizens in gaining knowledge that empowers them to use medicines safely and effectively.

1.4.2 A Call for Humanities and Epidemiology of Medicinal Product Risk Communication

This section of the chapter elaborates on why research on medicinal product risk communication should be further developed not only as part of pharmacovigilance (see Sect. 1.2.1), but also within wider contexts of the medical humanities as well as pharmacoepidemiology. The multilayered research framework (see Sect. 1.3.2) may prepare the ground for combining approaches and establishing a self-standing inclusive discipline of humanities and epidemiology of medicinal product risk communication.

Medical Humanities

The humane perspective to medicinal product risk communication (see Sect. 1.1.1) corresponds to the objectives of the medical humanities, which explore the world as it appears from the viewpoint of human experience and investigate, inter alia, aspects of patient-physician interactions, factors for healthy communities, social goods for wellbeing and the impact of regulation on the human side of medical practice. As an interdisciplinary field of medicine, it includes the humanities (e.g. linguistics, history, philosophy, ethics, religion), social sciences (e.g. anthropology, cultural studies, psychology, sociology, health geography) and the arts (e.g. literature, theatre, film, visual arts). The medical humanities draw on the creative and intellectual strengths of these diverse disciplines for their application to education of healthcare professionals and improving clinical practice (Aull 2011; Evans 2002; Evans and Greaves 2001; Greaves and Evans 2000; Kirklin 2003; Shankar 2014).

Medicinal products are a major medical intervention and as such are of interest to the medical humanities. For example, the following was presented at a medical humanities conference (Birkbeck Centre for Medical Humanities 2011): a US interview study in adolescents suffering chronic pain conditions showed that these girls and boys had developed their personal strategies for meeting their life challenges and planning for a fulfilled future. The prescribed medicines did not always help them and were sometimes taken only to please the parents. These adolescents found that healthcare professionals would not always believe them with regard to adverse events they experienced after taking their medicines, as expressed by this example quote: "They never admit they're wrong [but] they should take the patient's word". More generally dialogue seemed difficult according to these quotes: "They [healthcare professionals] don't understand; they think they understand. They put everything in the context of their own speciality", "They want to make you look even more like an idiot" and "They would only talk and talk and talk [without listening]" (Meldrun et al. 2009). The practical relevance of involving specialists from disciplines engaged with the medical humanities in preparing communication about disease, health behaviours and treatment options becomes obvious in the following two examples: In India, initiatives have been taken to overcome stigmatisation of those infected with HIV by deliberately applying positive language in public speaking (Finn and Sarangi 2009). In Guinea, anthropologists created a successful programme for communication with rebellious communities to fight the spread of Ebola virus disease in 2014 through socio-anthropological enquiry and participatory action research (Anoko 2014).

Communication occurring at interpersonal level, in particular between healthcare professionals and patients, is difficult to study through direct observation. Methods often used instead are surveys or medicines use studies at population level for studying outcomes of interpersonal communication. The research methods presented in this book are often more easily applicable to communication events targeting large audiences, mostly using data collected from these audiences, large data bases or observations of phenomena in the public domain. Nevertheless, linguistic discourse analysis investigates the use of language in its real-life social contexts and the meaning of communicative exchanges, and has been shown to be relevant to interpersonal communication in healthcare (Shaw and Bailey 2009). Video recordings or transcripts can be used (Shaw and Bailey 2009), or audio recordings of conversations, as has been done regarding human papillomavirus (HPV) vaccines

(HPV) vaccines (Sturm et al. 2017). Methods from the applied linguistics can create understanding of relationships between texts, talk and other modes of communication in interpersonal, intra-group or mass communication, and actions people take in relation to health and risks, including medicines (Jones 2013).

Humanities of Medicinal Product Risk Communication

The medical humanities remind us that good care for patients requires communication skills, empathy, self-awareness, judgement, professionalism and mastering the social and cultural context of personhood, illness and healthcare (Coulehan 2019). Medicinal product risk communication requires the same and research should generate the evidence necessary for communicating in a way that supports good patient care. Such evidence can be used for preparing communication events or training of communication skills. It is therefore suggested, as an outlook of this chapter to the future, to specifically establish humanities of medicinal product risk communication. In patient-centred care, the ultimate concern of researching and improving communication about medicines is the patient as an individual. It is however not only important to identify patient needs and preferences, but also how healthcare professionals feel and act about communication. The doctor who thinks the patient does not need or cannot understand medical information or who feels not to know how or when to provide understandable information is not a rare case. It is therefore hoped that establishing humanities of medicinal product risk communication can serve to shed more light on patient-healthcare professional interactions and support both parties in creating an effective and satisfying exchange. Likewise, the challenges those in regulatory or public health bodies feel when preparing statements for publication, responding to journalists, policy makers or parliamentarians, or engaging with patients and healthcare professionals at meetings or public hearings, and, vice-versa, the experiences of those interacting with regulatory or public health bodies or receiving information from them can be enlightened by the methods the medical humanities apply. For example, the finding of the words that adequately express the evidence, the uncertainty, the rationale for a regulatory decision, the advice for safe and effective use of the medicine and the respect for the patient, and, at the same time, address all information needs of patients and healthcare professionals and all legal requirements can be a challenge. Investigating the human experience of the words and the processes behind may be of research interest.

Humanities of medicinal product risk communication is proposed here to be defined as the application of the disciplines of humanities for studying medicinal product risk communication from the viewpoint of the human experience of patients, healthcare professionals and others involved in such communication, with the aim of practicing patient-centred care with shared therapeutic decision-making.

Pharmacoepidemiology

Another perspective on the future development of medicinal product risk communication research is offered by pharmacoepidemiology. This is the science that applies epidemiologic approaches to studying the use, effectiveness, value and safety of pharmaceuticals (International Society for Pharmacoepidemiology (ISPE) 2019) and investigates medicines as a determinant of health using data from populations (Spitzer 1991). Pharmacoepidemiological study designs are used to measure the impact of medicine-related communication events, such as changes to the product information or news media reports, on disease diagnoses, medicines use and subsequent health outcomes. Pharmacoepidemiology is a major contributor to research into medicinal product risk communication.

Epidemiology of Medicinal Product Risk Communication
As a focus of pharmacoepidemiology and at the same time an expansion in terms of data sources and multidisciplinary methods, it is suggested here to establish epidemiology of medicinal product risk communication. This is proposed as the application of epidemiological methods for studying medicinal product risk communication as a determinant of health with the aim of supporting evidence-based decisions on communication for patient safety and population health.

This acknowledges that the use and outcomes of a medicinal product can only be as good as the quality and adoption by patients and healthcare professionals of the information for the safe and effective use of the product, and this is influenced by many factors, risk perceptions in particular. However, epidemiology of medicinal product risk communication should not only study the communication materials belonging to the medicinal product. As far as epidemiological methods can, it should investigate structures and processes of any of the multiple omnipresent communication events (see Table 1.1), make use of a wide range of data and study all potential outcomes (see Table 1.2), to create understanding if and how these relate to health outcomes and are influenced by other factors, such as socio-economic ones. While pharmacoepidemiology has always been concerned with the use and effects of medicines in real world healthcare, routinely collected data relating to a patient's health status or the delivery of healthcare from a variety of sources (other than traditional clinical trials) are nowadays referred to as real world data (RWD). Evidence derived from the analysis of RWD is called real world evidence (RWE). This can benefit from the availability of larger, cross-linked and new data sources as a consequence of the ongoing digitalisation and increasing worldwide application of the internet. New data sources to highlight are mobile health apps and social media (Cave et al. 2019; Kholsa et al. 2018; United States Food and Drug Administration (US FDA) 2017b). The use of RWD and RWE offers opportunities for planning and evaluating communication events. Medicines use and other pharmacoepidemiological studies can identify patterns and influencing factors of medicines use as well as typical patient and prescriber profiles. The synergistic collaboration of pharmacoepidemiologists and social scientists for situation and audience analyses as well as for formulating and evaluating risk minimisation and communication strategies has already been called for (Radawski et al. 2015; Bahri 2010). This is supposed to help characterising audiences more comprehensively in terms of who they are, what they think and feel, and how they behave in terms of using medicines, as well as to understand communication flows, contents and outcomes. Beyond RWD on patient health status or delivery of healthcare, the large sets of data that are produced by people using the internet and that can only be stored and analysed computationally—especially in relation to human behaviour—are referred to as big data (Cambridge English Dictionary 2019). Online publishers use such data to inform their business development, and they may also be useful for medicinal product risk communication research, although care is warranted in interpreting findings (Edwards and Lindquist 2011). As has already been done for vaccines, media content analyses can shed light on public debates and concerns of patients and healthcare professionals and usefully inform communication strategies (Bahri et al. 2017; Larson et al. 2013). Ways for efficient and valid use of the new data sources have still to be developed.

Ways Forward

"Healthcare is a sacred mission ...
a moral enterprise and a scientific enterprise ...
We don't have a consumer who understands everything and
makes rational choices - and I include myself here ...
Ultimately the secret of quality is love ...
If you have love, you can then work backward
to monitor and improve the system."
Avedis Donabedian (Donabedian 2001)

This chapter takes a humane perspective on the triad of medicines, risks and communication with the goal to understand and improve communication for patient-centred care, enabling informed therapeutic decisions, preventing harm and hence contributing to patient and public health globally.

Medicinal product risk communication has become an essential process of pharmacovigilance, mainly through crises of safety concerns and recognition that product information and other risk minimisation measures are not as effective in healthcare as intended. Experience and research have shown that communicating about risks with medicines goes far beyond providing information on the evidence of risks and safe use advice. It includes detailing the underlying safety surveillance systems and methods, and their trustworthiness, in addition to listening to, collecting data from and engaging with patients and healthcare professionals. Information and exchanges about medicines and their potential risks are omnipresent in our lives, as experiences with medicines are frequently discussed in multiple spaces, in particular in healthcare as well as the news and social media. Certainly, responsible leaders are needed who connect those active in pharmacovigilance—whether in regulation, industry, research or healthcare—, with all healthcare professionals directly responsible for patient care as well as with patients, consumers and parents. Jointly, they should create common ground and motivation, and make patient empowerment and safe and effective use of medicines happen. Leadership is also needed to implement evidence-based communication practices, whether in healthcare, public bodies, or the media. In order to make these improvements, a comprehensive understanding of medicinal product risk communication is needed. As people, their interactions and media use change over time, this understanding also needs to be kept-to-date and requires continuous research.

This chapter therefore proposes the establishment of a self-standing inclusive discipline of humanities and epidemiology of medicinal product risk communication. When combining these two approaches of humanities and epidemiology, qualitative methods can generate hypotheses that can be tested through quantitative research, and quantified phenomena can be better interpreted by means of qualitative studies. Building on research that has been achieved to date, this discipline should apply a multilayered research framework. Such framework has been developed in this chapter to prepare a common platform for collaborations among researchers from a wide range of relevant disciplines, who will bring their own data sources, methods and expertise, and can create synergies and generate more complete evidence. This can consider the omnipresence of medicinal product risk communication in all social spheres of life as well as simultaneous, subsequent and interacting information flows between multiple parties. It is expected that multilayered research will provide for wider and deeper understanding of causal relationships, risk and success factors and pathways towards communication outcomes. The framework integrates participatory action research approaches for active roles of patients, healthcare professionals and journalists in data provision, calls for studies and even conduct of research. Connecting with those who require or transmit information is vital for medicinal product risk communication research, in order to achieve its full utility for individuals and society, in high and low resource settings alike.

Future multilayered research that aims for changes towards an informed, safe and effective use of medicines and patient-centred care in sustainable manner will have to especially incorporate design science as well as theories of implementation and realist evaluation. These can underpin and further develop a strategic approach to communication. Dissemination and implementation science was born out of the desire to achieve evidence-based best healthcare practices and investigates why implementation succeeds or fails (Nilsen 2015). The comprehensive question of realist evaluation is "What works, for whom, in what respects, to what extent, in what context, and how?". Its purpose is to explain how outcomes were caused by social and psychological factors that drive reasoning, emotions and behavioural responses in the given social and political context with many interwoven variables. This goes far beyond single pathways of cause and effect and looks for mechanisms of causal relationships within complex situations (Better Evaluation 2019), such as medicinal product risk communication. Which variables influence our choices most can be explored by methods using choice models (Ryan et al. 2001). Design science, informed by cognitive and behavioural sciences, will have to increasingly study so-called human factors as the discipline concerned with the interaction between humans and system elements. Human factors applies anatomical, physiological and psychological knowledge to designing systems that complement human ability, enhance safety, comfort and productivity, and reduce adverse incidences and human error. Human factors also apply methods like root-cause analysis (Tsukahara and Calil 2016). Relevant to healthcare are job-related, individual, organisational and environmental factors affecting healthcare professionals at work and equivalent factors for patients. They are important for interpersonal communication as well as for information technology (IT) systems, including prescribing and dispensing software, internet-based systems, mobile health apps and social media (Charted Institute of Ergonomics and Human Factors (CIEHF) 2019; Health and Safety Executive (HSE) 1999; National Center for Human Factors in Healthcare e.g.; World Health Organization (WHO) 2009). New IT tools can support patients and healthcare professionals, but there may also be threats to health equality due to algorithms of search engines or the dissemination of fake news. Human internet "trolls" and "chatbot" computer programmes that simulate human conversations through so-called artificial intelligence have lately become subject to health communication research (Jamison et al. 2019). Designing communication interventions with utility and effectiveness in mind right from the beginning, for avoiding errors and unintended outcomes, should benefit from a structured and culturally sensitive approach to messages and tools development, involving representatives from all target groups in formative research. Those with limited literacy or cognitive impairment have also to be catered for, e.g. by means of the FIP pictograms (International Pharmaceutical Federation (FIP) 2017b). Important to note, there are more and more calls from patients for visualisation of comparative risk quantification and warnings. For example, in the EU there was a major call from patients for a pictogram that warns about the teratogenic risk of valproate (European Medicines Agency (EMA) 2018c). Even the pros and cons of applying emoji in interpersonal healthcare communication and scientific articles has recently been discussed (Goodman 2019; O'Reilly-Shah et al. 2018). However, no matter which format of information, understandability of information is a key requirement, but not independent from the given level of health literacy of the target group. The scholarly body of knowledge in health literacy is considered still small (Aldoory 2017), but it is logical to see it as depending on the general literacy level. It is therefore worrying that in 2016 international research has shown that nowadays even in countries of high literacy like Germany almost 20% of 10-years-old schoolchildren have difficulties in deriving sense from reading (Boie 2018; TIMSS and PIRLS International Study Centre 2019). While this might possibly be addressed through audio and video product information for medicines, those deprived from literacy will be limited in proactively seeking health information and in participating in therapeutic decisions in a fully informed manner. No research and no improvement of medicinal product risk communication can remedy such inequality within or between countries. Researchers in medicinal product risk communication should therefore disseminate their findings and arguments widely and support general education and life-long learning as fundamental to health. Presenting medicines in a generally understandable manner will also face new challenges, as novel types of medicinal products are expected, such as advanced therapy products or so-called precision or personalised medicine that individualises products, for example through genetic tests (United States Food and Drug Administration (US FDA) 2018d). Apart from explaining such novel medical technologies, the personal and public dialogue for demonstrating the trustworthiness of the systems underpinning their safety, quality and efficacy will remain crucial. In addition to research into the ongoing digitalisation mentioned above, the interpersonal face-to-face communication requires research too. One can even argue that in times of high multiplicity of information flows due to the digitalisation with the potential to overwhelm, confuse and misinform, communicating with real trusted faces becomes more essential. This applies not only to healthcare but to communication of regulatory and public health bodies with stakeholders and the public too. Research from the humane perspective could embrace new ways of studying as well as training for patient-healthcare interactions. This includes role plays which are increasingly applied to prepare students for professional life. An example for a new way of training healthcare professionals is a workshop for pharmacists that applied Laban movement analysis to body exercises and role plays, in order to foster self-awareness when as a healthcare professional one starts feeling uncomfortable talking to a patient and to foster understanding the emotional impact of non-verbal communication on patients (Penfield and Bahri 2014). Importantly, these new ways provide a chance for healthcare professionals to gain embodied experiences of different mental states, both their own and of patients. This can inform managing one's own feelings and choosing the most effective communication behaviour in a given situation. Changing perspectives to understand better own and others' risk perceptions can also become subject of research for informing communication curricula and training events, or regulatory activities and communication. How uncertainty of evidence on a safety concern or lack of confidence in one's capacity to communicate influences the performance of communicators needs to be explored too. In this respect, the recent developments of cognitive psychology and neurosciences and how the cognitive-behavioural perspective and the biological, nervous system-focused perspective come together in cognitive neuropsychology raise expectations. This newly emerging approach studies brain functioning and perception across the life span (Vrije Universiteit Amsterdam (VU) 2019).

Last but not least, we should never forget that what is spoken, written or otherwise expressed, if heard, read, seen or felt, may have a long-lasting impact, or a short half-life; it can be replaced with a new message, but it can never be undone completely; it will stay forever, even if only in the faintest of someone's memory, even if only as the weakest trace in someone's behaviour that has the power to influence someone else. We should use the way we communicate, this behaviour of ours that connects us all, wisely—it is the key to so many things that we pursue in health and life.

Conclusions

- Given the major contribution of medicinal products to health benefits but also given that no medicine comes without risk, communication about medicines has become omnipresent in personal and public life.
- Communication about the risks of medicines and how to use them safely is essential for patient-centred care, shared therapeutic decision-making and avoiding harm; improving this communication is necessary due to recurrent problems with sustainable risk minimisation in healthcare and evolving expectations of patients.
- Beyond this pharmaceutical-medical perspective, communication is to be recognised as a vital human behaviour; such humane perspective has compassion and curiosity for how we seek understanding of the world and interact with each other within social spheres, how this relates to our perceptions and choices in life as well as our longings and goals, and how this may impact on our medicines use and health.
- With this wider perspective, medicinal product risk communication comprises the structures, processes and outcomes of information

exchanges about risks and any concerns people may have with medicines, about the measures to support safe use and minimise risks and about risk governance overall in private, community and society spheres.

- Research into medicinal product risk communication is so far limited in terms of medicinal products, outcomes and world regions studied as well as data sources and methods applied, and studies rarely conclude robustly on causality between a communication event and outcomes.
- With a view to gaining a wider and deeper understanding and instigating evidence-based improvements of communication, this chapter proposes a *multilayered research framework* that combines data types and methods from various scientific disciplines to establish causal relationships, risk and success factors and pathways towards communication outcomes; research objectives can be conceptual, generating basic and generally applicable understanding, formative, testing and evaluative.
- Multilayered research into medicinal product risk communication addresses the omnipresence, multitude and complexity of communication by studying situations before and after a communication event in the context of other simultaneous, subsequent or interacting communication in the various social spheres and at multiple levels, identifying immediate and far-reaching outcomes and analysing the multiple parties, flows and content of communication as well as structures of power and other influencing factors.
- This framework advocates for incorporating participatory action research with patients, healthcare professionals and journalists as partners in research and mutual learning.
- Those engaging in multidisciplinary research need to be aware of terminological discrepancies between disciplines and always clarify what is subject to their research and which terms they apply with which meanings; this chapter proposes typologies of communication events and their outcomes to promote collaborative research and convergence on concepts and terms needed for synthesising findings.
- The suggested *outcome categories* are (1) Exposure to messages; (2) Debate; (3) Risk knowledge and risk minimisation skills; (4) Attitudes; (5) Behaviours; (6) Health, quality of life and other benefits; (7) Trust, engagement and satisfaction; (8) Risk governance, management and communication systems; (9) Legal and other official procedures; and (10) Research.
- Based on the multilayered research framework, it is suggested to establish a research field dedicated to medicinal product risk communication that combines approaches from the humanities and epidemiology, defined by this chapter as:
  - *Humanities of medicinal product risk communication*: the application of the disciplines of humanities for studying medicinal product risk communication from the viewpoint of the human experience of patients,

healthcare professionals and others involved in such communication, with the aim of practicing patient-centred care with shared therapeutic decision-making;
  - *Epidemiology of medicinal product risk communication*: the application of epidemiological methods for studying medicinal product risk communication as a determinant of health with the aim of supporting evidence-based decisions on communication for patient and population health.
- A self-standing inclusive discipline of *humanities and epidemiology of medicinal product risk communication* is meant to support achieving the full potential of research into communication of risks with medicines for benefitting patients and societies worldwide.

Declarations The views expressed in this chapter are the author's personal views and may not be understood or quoted as being made on behalf of or reflecting the position of her employing organisation, i.e. the European Medicines Agency (EMA), or any of its committees or working parties. The work on this chapter and as editor of the whole book was undertaken in the author's free time outside EMA working hours, in accordance with the EMA policy on external activities. The author has not gained any profit from writing for this book and will not gain money through its sales.

References

Abalkhail MS, Alzahrany MS, Alghamdi KA, Alsoliman MA, Alzahrani MA, Almosned BS, Gosadi IM, Tharkar S (2017) Uptake of influenza vaccination, awareness and its associated barriers among medical students of a University Hospital in Central Saudi Arabia. J Infect Public Health 10:644–648

Ahlqvist-Radstad J, Andric A, Baldelli I, Buckley N, Coleman AM, Cupelli A, Escudero Y, Hearn J, Knudsen Y, Ángel MaciÁ M, Michan L, Montero D, Rodriguez A, Samdal H, Sipic I, Spooner A, Wennberg A (2016) SCOPE Work Package 6 survey report: patient and consumer consultation. Strengthening Collaboration for Operating Pharmacovigilance in Europe (SCOPE) Joint Action. http://www.scopejointaction.eu. Accessed 29 Dec 2017

Akl EA, Oxman AD, Herrin J, Vist GE, Terrenato I, Sperati F, Costiniuk C, Blank D, Schünemann H (2011a) Framing of the health information message in either negative or positive words. Cochrane Database Syst Rev (12):CD006777

Akl EA, Oxman AD, Herrin J, Vist GE, Terrenato I, Sperati F. Costiniuk C, Blank D, Schünemann H. Using alternative statistical formats for presenting risks and risk reductions. Cochrane Database Syst Rev. 2011b; 3: CD006776

Aldoory L (2017) The status of health literacy research in health communication and opportunities for future scholarship. Health Commun 32:211–218

Allport G (1935) Quoted in: Schwarz N and Bohner G (2001) The construction of attitudes. In: Tesser A and Schwarz N (eds) Intrapersonal processes (Blackwell Handbook of Social Psychology). Blackwell, Oxford, pp 436–457

Anderson T (2017) Curbing prescription opioid dependency. Bull World Health Organ 95:318–319

Andre FE, Booy R, Bock HL, Clemens J, Datta SK, John TJ, Lee BW, Lolekha S, Peltola H, Ruff TA, Santosham M, Schmitt HJ (2008) Vaccination greatly reduces disease, disability, death and inequity worldwide. Bull World Health Organ 86:140–146

Angamo MT, Chalmers L, Curtain CM, Bereznicki LRE (2016) Adverse-drug-reaction-related hospitalisations in developed and developing countries: a review of prevalence and contributing factors. Drug Saf 39:847–857

Anoko JN (2014) Communication with rebellious communities during an outbreak of Ebola Virus Disease in Guinea: an anthropological approach. Social Science for Emergency Response (online). http://www.ebola-anthropology.net/case_studies/communication-with-rebellious-communities-during-an-outbreak-of-ebola-virus-disease-in-guinea-an-anthropological-approach/. Accessed 18 June 2017

Aronson JK (2016) "Collaborative care" is preferable to "patient centred care". Br J Med 253:i2926

Atkins R, Bluebond-Langner M, Read N, Pittsley J, Hart D (2010) Adolescents as health agents and consumers: results of a pilot study of the health and health-related behaviors of adolescents living in a high-poverty urban neighborhood. J Pediatr Nurs 25:382–392

Aull F. Medical humanities. Medical Humanities Community, New York University School of Medicine, New York. Archived from the original on 18 May 2011. http://medhum.med.nyu.edu. Accessed 18 Jun 2017

Bahri P (2010) Public pharmacovigilance communication: a process calling for evidence-based, objective-driven strategies. Drug Saf 33:1065–1079

Bahri P, Harrison-Woolrych M (2012) Focusing on risk communication about medicines: why now? [editorial]. Drug Saf 35:971–975

Bahri P, Dodoo AN, Edwards BD, Edwards IR, Fermont I, Hagemann U, Hartigan-Go K, Hugman B, Mol PG, on behalf of the ISoP CommSIG (2015) The ISoP CommSIG for improving medicinal product risk communication: a new special interest group of the International Society of Pharmacovigilance. Drug Saf 38:621–627

Bahri P, Fogd J, Morales D, Kurz X (2017) ADVANCE consortium. Application of real-time global media monitoring and 'derived questions' for enhancing communication by regulatory bodies: the case of human papillomavirus vaccines. BMC Med 15:91

Bahri P, Rägo L, on behalf of the CIOMS Working Group on Vaccine Safety (2019) CIOMS guide to vaccine safety communication: executive summary. Vaccine 37:401–408

Banerjee AK, Zomerdijk IM, Wooder S, Ingate S, Mayall SJ (2014) Post-approval evaluation of effectiveness of risk minimisation: methods, challenges and interpretation. Drug Saf 37:33–42

BBC. A definition of information [archived webpage]. http://www.bbc.co.uk/schools/gcsebitesize/ict/databases/0datainforev2.shtml. Accessed 29 Dec 2017

Beck U (1986) Risikogesellschaft: Auf dem Weg in eine andere Moderne (Risk society: towards a new modernity). Suhrkamp, Frankfurt/Main

Better Evaluation. Triangulation [webpage]. Updated on 19 Nov 2018. https://www.betterevaluation.org/en/evaluation-options/triangulation. Accessed 13 Mar 2019

Better Evaluation. Realist evaluation [webpage]. https://www.betterevaluation.org/en/approach/realist_evaluation. Accessed 6 June 2019

Birkbeck Centre for Medical Humanities. The language of illness and pain identity, communication and the clinical encounter [conference]. Birkbeck College, London; 2–3 July 2011

Blendon RJ, Benson JM (2018) The public and the opioid-abuse epidemic. N Engl J Med 378:407–411

Blendon RJ, Benson JM, Hero JO (2014) Public trust in physicians: US medicine in international perspective. N Engl J Med:371–317

Boie K. Leseschwäche: Es ist zum Weinen. Zeit Online. 29 May 2018. https://www.zeit.de. Accessed 24 Mar 2019

Bongard V, Ménard-Taché S, Bagheri H, Kabiri K, Lapeyre-Mestre M, Montastruc JL (2002) Perception of the risk of adverse drug reactions: differences between health professionals and non health professionals. Br J Clin Pharmacol 54:433–436

Briesacher BA, Soumerai SB, Zhang F, Toh S, Andrade SE, Wagner JL, Shoaibi A, Gurwitz JH (2013) A critical review of methods to evaluate the impact of FDA regulatory actions. Pharmacoepidemiol Drug Saf 22:986–994

Bruns A. (2009) From prosumer to produser: understanding user-led content creation [presentation]. Transforming Audiences [conference], London; 3–4 September 2009

Brynner R, Stephens T (2001) Dark remedy: the impact of thalidomide and its revival as a vital medicine. Perseus, Cambridge

Cambridge English Dictionary. https://dictionary.cambridge.org/dictionary/english. Accessed 18 May 2019

Cave A, Kurz X, Arlett P (2019) Real-world data for regulatory decision making: challenges and possible solutions for Europe. Clin Pharmacol Ther 106(1):36–39

Charted Institute of Ergonomics & Human Factors (CIEHF). What is ergonomics: find out how it makes life better [webpage]. CIEHF, Birmingham. https://www.ergonomics.org.uk/Public/Resources/What_is_Ergonomics_/Public/Resources/What_is_Ergonomics_.aspx?hkey=2769db3e-4b5b-46c2-864c-dfcf2e44372d. Accessed 2 Sept 2019

Cheung K, Ho SMS, Lam W (2017) Factors affecting the willingness of nursing students to receive annual seasonal influenza vaccination: a large-scale cross-sectional study. Vaccine 35:1482–1587

Ciciriello S, Johnston RV, Osborne RH, Wicks I, deKroo T, Clerehan R, O'Neill C, Buchbinder R (2013) Multimedia educational interventions for consumers about prescribed and over-the-counter medications. Cochrane Database Syst Rev (4):CD008416

Cochrane Collaboration [website]. http://www.cochrane.org. Accessed 16 Jun 2018

Coulehan J. What is medical humanities and why? Lit Med Magazine. https://medhum.med.nyu.edu/magazine/?p=100. Accessed 11 May 2019

Council for International Organizations of Medical Sciences (CIOMS) (1999) Guidelines for preparing core clinical safety information on drugs: report of CIOMS working groups III and V, 2nd edn. CIOMS, Geneva

Council for International Organizations of Medical Sciences (CIOMS) (2010) Practical aspects of signal detection in pharmacovigilance: report of CIOMS working group VIII. CIOMS, Geneva

Council for International Organizations of Medical Sciences (CIOMS) (2014) Practical approaches to risk minimisation for medicinal product: report of CIOMS working group IX. CIOMS, Geneva

Council for International Organizations of Medical Sciences (CIOMS) (2018) CIOMS guide on vaccine safety communication. CIOMS, Geneva. (includes references to regional and global guidance)

Council for International Organizations of Medical Sciences (CIOMS), World Health Organization (WHO) (2012) Definition and application of terms of vaccine pharmacovigilance: report of CIOMS/WHO working group on vaccine pharmacovigilance. CIOMS, Geneva

Council of Canadian Academies (2015) Health product risk communication: is the message getting through? The Expert Panel on the Effectiveness of Health Product Risk Communication, Council of Canadian Academies, Ottawa

Cox AT, Butt TF (2012) Adverse drug reactions: when the risk becomes a reality for patients. Drug Saf 35:977–981

Daly A (1998) Thalidomide: was the tragedy preventable? Lancet 351:1197–1199

Dana Centre (host) (2006) When science hits the headlines [public discussion with panelists: F Mellor (Imperial College London), N Mendoza (science media Centre), J Perry (the sun), D Vaughan (British Antarctic survey)]. Dana Centre, London

Dante or Die (1 Mar 2011) Side effects [dance theatre performance]. Trinity Laban Conservatoire of Music and Dance, London. Information on the performance accessible at: http://www.danteordie.com/side_effects.html0. Accessed 29 Dec 2017

Dean AJ, Hendy A, McGuire T (2007) Antidepressants in children and adolescents: changes in utilisation after safety warnings. Pharmacoepidemiol Drug Saf 16:1048–1053

DeFrank JT, McGormack L, West SL, Lefebvre C, Burrus O (2019) Unintended effects of communicating about drug safety issues: a critical review of the literature. Drug Saf 42: 1125–1134

Demicheli V, Rivetti A, Debalini MG, Di Pietrantonj C (2012) Vaccines for measles, mumps and rubella in children. Cochrane Database Syst Rev (2):CD004407

Deming WE (1982) Out of the crisis. Massachusetts Institute of Technology, Cambridge

Dodoo A, Adjei S, Couper M, Hugman B, Edwards R (2007) When rumours derail a mass deworming exercise. Lancet 370:465–466

Donabedian A (1966) Evaluating the quality of medical care. Milbank Q 44:166–203

Donabedian A (1988) The quality of care: how can it be assessed? J Am Med Assoc 260:1743–1748

Donabedian A (2001) A founder of quality assessment encounters a troubled system first-hand: interview by Fitzhugh Mullan. Health Aff (Millwood) 20:137–141

Douglas J (regional representative of the UN Office on Drugs and Crime (UNODC) to Southeast Asia and the Pacific), Holpuch A (18 Aug 2017) Synthetic opioid crisis in US serves as warning for the world, says UN. Guardian [online news]. https://www.theguardian.com/us-news/2017/aug/18/un-synthetic-opioid-crisis-uk-australia-deaths. Accessed 18 Aug 2017

Downs JS (2011) Evaluation (chapter 3). In: Fischhoff B, Brewer NT, Downs JS (eds) Communicating risks and benefits: an evidence-based user's guide. US Food and Drug Administration, Silver Spring, pp 11–18

Dragoman MV, Tepper NK, Fu R, Curtis KM, Chou R, Gaffield ME (2018) A systematic review and meta-analysis of venous thrombosis risk among users of combined oral contraception. Int J Gynaecol Obstet 141(3):287–294

Dulicek P, Ivanova E, Kostal M, Sadilek P, Beranek M, Zak P, Hirmerova J (2018) Analysis of risk factors of stroke and venous thromboembolism in females with oral contraceptives use. Clin Appl Thromb Hemost 24(5):797–802

Dusetzina SB, Higashi AS, Dorsey ER, Conti R, Huskamp HA, Zhu S, Garfield CF, Alexander GC (2012) Impact of FDA drug risk communications on health care utilization and health behaviors: a systematic review. Med Care 50:466–478

Edwards B, Chakraborty S (2012) Risk communication and the pharmaceutical industry. Drug Saf 35:1027–1040

Edwards IR, Lindquist M (2011) Social media and networks in pharmacovigilance: boon or bane. Drug Saf 34:267–271

Elias C, Fournier A, Vasiliu A, Beix N, Demillac R, Tillaut H, Guillois Y, Eyebe S, Mollo B, Crépey P (2017) Seasonal influenza vaccination coverage and its determinants among nursing homes personnel in western France. BMC Public Health 17:634

Encyclopedia of Sociology (2001) Sentiment. https://www.encyclopedia.com/social-sciences/encyclopedias-almanacs-transcripts-and-maps/sentiments. Accessed 30 Dec 2018

Erice (2017) A new Erice report considering the safety of medicines in the 21st century (report of a meeting held in Erice, 25–29 September 2016, organised by professor Giampaolo Velo, the International School of Pharmacology at the Ettore Majorana Foundation and Centre for Scientific Culture in Erice, Italy, in collaboration with the Uppsala Monitoring Centre (UMC)). UMC, Uppsala

Erice Declaration (1997) Effective communications in pharmacovigilance (report of the international conference on developing effective communications in pharmacovigilance held in Erice, 24–27 September 1997, organised by the Uppsala monitoring Centre (UMC), the clinical pharmacology unit of Verona University, the International School of Pharmacology of the Ettore Majorana Centre for Scientific Culture in Erice, Italy and the World Health Organisation, and supported by EQUUS Communications, London). UMC, Uppsala

European Centre for Disease Prevention and Control (ECDC) (2017) Measles [webpage]. ECDC, Stockholm. https://ecdc.europa.eu. Accessed 6 Apr 2019

Pharmacoepidemiological Research on Outcomes of Therapeutics by a European Consortium (PROTECT) [website]. European Medicines Agency: PROTECT; 2009–2017. www.imi-protect.eu. Accessed 6 Apr 2019

European Medicines Agency (EMA) (2005) European medicines agency finalises review of antidepressants in children and adolescents [media release]. EMA, London

European Medicines Agency (EMA) (2008) Assessment report for thalidomide pharmion. EMA, London

European Medicines Agency (EMA) (2011) Pandemic report and lessons learned: outcome of the European medicines Agency's activities during the 2009 (H1N1) flu pandemic. EMA, London

European Medicines Agency (EMA) (2013) Combined hormonal contraceptives [webpage]. EMA, London. https://www.ema.europa.eu. Accessed 29 Dec 2017

European Medicines Agency (EMA) (2015) EMA-PRAC good practice guide on recording, coding, reporting and assessment of medication errors. EMA, London
European Medicines Agency (EMA) (10 Aug 2018a). Update on review of valsartan medicines due to detection of NDMA [press release]. EMA, London. https://www.ema.europa.eu. Accessed 27 Aug 2018
European Medicines Agency (EMA) (13 Sept 2018b) Update on review of valsartan medicines: risk from NDMA remains low, a related substance NDEA also being investigated [press release]. EMA, London. https://www.ema.europa.eu. Accessed 3 Sept 2019
European Medicines Agency (EMA) (2018c) Valproate and related substances [webpage]. EMA, London. https://www.ema.europa.eu. Accessed 6 Apr 2019
European Medicines Agency (EMA), Heads of Medicines Agencies. Guideline on good pharmacovigilance practices (EU-GVP). EMA (2012–2019), London; EMA (2019–), Amsterdam
European Medicines Agency (EMA), Heads of Medicines Agencies (2013) Guideline on good pharmacovigilance practices - product- or population-specific considerations I: vaccines for prophylaxis against infectious diseases. EMA, London
European Medicines Agency (EMA), Heads of Medicines Agencies (2017) Guideline on good pharmacovigilance practices - module XVI on risk minimisation measures: selection of tools and effectiveness indicators, Rev 2. EMA, London
European Medicines Agency (EMA), Heads of Medicines Agencies (9 Oct 2017) Guideline on good pharmacovigilance practices – annex II – templates. Communication Plan for Direct Healthcare Professional Communication (CP DHPC), London (following informal use for a number of years, the template was formalised as regulatory guidance in 2017)
European Medicines Agency (EMA), Pharmacovigilance Risk Assessment Committee (PRAC) (30 Nov 2017) PRAC strategy on measuring the impact of pharmacovigilance activities, Rev 1. EMA, London
European Network of Centres for Pharmacoepidemiology and Pharmacovigilance (ENCePP) (4 Jul 2018) Guide on methodological standards in pharmacoepidemiology, Rev 7. EMA, London
European Union (28 Nov 2004a) Directive 2001/83/EC of the European parliament and of the council of 6 November 2001 on the community code relating to medicinal products for human use as amended. Off J Eur Commun L 311:67–128. Amended by: European Union (31 Dec 2010). Directive 2010/84/EU of the European parliament and of the council of 15 December 2010 amending, as regards pharmacovigilance Directive 2011/83/EC. Off J Eur Commun L 348:74–99, Article 1(2)
European Union (28 Nov 2004b) Directive 2001/83/EC of the European parliament and of the council of 6 November 2001 on the community code relating to medicinal products for human use as amended. Off J Eur Commun L 311:67–128. Amended by: European Union (31 Dec 2010) Directive 2010/84/EU of the European parliament and of the council of 15 December 2010 amending, as regards pharmacovigilance Directive 2011/83/EC. Off J Eur Commun L 348:74–99: Article 1(3)
Evans M (2002) Reflection on the humanities in medical education. Med Educ 36:508–513
Evans M, Greaves D (2001) 'Developing the medical humanities': report of a research colloquium, and collected abstracts of papers. Med Humanit 27:93–98
Fernández-Villa T, Molina AJ, Torner N, Castilla J, Astray J, García-Gutiérrez S, Mayoral JM, Tamames S, Domínguez Á, Martín V, CIBERESP Working Group for the Survey on Influenza Vaccination in Primary Health Care Workers (2017) Factors associated with acceptance of pandemic flu vaccine by healthcare professionals in Spain, 2009–2010. Res Nurs Health 40:435–443
Finn M, Sarangi S (2009) Humanizing HIV/AIDS and its (re)stigmatizing effects: HIV public 'positive' speaking in India. Health (London) 13:47–65
Fischhoff B, Brewer NT, Downs JS (eds) (2011) Communicating risks and benefits: an evidence-based user's guide. US Food and Drug Administration, Silver Spring
Freeman S, Critchley D, Lee L (2010) Pharmacopoeia medical-art collaboration. Cradle to grave [art installation]. 2003. Exhibited at: British museum, London. (cradle to grave [epilogue]). In: Wynants M (ed) In sickness and in health: the future of medicine - added value and global access. ASP, Brussels. http://www.pharmacopoeia-art.net/articles/in-sickness-and-in-health/. Accessed 29 Dec 2017

Frewer LJ (1999) Public perceptions and risk communication. In: Bennett P, Calman K (eds) Risk communication and public health. Oxford University Press, Oxford, pp 20–32

Friedman RA (2014) Antidepressants' black-box warning: 10 years later. N Engl J Med 371:1666–1668

GBD 2016 Disease and Injury Incidence and Prevalence Collaborators (2017) Global, regional, and national incidence, prevalence, and years lived with disability for 328 diseases and injuries for 195 countries, 1990-2016: a systematic analysis for the global burden of disease study 2016. Lancet 390:1211–1259

Giddens A (1998) The third way: the renewal of social democracy. Polity, Blackwell, Cambridge

Goedecke T, Morales D, Pacurariu A, Kurz X (2018) Measuring the impact of medicines regulatory interventions: systematic review and methodological considerations. Br J Clin Pharmacol 84:419–433

Goldacre B (2009) Bad science. Fourth Estate, London

Goodman JR (2019) Reliance on emoji may push as back towards cave drawings. Br Med J 364:l264

Govender E (2013) Working in the greyzone: exploring education-entertainment in Africa. Afr Commun Res 6:5–32

Grainger D, Lead Investigator. EDURANT/EVIPLERA health care professional survey (rilpivirine). The European Union Electronic Register of Post-Authorisation Studies (EU PAS Register), London (EU PAS Register Number EUPAS5565, last updated on 2 Aug 2017). http://www.encepp.eu/encepp/viewResource.htm?id=20230. Accessed 29 Dec 2017

Greaves D, Evans M (2000) Medical Humanities. Med Humanit 26:1–2

Grilli R, Ramsay C, Minozzi S (2002) Mass media interventions: effects on health services utilisation. Cochrane Database Syst Rev (1):CD000389

Grunig JE, National Academies of Sciences, Engineering, and Medicine (2015) Trust and confidence at the interfaces of the life sciences and society: does the public trust science? [workshop summary]. The National Academies Press, Washington, DC, p 7

Habib S, Rishpon S, Grotto I, Afek A (2017) Influenza vaccination among healthcare workers: the data and the duty [in Hebrew; abstract in English]. Harefuah 156:4–7

Hagemeister MH, Stock NK, Ludwig T, Heuschmann P, Vogel U (2018) Self-reported influenza vaccination rates and attitudes towards vaccination among health care workers: results of a survey in a German university hospital. Public Health 154:102–109

Hallgreen CE, Mt-Isa S, Lieftucht A, Phillips LD, Hughes D, Talbot S, Asiimwe A, Downey G, Genov G, Hermann R, Noel R, Peters R, Micaleff A, Tzoulaki I, Ashby D, on behalf of PROTECT Benefit-Risk Group (2016) Literature review of visual representation of the results of benefit–risk assessments of medicinal products. Pharmacoepidemiol Drug Saf 25:238–250

Health and Safety Executive (HSE) (1999) Reducing error and influencing behaviour. HSG48. HSE, London

Health Canada (2015) Guide for using the standardized health product risk communication template. Health Canada, Ottawa

Health Communication Partnership (HCP) (2003) The new P-process: steps in strategic communication. HCP at Johns Hopkins Bloomberg School of Public Health, Center for Communication Programs, Baltimore

Hernandez JF, van Thiel GJMW, Mantel-Teeuwisse AK, Raaijmakers JA, Pieters T (2014) Restoring trust in the pharmaceutical sector on the basis of the SSRI case. Drug Discov Today 19:523–527

Hickler B (2015) Vaccine special issue on vaccine hesitancy [editorial]. Vaccine 33:4155–4156

Higgins O, Sixsmith J, Barry MM, Domegan C (2011) A literature review on health information-seeking behaviour on the web: a health consumer and health professional perspective. ECDC, Stockholm

Hirst D (1992) Pharmacy [art installation]. Exhibited at: Cohen Gallery, New York, Tate Modern, London. Information on the exhibition in: Manchester E. Damien Hirst, Pharmacy, 1992, 2000, revised 2009. http://www.tate.org.uk/art/artworks/hirst-pharmacy-t07187. Accessed 29 Dec 2017

Hotez PJ (2018) Vaccines did not cause Rachel's autism. Johns Hopkins University Press, Baltimore

Hugman B (2009) Healthcare communication. Pharmaceutical Press, London, Chicago
Hugon-Rodin J, Horellou MH, Conard J, Flaujac C, Gompel A, Plu-Bureau G, for the COntraception, REcurrent Venous Event (COREVE) investigators (2017a) First venous thromboembolism and hormonal contraceptives in young French women. Medicine (Baltimore) 96:e7734
Hugon-Rodin J, Horellou MH, Conard J, Gompel A, Plu-Bureau G (2017b) Combined hormonal contraceptives and first venous thrombosis in young French women: impact of thrombotic family history. J Endocr Soc 1:762–771
ICH Secretariat (2003) International conference on harmonisation of technical requirements for registration of pharmaceuticals for human use (ICH). ICH-E2D guideline: post-approval safety data management - definitions and standards for expedited reporting. ICH Secretariat, Geneva
ICH Secretariat (2010) International conference on harmonisation of technical requirements for registration of pharmaceuticals for human use (ICH). ICH-E2F guideline: development safety update report. ICH Secretariat, Geneva
ICH Secretariat (2013) International conference on harmonisation of technical requirements for registration of pharmaceuticals for human use (ICH). ICH-E2C (R2) guideline: periodic benefit-risk evaluation report (PBRER). ICH Secretariat, Geneva
Illman J (2013) MMR and the media: a historical perspective. Society of Applied Microbiology, London
Institute of Development Studies, United Kingdom. Participatory action research [webpage]. https://www.participatorymethods.org/glossary/participatory-action-research. Accessed 30 Mar 2019
International Pharmaceutical Federation (FIP) (2017a) Medicines information: strategic development. FIP, The Hague
International Pharmaceutical Federation (FIP) (2017b) Pictogram software (last update: 7 February 2017). FIP, Den Haag. https://www.fip.org/pictograms. Accessed 28 Jun 2017
International Society for Pharmacoepidemiology (ISPE). Pharmacoepidemiology [definition]. https://www.pharmacoepi.org/about-ispe/overview/. Accessed 11 May 2019
Jacobs W, Amuta AO, Jeon KC (2017) Health information seeking in the digital age: an analysis of health information seeking behavior among US adults. Cogent Soc Sci 3:1302785
Jamison AM, Broniatowski DA, Quinn SC (2019) Malicious actors on twitter: a guide for public health researchers. Am J Public Health 109:688–692
Jarosch J, Allhoff F (2006) Ethics and patient-centered communication. Appendix B to: improving communication-improving care: an ethical force program consensus report. American Medical Association, Chicago
Jarret C, Wilson R, O'Leary M, Eckersberger E, Larson HJ, SAGE Working Group on Vaccine Hesitancy (2015) Strategies for addressing vaccine hesitancy: a systematic review. Vaccine 33:4180–4190
Johns Hopkins Medical Institutions (JHMI) (24 June 2008) Mendel didn't have the whole picture: our genome changes over lifetime, Johns Hopkins experts say [media release]. JHMI, Baltimore
Jones RH (2013) Health and risk communication: an applied linguistic perspective. Routledge, Abingdon
Jordan T (2008) Addition [novel]. Sceptre, London
van Mill JWF (ed) (1997–) International journal of clinical pharmacy. Springer, Basel
Karafillakis E, Larson H, on behalf of the ADVANCE Consortium (2017) A systematic literature review of perceived risks of vaccines in European populations. Vaccine 35:4840–4850
Kasperson RE, Renn O, Slovic P, Brown HS, Emel J, Goble R et al (1988) The social amplification of risk: a conceptual framework. Risk Anal 8:177–187
Katz LY, Kozyrskyj AL, Prior HJ, Enns MW, Cox BJ, Sareen J (2008) Effect of regulatory warnings on antidepressant prescription rates, use of health services and outcomes among children, adolescents and young adults. Can Med Assoc J 178:1005–1011
Kaufman J, Synnot A, Ryan R, Hill S, Horey D, Willis N, Lin V, Robinson P (2013) Face to face interventions for informing or educating parents about early childhood vaccination. Cochrane Database Syst Rev (5):CD010038

Kesselheim AS (2012) Pharmacoepidemiology and the law. In: Strom BL, Kimmel SE, Hennessy S (eds) Pharmacoepidemiology, 5th edn. Wiley, Chichester, pp 117–134

Kesselheim AS, Campbell EG, Schneeweiss S, Rausch P, Lappin BM, Zhou EH, Seeger JD, Brownstein JS, Woloshin S, Schwartz LM, Toomey T, Dal Pan GJ, Avorn J (2015) Methodological approaches to evaluate the impact of FDA drug safety communications. Drug Saf 38:565–575

Kesselheim AS, McGraw AS, Dejene SZ, Rausch P, Dal Pan GJ, Lappin BM, Zhou EH, Avorn J, Campbell EG (2017) Patient and physician perceptions of drug safety information for sleep aids: a qualitative study. Drug Saf 40:531–542

Kesselheim AS, Sinha MS, Campbell EG, Schneeweiss S, Rausch P, Lappin BM, Zhou EH, Avorn J, Dal Pan GJ (2019) Multimodal analysis of FDA drug safety communications: lessons from zolpidem. Drug Saf 42:1287–1295

Kholsa S, White R, Medina J, Ouwens M, Emmas C, Koder T, Male G, Leonard S (2018) Real world evidence (RWE): a disruptive innovation or the quiet evolution of medical evidence generation? F1000Res 7:111

Kirklin D (2003) The Centre for Medical Humanities, Royal Free and university college medical school, London, England. Acad Med 78:1048–1053

Ko K, Kim S, Kim SH, Son KY, Lee J, Lee DR (2017) Knowledge, current status, and barriers toward healthcare worker vaccination among family medicine resident participants in a web-based survey in Korea. Korean J Fam Med 38:21–27

Kobayashi T, Sugiura K, Ojima T (2017) Risks of thromboembolism associated with hormone contraceptives in Japanese compared with Western women. J Obstet Gynaecol Res 43:789–797

Kotler P, Roberto N, Lee N (2002) Social marketing: improving the quality of life. Sage, Thousand Oaks

Lancet (eds) (2010) Retraction: ileal-lymphoid-nodular hyperplasia, non-specific colitis, and pervasive developmental disorder in children. Lancet 375:445. (retraction of: Wakefield AJ, Murch SH, Anthony A, Linnell J, Casson DM, Malik M, Berelowitz M, Dhillon AP, Thomson MA, Harvey P, Valentine A, Davies SE, Walker-Smith JA (1998) Ileal-lymphoid-nodular hyperplasia, non-specific colitis, and pervasive developmental disorder in children. Lancet 351:637–741)

Lancet (eds) (2017) Untangling the web of opioid addictions in the USA. Lancet 389:2443

Lancet Respiratory Medicine (eds) (2018) Fake medicines: fighting on all fronts. Lancet Respir Med 6:315

Larivée N, Suissa S, Coulombe J, Tagalakis V, Filion KB (2017a) Drospirenone-containing oral contraceptive pills and the risk of venous thromboembolism: an assessment of risk in first-time users and restarters. Drug Saf 40:583–596

Larivée N, Suissa S, Khosrow-Khavar F, Tagalakis V, Filion KB (2017b) Drospirenone-containing oral contraceptive pills and the risk of venous thromboembolism: a systematic review of observational studies. BJOG 124:1490–1499

Larson HJ, Brocard P, Garnett G (2010) The India HPV-vaccine suspension. Lancet 376:572–573

Larson HJ, Smith DMD, Paterson P, Cumming M, Eckersberger E, Freifeld CC, Ghinai I, Jarrett C, Paushter L, Brownstein JS, Madoff LC (2013) Measuring vaccine confidence: analysis of data obtained by a media surveillance system used to analyse public concerns about vaccines. Lancet Infect Dis 13:606–613

Larson HJ, Karafillakis E, Yiangou A, Bahri P, Fogd J, Kurz J, Świerzewski R, Bauchau V, Derrough T, Plebani B, Nohynek H, Mollema L, Sturkenboom M, Myint T-T H, Perez Gomez J, ADVANCE Consortium (4 Oct 2017) Developing communication strategies on vaccine benefits and risks: Guidance for public-private collaborations. Accelerated Development of VAccine beNefit-risk Collaboration in Europe (ADVANCE). http://www.advance-vaccines.eu. Accessed 29 Dec 2017

Lazer DMJ, Baum MA, Benkler Y, Berinsky AJ, Greenhill KM, Menczer F, Metzger MJ, Nyhan B, Pennycook G, Rothschild D, Schudson M, Sloman SA, Sunstein CR, Thorson EA, Watts DJ, Zittrain JL (2018) The science of fake news: addressing fake news requires a multidisciplinary effort. Science 359:1094–1096

Légaré F, Stacey D, Turcotte S, Cossi MJ, Kryworuchko J, Graham ID, Lyddiatt A, Politi MC, Thomson R, Elwyn G, Donner-Banzhoff N (2014) Interventions for improving the adop-

tion of shared decision making by healthcare professionals. Cochrane Database Syst Rev (9):CD006732
Littlejohn SW, Foss KA, Oetzel JG (2016) Theories of human communication, 11th edn. Long Grove, Waveland
Löfstedt RE (2005) Risk management in post-trust societies. Palgrave Macmillan, New York
Löfstedt RE (2007) The impact of the cox-2 inhibitor issue on perceptions of the pharmaceutical industry: content analysis and communication implications. J Health Commun 12:471–491
Looijmans-van den Akker I, van Delden JJ, Verheij TJ, van Essen GA, van der Sande MA, Hulscher ME, Hak E (2009) Which determinants should be targeted to increase influenza vaccination uptake among health care workers in nursing homes? Vaccine 27:4724–4730
Lu CY, Zhang F, Lakoma MD, Madden JM, Rusinak D, Penfold RB, Simon G, Ahmedani BK, Clarke G, Hunkeler EM, Waitzfelder B, Owen-Smith A, Raebel MA, Rossom R, Coleman KJ, Copeland LA, Soumerai SB (2014) Changes in antidepressant use by young people and suicidal behavior after FDA warnings and media coverage: quasi-experimental study. Br Med J 348:g3596
Maasen S, Weingart P (eds) (2006) Democratization of expertise?: exploring novel forms of scientific advice in political decision-making. Springer, Dordrecht
MacDonald NE, SAGE Working Group of Vaccine Hesitancy (2015) Vaccine hesitancy: definition, scope and determinants. Vaccine 33:4161–4164
Maridor M, Ruch S, Bangerter A, Emery V (2017) Skepticism toward emerging infectious diseases and influenza vaccination intentions in nurses. J Health Commun 22:386–394
Marshall E, Salmon D, Bousfiha N, Togola Y, Ouedraogo F, Santantonio M, Dieng CK, Tartière S, Emmanuelli X (2017) Vaccination coverage among social and healthcare workers in ten countries of Samu-social international sites. Vaccine 35:5291–5296
Mass YS (2017) Lawmaker urges World Health Organization to stop 'aggressive' opioid marketing overseas. masslive.com
Mazzaglia G, Straus SMJ, Arlett P, da Silva D, Janssen H, Raine J, Alteri E (2018) Study design and evaluation of risk minimization measures: a review of studies submitted to the European medicines agency for cardiovascular, endocrinology, and metabolic drugs. Drug Saf 41:191–202
McDaid A, Logette E, Buchillier V, Muriset M, Suchon P, Pache TD, Tanackovic G, Kutalik Z, Michaud J (2017) Risk prediction of developing venous thrombosis in combined oral contraceptive users. PLoS One 12:e0182041
McGreal C (13 Aug 2017) Don't blame addicts for America's opioid crisis: here are the real culprits. The Guardian [online news]. https://www.theguardian.com. Accessed 13 Aug 2017
McKee C, Bohannon K (2016) Exploring the reasons behind parental refusal of vaccines: brief review article. J Pediatr Pharmacol Ther 21:104–109
McLuhan M (1964) Understanding media: the extensions of man. Routledge, London, New York
Meldrun ML, Tsao JC-I, Zeltzer LK (2009) "I can't be what I want to be": children's narratives of chronic pain experiences and treatment outcomes. Pain Med 10:1018–1034
Merriam-Webster Dictionary. https://www.merriam-webster.com. Accessed 29 Dec 2017
Minister of Health, Canada (2006) Strategic risk communications framework and handbook. Minister of Health, Canada, Ottawa
Ministry of Health, Labour and Welfare (MHLW) (2006) Q&A on early post-marketing phase vigilance for prescription drugs. MHLW, Tokyo
Ministry of Health, Labour and Welfare (MHLW) (2009) Q&A on use-results surveys conducted as all-case surveillance and early post-marketing phase vigilance (EPPV) for prescription drugs. PMDA, Tokyo
Morgan MG, Fischhoff B, Bostrom A, Atman CJ (2002) Risk communication: a mental models approach. Cambridge University Press, Cambridge
Murthy VH (2016) Ending the opioid epidemic: a call to action. N Engl J Med 375:2413–2415
Mustafa M, Al-Khal A, Maslamani M, Al Soub H (2017) Improving influenza vaccination rates of healthcare workers: a multipronged approach in Qatar. East Mediterr Health J 23:303–310
National Center for Human Factors in Healthcare (n.d.) What is human factors in healthcare? [webpage]. Washington, DC: National Center for Human Factors in Healthcare

National Health Service (NHS) Childhood vaccination coverage statistics, England, 2016–2017 [webpage]. https://digital.nhs.uk. Accessed 1 May 2018

New England Journal of Medicine (NEJM) Catalyst (2017) What is patient-centred care? NEJM Catalyst. https://catalyst.nejm.org/what-is-patient-centered-care/. Accessed 1 May 2018

Nicolson DJ, Knapp P, Raynor DK, Spoor P (2009) Written information about individual medicines for consumers. Cochrane Database Syst Rev (2):CD002104

Nilsen P (2015) Making sense of implementation theories, models and frameworks. Implement Sci 10:53

Nilsen ES, Myrhaug HT, Johansen M, Oliver S, Oxman AD (2006) Methods of consumer involvement in developing healthcare policy and research, clinical practice guidelines and patient information material. Cochrane Database Syst Rev (3):CD004563

O'Reilly-Shah VN, Lynde GC, Jabaley CS (2018) Is it time to start using emoji in biomedical literature? Br Med J 363:k5033. Online comments accessible at https://www.bmj.com. Accessed 6 Jun 2019

O'Sullivan GA, Yonkler JA, Morgan W, Merritt AP (2003) A field guide to designing a health communication strategy. Johns Hopkins Bloomberg School of Public Health, Center for Communication Programs, Baltimore

Olsson S, Pal SN, Dodoo A (2015) Pharmacovigilance in resource-limited countries. Expert Rev Clin Pharmacol 8:449–460

Organisation for Economic Co-operation and Development (OECD) (2019) Addressing problematic opioid use in OECD countries. OECD, Paris

Oxford Dictionary. https://en.oxforddictionaries.com. Accessed 29 Dec 2017

Pang A (2013) Dealing with external stakeholders during the crisis: managing the information vacuum. In: DuBrin AJ (ed) Handbook of research on crisis leadership in organizations. Elgar, Cheltenham, pp 209–230

Penfield K, Bahri P. Kommunikation zwischen Patient und Apotheker: Trainingsvorschlag basierend auf der Bewegungsanalyse nach Laban [workshop abstract]. Hamburg: 22. Norddeutscher Zytostatikaworkshop (NZW); 24–26 January 2014

Pharmaceutical Group of European Union (PGEU) (2017) PGEU best practice paper: pharmacovigilance and risk minimisation. PGEU, Brussels

Piening S, Haaijer-Ruskamp FM, de Vries JTN, van der Elst ME, de Graeff PA, Straus SMJM, Mol PGM (2012) Impact of safety-related regulatory action on clinical practice: a systematic review. Drug Saf 35:373–385

Practice Committee of the American Society for Reproductive Medicine (2017) Combined hormonal contraception and the risk of venous thromboembolism: a guideline. Fertil Steril 107:43–51

Rabensteiner A, Buja A, Regele D, Fischer M, Baldo V (2018) Healthcare worker's attitude to seasonal influenza vaccination in the South Tyrolean province of Italy: barriers and facilitators. Vaccine 36:535–544

Radawski C, Morrato E, Hornbuckle K, Bahri P, Smith M, Juhaeri J, Mol P, Levitan B, Huang H-Y, Coplan P, Li H, on behalf of the ISPE BRACE SIG (2015) Benefit-risk assessment, communication and evaluation (BRACE) throughout the life cycle of therapeutic products: overall perspective and role of the pharmacoepidemiologist. Pharmacoepidemiol Drug Saf 24:1233–1240

Raine J, Wise L, Blackburn S, Eichler HG, Breckenridge A (2011) European perspective on risk management and drug safety. Clin Pharmacol Therapeutics 89:650–654

Renn O (2015) Stakeholder and public involvement in risk governance. Int J Disaster Risk Sci 6:8–20

Renn O, Levine D (1991) Credibility and trust in risk communication. In: Kasperson R, Stallen P (eds) Communicating risks to the public. Kluwer Academic Publishers, Boston, pp 175–218

Riedel G (2017) Influenza vaccination of healthcare personnel by work setting and occupation [in Spanish]. Rev Chil Infectol 34:294 (abstract in English)

Rimon JG (2007) Strategic communication in public health [lecture at training course "leadership in strategic health communication"]. Johns Hopkins Bloomberg School of Public Health, Center for Communication Programs, Baltimore

Rolfe A, Cash-Gibson L, Car J, Sheikh A, McKinstry B (2014) Interventions for improving patients' trust in doctors and groups of doctors. Cochrane Database Syst Rev (3):CD004134

Ropeik D (15 Dec 2002) Journalists can be seduced by aspects of risk. Nieman Reports

Rosenbaum L (2017) The march of science: the true story. N Engl J Med 377:188–191

Ryan M, Bate A, Eastmond CJ, Ludbrook A (2001) Use of discrete choice experiments to elicit preferences. Qual Health Care 10(Suppl I):i55–i60

Ryan R, Santesso N, Lowe D, Hill S, Grimshaw JM, Prictor M, Kaufman C, Cowie G, Taylor M (2014) Interventions to improve safe and effective medicines use by consumers: an overview of systematic reviews. Cochrane Database Syst Rev (4):CD007768

Saeterdal I, Lewin S, Austvoll-Dahlgren A, Glenton C, Munabi-Babigumira S (2014) Interventions aimed at communities to inform and/or educate about early childhood vaccination. Cochrane Database Syst Rev (11):CD010232

Salisbury D, Council for International Organizations of Medical Sciences (CIOMS) (2018) CIOMS guide on vaccine safety communication. CIOMS, Geneva

Schwartz JL (2012) New media, old messages: themes in the history of vaccine hesitancy and refusal. Virtual Mentor 14:50–55

Schwarz N, Bohner G (2001) The construction of attitudes. In: Tesser A, Schwarz N (eds) Intrapersonal processes (Blackwell handbook of social psychology). Blackwell, Oxford, pp 436–457

Schwitzer G (2008) How do US journalists cover treatments, tests, products, and procedures?: an evaluation of 500 stories. PLoS Med 5:e95

Schwitzer G, Mudur G, Henry D, Wilson A, Goozner M, Simbra M, Sweet M, Baverstock KA (2005) What are the roles and responsibilities of the media in disseminating health information? PLoS Med 2(7):e215

Shankar PR (2014) Medical humanities. Ann Commun Health 2:18–20

Shaw SE, Bailey J (2009) Discourse analysis: what is it and why is it relevant to family practice? Fam Pract 26:413–419

Sinha MS, Freifeld CC, Brownstein JS, Donneyong MM, Rausch P, Lappin BM, Zhou EH, Dal Pan GJ, Pawar AM, Hwang TJ, Avorn J, Kesselheim AS (2018) Social media impact of the Food and Drug Administration's drug safety communication messaging about zolpidem: mixed-methods analysis. JMIR Public Health Surveill 4:e1

Slovic P (2010) The feeling of risk: new perspectives on risk perception. Earthscan, London, Washington, DC

Smith MY, Russel A, Bahri P, Mol PGM, Frise S, Freeman E, Morrato EH (2018) The RIMES statement: a checklist to assess the quality of studies evaluating risk minimization programs for medicinal products. Drug Saf 41:389–401

Soderbergh S (director), Burns SZ (screenplay writer) (2013) Side effects [movie website]. http://sideeffectsmayvary.com. Accessed 29 Dec 2017

Soumerai SB. In: Gallaghar J (19 June 2014) Antidepressant suicide warnings 'may have backfired'. BBC [online news]. http://www.bbc.co.uk/news/health-27904749. Accessed 23 Jun 2014

Soumerai SB, Avron J (1990) Principles of educational outreach ("academic detailing") to improve clinical decision making. J Am Med Assoc 263:549–556

Speers T, Lewis J (2004) Journalists and jabs: media coverage of the MMR vaccine. Commun Med 1:171–181

Spiewak M (23 Aug 2017) Forscherfeindlichkeit? Autoritätsverlust? Unsinn!: Der deutschen Wissenschaft geht es so gut wie nie zuvor. Zeit [online news]. http://www.zeit.de/2017/35/deutsche-wissenschaft-forschung-studien/komplettansicht. Accessed 23 Aug 2017

Spitzer WO (1991) Drugs as determinants of health and disease in the population: an orientation to the bridge science of pharmacoepidemiology. J Clin Epidemiol 44:823–830

Squiers L, Peinado S, Berkman N, Boudewyns V, McCormack L (2012) The health literacy skills framework. J Health Comm 17:30–54

Stacey D, Légaré F, Col NF, Bennett CL, Barry MJ, Eden KB, Wu JH (2014) Decision aids for people facing health treatment or screening decisions. Cochrane Database Syst Rev (1):CD001431

Stone MB (2014) The FDA warning on antidepressants and suicidality: why the controversy? N Engl J Med 371:1668–1671

Storey D, Figueroa ME (2012) Toward a global theory of health behaviour and social change. In: Obregon R, Waisbord S (eds) The handbook of global health communication. Wiley-Blackwell, Oxford, pp 70–94

Sturm L, Donahue K, Kasting M, Kulkarni A, Brewer NT, Zimet GD (2017) Pediatrician-parent conversations about human papillomavirus vaccination: an analysis of audio recordings. J Ado Health 61:246–251

Taylor BJ, Killick C, McGlade A (2015) Understanding and using research in social work. Sage, London

Thom DH, Ribisl KM, Stewart AL, Luke DA (1999) Further validation and reliability testing of the Trust in Physician Scale. The Stanford trust study physicians. Med Care 37:510–517

TIMSS & PIRLS International Study Centre. PIRLS 2016 International study results in reading. http://timssandpirls.bc.edu. Accessed 8 Jun 2019

Trevena LJ, Davey HM, Barratt A, Butow P, Caldwell P (2004) A systematic review on communicating with patients about evidence. J Eval Clin Pract 12:13–23

Tsintis P, La Mache E (2004) CIOMS and ICH initiatives in pharmacovigilance and risk management: overview and implications. Drug Saf 27:509–517

Tsukahara VHB, Calil SJ (2016) Root cause analysis combined with human factors engineering tools for adverse events investigation in healthcare. In: Kyriacou E, Christofides S, Pattichis C (eds) XIV Mediterranean conference on medical and biological engineering and computing 2016 (IFMBE proceedings), vol 57. Springer, Basel

United Nations (UN) Commission on Life-Saving Commodities (2012) Commissioners' report. UN, New York

United Nations Children's Fund (UNICEF). What are the social ecological model (SEM), and communication for development (C4D)? UNICEF, New York. https://www.unicef.org/cbsc/files/Module_1_SEM-C4D.docx. Accessed 30 Jul 2017

United States Centers of Disease Control (US CDC) (2019) Measles: cases and outbreaks [webpage]. US CDC, Atlanta. https://www.cdc.gov. Accessed 6 Apr 2019

United States Food and Drug Administration (US FDA). FDA approved drug products: Thalomid [webpage] (updated in January 2017a). US FDA, Silver Spring. https://www.fda.gov. Accessed 29 Dec 2017

United States Food and Drug Administration (US FDA) (2017b) Use of real-world evidence to support regulatory decision-making for medical devices: guidance for Industry and Food and Drug Administration staff. US FDA, Silver Spring

United States Food and Drug Administration (US FDA). FDA updates on valsartan recalls. https://www.fda.gov/Drugs/DrugSafety/ucm613916.htm. Accessed 27 Aug 2018a

United States Food and Drug Administration (US FDA) (26 Jan 2018b) What's in a REMS? [webpage]. US FDA, Silver Spring. https://www.fda.gov. Accessed 1 May 2018

United States Food and Drug Administration (US FDA) Class suicidality labeling language for antidepressants. US FDA, Silver Spring. https://www.accessdata.fda.gov/drugsatfda_docs/label/2005/20031s045,20936s020lbl.pdf. Accessed 4 Mar 2018c

United States Food and Drug Administration (US FDA) (27 Sept 2018d) Precision medicine [webpage]. US FDA, Silver Spring. https://www.fda.gov. Accessed 12 May 2019

Uppsala Monitoring Centre (UMC) (15 Mar 2018) Glossary of pharmacovigilance terms. UMC, Uppsala. https://www.who-umc.org. Accessed 1 May 2018

van Amsterdam J, van den Brink W (2015) The misuse of prescription opioids: a threat for Europe? Curr Drug Abuse Rev 8:3–14

Velo G (2010) Erice statement 2009: communication, medicines and patient safety (report of the workshop on drug risk communication held in Erice, 3-8 July 2009, organised by the International School of Pharmacology at the Ettore Majorana Foundation and Centre for Scientific Culture in Erice, Italy, in collaboration with the International Society of Pharmacovigilance (ISoP), the SK Foundation and the Uppsala Monitoring Centre (UMC)). Br J Clin Pharmacol 69:207–208

Venkatraman A, Garg N, Kumar N (2015) Greater freedom of speech on web 2.0 correlates with dominance of views linking vaccines to autism. Vaccine 33:1422–1425

Venulet J, Helling-Borda M (2010) WHO's international drug monitoring: the formative years, 1967-1975. Drug Saf 33:e1–e23

Vicusi WK (1994) Efficacy of labeling of foods and pharmaceuticals. Annu Rev Public Health 15:325–343

Vollman AR, Anderson ET, McFarlane J (2004) Canadian community as partner. Lippincott Williams & Wilkins, Philadelphia

Vosoughi S, Roy D, Aral S (2018) The spread of true and false news online. Science 359:1146–1151

Vrije Universiteit Amsterdam (VU). Neuropsychology [master's degree webpage]. VU, Amsterdam. https://masters.vu.nl/en/programmes/cognitive-neuropsychology/index.aspxrrd. Accessed 11 May 2019

Waisbord S. Watchdog journalism. Wiley Online Library. https://onlinelibrary.wiley.com/doi/pdf/10.1002/9781118541555.wbiepc046. Accessed 5 Jun 2019

Waller P, Harrison-Woolrych M (2017) An introduction to pharmacovigilance, 2nd edn. Wiley Blackwell, Chichester

Waller PC, Evans SJW, Beard K (2005) Drug safety and the media. Br J Clin Pharmacol 61(2):123–126

Way D, Blazsin H, Löfstedt R, Bouder F (2017) Pharmaceutical benefit-risk communication tools: a review of the literature. Drug Saf 40:15–36

West SL, Squiers LB, McCormack L, Southwell BG, Brouwer ES, Ashok M, Lux L, Boudewyns V, O'Donoghue A, Sullivan HW (2013) Communicating quantitative risks and benefits in promotional prescription drug labeling or print advertising. Pharmacoepidemiol Drug Saf 22:447–458

Wikipedia. Wit (film) (director: Mike Nichols; play writer: Margaret Edson). Edited on: 7 May 2018a. https://en.wikipedia.org/wiki/Wit_(film). Accessed 1 Jun 2018

Wikipedia. BPM (film) (director: Robin Campillo; co-screenwriter: Philippe Mangeot). Edited on: 27 May 2018b. https://en.wikipedia.org/wiki/BPM_(Beats_per_Minute). Accessed on: 1 June 2018

Williams J. Strategy development for communication development [lecture]. Baltimore, MD; 12 June 2007 (the lecture was part of the training course "Leadership in Strategic Health Communication" provided by Johns Hopkins Bloomberg School of Public Health, Center for Communication Programs in Baltimore, MD: 4–22 June 2007)

Woloshin S, Schwartz LM, Dejene S, Rausch P, Dal Pan GJ, Zhou EH, Kesselheim AS (2017) Media coverage of FDA drug safety communications about zolpidem: a quantitative and qualitative analysis. J Health Commun 22:365–372

World Health Organization (WHO) (2002) The importance of pharmacovigilance: safety monitoring of medicinal products. WHO, Geneva

World Health Organization (WHO) (2009) Human factors in patient safety: review of topics and tools. WHO, Geneva

World Health Organization (WHO) (2014) EMP thalidomide is back: are we ready for it? [news release]. WHO, Geneva

World Health Organization (WHO) (2014–2017) Community engagement in the Ebola response [webpage]. WHO, Geneva. http://www.who.int. Accessed 29 Dec 2017

World Health Organization (WHO) (2015) Global action plan on antimicrobial resistance. WHO, Geneva

World Health Organization (WHO) (2016a) Final trial results confirm Ebola vaccine provides high protection against disease [news release]. WHO, Geneva

World Health Organization (WHO) (2016b) Antimicrobial resistance [fact sheet]. WHO, Geneva

World Health Organization (WHO) (2017a) Leprosy [fact sheet]. WHO, Geneva

World Health Organization (WHO) (2017b) MMR and autism [webpage]. WHO, Geneva. http://www.who.int. Accessed 29 Dec 2017

World Health Organization (WHO) (2017c) Measles [fact sheet]. WHO, Geneva

World Health Organization (WHO) (2017d) Mental health [webpage]. WHO, Geneva. http://www.who.int. Accessed 29 Dec 2017

World Health Organization (WHO) (2017e) Depression [fact sheet]. WHO, Geneva

Part I

Medicines in Real Life as Communication Challenges

Hormonal Contraceptives: Communication for Risk Awareness and Informed Choice, or a Public Scare?

2

Barbara Mintzes and Teresa Leonardo Alves

Abstract

This chapter discusses oral contraceptives as a special case in risk communication on medicines, as they are provided to large populations of young, healthy people and the tolerance for risks is therefore low. All combined oestrogen–progestin containing oral contraceptives have similar effectiveness in preventing pregnancy, but carry different risks for rare but serious venous thromboembolism (VTE), i.e. blood clots that are potentially fatal if they travel to the lungs. In 1995, large-scale studies indicated a higher VTE frequency with newer "third-generation" contraceptives, and in 2009, with drospirenone-containing contraceptives. This chapter describes the challenges and outcomes of the related communication events and discusses the media representation of the "pill scare" in the United Kingdom in 1995. This had an immediate impact, leading to worldwide recognition of the need for effective communication of risks of medicines as a crucial task, with a profound effect on regulatory risk communication that is still haunting us today. The chapter further examines the role of financial conflicts of interests of medical journal authors in the interpretation and wider dissemination of research evidence.

A contribution from the author Priya Bahri is included in this chapter as Appendix 2.1.

B. Mintzes (✉)
School of Pharmacy and Charles Perkins Centre, The University of Sydney, Camperdown, NSW, Australia
e-mail: barbara.mintzes@sydney.edu.au

T. L. Alves
Division of Pharmacoepidemiology and Clinical Pharmacology, Utrecht Institute for Pharmaceutical Sciences, Utrecht University, Utrecht, Netherlands

© Springer Nature Singapore Pte Ltd. 2020

P. Bahri (ed.), *Communicating about Risks and Safe Use of Medicines*,
https://doi.org/10.1007/978-981-15-3013-5_2

2.1 Situation: The Safety Concerns with Hormonal Contraceptives and Communication Challenges

When the first oral combined hormonal contraceptive (CHC), commonly called "the pill", was introduced onto the market in the United States (US) in 1960, it represented a major shift in the use of medicinal products. This was the first product with the intended effect of altering a normal physiological process, i.e. to suppress monthly ovulation for the prevention of pregnancy. While CHCs were celebrated by many as key to women's right to take control of their fertility and whether and when to have a child as well as women's liberation to enjoy sexuality without aiming for or fearing pregnancy, others condemned CHCs as being against the natural or moral order (Dhont 2010; Kruvand 2012). These controversies highlight the fact that medicines may not only be a medical intervention but also of broader societal concern tied to individual life choices, gender equity, and morality. Since the 1960s, CHCs have become widely available and used in most countries, and have been included in the *Essential Medicines List* issued by the World Health Organization (WHO) (World Health Organization 2017). Over 100 million women worldwide use CHCs (Brynhildsen 2014; United Nations, Department of Economic and Social Affairs, Population Division 2015).

Given that contraceptives are used, often for many years, by large populations of generally young, healthy people, safety standards need to be particularly high. Tolerance for risks of rare, serious harmful effects is lower than for a medicine used to treat or prevent disease. Risk assessment of CHCs therefore differs fundamentally from that of other medicinal products, because risks are not being weighed against the harmful effects of a disease process. The level of risk that a contraceptive user judges to be acceptable also differs depending on a woman's life circumstances and can involve a trade-off of acceptance of higher risks in exchange for higher effectiveness. This can be especially acute in countries where there is limited access to therapeutic or elective pregnancy termination, in particular for women in lower income-settings or where religious or moral beliefs make this option unacceptable. When CHCs were first marketed in the 1960s, pregnancy termination was illegal in most countries and deaths from unsafe illegal terminations were a frequent cause of death in women of reproductive age; this situation continues in countries with restrictive laws in Africa, Latin America, and Asia (Haddad and Nour 2009). Gender inequity can also play a role, for example, in relation to employment conditions and financial insecurity associated with pregnancy, inability to negotiate condom use, or where women's contraceptive use must remain hidden. Additionally, some women have health conditions that make pregnancy riskier. These factors provide an important role in women users' and physicians' judgments of the acceptability of risks of harm and contraceptive choice.

It is therefore no wonder that the way that safety and harmful effects are communicated for CHCs has been fraught with controversy. Among CHCs there is no reliable evidence of differences in effectiveness with appropriate use (Lopez et al. 2013). This includes low-oestrogen-dose CHCs with less than 20 μg per day, which are equally effective as products containing more than 20 μg (Gallo et al. 2011). Against this backdrop of similar effectiveness in preventing pregnancy, there are however differences in the safety profile of different formulations. Two main "waves" of pharmacoepidemiological research have identified risk differences between CHCs, the first beginning in 1995, and the second nearly 25 years later, in 2009. Although the specific products involved differed, a common theme runs through both waves in relation to risk communication. In both cases, the newer, heavily promoted CHCs were found to be riskier than older products with a longer history of use, flying in the face of a common assumption among physicians and the public that "newer is better". In both cases, increased risks of the newer products have been hotly contested, with contradictory messages in both the medical and general media. The extensive media coverage included personal stories of young women who died or suffered serious harm.

This chapter describes the communication events surrounding CHCs and the differences in risks of blood clots, or venous thromboembolic events (VTE), of different lower dose (≤50 μg oestrogen) formulations and examines two major aspects of risk evaluation and communication:

1. communication regarding the regulatory response to the scientific evidence of differing risks and sometimes conflicting roles of the general media in representing these risk differences, and
2. the potential role of conflict of interests in the dissemination of scientific evidence to healthcare professionals in medical journals as a major communication type and information source for healthcare professionals.

The Safety Concerns

CHCs consist of an oestrogen and a progestin, two synthetic hormones similar to the natural female sexual hormones. They prevent the release of egg cells from the ovaries (ovulation) through a number of interacting hormonal feedback loops. They are now available for oral use, as a vaginal ring, and as a patch, but oral preparations are by far the most commonly used.

While CHCs are generally safe, there are some rare risks associated with their use, as with all other medicinal products. Amongst those, VTE is the most important serious adverse event which may be caused by CHCs. VTE is caused by blood clots in the deep veins, e.g. in the leg, that may travel to the lungs. VTE can lead to severe harm with irreversible disabilities and even death. According to a comprehensive review of the evidence, conducted by the European Medicines Agency (EMA) in 2013, the risk of blood clots in the veins varies between CHCs, depending on the oestrogen dose and the type of progestin they contain, and ranges from "5 to 12 cases of blood clots per 10,000 women who use them for a year". This compares with "2 cases of blood clots in the veins each year per 10,000 women who are not using CHCs" (European Medicines Agency 2014).

The first report in the medical literature of a link between CHCs and increased risk of VTE dates from 1961, with a case report published in the *Lancet* of a woman who experienced a pulmonary embolism following CHC use (Jordan 1961). By 1962, the manufacturer of the first marketed CHC, Searle, had received reports of

132 cases of VTE in CHC users, 11 of which were fatal (Geampana 2016). In 1967, the Medical Research Council in the United Kingdom (UK) published a preliminary report of the results of three case–control studies, all indicating a higher rate of blood clots with CHC use (Anonymous 1967), and in 1969 the UK Committee on Safety of Medicines (CSM) warned of higher risks with CHCs containing more than 50 μg of oestrogen (Lackie and Fairchild 2016). The research had indicated risk differences based on the oestrogen dose, with CHCs containing 50 μg or more of oestrogen associated with higher risks.

The Increased VTE Risk of "Third-Generation" Contraceptives

The first large-scale evidence of differences in risk of blood clots in women using CHCs containing different progestins dates from late 1995, when three case–control studies found evidence of higher VTE risks among newer "third-generation" CHCs containing the progestins desogestrel or gestodene, as compared with older "second-generation" CHCs containing the progestins levonorgestrel or norethindrone (Anonymous 1995; Jick et al. 1995; Spitzer et al. 1996). One of these studies was sponsored by the WHO (World Health Organization Collaborative Study of Cardiovascular Disease and Steroid Hormone Contraception 1995), another instigated by the UK CSM (Jick et al. 1995), and the third conducted by the Transnational Research Group on Oral Contraceptives and the Health of Young Women and funded by a manufacturer of a "third-generation" CHC (Spitzer et al. 1996). These studies constitute the first large-scale research indicating that the progestin component of a CHC was also an important determinant of VTE risk, in addition to the oestrogen dose. The riskier "third-generation" products were also newer and had been heavily promoted to physicians as having a more favourable side effect profile than older CHCs.

The Increased VTE Risk of Drospirenone-Containing Contraceptives

In 2001, the first CHC containing the progestin drospirenone was approved, under the trade name of Yasmin® (drospirenone 3 mg/ethinylestradiol 0.03 mg). This was the first novel progestin to be included in a CHC for many years. When this product was first marketed, it was not clear how its risk of blood clotting compared with that of other oral contraceptives, as too few women had been exposed in pre-market studies to characterise this infrequent risk (Pearce et al. 2005). This is similar to the situation faced with "third-generation" products when they first came to market. The first population-based studies to indicate an increased VTE risk with drospirenone were published in the *British Medical Journal* (*BMJ*) in 2009. These included a Dutch case–control study of patients in VTE treatment centres (Vlieg et al. 2009) and a Danish population-based study (Lidegaard et al. 2009). These studies came to differing conclusions from two earlier manufacturer-sponsored studies, both published in 2007 (Dinger et al. 2007; Seeger et al. 2007) and carried out at the request of the EMA(Dinger et al. 2007) and the US Food and Drug Administration (US FDA) (Seeger et al. 2007). Another manufacturer-sponsored study published in 2010 also failed to find increased risks (Dinger et al. 2010). These conflicting results likely reflect differences in research methods, including how exposures and health outcomes were defined and which types of oral contraceptives were chosen as a comparison group (Jick 2015).

In 2011, four additional studies confirmed drospirenone's higher VTE risks (Gronich et al. 2011; Jick and Hernandez 2011; Lidegaard et al. 2011; Parkin et al. 2011). The US FDA carried out its own study, published in 2013, also confirming these increased risks (Sidney et al. 2013). When all studies were combined in a Cochrane systematic review published in 2014, the magnitude of increased risk of blood clotting with drospirenone was similar to that of "third-generation" CHCs (de Bastos et al. 2014).

The Communication Challenges

Following the initial evidence of increased VTE risks for "third-generation" and drospirenone-containing CHCs, an ongoing controversy affected interpretation of the risk evidence and its communication. Major challenges in communicating the evidence arise from what has already been discussed or will be elaborated further on in this chapter, in summary:

- the need for an informed choice to use a medicinal product by healthy individuals;
- social tensions regarding the morality of contraceptive use;
- accumulating and controversial evidence about differences in VTE risk between the different CHC products;
- ongoing court cases;
- commercial interests of the manufacturers; and
- the role of the media in social amplification of risk perception.

From very early in the history of CHCs, there has been a tension between an interpretation of "the pill" as a source of liberation on the one hand and, on the other hand, considerations that women were not adequately warned about evidence of harm. Barbara Seaman, in her book *The Doctor's Case Against the Pill* of 1969, critiqued medical paternalism and argued that women were being kept in the dark about serious risks, including deaths from VTE (Seaman 1969). In 1970, a year after the launch of this book, US Senate Subcommittee hearings were held on the safety of CHCs which led to a recommendation that all CHCs to be accompanied by a patient package insert in order for women to be informed of potential risks. The package insert was based on the approved product information but written in lay language, the first such requirement for a pharmaceutical product in the US (Lackie and Fairchild 2016). Public attention to VTE risks also likely helped to stimulate the research leading to a reduction in both the oestrogen and progestin dose in CHCs and to the development of safer formulations widely available since the early 1980s.

A related communication issue is the advertising of CHCs to the public, especially in the US, which allows direct-to-consumer advertising (DTCA) of prescription-only medicines. Between 2005 and 2010, overlapping the period in which the risk controversy described above was unfolding, the manufacturer of the drospirenone-containing CHCs Yasmin® and Yaz® (another trade name for a drospirenone-containing CHC) spent US $404 million advertising these brands to the US public. This was 56% of the US $717 million spent on advertising of all CHCs to the US public during this 6-year period (Wu et al. 2016). In 2003, the US FDA judged

Yasmin® television advertisements and in 2008 Yaz® advertisements to contravene US regulations (Abrams 2008; Hankin 2003), in both cases partly due to minimisation of information on serious risks.

2.2 Events: The Communication Experiences

The so-called VTE pill scare of 1995 in the UK was a major event in medicinal risk communication affecting regulators' understanding of potential pitfalls in the communication of emergent evidence on harmful effects of products that are already on the market (see Chap. 1). This chapter describes the "VTE pill scare" and reflects on why it led to divided responses.

The "VTE Pill Scare" in the United Kingdom

In October 1995, the UK CSM issued a warning on the increased risks of blood clots with desogestrel- and gestodene-containing CHCs in a direct health professional communication (DHPC) (also called a "Dear Doctor" letter), advising physicians to switch women using these CHCs to lower risk products (UK Committee on the Safety of Medicines 1995). Similar warnings were issued concurrently by regulatory authorities in Germany and Norway. All of these warnings were issued "pre-publication", i.e. when the studies (see Sect. 2.1) had been seen by the regulators but were not yet publicly available. The fact that the studies had not yet undergone the peer-review process for publication in a medical journal was highlighted in critiques of the public CSM warning (Spitzer 1997).

Recommendations in other countries varied. The Netherlands issued a more restrictive warning, recommending switching to a product with lower VTE risk in women with risk factors, and avoiding initiation of "third-generation" CHCs in first-time contraceptive users (de Vries et al. 1998). Neither the US FDA nor Health Canada issued similar advisories (Geampana 2016). The CSM warning is referred to as having caused the UK "VTE pill scare" because of its extensive press coverage and implications, which are discussed later in this chapter.

Following these regulatory warnings and publication of the underlying studies, a scientific controversy arose about whether VTE risks were truly higher with "third-generation" CHCs. This was based on extensive critique of the methods used in the 1995 studies and in additional studies published following the CSM warning. One of the 1995 studies had been carried out in the UK General Practice Research Database (GPRD) (Jick et al. 1995), and a second analysis, carried out of the same database and funded by manufacturers of "third-generation" CHCs, was published in 1997 (Farmer et al. 1997). This second study did not find increased risks with use of "third-generation" CHCs (Farmer et al. 1997). Similarly, the 1995 Transnational Study (Spitzer et al. 1996) was re-analysed—this time with only manufacturer funding—and this analysis failed to find a risk difference and blamed earlier results on methodological shortcomings (Lewis 1999; Loder et al. 2015). This re-analysis of the Transnational Study was influential in sowing doubt in a UK legal case against the three manufacturers of "third-generation" CHCs by women who had suffered blood clots (Skegg 2000). A second reason this legal case failed to find the manufacturers liable is that the most reliable estimate of the relative risk of VTE with "third-generation" versus other CHCs was 1.7 (Kemmeren et al. 2001). This was below a threshold set by the court of a doubling of risk (Skegg 2000). In his July 2002 decision, the presiding judge, Mackay agreed with the 1.7 relative risk, but found it below the threshold required for liability, stating: "I would incline to a finding that there is an underlying causal connection at about that level of increased risk" (Ashraf 2002).

Beforehand, in July 2001, the first systematic review had been published in the *British Medical Journal* synthesising all research evidence to date in a meta-analysis of the results of the 13 included studies and confirming an overall odds ratio of 1.7 (95% CI 1.4–2) for blood clots in users of "third-generation" versus "second-generation" CHCs (Kemmeren et al. 2001). This research team also carried out a separate analysis by industry funding and found an odds ratio of 1.3 (95% CI 1.0–1.7) of increased risk for "third-generation" CHCs in studies funded by the pharmaceutical industry, as compared with 2.3 (95% CI 1.7–3.2) in non-industry-funded research (Kemmeren et al. 2001). The authors further examined the methods used to evaluate risks and suspected biases that had been cited to refute study results, such as a potential healthy user bias, biases due to recency of product introduction, duration of use, diagnostic suspicion and referral biases, prescribing bias and effects of switching (Suissa et al. 2000). The observed risk differences stood up to scrutiny in sensitivity analyses taking these factors into account. For example, the odds ratio among first-time contraceptive users was 3.1 (95% CI 2.0–4.6), among short-term users 2.5 (95% CI 1.6–4.1), and longer-term users 2.0 (95% CI 1.4–2.7) (Kemmeren et al. 2001), suggesting that taking these factors into consideration strengthened rather than weakened the evidence of increased risk.

Intense methodological criticism has been a consistent feature of the research literature on VTE risks of CHCs. As this case highlights, scientific controversies had important legal, medical, commercial, and communication consequences. Within this controversy, medicines regulators needed to decide when and how to respond, what to communicate to the public, and whether any limits on prescribing should be imposed, such as restricting use of riskier products to second-line use for women who cannot tolerate less risky products. As is described below, the experience with the "VTE pill scare" has no doubt had a chilling effect on risk communication.

Alarmist press coverage of the CSM warnings has been blamed for the "VTE pill scare" in the UK in 1995, but the potential for alarm may have also rested on lack of prior knowledge and awareness, and may have affected non-users more than users (Jick et al. 1998; Martin et al. 1997). Secondly, the nearly mythic status of this "scare" might not necessarily have been a neutral communication event. The two progestin components of lower risk products, levonorgestrel and norethisterone, were no longer under patent protection and thus less expensive generic products could be produced, whereas the progestin components of the riskier "third-generation" CHCs were still under patent protection. Researchers have highlighted the influence of commercial pressures on patterns of risk communication (Pearce 2008), and on a muddying of the waters concerning the scientific evidence that has left physicians and the public unsure what and whom to believe (Dukes 2011).

The implications of the "VTE pill scare" (see Sect. 2.3) are in many ways extraordinary. The first question it poses is why is this described as a UK "pill scare" given that CHCs were being used globally? Were there specific features of risk communication in the UK that contributed to this view? As is noted above, regulators differed in their responses, and in North America were notably silent. The second question is, why did a sedate, practical warning for women using certain types of CHCs to switch to another type with lower VTE risks, unless they had specific reasons to stay on a "third-generation" CHC, lead to a scare? The wide availability of equally effective yet safer CHCs through a universal public healthcare system in the UK greatly simplified the message and should have provided reassurance, not fear.

When drospirenone-containing oral contraceptives were also associated with increased VTE risks over 10 years later, again a similar pattern occurred of dismissal of evidence of risk differences as being due to methodological weaknesses and biases in studies indicating increased harm (Shapiro 2013). Given the similarities in these two events, we were interested to examine whether financial conflicts of interest might influence key messages about risk differences communicated to physicians in medical journals, and conducted the study described in Sect. 2.2.1.

2.2.1 Study of the Impact of Conflicts of Interests on the Dissemination of Evidence on Risk Differences Between Hormonal Contraceptives in Medical Journals

Objectives and Methods In order to examine whether conflicts of interests played a role in the interpretation and communication of evidence on relative safety of different CHCs in medical journals, we carried out an analysis of articles published from 2010 until the end of 2016 that cited one or more of the studies that compared drospirenone-containing CHCs with levonorgestrel- or norethindrone-containing ("second generation") CHCs (Dinger et al. 2007, 2010, 2016; Gronich et al. 2011; Jick and Hernandez 2011; Lidegaard et al. 2011; Parkin et al. 2011; Sidney et al. 2013; Bird et al. 2013; van Hylckama Vlieg et al. 2009; Vinogradova et al. 2015; Ziller et al. 2014). Some of these studies also included a comparison of desogestrel- and gestodene- containing ("third generation") pills. We used Web of Science Core Collection (Clarivate Analytics, December 2017) to carry out a cited reference search, identifying all citing articles ($n = 481$). We eliminated duplicates and selected citing articles for inclusion if they met the following three criteria: (1) they were reviews (systematic or narrative), commentaries, letters to the editor, clinical guidelines, or original empirical studies; (2) they were about women of reproductive age; and (3) they addressed VTE risks associated with CHCs as a key focus, which was operationally defined as either discussing these risks in the article abstract or, in the absence of an abstract, devoting at least 50% of the full text article content on this topic.

We focused on this secondary literature because of its role in synthesising and interpreting the evidence for use by physicians in healthcare. The start date of 2010 was chosen because the first studies indicating higher risks for drospirenone-containing CHCs were published in 2009 (Lidegaard et al. 2009; van Hylckama Vlieg et al. 2009). We classified authors' expressed positions regarding risk differences with drospirenone and "third-generation" CHCs versus "second-generation" CHCs as "higher", "equivalent", or "neutral/unsure" and examined these expressed positions in relation to whether authors had declared financial links with pharmaceutical companies.

Findings In total, 148 articles met our inclusion criteria (see Appendix 2.2). Of these 148, 62 (42%) had one or more authors with declared pharmaceutical industry financing, 67 (45%) had no industry financing, and 19 (13%) failed to disclose any information on conflicts of interests. In total, 136 (92%) of the 148 articles included a stated position on drospirenone's VTE risks. Of these, 59 (43%) included authors with pharmaceutical industry financing, 59 (43%) had no such financing, and 18 (13%) with no financial disclosures.

Among those with declared industry financing, 36/59 (61%) asserted that drospirenone had similar VTE risk levels to other contraceptives (e.g. no increased risk in comparison to levonorgestrel-containing/"second-generation" CHCs). In contrast, only 5 of the 59 (9%) of articles in which no author had a declared conflict judged risks for drospirenone-containing CHCs to be no higher. The relative risk (RR) of a position that drospirenone's risks were no higher to those of "second-generation" CHCs among conflicted versus non-conflicted authors was 7.2 (95% CI 3.0–17.1). For "third-generation" CHCs, a similar strongly skewed pattern exists: 27/47 authors (57%) with conflicts judged "third-generation" CHCs to have no higher VTE risks than "second-generation" CHCs, as compared with only 4/56 (12%) with no conflicts, and the RR was 8.0 (95% CI 3.0–21.3). Hence authors' conflicts of interest and their positions were closely associated. There was also strong consistency in authors' interpretation of relative VTE risks for "third-generation" and drospirenone-containing CHCs. Of the 109 articles that commented on both risk comparisons, 104 came to similar conclusions: 71 (65%) stated that both types of products had higher VTE risks than levonorgestrel-containing CHCs and 31 (28%) argued against risk differences for both types of products.

Figure 2.1 lists the numbers of articles per year concluding that drospirenone-containing CHCs have higher VTE risks ($n = 74$) or no higher VTE risks ($n = 41$) than "second-generation" CHCs in relation to article authors' pharmaceutical industry funding. Conflicted authors were especially likely to state that drospirenone-containing CHCs were not riskier than levonorgestrel-containing CHCs during the first 2 years of this analysis of citing articles, e.g. 2010 and 2011. Figure 2.2 presents an overview of positions for all authors with and without declared conflicts over the entire 7-year study period.

Comparing timing of these messages with risk communication by regulators, the US FDA published a safety communication supporting increased VTE risks for drospirenone-containing products and required changes to product information in April 2012 (US Food and Drug Administration 2012). In Europe, a series of reviews were carried out as the evidence on VTE risks evolved over time. In May 2010, the EMA published its first review of the risks of the

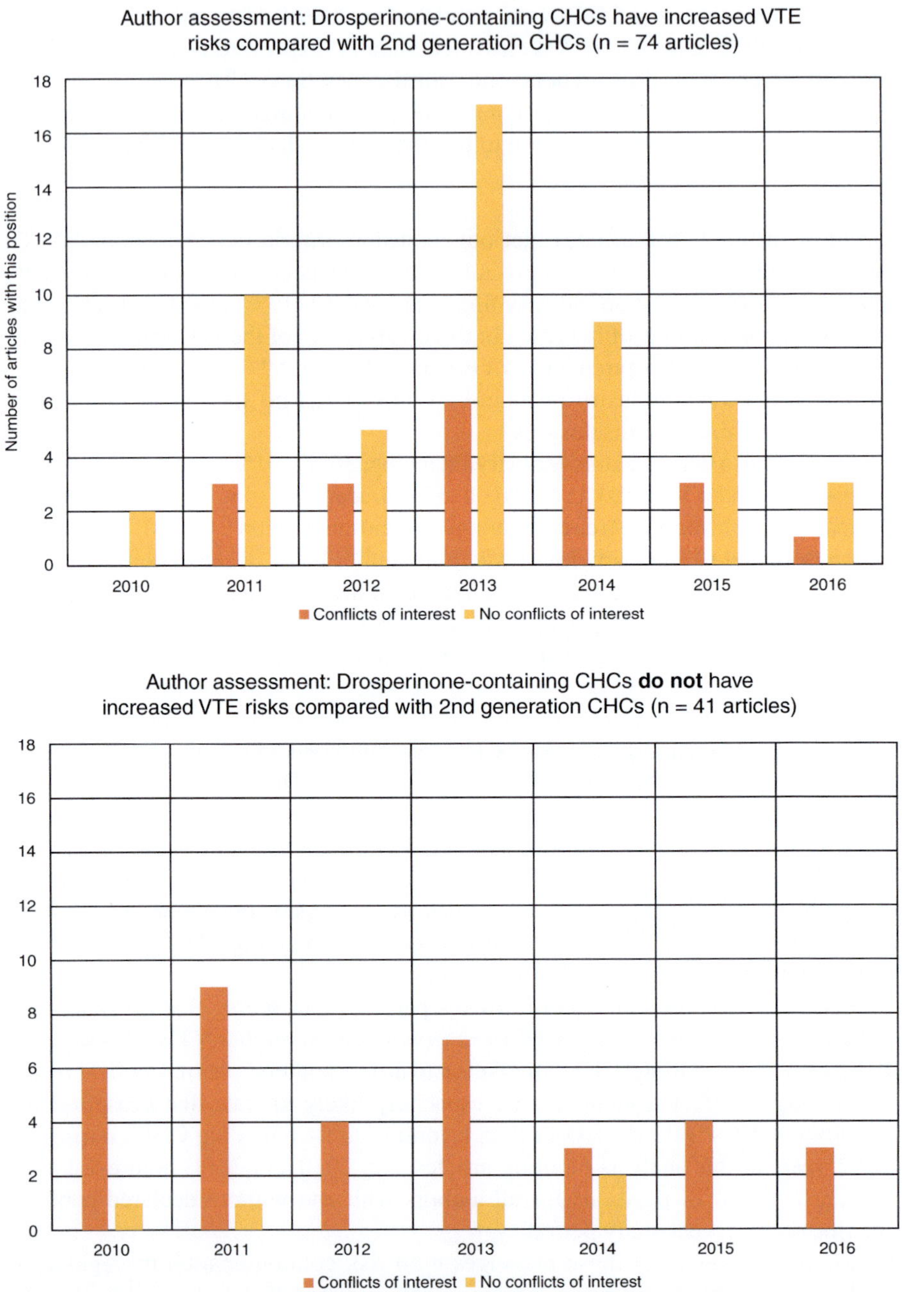

Fig. 2.1 Numbers of articles per year concluding that drospirenone-containing CHCs have higher VTE risks ($n = 74$) or no higher VTE risks ($n = 41$) than "second-generation" CHCs in relation to article authors' pharmaceutical industry funding

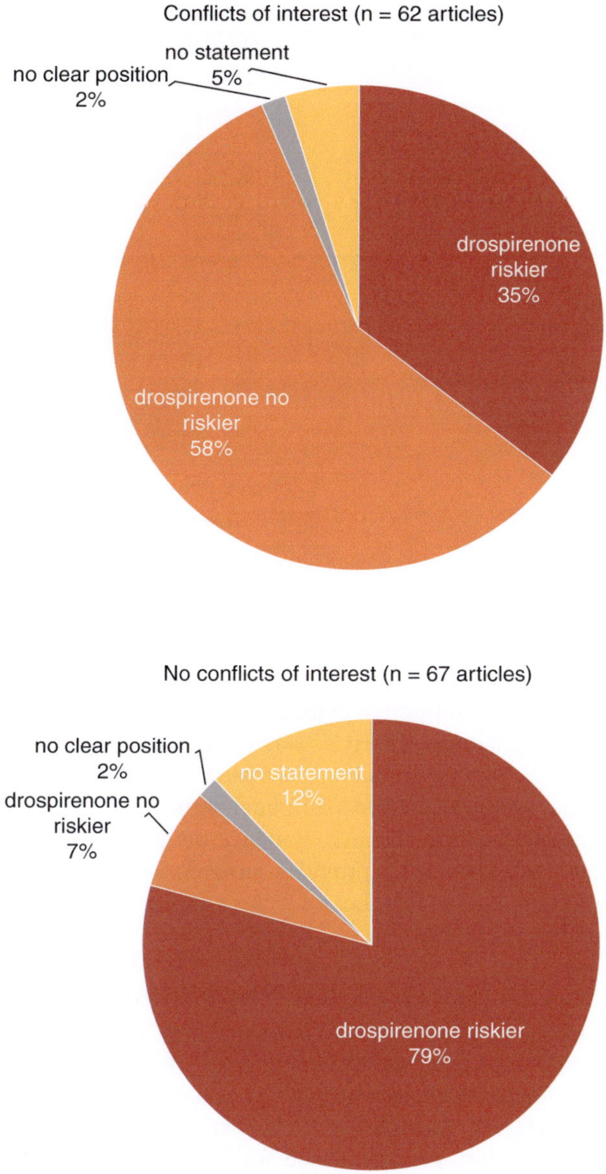

Fig. 2.2 Overview of article authors' opinions over the 7-year period

drospirenone-containing CHC Yasmin, finding an intermediate VTE risk level, between those of "second-" and "third-generation" CHCs (European Medicines Agency Pharmacovigilance Working Party (PhVWP) 2010). In May 2011, the EMA concluded that drospirenone CHC risks were similar to "third-generation" CHCs (European Medicines Agency Pharmacovigilance Working Party (PhVWP) 2011), a position they confirmed in January 2012 (European Medicines Agency Pharmacovigilance Working Party (PhVWP) 2012). The EMA's review on VTE

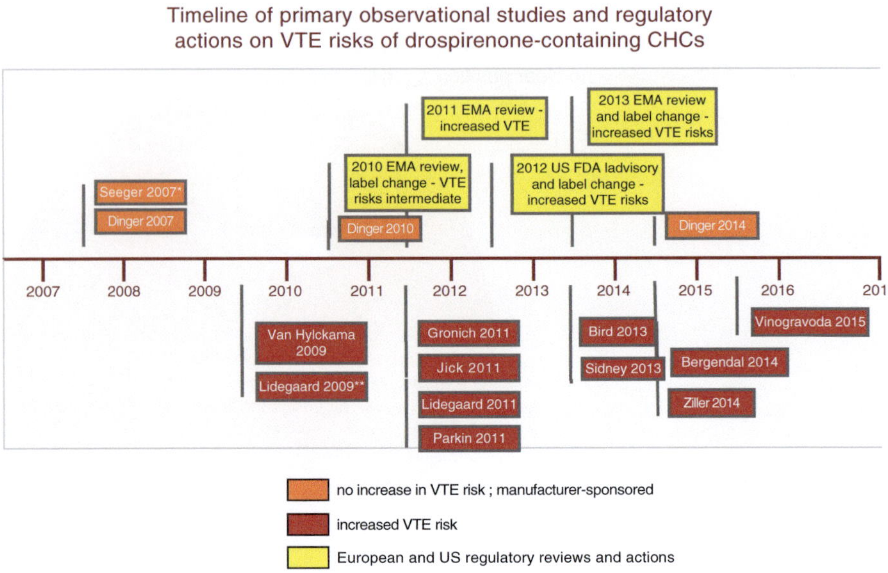

Fig. 2.3 Timeline of primary observational studies and regulatory actions by the EMA and US FDA

risks, which supported evidence of increased risk levels for both drospirenone and "third-generation" CHCs, was completed and published in late 2013, requiring updates to the product information (European Medicines Agency 2014). This series of reports reflects a radical shift in the EMA's position from early 2011 to late 2013 as the research evidence on drospirenone's increased VTE risks accumulated. Figure 2.3 provides an overview of the timeline of publication of the primary studies that these articles cited, as well as regulatory actions by the EMA and the US FDA.

Discussion and Conclusions Despite the considerable body of evidence since 1995 indicating an increased VTE risk among "third-generation" and later drospirenone-containing CHCs, authors with industry financing continued to dismiss differences in risk levels when citing the studies and interpreting the scientific evidence in medical journals. For example, in 2015, Han and Jensen wrote that, "Whether VTE rates in users of third-generation and fourth-generation CHCs are increased in relation to "second-generation" pills remains highly controversial. At this time, the best prospective literature does not show an increased risk…" (*note*: more recently developed CHCs, including drospirenone, are also referred to as "fourth-generation" CHCs) (Han and Jensen 2015). This statement is only possible if cohort studies using existing health records data are dismissed as "retrospective" although they are prospective in their analytical approach (i.e. people are enrolled at first exposure and are followed over time). Despite advances in the science of pharmacoepidemiology (see Chap. 14) and extensive replication of results in different studies and by different study authors indicating risk increases, the most frequently cited reason to dismiss the evidence was on methodological grounds. Foran characterised the situation in this way: "In a case of duelling epidemiologists, one side stands accused of potential commercial bias and the other of poor control selection, non-significance, missing data and neglecting the effect of bias and confounders" (Foran 2014). This statement appears to reflect an assumption that studies without industry funding are generally of poorer methodological quality than those with commercial support. This assumption is not supported by systematic reviews of the research evidence (de Bastos et al. 2014; Kemmeren et al. 2001; Wu et al. 2013). One measure of a study's rigour, for example, is objective confirmation of VTE, as this ensures that a common standard for VTE diagnosis is applied within all comparison groups, regardless of whether they are exposed to CHCs or which product they were using, eliminating expectation biases among ambiguous diagnoses, which could artificially inflate VTE rates among women taking CHCs believed to be higher risk. Increased diagnostic accuracy is a feature of more, not less rigorous methodology (Jick 2015). Risk differences between CHCs might therefore be expected to be higher in studies without objectively confirmed VTE if this bias exaggerated risk estimates. In contrast, the Cochrane systematic review on VTE risks of CHCs by de Bastos et al. found that risk estimates were higher in all studies with objectively confirmed VTE, none of which were industry-sponsored (de Bastos et al. 2014).

In our 7-year analysis of communication on relative VTE risks of different contraceptives in secondary literature, we found a sevenfold increased likelihood that conflicted authors, as compared with non-conflicted authors, would judge the risks of drospirenone-containing contraceptives to be equivalent to those of levonorgestrel-containing contraceptives, and an eightfold likelihood that conflicted authors would judge desogestrel- and gestodene-containing contraceptives to be equivalent to levonorgestrel-containing contraceptives. Our results support the decisions of some journal editors, such as the *British Medical Journal*, to have a "zero tolerance policy on education pieces by authors with industry ties" in order to prioritise independent assessments of treatment benefits and harms (Loder et al. 2015).

The judgments of authors who concluded that the risks of drospirenone and "second-generation" CHCs were equivalent were often based on claims of methodological weaknesses of administrative databases analyses and a claim that prospectively collected data in a cohort developed specifically for research purposes is methodologically superior (Society of Obstetricians and Gynaecologists of Canada (SOGC) 2013). They also tended to reflect a lack of attention to issues such as how exposure periods and health outcomes were defined, and whether women at high VTE risk due to cancer, surgery, major trauma, or even pregnancy were included in outcome assessments (Jick 2015). The critique of analyses based on administrative health records is at odds with current "state of the art" approaches to pharmacoepidemiology that rely on large-scale population-based administrative databases to assess rare harmful effects of medicines (Suissa et al. 2012).

The continued scientific controversy created in the medical literature is highly relevant to risk communication, as controversy and perceived uncertainties are one of the major factors altering risk perception and trust in scientific assessments (see Chap. 7).

2.3 Evaluation: Feedback, Outcomes and Lessons Learnt

A key critique of many of the warnings about increased VTE risks with either "third-generation" or drospirenone-containing CHCs is of inadequate communication of either the magnitude of the risk in absolute or relative terms, or of the context, for example, how risks of CHCs compared with VTE risks associated with alternative contraceptive methods, pregnancy, and the post-partum period or pregnancy termination.

Researchers in the UK tested how well a convenience sample of university students understood revised wording on VTE risks included in CHC package leaflets in 1999 at the UK CSM's request (n = 186). They found that 80% of the women could not translate information presented as number of events per 100,000 women per year into a probability they would experience a thromboembolic event, expressed as a percentage. Most provided overestimates. A key factor in misinterpretation was the need to translate a number per 100,000 into a percentage. If asked the same question in a way that was more closely tied to how the information had been presented to them (e.g. numbers of people out of 100,000), around two-thirds answered correctly (Berry et al. 2002).

Similarly, a study carried out by Machado and colleagues at the Jundiai Medical Faculty in Brazil examined the response of women students attending a family practice clinic (n = 159) to different framing of risks of blood clotting with CHCs (Machado et al. 2015). The survey respondents were all women who were either current CHC users or who were initiating use. If risks of clotting were presented as a twofold greater risk of "third-generation" over "second-generation" CHCs, 68% of the women agreed with a statement that the risks concerned them; if presented in absolute risk levels (9 cases of VTE per 10,000 women taking a pill) only 12% agreed with a statement of concern, and if presented as a risk difference versus no exposure (an additional 4 cases per 10,000 women per year), 9% agreed.

These studies of the effects of different forms of risk communication highlight the importance of providing information on the absolute level of risk, and not just relative risks, in order for women to be adequately informed of the risks of CHC use.

As re-analyses and new studies provided evidence following the initial studies of 1995, the EMA coordinated and published two assessments of "second-" and "third-generation" CHCs at EU level, one in 2001 and one in 2013. Appendix 2.1 describes how the EMA planned communication while being mindful of the need to avoid inappropriate risk perceptions and possible new scares. This illustrates the long-term haunting effect the "VTE pill scare" has had, and still has, on regulatory risk communication.

The effect on regulatory risk communication, as is described below, is one of caution to avoid negative consequences of alarmist media attention. The medical literature almost entirely characterised media attention to warnings of increased VTE risks associated with the use of specific contraceptives as negative or alarmist, e.g. provoking a "pill scare". This is at odds with a potential positive role for the media in broadly disseminating messages aiming to improve the safety of contraceptive use. A notable exception to this negative characterisation of media attention is a study of pulmonary embolism hospitalisations in France in 2013, after a shift in reimbursement. This study focused on the positive role played by the media: "The media attention regarding the risks associated with contraceptive pills and the subsequent reinforcement of pre-existing health recommendations to use the safest COC have led women to modify their methods of contraception". (*note*: COC stands for combined oral contraceptive, another abbreviation for CHC) (Tricotel et al. 2015).

The "VTE Pill Scare": Did Women Really Panic and Abandon Contraceptive Use? Relating the UK CSM warnings of October 1995 on risks of "third-generation" contraceptives to a "VTE pill scare" implies that this warning led women to become fearful about risks of contraceptive use, leading to discontinuations. A number of analyses have been carried out on the rates of contraceptive switching or stopping, pregnancy, and pregnancy termination following the regulatory announcements of the UK CSM (Lackie and Fairchild 2016). These have differed in terms of strength of evidence and reported results. The most dramatic evidence of an increase in pregnancy rates has come from studies with weaker methodology. For example, the British Pregnancy Advisory Service (BPAS), a charity that carried out 18% of UK pregnancy terminations, reported that it had provided 823 more terminations from December 1995 to the end of January 1996 than during the same period in the previous year (Ramsay 1996). This analysis was limited to a 2-month period per year; longer-term annual variation should have been assessed. The BPAS also surveyed 300 women with unplanned pregnancies that the women believed were due to a change in their contraception: 41% reported stopping their pills immediately after the warning, and 61% not finishing their current course. This was a non-representative sample, with selection based on women's belief that her pregnancy was due to a method change, thus cannot be assumed to reflect broader trends.

A study in Grampian (Aberdeen and Aberdeenshire in the UK) illustrates the difference that longer-term data can make (Flett et al. 1998). The authors compared pregnancy termination rates from November 1995 to 30 April 1996 with the same period in the previous year. There were 728 terminations in 1995–1996, compared with 723 in 1994–1995, and also no significant difference in pregnancies taken to term; the proportion of women taking oral contraceptives prior to a termination was also stable, at 14%. This contrasts with statistics on pregnancy termination in England and Wales in 1996 and 1997 indicating an 8.8% increase in the termination rate, or in absolute terms, 13,604 additional women obtaining terminations (Furedi 1999). Regional variations may have existed. Terminations also represent a subset of pregnancies, both planned and unplanned: a study in Oxford found that terminations increased by 9.9% compared with the previous 2 years but live births decreased by 5.6% (Child et al. 1996). As the authors note, these findings were at odds with claims of an increase in both terminations and unplanned deliveries.

Jick et al. carried out an analysis of health records data in the UK General Practice Research Database (GPRD), including over 31,000 users of CHCs, about 17,000 of whom took "third-generation" contraceptives (Jick et al. 1998). They compared rates of CHC switching and stopping as well as pregnancy terminations from October 1994 to the end of September 1995, before the CSM warning, with the following year. Consistent with the warning, most users of "third-generation" CHCs (68%) switched to a "second-generation" product after the warning, but there was no difference in the proportion of women who stopped using CHCs between the 2 years, or between "second-" and "third-generation" CHCs users. For all women in the UK GPRD, pregnancy frequencies did not differ significantly in the 12 months before and after the warning (30.7 versus 31.4 per 1000, respectively), nor did pregnancy terminations (9.4 and 9.1 per 1000, respectively). For "third-generation" CHCs users, similarly, pregnancy termination rates did not differ between the two periods. An analysis of a network of 100 general practices (GPs) (n = 372 GPs; n = 34,791 CHC users) similarly found extensive switching to "second-generation" contraceptives, but very little difference in total CHC use: from 19.7% of women of reproductive age to 19.0% in the 6 months after the warning (Martin et al. 1997).

These studies differ in two ways from studies of national pregnancy termination and birth statistics that indicated a temporary increase in terminations and that have been cited to suggest that many women panicked and stopped using CHC's and other effective contraceptives as a result of the CSM warning. First, the studies that did not find an increase in CHC discontinuations, pregnancies, or pregnancy terminations followed individual women, rather than looking only at aggregated statistics. The former is considered a more rigorous approach to examining health outcomes than an "ecological approach", as it allows women with specific characteristics, in this case use of "third-generation" CHCs, to be assessed. Secondly, the studies that did not find a "VTE pill scare" effect focused on examining pregnancy rates in the women expected to be directly affected by the warning, i.e. CHC users. Reasons for the difference between these findings and broader national or regional birth statistics warrant further exploration.

An interrupted time series analysis examining rates of pregnancy terminations and births in the UK in the period following the October 1995 warning provides some clues to this difference (Del Bono et al. 2011). Del Bono et al. found that significant increases in pregnancy rates were limited to younger women, aged 18–25 years, and to women of lower socioeconomic status. This was based on aggregated data, so individual women's prior CHC use could not be examined, but it suggests an effect on initiation of CHC's, rather than ongoing use. The social class differences also warrant further investigation, in that they could reflect differences in types of media exposure or differences in prior knowledge of a clotting risk with CHC use.

Despite a similar regulatory warning to switch to lower risk CHCs, Norway did not appear to experience an increase in birth and pregnancy termination rate. Iversen and Nilsen carried out an analysis of pregnancy termination rates in the nine largest hospitals in Norway, representing around half of all terminations in the country, before and after the November 2015 regulatory agency's warning, which was similar to that of the UK CSM (Iversen and Nilsen 1996). Over a two-month period, January to February 1996, they found an increase of 104 terminations (7.7%). Another Norwegian study examined rates from 1992 to 1996 in the county of Sor-Trondelag, representing 6–7% of women of reproductive age in Norway, and found a barely significant increase in the first quarter of 1996 in the pregnancy termination rate among women aged 15–24 years compared with the first quarter of 1995 ($p = 0.050$) (Skjeldestad 1997). Longer-term and full population trends did not indicate any significant differences.

The general media issued headlines on the implications of the VTE warning that were inconsistent with the more nuanced and conflicting study results discussed above. In 2001, *The Scotsman* reported that, "The Pill scare was responsible for 29,000 extra abortions—an increase of eight per cent—and did untold damage to women's confidence" (Veitch 2001). A 2012 article in *The Independent* states that the "pill scare" "led to a 25 per cent drop in use" (Laurance 2012). The CSM warning was also characterised as feeding into more general anti-pill sentiments. On 20 October 1995—days after the CSM warning—an editorial in *The Independent* blamed the "pill panic" on the view that "In the darker corners of our cultural undergrowth… a powerful puritanical instinct, eager to believe that the pill is bad for you, it will kill you—in effect, you will die of the promiscuity that the pill precipitated in the Sixties" (Toynbee 1995).

Only one press commentary, by Dr. Trisha Greenhalgh, congratulated Professor Michael Rawlins, Chair of the CSM, for engaging with the press at a press conference and described television appearances, as representing "indelicate but entirely laudable attempts to operate in a culture of openness" (Greenhalgh 1995). In an editorial in *The Times*, Dr. Greenhalgh refers to her patients who sought extra information as "certainly not hysterical… They simply wanted my help in converting the warning, which was couched in general terms, into a decision about their personal contraceptive choices. Most of them spent less than three minutes in my surgery or on the phone to me. Dealing with problems like this is exactly what I and my fellow GPs are paid for". (*note*: GP stands for general practitioner). She may have been responding to the statement published a couple of days earlier by a staff member at a family planning clinic, the Margaret Pyke Centre, who said, "There are people out there who are worried they might die. We have had some hysterical calls from people who are very distressed" (Milton 1995).

Lessons Learnt from the "VTE Pill Scare"

To conclude, the available data strongly support a hypothesis that the October 1995 warning led to extensive switching from "second-" to "third-generation" CHCs. This is documented in the Netherlands as well as in the UK (de Vries et al. 1998), and is consistent with intended consequences of this warning. Study outcomes concerning discontinuations in CHC use and rates of pregnancy and pregnancy termination conflict, with the largest effect sizes reported in studies that depended on convenience samples or only reported short-term outcomes. Prescribing data based on large samples of GP practices fail to support the results of smaller survey data. Studies that followed individual women's prescribing records over time did not find evidence that they stopped using CHCs to a greater extent following the CSM warning. National statistics do suggest higher pregnancy and pregnancy termination rates in the year following the warning, but these fail to suggest immediate effects in late 1995; 1996 increases should also be examined in light of longer-term trends.

Taken as a whole, the evidence suggests that the unintended consequences of this warning are likely to have been exaggerated in the general media and may have resulted in amplified perception of negative consequences of the CSM warning both among the general public and experts. Undoubtedly, there was some sensationalised media reporting of the CSM warning that failed to provide adequate context, especially on the rarity of clotting risks. However, there also appears to have been some one-sided reporting of the effects of this warning on women's and couple's contraceptive choices. The invisibility of male partners of CHC users in the discussion of the "pill scare" is also notable, as is the characterisation of women as "scared" or "panicked". It remains an open question whether the public's response would have been framed as paternalistically if men, not women, had been at risk.

As is noted above, the characterisation of media attention to regulatory warnings on CHC clotting risks in the medical literature is almost entirely negative. This is remarkable because a major objective of risk communication should be to support well-informed choices and safer use of medicinal products. The negative attention on media coverage has focused entirely on media alarmism and exaggeration of clotting risks. There has been little to no commentary in the medical literature on the accuracy of media messages about the "VTE pill scare" itself.

As presented in Sect. 2.2.1, we found a strong association between authors' stated opinions on clotting risks of different contraceptives in medical journal articles that cited the primary research studies, and whether or not they had financial links to manufacturers. This pattern continued after regulators in the EU and the US had reviewed the research evidence and concluded that desogestrel-, and gestodene-containing CHCs ("third-generation" products) and drospirenone-containing CHCs had higher risks of clotting, compared with levonorgestrel-containing products. It also continued after meta-analyses of the research evidence in good quality systematic reviews had reached similar conclusions (de Bastos et al. 2014; Kemmeren et al. 2001; Wu et al. 2013; Martinez et al. 2012).

Communication about the effectiveness and risks of CHCs and other contraceptive methods continues to be of major global importance for both women and men. The controversy over how best to understand and communicate the clotting risks of contraceptives following the "VTE pill scare" of 1995 led to important changes in regulatory risk communication. The experiences with communicating risk differences of infrequent but still relevant risks of different CHCs led to worldwide recognition that effective communication of risks and advice for safe use of medicines is a crucial task of regulators (see Chap. 1). If there is one "take-home message", it is the importance of the medical and general media in risk communication on medicinal products. The sense of "déjà vu" in the unfolding communication and perceptions of scientific uncertainty around clotting risks of drospirenone-containing contraceptives more than a decade after the "VTE pill scare" highlights the need for a rethink of lessons learnt. The UK CSM and other regulators were not wrong to warn physicians and the public. Better communication of messages was needed, and ongoing engagement with the general and medical media to support accurate, informed, and balanced information.

Conclusions

- The first hormonal contraceptive became available to women in 1960 and various types have been developed since then, which combine different doses of an oestrogen component and different progestin components.
- All these combined hormonal contraceptives (CHCs) carry a risk of blood clotting, or venous thromboembolism (VTE), which is rare but may be serious, potentially leading to life-long disabilities or even death; frequencies of VTE events differ between progestin components.
- Communicating these risk differences for informed contraceptive choices has been challenging for various reasons, including scientific controversy around the research evidence, ongoing court cases, commercial interests of the manufacturers as well as the use of CHCs by a healthy rather than ill population group and societal controversy around separating women's sexuality from aims or fears of pregnancy.
- Within the medical literature, interpretation of the research evidence on clotting risks of different types of contraceptives has differed considerably between authors, leading to inconsistent risk communication messages. We found a strong association between authors' financial links with pharmaceutical manufacturers and their interpretation of the evidence on risk differences, with those with financial links much more likely to consider risks to be equivalent.
- The warning about the differential risk by UK regulators in 1995 had a profound effect on regulatory risk communication, in part due to its representation in the general media as the UK "VTE pill scare" with claims of widespread panic among CHC users resulting in stopping CHC use, unwanted pregnancies, and pregnancy terminations.
- Research on the actual impact of the warning has a number of limitations, but evidence from those using more appropriate methods suggest that its unintended consequences are likely to have been exaggerated in both the general and medical media at the time.

Appendix 2.1: Impact of Stakeholder Consultations on Audience-Tailoring of Risk Communication and Implications for Pharmacoepidemiology and Real World Evidence Generation—The Case of Venous Thromboembolism with Combined Hormonal Contraceptives in the European Union[1]

Priya Bahri

1. Background

The risk of venous thromboembolism (VTE) of certain combined hormonal contraceptives (CHCs) was assessed as a medicines class review at the European Medicines Agency (EMA) three times, in 1995, 2001, and 2013. Each review assessed recent studies and their impact on marketing authorisations and safe use advice, comparing risks between CHCs containing newer progestins (the "third-generation" CHCs) versus those containing levonorgestrel or other "older" progestins (the "second-generation" CHCs). Emerging drospirenone-containing CHCs were also closely monitored, and accumulating evidence was assessed between 2010 and 2012, and then again within the review of CHCs in 2013. This latest review was a referral procedure under new legislation of the European Union (EU) for which the then newly (2012) established Pharmacovigilance Risk Assessment Committee (PRAC) at the EMA took the opportunity to consult patients/consumers (P/Cs) and healthcare professionals (HPs).

The 2013 Review of CHCs and Communication Preparations

This procedure was concluded as follows:

- The risk-benefit balance was considered positive for all assessed CHCs;
- Updated and strengthened risk information was agreed to be included in the legally required product information (the summary of product characteristics (SmPC) targeting HPs and the package leaflet (PL) targeting P/Cs) to clarify risk differences between products, contraindications as well as signs and symptoms of VTE, and to allow P/Cs and HPs to make informed contraceptive choices;
- Additional proactive communication materials should include a questions & answers document (Q&A) for women and a direct healthcare professional communication (DHPC) (to be agreed with the authorities in EU member states (MS) in the applicable language(s) and disseminated by the pharmaceutical companies individually to all HPs of defined specialities) (European Medicines Agency (EMA) 2014a).

---

[1] The views expressed in this case study are the author's personal views and may not be understood or quoted as being made on behalf of or reflecting the position of her employing organisation, i.e. the European Medicines Agency (EMA), or any of its committees or working parties.

Right from the beginning of this review, the EMA was mindful of the concerns that women using CHCs might have and of possible amplification of public risk perception through debate in the media, as had been claimed for the so-called "VTE pill scare" in the United Kingdom in 1995 after emerging studies on increased VTE risks with "third-generation" CHCs. The EMA considered that communication with the public had to be especially proactive and well-planned and to address the information needs of P/Cs and HPs, in order to avoid undue scare with using CHCs.

Therefore, the EMA created, immediately when the procedure had started, a special webpage summarising all previous reviews of CHCs at the EMA. Creating a webpage dedicated to a specific risk and pulling together assessments from previous reviews under different legal frameworks was at the time unique for the EMA. The aim of this webpage was to proactively provide P/Cs, HPs, and journalists with an information resource in a "one stop shop" approach while the review was ongoing. The webpage was also used by the EMA media office to provide complete and consistent responses and references to persons who enquired about what evidence had been established to date and how to use CHCs safely. After the procedure, this special webpage was updated with the latest CHCs review outcome and a section tailored for women using CHCs. The webpage was hyperlinked on the procedure webpage, i.e. a webpage type routinely set up for all EU referral procedures (European Medicines Agency (EMA) 2014b). Such a procedure webpage includes, in an online format, an overview on the review outcome with a summary and expandable sections with information for P/Cs and HPs, more details on the medicine, and more details on the procedure (all sections are visible at once in the pdf format of this overview). Through the procedure webpage the public can also access the documents with the notification of the procedure, its scope, the concerned products, the timetable, questions to the pharmaceutical companies holding a marketing authorisation, the committee assessment reports, the official decision of the European Commission (EC), the updated product information, and any other conditions of the marketing authorisations.

Further, planning for communication of the review outcome became a prioritised task at the EMA, while the procedure was still ongoing. In order to obtain input from P/Cs and HPs to support regulatory decision-making on risk minimisation measures and identify their information needs and communication preferences, the PRAC carried out stakeholder consultations. This happened in addition to the standing P/C and HP representations at the PRAC. Two forms of consultation were used: an ad hoc group meeting in July and a written consultation in October 2013. The European Institute of Women's Health sent a P/C representative to the ad hoc meeting. HPs at the ad hoc meeting were mostly physicians from clinical-academic institutions, and the midwife organisation sent a representative too. Representatives from patient, women's health, and consumer advocacy organisations and HPs from general practitioner and gynaecologist organisations responded to the written consultation.

The questions the PRAC posed to the ad hoc group related to:

– Differential prescribing based on differences in tolerability (and evidence of tolerability differences);

- Perceptions of risk and risk factors and their influence on prescribing;
- Attitude towards prescribing of products with lack of pharmacoepidemiological data;
- Knowledge of VTE risk, diagnosis, and management;
- Product information and risk minimisation, including in women at risk for VTE;
- Preferences for expression of risk characteristics and magnitude;
- Audiences, routes, means, and messages of communication.

The questions to P/C representatives during the written consultation related to:

- Preferred option for presenting the information in the PLs in text and visual ways, e.g. in the format of a table, bar graph, or Paling palette (Paling 2003), or other useful ways of presenting risk information;
- Comparison between VTE risk of CHCs and VTE risk with pregnancy, to help putting the magnitude of risk with CHCs into perspective, or other risk comparisons.

The questions to HP representatives during the written consultation related to:

- Preferred option for presenting the information in the SmPCs and the DHPC in visual ways, e.g. in the format of a table, bar graph, or Paling palette, also considering utility as aid for discussions with women, or other useful ways of presenting risk information;
- Comparison between VTE risk of CHCs and VTE risk with pregnancy, to help putting the magnitude of risk with CHCs into perspective, or other risk comparisons.

The feedback from the consultations was taken into account by the PRAC and the EMA for audience-tailoring the product information legally binding in all MS, as well as for audience-tailoring of the other communication tools specifically requested through the procedure outcome (see above) and the regular EMA communication announcing the outcome. MS authorities usually base their communication on materials agreed at EU level.

Considering Previous Experience: The 2001 Review of CHCs and Communication Preparations

Mechanisms and stakeholder networks for consultations had not yet been established in 2001, when the previous review was conducted under the then applicable legal framework. This review concluded on a differential risk estimate for “third-” versus “second-generation” CHCs and updated product information as a recommendation directly to MS authorities (i.e. not submitted to the EC for an official decision legally binding in all MS). As in 2013, the EMA in 2001 (then the EMEA) was mindful of a potential public scare and therefore issued an unprecedented set of audience-tailored documents on its website: a position statement, a public assessment report (PAR), a DHPC, and an information sheet for women. A position statement was a regular document at the time for major safety concerns, mainly targeted at the general and medical-scientific media. The PAR was the first one from the EMA for products which had been authorised nationally by MS authorities (while it was EMA practice to publish

European public assessment reports (EPARs) for all products authorised by the EC centrally for all MS). The PAR included the recommended SmPC updates, but no PL wordings. Likewise, the publication of a DHPC by the EMA (in addition to its dissemination by the pharmaceutical companies individually to all HPs of defined specialities) was special at the time, as DHPCs have only started to be published on the EMA website on a regular basis in 2020. The information sheet for women was a first-time tool specifically designed for P/Cs, worded with care and spontaneously tested with non-medical female EMA staff members (European Medicines Agency (EMA) 2001).

2. Objective and Methods

As in both reviews the EMA made special efforts to serve audiences and in 2013 applied new mechanisms for stakeholder consultation, it seemed worth assessing the impact of the consultations on audience-tailoring by comparing the two communication events.

Therefore, this study analysed how the input gained from the consultations of P/C and HP representatives in 2013 affected EMA's communication of the review outcome to public audiences (European Medicines Agency (EMA) 2014b) and the revision of the product information (European Medicines Agency (EMA) 2014c), and compared this 2013 communication with the 2001 communication (European Medicines Agency (EMA) 2001). Further, the P/C and HP input was compared with best risk communication practices that were established in 2011 mainly on the basis of evidence that had accumulated after 2001 (Fischhoff et al. 2011, Brewer NT, Downs JS (eds) 2011), in order to assess the synergistic value of stakeholder consultations in addition to relying on established evidence-based best practices. The comparisons focused on the major points raised in the 2013 consultations in response to the questions posed by the PRAC.

3. Analysis and Findings

The analysis is presented in Table 2.1 and yields the following findings:

Fundamentally the EMA made similar communication choices in 2001 and 2013: VTE with CHCs was characterised as a rare risk requiring urgent action if it occurs, i.e. there was a focus on risk management behaviours and problem solution. Relative risk quantifications like "doubled" and words like "serious" with a potential to create alarm were avoided in the documents targeted at the media and the wider public (while explaining the seriousness in the PLs, SmPCs, and DHPCs and providing relative risk quantification in documents targeted at HPs). A second choice was in the contextualisation of the risk with the benefits of CHCs. These choices are in line with the evidence from communication research.

However, three differences between 2013 and 2001were identified:

First, visualisation of risk differences was only considered in 2013, given advances in information provision through digitalisation and nowadays widespread usage of visuals and respective audience expectations.

Table 2.1 Analysis of the impact of the stakeholder consultation on communication of VTE risk with CHCs (quotation marks indicate quotes)

1. *Risk characterisation*	
Consultation input from P/Cs and HPs	Communication should stress that "the actual VTE risk is not large" and "that all CHCs are very safe with many non-contraceptive and non-contraceptive benefits". A P/C representative asked for explanations what blood clots with VTE are and where in the body they occur
Impact of consultations on public communication of 2013 review outcome and updates to the product information	Accordingly, the EMA overview statement on the review outcome stated that "benefits of CHCs in preventing unwanted pregnancies continue to outweigh their risks, and that the well-known risk of VTE with all CHCs is small" and did not mention the seriousness of VTE (however, more practically it stressed the need for immediate medical care, should signs and symptoms of VTE occur) (European Medicines Agency (EMA) 2014d) The SmPCs were strengthened; however, no characterisation of the risk as small or contextualisation of the risk with benefits was included, as is considered inappropriate in accordance with the applicable guideline on SmPCs (European Commission (EC) 2009). The seriousness was expressed in the SmPC with reference to VTE fatality (European Medicines Agency (EMA) 2014c) At the top of the PLs, the following new statement was introduced: "***Important things to know about combined hormonal contraceptives (CHCs)***: – They are one of the most reliable reversible methods of contraception if used correctly; – They slightly increase the risk of having a blood clot in the veins and arteries, especially in the first year or when restarting a combined hormonal contraceptive following a break of 4 or more weeks; – Please be alert and see your doctor if you think you may have symptoms of a blood clot (see Sect. 2 "Blood clots")" (European Medicines Agency (EMA) 2014c) The seriousness, including fatality, was stated later in the warning and adverse reaction sections of the PLs, where a special boxed warning, an advice statement, and explanations on where in the body blood clots occur and how to recognise them were inserted too
Comparison of 2013 public communication with public communication of 2001 review outcome	The comparison showed similarity in the two communication approaches, as the 2001 position statement focused on the favourable benefit-risk balance of all CHCs and the low frequency of VTE, and did not mention the seriousness. The information sheet for women started with the low frequency and also described upfront the effectiveness of CHCs in preventing pregnancy, and only later mentioned the seriousness, including reference to "potentially life-threatening condition". The DHPC highlighted the rare occurrence of VTE with CHCs and the seriousness (however, without reference to life-threatening or fatal risk) as well as the favourable benefit-risk balance. In the SmPC, the seriousness was expressed with reference to VTE fatality (European Medicines Agency (EMA) 2001)
Comparison of P/Cs and HP input with communication research evidence	The consultation input was in accordance with evidence-based best communication practices, as these advise that communication must enable informed choices and hence address the outcomes of interest to the audiences, including both risks and benefits (Fischhoff et al. 2011, Brewer NT, Downs JS (eds) 2011)

2. *Risk quantification*	
Consultation input from P/Cs and HPs	Risk magnitude should be expressed in a "simple manner", understandable language, in absolute terms as incidence rates with natural numbers and in relative terms. One HP suggested "incidence rates in percentages". In particular HPs were interested in both absolute and relative risks, and one P/C representative asked for text on doubled risk of "second-generation" CHC versus non-CHC use and doubled risk of newer versus "second-generation" CHC use. Risks should also be described for different age groups of CHC users and with information on the VTE risk in non-CHC users and changes of VTE risk levels with CHC use over time. For CHCs containing a progestin other than levonorgestrel, the lower risk for levonorgestrel-containing CHCs should be provided as a reference
Impact of consultations on public communication of 2013 review outcome and updates to the product information	Accordingly, the EMA overview statement on the review outcome presented, in the online format in the expandable section for P/Cs, incidence rates as the range for all CHCs as follows: "5–12 cases of blood clots per 10,000 women who use them for a year", together with the baseline risk level of "2 cases of blood clots in the veins each year per 10,000 women who are not using CHCs" and the statement that the "risk of a blood clot is also higher in the first year of using a CHC". Differential incident rates by progestin component were presented in a table in the expandable section for HPs (or immediately visible in the pdf format), together with the statement that "because a woman's individual risk factors will change over time, there is a need to regularly re-assess the suitability of her contraceptive". Relative risks were not quantified (European Medicines Agency (EMA) 2014d) The SmPCs contained the risk quantification in the incidence rate format for the progestin component contained in a given CHC, the baseline risk level and the risk level for levonorgestrel-containing CHCs if the given CHC has a higher risk. The relative risk was verbalised and quantified as "up to twice" for the concerned CHCs. The increased risks in the first year of or after a break from CHC use were included too. The recommendation for re-assessment of a woman's suitability for a CHC noted on (European Medicines Agency (EMA) 2014d) was not included in the SmPCs (European Medicines Agency (EMA) 2014c) The PLs were revised to include, in the new statement at the top of the PLs, the increased risk "especially in the first year or when restarting […] following a break of 4 or more weeks", and in the warning and adverse reaction sections, the incidence rates applicable to the progestin component contained in a given CHC and the baseline risk level. The need to notify the physician of changes in risk factors was included too. Relative risks were not quantified; however, the risk for levonorgestrel-containing CHCs was included as a lower reference risk level in the PLs of all CHCs with higher risk levels (European Medicines Agency (EMA) 2014c)

(continued)

Table 2.1 (continued)

Comparison of 2013 public communication with public communication of 2001 review outcome	The comparison showed similarity in the two communication approaches, as in 2001 risk differences were verbalised but reference to a doubled relative risk was avoided in the public statement and the information sheet for women; however, the "best estimate of the relative risk" as "in the range of 1.5–2.0" was included in the DHPC. The risk levels for "third-" and "second-generation" CHCs were quantified in the DHPC and in the information sheet for women. The baseline risk for VTE without CHC use was only mentioned in the position statement and the DHPC. The increased risk in the first year of use was mentioned in all three of these audience-tailored documents. A major difference was however in the numerical risk expression. The 2001 communication describes this as an incidence density rate (rather than an incidence rate) with a denominator of women-years of use (e.g. for levonorgestrel: "20 cases per 100,000 women-years of use"), i.e. the incidence measure used in the assessed studies. In the SmPCs for all CHCs the risk for the given CHC was included in the same incidence density format, and for CHCs with a progestin that carries a higher risk than levonorgestrel in addition the risk of the latter as a lower risk reference, together with best relative risk estimate and the excess risk expressed as the number of additional VTE cases per 10,000 women-years of use. However, the baseline risk level in women not using a CHC was not quantified in the SmPCs. The SmPCs also included the increased risk in the first year of CHC use (European Medicines Agency (EMA) 2001)
Comparison of P/Cs and HP input with communication research evidence	The consultation input was in accordance with the evidence-based best communication practices, as these advise to describe risks in incidence rates or natural frequencies. Communication research has also established that relative risk expressions may distort risk perceptions and amplify perceptions of rare risks, potentially leading to undue scare, and hence have to be used in communication documents with caution (Fischhoff et al. 2011, Brewer NT, Downs JS (eds) 2011)
3. *Visualisation of risk differences*	
Consultation input from P/Cs and HPs	HPs favoured bar graphs or even tables to visualise risk differences for themselves, but considered bar graphs too abstract to support their communication with P/Cs. Most P/C representatives found bar graphs and Paling palettes not understandable without an explanation (as would be the case on a website without personal interaction) and preferred a table as more understandable. P/Cs also preferred providing the high denominator (i.e. 10,000) first, to enable readers to perceive immediately that the risk frequency was low. One P/C representative doubted the user-friendliness of the table, but found the comparative text essential and suggested testing the Paling palette
Impact of consultations on public communication of 2013 review outcome and updates to the product information	Accordingly, the proposed table was added to the PLs, while the bar graph was included instead in the SmPCs for those CHC products with known VTE incidence rates (European Medicines Agency (EMA) 2014c). The table was also included in the online version of the EMA overview of the review outcome in the section addressed to HPs. However, in the section for P/Cs there was only a mention of the table without including it (however, the table is visible to all website visitors when expanding the HP section and in any case in the pdf version) (European Medicines Agency (EMA) 2014d). The table was also included in the P/C section of the special CHC webpage. The table provided the numerator before the denominator as incidence rates, but the PLs provided additional sentences starting with the denominator "out of 10, 000…" (European Medicines Agency (EMA) 2014c)

Comparison of 2013 public communication with public communication of 2001 review outcome	In 2001, no thought was given to a visualisation, but at least the DHPC contained an indented overview of the different risks by progestin component (European Medicines Agency (EMA) 2001)
Comparison of P/Cs and HP input with communication research evidence	Evidence-based best risk communication practices have recommended graphs in addition to presenting risk in numerical format. Pictographs highlighting the number of people affected and not affected by a risk, like, e.g. a Paling palette, have been evidenced as decreasing risk-avoidant behaviours, which will be judged positively for rare risks and important benefit of a medical intervention. For risk comparisons, bar graphs have been shown useful (Fischhoff et al. 2011, Brewer NT, Downs JS (eds) 2011). The preference of HP representatives for a bar graph was in line with this evidence. The preference of most P/C representatives for a table rather than any visual risk expression in settings other than one-to-one communication with a HP may reflect their uncertainty about interpreting graphic representations correctly on their own without the opportunity to check their interpretation with a HP (e.g. when reading a PL or viewing websites at home)
4. *Risk comparisons (other than between CHCs)*	
Consultation input from P/Cs and HPs	The ad hoc group concluded that providing a comparison of the risk with VTE in/after pregnancy in communication materials was not relevant because of the difference in risk time windows (i.e. during and 6 weeks following a pregnancy versus any time during CHC use (albeit higher in the first year of use or when restarting after a break)). However, HP representatives still favoured pregnancy as a helpful comparator, because of the oestrogen-mediated VTE aetiology and because it was thought to facilitate "immediate perception of risk". During the written consultation the majority of P/C representatives considered pregnancy as an inappropriate comparator, because the objectives, choices, and life situations of CHC use and pregnancy are different and so are the risk acceptance, and because pregnancy is a shorter event than CHC use and the comparison may lead to perception of a too low risk ("underestimation"), and because such comparison may be "confusing". Some P/Cs however supported the comparison with pregnancy if provided in the context of other comparisons, like post-partum period, non-CHC use, and (car) accidents. Smoking was also considered a possibly suitable comparator (Sundseth H, President of the European Institute of Women's Health, personal communication with the author in 2014)

(continued)

Table 2.1 (continued)

Impact of consultations on public communication of 2013 review outcome and updates to the product information	Accordingly, the SmPCs included a statement that "the number of VTEs per year with low dose [relating to the oestrogen component] CHCs is fewer than the number expected in women during pregnancy or in the post-partum period", while this comparison was left out in the PL (however, the post-partum period was included as an unquantified general risk factor for VTE, as was smoking) (European Medicines Agency (EMA) 2014c). The EMA overview of the review outcome also omitted any comparison with VTE in pregnancy (European Medicines Agency (EMA) 2014d)
Comparison of 2013 public communication with public communication of 2001 review outcome	In 2001, it was decided to put more emphasis on the risk comparison with pregnancy. The DHPC had a quantified risk comparison as follows: "It should however be noted that the risk associated with all COCs [combined oral contraceptives] is lower than in pregnancy which is around 60 per 100,000 pregnancies" and the SmPC wording was similar. The position statement and the information sheet for women included an unquantified statement on the lower VTE risk of CHCs than associated with pregnancy (European Medicines Agency (EMA) 2001)
Comparison of P/Cs and HP input with communication research evidence	Looking at best risk communication practices, caution with risk comparisons, as exercised in 2013, is indeed warranted, as the lead editor of (Fischhoff et al. 2011, Brewer NT, Downs JS (eds) 2011) advises elsewhere that "risk comparisons should not be made, unless they are developed in a scientifically sound way, addressing all recipients" values and circumstances, and are empirically "evaluated" (Fischhoff 2006)

Second, the expression of the risk magnitude differed. In 2001, a person-time denominator reported the risks as quantified in the reviewed studies. As these incidence density rates are abstract parameters that do not describe anything tangible or imaginable, even for pharmacoepidemiological experts, P/C as well as HP representatives in 2013 understandably asked for incidence rates with a standardised denominator of CHC users (i.e. 10,000). According to communication research, incident rates with natural numbers are more easily understood by members of the public than percentages and relative risks. In 2013, incidence rates with a person denominator for communication purposes had therefore to be derived from the available data with a person-time denominator. As the SmPCs explain, incidence rates were estimated using baseline VTE incidence rates and the relative risks for use of levonorgestrel-containing CHCs versus CHC non-use and for use of levonorgestrel-containing versus other CHCs (European Medicines Agency (EMA) 2014c).

Third, the impact of the 2013 consultations with women P/C representatives that could not be extracted from existing communication research consisted in abandoning in the PL the comparison of CHC VTE risks with pregnancy-associated VTE risks. This comparison however continued to be included in the materials for HPs, because HP representatives found this comparator useful. Already during the 2001 review, it was raised whether this comparison would be appropriate from a woman's perspective, but the expert group in charge of the review (consisting of male HPs) recommended to include the comparison not only in the materials for HPs, but also in the PL. Considering that in 2013 male and female HPs supported the comparison with pregnancy at least for their own materials, it seems that HPs' communication preferences are more shaped by their medical perspective than by considering the (female) life-choice perspective.

4. Discussion and Conclusions

This study compares the EMA's approaches to communicating the outcomes of two reviews of CHCs, in 2001 and in 2013. The communication materials in 2013 benefited from revisiting the careful considerations given to communication in 2001 and from new consultations with P/C and HP representatives. Many aspects could have been analysed in this case study, but the study focused on the major points raised in the 2013 stakeholder consultations in response to the questions posed by the PRAC.

The key principle at both occasions was how to inform people, in audience-tailored ways, about risks in an honest manner and in accordance with legal obligations, with the aim of contributing to informed contraceptive choices, safe use of CHCs and harm reduction, and without creating undue scare in those using or intending to use these products.

The analysis shows that applying this principle resulted in similarity of fundamental communication choices in 2001 and 2013 regarding risk characterisation, relative risk quantification only in HP-targeted materials, and contextualisation of the risk with CHC benefit. Risk management, i.e. advice to consider risk differences between CHCs when prescribing and to seek urgent care in the case of VTE signs, was prioritised at both occasions, and strengthened in 2013. The inclusion of risk comparisons between products of a whole medicines class in the product information of higher risk products was exceptional, as SmPCs and PLs usually contain only data for the given product (apart from data on clinical trial comparators in SmPCs) and usually do not provide guidance on the place of a product in its medicines class.

Also, as part of risk management strengthening in 2013, a new statement was introduced at the top of the PLs (see Table 2.1, point 1). While warning statements at the top of PLs are usually included when warranted (in addition to appearing in the warning section of a PL), the statement at the top of PLs for CHCs was likewise exceptional for two reasons: First, warning statements at the top of PLs are usually reserved for serious risks, and while the VTE risk is serious and potentially fatal, the CHC statement as worded did not explicitly state the seriousness. It highlighted instead (with the words “slightly increase”) that the risk is rare and, importantly, stressed clearly the medical urgency of VTE. Second, the statement referred to the benefits of the product, which are usually given less prominence in PLs, to avoid promoting overuse of medicinal products. Including prominent benefit information however responded to the consultation feedback.

Further, the analysis shows differences between the communication choices in 2001 and 2013, mainly regarding the expression of risk magnitude (in 2013 in incidence rates, in 2001 as incidence density rates), the visualisation of risk differences (new in 2013), and the comparison of VTE associated with pregnancy (abandoned in 2013 with good reasoning in materials targeted at P/Cs and the wider public).

Overall, the stakeholder input was in line with evidence from communication research that has been accumulating mainly after 2001; however, it was more specific to the case.

Implications for Medicinal Product Risk Communication

This study provides two lessons for those preparing risk communication interventions: First, relying on validated evidence from communication research is justified for communication planning. Second, the participation of information users in designing communication materials is additionally required to confirm the applicability of existing communication research findings in the given situation and to obtain feedback on situation-specific aspects of communication. Such aspects may include e.g. meaningful risk comparisons and understandable graphical presentations, in particular when specific audiences by, e.g. sex, age, or culture are to be addressed. However, assuring the representativeness of P/Cs and HPs may be a challenge, as those who participate in consultations do so in self-selected manner and may be highly experienced in healthcare and medical sciences and hence be different from the typical audience member. Communication research may investigate bigger populations and have higher representativeness. Hence, reviewing communication research and conducting stakeholder consultations as well as user testing of draft communication materials can be seen as synergistic.

Implications for Pharmacoepidemiology and Real World Evidence Generation

The study has also identified wider implications. The current model of researching and assessing risks and safety of medicines and afterwards considering how the results can be best communicated to broader audiences can make communication very challenging. In this case, the data from studies were not directly suitable for communication. As their results were reported as incidence density rates, more audience-understandable incidence rates had to be estimated using baseline incidence rates and relative risks. Ideally, such estimates would have been cross-checked with estimates using incidence density rates and average/typical length of CHC use in the study population, had these data been available. Therefore, this study provides two lessons for those in charge of pharmacoepidemiological research and real world evidence (RWE) generation: First, research should be planned to include generating data that support expressing risks in generally understandable ways, in particular as incidence rates. Second, there is a need for more pharmacoepidemiological research on medicine use, including typical duration of use and use among people with risk factors, and on the relationship of prescribing and use of medicines with risk perceptions. Moreover, real world healthcare research into P/C values and choices, risk perceptions, risk acceptability, information needs, and communication preferences of both P/Cs and HPs as well as delivery of communication at population and personal level within healthcare is crucial for audience-tailoring and optimising medicinal product risk communication.

Regulatory Evaluation of the 2001 and 2013 Communication Preparations

Of course, the EMA has been interested in understanding the impact of their efforts of audience-tailoring. At both occasions, in 2001 and 2013, the EMA did not experience any exceptionally high media interest or even a "media crisis", or became aware of any other sign of a public scare. For the 2001 review, it has to be noted that the communication occurred on 28 September 2001 and media were focused on the aftermath of the September 11 attacks.

After the 2013 CHC review, the EMA commissioned a mixed-methods evaluation of the impact of the regulatory action in several MS (Denmark, Germany, Netherlands, Slovakia, Spain, United Kingdom), involving a literature review, surveys of P/Cs and HPs, an interview study with P/Cs and HPs, and a content analysis of information on the internet. It was found that HPs and P/Cs tended to consider VTE following CHC use an unlikely event. Overall, HPs reported being satisfied with the amount of information they received from regulatory bodies. Fifty-three percent of the HP sample was aware of the review outcome, even though most HPs did not report using this safe use advice in practice. They highlighted their lack of time to read updates from regulatory bodies. One-third of women did not seek any information about CHCs before deciding to take them. Although most women tended to seek information beforehand, most had never heard about regulatory bodies. When prompted, most women tended to identify national health organisations, but not the EMA, and reported regulatory authorities to be one of the least important and/or least interesting information sources for them. If they had heard about regulators, this tended to be via the media. The studied women generally considered CHCs to be safe, but felt the need to receive more information about possible risks during consultations with their HPs. However, HPs considered communicating CHC risks to women challenging, particularly during short appointments. This led the study to conclude that research should be conducted to support HPs in this task. The internet content analysis simulated search strategies women would commonly use in their local languages and concluded that despite the large number of websites containing information about CHCs and their risks, particularly VTE, only a limited number referred to accredited sources. In particular, citation of either the MS regulatory body or the EMA was limited (Stevenson F 2017; Alves PG, Petersen I, Stevenson F 2019).

Reflecting on these findings, the P/Cs' and HPs' perception that VTE following CHC use is an unlikely event corresponds with the EMA message on the rare frequency of VTE with CHCs; however, it seems that for P/Cs this perception is not so much knowledge-based. The finding that the EMA is not widely known is less worrying than that the information materials from the better known MS regulatory bodies—which were based on the EU review—were not read or searched for as much as the regulators had aimed or wished for.

Further, it remains uncertain whether the VTE risk differences between different CHCs are commonly known and taken into account when prescribing and deciding to take a CHC (as is advised in the SmPC). Prescription data analyses can possibly help to answer this. For Germany, a study of 2019 demonstrated a continued decrease in prescriptions of CHCs with higher VTE risk after the 2013 review (Krulichova S et al. 2019). Studies in other MS could not be identified from the scientific literature to date (2019). The authors of the German study concluded that, although the evidence for a causal association between the communication of the review outcome and the change in prescribing is only indirect, their study showed that routine health and prescription data are suitable for impact analyses of regulatory interventions.

As the EMA-commissioned study (Stevenson F 2017) did not succeed in recruiting survey participants from Germany and did not conduct interviews in Germany, no discussion can be offered here on how surveys or interviews of HPs or P/Cs could support investigating whether a change in prescribing as identified in Germany (Krulichova S et al. 2019) has possibly been caused by the CHCs review outcome or whether other influential factors were present. However, the application of various approaches to evaluating the impact of regulatory communication in this case can still serve as an example for how methods from different disciplines could complement each other for gaining a better understanding of the impact of communication events, as suggested by the multilayered research framework in Chap. 1.

Outlook

Overall, this study shows that regulators can be flexible in their communication choices and put major effort into preparing for communication, including through stakeholder consultation. Conducting the case study revealed once more how work-intensive and complex regulatory communication is, given that the legally required SmPCs and PLs, all documents on a review procedure and assessment to be published under legal transparency provisions, as well as the materials communicating the review outcomes to different audiences must be prepared, checked for accuracy and consistency, and released under the constraints of short timelines, demanded by legislation or self-imposed by policies for timeliness. While audience-tailoring of information can be seen as mandatory for a public body that provides for and is accountable to all citizens, the impact of these communication efforts may still be limited. This may be due to incomplete reach of audiences, even if information has been audience-tailored. Therefore, in addition to benefitting from available communication research and promoting pharmacoepidemiological and broader real world evidence generation for audience-tailoring of communication, medicinal product regulators need to continue their efforts in disseminating information and to engage with leaders in patient advocacy and healthcare quality management for the implementation of pharmaceutical risk management and safe use behaviours.

References for Appendix 2.1

Alves et al (2019) Searching for information on the risks of combined hormonal contraceptives on the internet: a qualitative study across six European countries. J Med Internet Res 21:e10810

European Commission (EC) (2009) Guideline on summary of product characteristics (SmPC). Rev 2. EC, Brussels. In: EC. Rules governing medicinal products in the European Union, Notice to Applicants, Volume 2C

European Medicines Agency (EMA) (2001) Position statement on combined oral contraceptives (COCs), CPMP public assessment report, Dear healthcare professional letter on 3rd generation COCs, Information for women using oral contraceptives. EMA, London

European Medicines Agency (EMA) (2014a) Assessment report for combined hormonal contraceptives containing medicinal products. EMA, London. Accessible at: European Medicines Agency (EMA) (2014b)

European Medicines Agency (EMA) (2014b) Combined hormonal contraceptives [webpage for Article 31 referral procedure]. EMA, London. https://www.ema.europa.eu/en/medicines/human/referrals/combined-hormonal-contraceptives#all-documents-sectionke. Last updated on 16 Jan 2014

European Medicines Agency (EMA) (2014c) Combined hormonal contraceptives Article 31 referral – Annex III. EMA, London. Accessible at: European Medicines Agency (EMA) (2014b)

European Medicines Agency (EMA) (2014d) Overview on review outcome of Article 31 referral procedure on combined hormonal contraceptives [online format and pdf format]. EMA, London. Accessible at: European Medicines Agency (EMA) (2014b)

Fischhoff (2006) Problems with risk comparisons. Carnegie Mellon University, Pittsburgh. https://www.cmu.edu/epp/people/faculty/research/Fischhoff-Risk-Comparisons.pdf

Fischhoff et al (2011) Communicating risks and benefits: an evidence-based user's guide. US Food and Drug Administration, Silver Spring

Krulichova S, Selke GW, Eichler U, Lappe V. Godman B, Schubert I (2019) Impact of EU risk assessment process and administrative regulations for manufacturers of combined hormonal contraceptive prescribing: an analysis of developments in Germany and the implications. Curr Med Res Opin 35:697–704

Paling J (2003) Strategies to help patients understand risks. Br Med J 327:745–748

Stevenson F (2017) Study of regulatory communication and risk awareness following the Article 31 referral of combined hormonal contraceptives in relation to thromboembolism [final report]. http://www.encepp.eu/encepp/openAttachment/studyResultLatest/26585;jsessionid=EzL6TfhMqMAlHzAd_gdP098l1m78KSv9WVcburEixcDywPTDa89B!693664918

Appendix 2.2: References for the Study Presented in Sect. 2.2.1

Articles citing primary studies comparing venous thromboembolic risks of drospirenone-containing vs. "second-generation" oral contraceptives:

Allan GM, Koppula S (2012) Risks of venous thromboembolism with various hormonal contraceptives. Can Fam Physician 58(10):1097

Archer DF, Lasa IL (2011) Tailoring combination oral contraceptives to the individual woman. J Womens Health 20(6):879–891

Arie S (2013) French doctors are told to restrict use of third and fourth generation oral contraceptives. BMJ 346

Banerjee C (2016) Obesity, oral contraceptive use, and cerebral venous thrombosis in women. JAMA Neurol 73(5):512–513

Barsoum MK, Heit JA, Ashrani AA, Leibson CL, Petterson TM, Bailey KR (2010) Is progestin an independent risk factor for incident venous thromboembolism? A population-based case-control study. Thromb Res 126(5):373–378

Bateson D, Butcher BE, Donovan C, Farrell L, Kovacs G, Mezzini T et al (2016) Risk of venous thromboembolism in women taking the combined oral contraceptive: a systematic review and meta-analysis. Aust Fam Physician 45(1–2):59

Bergendal A, Persson I, Odeberg J, Sundstrom A, Holmstrom M, Schulman S et al (2015) Association of venous thromboembolism with hormonal contraception and thrombophilic genotypes (vol 124, pg 600, 2014). Obstet Gynecol 125(2):495

Bergendal A, Persson I, Odeberg J, Sundstrom A, Holmstrom M, Schulman S et al (2014) Association of venous thromboembolism with hormonal contraception and thrombophilic genotypes. Obstet Gynecol 124(3):600–609

Bird ST, Delaney JAC, Etminan M, Brophy JM, Hartzema AG (2013a) Drospirenone and non-fatal venous thromboembolism: is there a risk difference by dosage of ethinyl-estradiol? J Thromb Haemost 11(6):1059–1068

Bird ST, Hartzema AG, Brophy JM, Etminan M, Delaney JAC (2013b) Risk of venous thromboembolism in women with polycystic ovary syndrome: a population-based matched cohort analysis. Can Med Assoc J 185(2):E115–EE20

Bitzer J, Amy JJ, Beerthuizen R, Birkhauser M, Bombas T, Creinin M et al (2013) Statement on combined hormonal contraceptives containing third- or fourth-generation progestogens or cyproterone acetate, and the associated risk of thromboembolism. Eur J Contracept Reprod Health Care 18(3):143–147

Bitzer J (2013) Statement on combined hormonal contraceptives containing third- or fourth-generation progestogens or cyproterone acetate, and the associated risk of thromboembolism. J Fam Plann Reprod Health Care 39(3):156–159

Bleker SM, Coppens M, Middeldorp S (2014) Sex, thrombosis and inherited thrombophilia. Blood Rev 28(3):123–133

Brown DA, Vartan CM (2011) Risk of venous thromboembolism with drospirenone-containing oral contraceptives. Am J Health Syst Pharm 68(11):1003–1010

Burkman R, Bell C, Serfaty D (2011) The evolution of combined oral contraception: improving the risk-to-benefit ratio. Contraception 84(1):19–34

Buzney E, Sheu J, Buzney C, Reynolds RV (2014) Polycystic ovary syndrome: a review for dermatologists: part II. Treatment. J Am Acad Dermatol 71(5):859.e1–859.e859859

Carmina E (2013) Oral contraceptives and cardiovascular risk in women with polycystic ovary syndrome. J Endocrinol Investig 36(5):358–363

Casey PM, Files JA, Mayer AP (2013) Drospirenone-related venous thromboembolism risk: "the rest of the story". J Womens Health 22(5):467–468

Chabbert-Buffet N, Gerris J, Jamin C, Lello S, Lete I, Lobo P et al (2013a) Toward a new concept of "natural balance" in oral estroprogestin contraception. Gynecol Endocrinol 29(10):891–896

Chabbert-Buffet N, Guigues B, Trillot N, Biron C, Morange P, Pernod G et al (2013b) DVT and combined oral contraceptives: update of the pluridisciplinary CNGOF-FNCGM-GEHT-SFMV group. J Gynecol Obstet Biol Reprod 42(4):309–315

Chadwick KD, Burkman RT, Tornesi BM, Mahadevan B (2012) Fifty years of "the pill": risk reduction and discovery of benefits beyond contraception, reflections, and forecast. Toxicol Sci 125(1):2–9

(2015) Choice of contraceptives. Med Lett Drugs Ther 57(1477):127–132

(2010) Combination oral contraceptives and the risk of venous thromboembolism. Med Lett Drugs Ther 52(1334):23–24

Costescu DJ, Waddington A (2013) Hormonal contraception and thrombosis. Any review must carefully weigh the available evidence. BMJ 346

Cox L (2015) The bitter pill. J Fam Plann Reprod Health Care 41(2):81–83

Cremer M, Phan-Weston S, Jacobs A (2010) Recent innovations in oral contraception. Semin Reprod Med 28(2):140–146

de Bastos M, Stegeman BH, Rosendaal FR, Vlieg AV, Helmerhorst FM, Stijnen T, et al (2014) Combined oral contraceptives: venous thrombosis. Cochrane Database Syst Rev (3):CD010813

Debarre JM (2013) Suspension of Diane35 (R) and its generics: an over-reaction by the French National Medicines Agency (ANSM) unfounded in the light of proven or accepted medical knowledge. Ann Dermatol Venereol 140(6–7):474–478

DeLoughery TG (2011) Estrogen and thrombosis: controversies and common sense. Rev Endocr Metab Disord 12(2):77–84

Dinger J, Assmann A, Mohner S, Minh TD (2010) Risk of venous thromboembolism and the use of dienogest- and drospirenone-containing oral contraceptives: results from a German case-control study. J Fam Plann Reprod Health Care 36(3):123–129

Dinger J, Bardenheuer K, Heinemann K (2014) Cardiovascular and general safety of a 24-day regimen of drospirenone-containing combined oral contraceptives: final results from the International Active Surveillance Study of Women Taking Oral Contraceptives. Contraception 89(4):253–263

Dinger J, Mohner S, Heinemann K (2016) Cardiovascular risks associated with the use of drospirenone-containing combined oral contraceptives. Contraception 93(5):378–385

Dinger J, Shapiro S (2012) Combined oral contraceptives, venous thromboembolism, and the problem of interpreting large but incomplete datasets. J Fam Plann Reprod Health Care 38(1):2–6

Dinger J (2010) OCs and VTE: a practical answer to an old question reply. J Fam Plann Reprod Health Care 36(1):44

Dinger J (2016) Reply to letter to the editor: "questions to the LASS study group". Contraception 94(4):381–383

Dinger J (2014) Reply to letter to the editor: "the INTAS-OC study". Contraception 90(6):618–621

Domecq JP, Prutsky G, Mullan RJ, Sundaresh V, Wang AT, Erwin PJ et al (2013) Adverse effects of the common treatments for polycystic ovary syndrome: a systematic review and meta-analysis. J Clin Endocrinol Metabol 98(12):4646–4654

Dragoman MV (2014) The combined oral contraceptive pill- recent developments, risks and benefits. Best Pract Res Clin Obstet Gynaecol 28(6):825–834

Dunn N (2011) The risk of deep venous thrombosis with oral contraceptives containing drospirenone. Br Med J 342

Ehspre Capri working Group (2013) Venous thromboembolism in women: a specific reproductive health risk. Hum Reprod Update 19(5):471–482

Foran TM (2014) The newer contraceptive pills and venous thromboembolism risk. Med J Aust 200(7):376–377

Gigerenzer G, Wegwarth O, Feufel M (2010) Misleading communication of risk. Br Med J 341

Gourbil M, Grandvuillemin A, Beyens MN, Massy N, Gras V, D'Amico A et al (2014) Thromboembolic events in women exposed to hormonal contraception or cyproterone acetate in 2012: a cross-sectional observational study in 30 French public hospitals. Drug Saf 37(4):269–282

Gourdy P, Bacheloth A, Catteau-Jonard S, Chabbert-Buffet N, Christin-Maitre S, Conard J et al (2012) Hormonal contraception in women at risk of vascular and metabolic disorders: guidelines of the French Society of Endocrinology. Ann Endocrinol 73(5):469–487
Grimes D (2011) Epidemiologic research using administrative databases: garbage in, garbage out. Obstet Gynaecol 117(2):411
Grimes DA (2015) Epidemiologic research with administrative databases: red herrings, false alarms and pseudo-epidemics. Hum Reprod 30(8):1749–1752
Gronich N, Lavi I, Rennert G (2011) Higher risk of venous thrombosis associated with drospirenone-containing oral contraceptives: a population-based cohort study. Can Med Assoc J 183(18):E1319–E1E25
Gronier-Gouvernel H, Robin G (2014) Cardiovascular risks of combined oral contraceptives - beyond the French controversy. Gynecol Obstet Fertil 42(3):174–181
Gundert-Remy U, Stammschulte T (2011) Risk of venous thromboembolism. Dtsch Arztebl Int 108(45):768
Han L, Jensen JT (2015) Does the progestogen used in combined hormonal contraception affect venous thrombosis risk? Obstet Gynecol Clin N Am 42(4):683
Hannaford PC (2011a) Epidemiology of the contraceptive pill and venous thromboembolism. Thromb Res 127:S30–SS4
Hannaford PC (2011b) The progestogen content of combined oral contraceptives and venous thromboembolic risk. Br Med J 343
Hannaford PC (2016) The vascular risks associated with combined oral contraceptives. BMJ 353
Harper JC (2016) Use of oral contraceptives for management of acne vulgaris practical considerations in real world practice. Dermatol Clin 34(2):159
Harrison-Woolrych M, Woolley J (2015) Combined oral contraceptives and venous thromboembolism. New study supports MHRA advice on combined oral contraceptives. BMJ 350
Heinemann K, Heinemann LAJ (2011) Comparative risks of venous thromboembolism among users of oral contraceptives containing drospirenone and levonorgestrel. J Fam Plann Reprod Health Care 37(3):132–135
Heinemann LAJ, Dinger JC, Assmann A, Do Minh T (2010) Use of oral contraceptives containing gestodene and risk of venous thromboembolism: outlook 10 years after the third-generation "pill scare". Contraception 81(5):401–407
Helmerhorst FM, Rosendaal FR (2013) Is an EMA review on hormonal contraception and thrombosis needed? BMJ 346
Helvaci N, Yildiz BO (2014) Oral contraceptives in polycystic ovary syndrome. Minerva Endocrinol 39(3):175–187
Hugon-Rodin J, Gompel A, Plu-Bureau G (2014) Epidemiology of hormonal contraceptives-related venous thromboembolism. Eur J Endocrinol 171(6):R221–RR30
Idota N, Kobayashi M, Miyamori D, Kakiuchi Y, Ikegaya H (2015) Drospirenone detected in postmortem blood of a young woman with pulmonary thromboembolism: a case report and review of the literature. Legal Med 17(2):109–115
Jacobsen AF, Sandset PM (2012) Venous thromboembolism associated with pregnancy and hormonal therapy. Best Pract Res Clin Haematol 25(3):319–332
Jamin C (2016) Combined hormonal contraceptives and the subsequent risk of a venous thromboembolism. Phlebolymphology 23(1):31–36
Jamin CG (2013) "All that fuss for what?" (C. Lelouch) or worse "Much ado about nothing" (W. Shakespeare). Gynecol Obstet Fertil 41(12):679–680
Jensen JT, Trussell J (2012) Communicating risk: does scientific debate compromise safety? Contraception 86(4):327–329
Jick S, Parkin L, Hernandez R, Sharples K (2011) The pill and thrombosis. Authors' reply. Br Med J 342
Jick SS, Hernandez RK (2011) Risk of non-fatal venous thromboembolism in women using oral contraceptives containing drospirenone compared with women using oral contraceptives containing levonorgestrel: case-control study using United States claims data. Br Med J 342
Kaminski P, Szpotanska-Sikorska M, Wielgos M (2013) Cardiovascular risk and the use of oral contraceptives. Neuroendocrinol Lett 34(7):585–589

Lackie E, Fairchild A (2016) The birth control pill, thromboembolic disease, science and the media: a historical review of the relationship. Contraception 94(4):295–302

Leppee M, Culig J, Eric M (2010) Consumption of combined oral contraceptives and venous thromboembolism in Zagreb, Croatia. Eur J Contracept Reprod Health Care 15(6):445–446

Lete I, Chabbert-Buffet N, Jamin C, Lello S, Lobo P, Nappi RE et al (2015) Haemostatic and metabolic impact of estradiol pills and drospirenone-containing ethinylestradiol pills vs. levonorgestrel-containing ethinylestradiol pills: a literature review. Eur J Contracept Reprod Health Care 20(5):329–343

Levesque H, Hanslik T (2013) Combined hormonal pills and thrombosis: from clinical data to media consequences. Rev Med Interne 34(8):453–455

Lidegaard O, Milsom I, Geirsson RT, Skjeldestad FE (2012) Hormonal contraception and venous thromboembolism. Acta Obstet Gynecol Scand 91(7):769–778

Lidegaard O, Nielsen LH, Skovlund CW, Skjeldestad FE, Lokkegaard E (2011) Risk of venous thromboembolism from use of oral contraceptives containing different progestogens and oestrogen doses: Danish cohort study, 2001–9. Br Med J 343

Lidegaard O (2011) Epidemiologic research using administrative databases: garbage in, garbage out. Obstet Gynecol 117(2):410–411

Lidegaard O (2014) Hormonal contraception, thrombosis and age. Expert Opin Drug Saf 13(10):1353–1360

Lidegaard O (2016) Questions to the LASS study group. Contraception 94(4):379–381

Lobert M, Pigeyre M, Gronier H, Catteau-Jonard S, Robin G (2015) Contraception and obesity. Gynecol Obstet Fertil 43(11):740–747

Machado RB, Morimoto M, Santana N, Arruda LF, Bernardes CR, de Souza IM (2015) Effect of information on the perception of users and prospective users of combined oral contraceptives regarding the risk of venous thromboembolism. Gynecol Endocrinol 31(1):57–60

Manzoli L, De Vito C, Marzuillo C, Boccia A, Villari P (2012) Oral contraceptives and venous thromboembolism: a systematic review and meta-analysis. Drug Saf 35(3):191–205

Martinez F, Latorre K, Ramirez I, Perez-Campos E, Lete I (2013) Can a meta-analysis that included articles with high heterogeneity appropriately evaluate the risk of venous thromboembolism in users of combined hormonal contraceptives containing drospirenone or desogestrel? A reply to Rosa et al. Eur J Contracept Reprod Health Care 18(2):139–142

Martinez F, Ramirez I, Perez-Campos E, Latorre K, Lete I (2012) Venous and pulmonary thromboembolism and combined hormonal contraceptives. Systematic review and meta-analysis. Eur J Contracept Reprod Health Care 17(1):7–29

Merki-Feld GS, Skouby S, Serfaty D, Lech M, Bitzer J, Crosignani PG et al (2015) European society of contraception statement on contraception in obese women. Eur J Contracept Reprod Health Care 20(1):19–28

Merviel P (2013) Lamb to the slaughter. Gynecol Obstet Fertil 41(4):211–212

O'Brien SH (2014) Contraception-related venous thromboembolism in adolescents. Semin Thromb Hemost 40(1):66–71

Reid R et al (2011) Oral contraceptives and the risk of venous thromboembolism: an update no. 252, December 2010. Int J Gynecol Obstet 112(3):252–256

Parkin L, Sharples K, Hernandez RK, Jick SS (2011) Risk of venous thromboembolism in users of oral contraceptives containing drospirenone or levonorgestrel: nested case-control study based on UK General Practice Research Database. Br Med J 342

Plu-Bureau G, Maitrot-Mantelet L, Hugon-Rodin J, Canonico M (2013) Hormonal contraceptives and venous thromboembolism: an epidemiological update. Best Pract Res Clin Endocrinol Metab 27(1):25–34

Pries J (2011) Serious concerns. Dtsch Arztebl Int 108(45):769

Raps M, Curvers J, Helmerhorst FM, Ballieux B, Rosing J, Thomassen S et al (2014) Thyroid function, activated protein C resistance and the risk of venous thrombosis in users of hormonal contraceptives. Thromb Res 133(4):640–644

Raps M, Helmerhorst F, Fleischer K, Thomassen S, Rosendaal F, Rosing J et al (2012) Sex hormone-binding globulin as a marker for the thrombotic risk of hormonal contraceptives. J Thromb Haemost 10(6):992–997

Raps M, Helmerhorst FM, Fleischer K, Dahm AEA, Rosendaal FR, Rosing J et al (2013a) The effect of different hormonal contraceptives on plasma levels of free protein S and free TFPI. Thromb Haemost 109(4):606–613

Raps M, Rosendaal F, Ballieux B, Rosing J, Thomassen S, Helmerhorst F et al (2013b) Resistance to APC and SHBG levels during use of a four-phasic oral contraceptive containing dienogest and estradiol valerate: a randomized controlled trial. J Thromb Haemost 11(5):855–861

Raymond EG, Burke AE, Espey E (2012) Combined hormonal contraceptives and venous thromboembolism: putting the risks into perspective. Obstet Gynecol 119(5):1039–1044

Reid RL, Westhoff C, Mansour D, de Vries C, Verhaeghe J, Boschitsch E et al (2010) Oral contraceptives and venous thromboembolism consensus opinion from an international workshop held in Berlin, Germany in December 2009. J Fam Plann Reprod Health Care 36(3):117–122

Reid RL (2014) Oral hormonal contraception and venous thromboembolism (VTE). Contraception 89(4):235–236

Rosa MI, Madeira K, Medeiros LR (2013) Can a meta-analysis that included articles with high heterogeneity appropriately evaluate the risk of venous thromboembolism in users of combined hormonal contraceptives containing drospirenone or desogestrel? Eur J Contracept Reprod Health Care 18(2):137–139

Rosendaal FR, Helmerhorst FM (2013) Hormonal contraception and thrombosis. Authors' reply to Costescu and Waddington. BMJ 346

Rott H (2013) Contraception, venous thrombosis and biological plausability. Minerva Med 104(2):161–167

Rott H (2012a) Hormonal contraception in thrombophilic adolescents. Risk of thrombosis and recommendations. Hamostaseologie 32(1):15–21

Rott H (2012b) Thrombotic risks of oral contraceptives. Curr Opin Obstet Gynecol 24(4):235–240

Sandset PM (2013) Mechanisms of hormonal therapy related thrombosis. Thromb Res 131: S4–S7

Santosa F, Moysidis T, Moerchel C, Kroger K, Bufe A (2014) Pulmonary embolism in young people. Trends in Germany from 2005 to 2011. Hamostaseologie 34(1):88–92

Scala C, Maggiore ULR, Remorgida V, Venturini PL, Ferrero S (2013) Drug safety evaluation of desogestrel. Expert Opin Drug Saf 12(3):433–444

Sehovic N, Smith KP (2010) Risk of venous thromboembolism with drospirenone in combined oral contraceptive products. Ann Pharmacother 44(5):898–903

Shapiro S, Dinger J (2010a) Critique of a Danish cohort study on hormonal contraception and VTE reply. J Fam Plann Reprod Health Care 36(2):104–105

Shapiro S, Dinger J (2010b) Risk of venous thromboembolism among users of oral contraceptives: a review of two recently published studies. J Fam Plann Reprod Health Care 36(1):33–38

Shapiro S, Dinger J (2010c) Risk of VTE among users of oral contraceptives. J Fam Plann Reprod Health Care 36(2):103

Shapiro S (2013) Combined hormonal contraceptives and the risk of venous and arterial thromboembolism and cardiovascular death: misuse of automated databases. J Fam Plann Reprod Health Care 39(2):89–96

Shapiro S (2011) The pill and thrombosis. Venous thromboembolism is egregiously underestimated. Br Med J 342

Shulman LP (2011) The state of hormonal contraception today: benefits and risks of hormonal contraceptives: combined estrogen and progestin contraceptives. Am J Obstet Gynecol 205(4):S9–S13

Sidney S, Cheetham TC, Connell FA, Ouellet-Hellstrom R, Graham DJ, Davis D et al (2013) Recent combined hormonal contraceptives (CHCs) and the risk of thromboembolism and other cardiovascular events in new users. Contraception 87(1):93–100

Sidney S (2013) Another flawed database study response. Contraception 87(4):506–507

Sitruk-Ware R (2016) Hormonal contraception and thrombosis. Fertil Steril 106(6):1289–1294

Solymoss S (2011) Risk of venous thromboembolism with oral contraceptives. Can Med Assoc J 183(18):E1278–E12E9

Stam-Slob MC, Lambalk CB, van de Ree MA (2015) Practice pointer. Contraceptive and hormonal treatment options for women with history of venous thromboembolism. BMJ 351
Stanczyk FZ, Archer DF, Bhavnani BR (2013) Ethinyl estradiol and 17 beta-estradiol in combined oral contraceptives: pharmacokinetics, pharmacodynamics and risk assessment. Contraception 87(6):706–727
Stegeman BH, de Bastos M, Rosendaal FR, Vlieg AV, Helmerhorst FM, Stijnen T et al (2013) Different combined oral contraceptives and the risk of venous thrombosis: systematic review and network meta-analysis. BMJ 347
Stewart M, Black K (2015) Choosing a combined oral contraceptive pill. Aust Prescr 38(1):6–11
Stocco B, Fumagalli HF, Franceschini SA, Martinez EZ, Marzocchi-Machado CM, Felipe M et al (2015) Comparative study of the effects of combined oral contraceptives in hemostatic variables: an observational preliminary study. Medicine 94(4):e385
Suchon P, Al Frouh F, Henneuse A, Ibrahim M, Brunet D, Barthet MC et al (2016) Risk factors for venous thromboembolism in women under combined oral contraceptive. The PILl Genetic RIsk Monitoring (PILGRIM) Study. Thromb Haemost 115(1):135–142
Sugiura K, Kobayashi T, Ojima T (2016) Risks of thromboembolism associated with hormonal contraceptives related to body mass index and aging in Japanese women. Thromb Res 137:11–16
Sugiura K, Kobayashi T, Ojima T (2015) Thromboembolism as the adverse event of combined oral contraceptives in Japan. Thromb Res 136(6):1110–1115
Swanepoel AC, Visagie A, Pretorius E (2016) Synthetic hormones and clot formation. Microsc Microanal 22(4):878–886
Szarewski A, Mansour D, Shapiro S (2013) Another flawed database study. Contraception 87(4):505–506
Tchaikovski SN, Rosing J (2010) Mechanisms of estrogen-induced venous thromboembolism. Thromb Res 126(1):5–11
Tchaikovski SN, Thomassen M, Costa SD, Bremme K, Rosing J (2014) Changes in haemostatic parameters during the menstrual cycle and subsequent use of drospirenone-containing oral contraceptives. Thromb Res 134(5):1032–1037
Terplan M, Zuckerman D (2013) Comment on 'Statement on combined hormonal contraceptives containing third- or fourth-generation progestogens or cyproterone acetate, and the associated risk of thromboembolism' reply. J Fam Plann Reprod Health Care 39(4):304–305
Trenor CC, Chung RJ, Michelson AD, Neufeld EJ, Gordon CM, Laufer MR et al (2011) Hormonal contraception and thrombotic risk: a multidisciplinary approach. Pediatrics 127(2):347–357
Tricotel A, Collin C, Zureik M (2015) Impact of the sharp changes in the use of contraception in 2013 on the risk of pulmonary embolism in France. J Thromb Haemost 13(9):1576–1580
Tricotel A, Raguideau F, Collin C, Zureik M (2014) Estimate of venous thromboembolism and related-deaths attributable to the use of combined oral contraceptives in France. PLos One 9(4):e93792
Trigg DE, Wood MG, Kouides PA, Kadir RA (2011) Hormonal influences on hemostasis in women. Semin Thromb Hemost 37(1):77–86
van Grootheest K, Harmark L, van Puijenbroek E (2011) Pharmacovigilance of contraceptives: why does it take so long to take action? Drug Saf 34(10):901
Verhaeghe J (2012) Clinical practice: contraception in adolescents. Eur J Pediatr 171(6):895–899
Vinogradova Y, Coupland C, Hippisley-Cox J Authors' reply to Zagarella. BMJ 350:h3308
Vinogradova Y, Coupland C, Hippisley-Cox J (2014) Exposure to combined oral contraceptives and risk of venous thromboembolism: a protocol for nested case-control studies using the QResearch and the CPRD databases. BMJ Open 4(4):e004499
Vinogradova Y, Coupland C, Hippisley-Cox J (2015a) New study supports MHRA advice on combined oral contraceptives. Authors' reply to Zagarella. BMJ 350
Vinogradova Y, Coupland C, Hippisley-Cox J (2015b) Use of combined oral contraceptives and risk of venous thromboembolism: nested case-control studies using the QResearch and CPRD databases. BMJ 350
Vlieg AV, Middeldorp S (2011) Hormone therapies and venous thromboembolism: where are we now? J Thromb Haemost 9(2):257–266

Voelker R (2011) Risk of blood clots higher for oral contraceptives with certain progestins. JAMA 306(20):2206
Weill A, Dalichampt M, Raguideau F, Ricordeau P, Blotiere PO, Rudant J et al (2016) Low dose oestrogen combined oral contraception and risk of pulmonary embolism, stroke, and myocardial infarction in five million French women: cohort study. BMJ 353
Wiegratz I, Thaler C (2011) Serious concerns reply. Dtsch Arztebl Int 108(45):769–770
Williams DJP (2016) Commentary on hormonal contraceptive use in Ireland: trends and co-prescribing practices. Br J Clin Pharmacol 81(4):587–588
Woods GM, Kerlin BA, O'Brien SH, Bonny AE (2016) A review of hormonal contraception and venous thromboembolism in adolescents. J Pediatr Adolesc Gynecol 29(5):402–408
Wu CQ, Grandi SM, Filion KB, Abenhaim HA, Joseph L, Eisenberg MJ (2013) Drospirenone-containing oral contraceptive pills and the risk of venous and arterial thrombosis: a systematic review. BJOG Int J Obstet Gynaecol 120(7):801–811
Zagarella SS (2015) Combined oral contraceptives and venous thromboembolism. Oral contraceptive study omitted several confounders. BMJ 350
Zakharova MY, Meyer RM, Brandy KR, Datta YH, Joseph MS, Schreiner PJ et al (2011) Risk factors for heart attack, stroke, and venous thrombosis associated with hormonal contraceptive use. Clin Appl Thromb Hemost 17(4):323–331
Ziller M, Ziller V, Haas G, Rex J, Kostev K (2014) Risk of venous thrombosis in users of hormonal contraceptives in German gynaecological practices: a patient database analysis. Arch Gynecol Obstet 289(2):413–419

References

Abrams T (2008) Letter to Reinhard Franzen, Bayer Healthcare Pharmaceuticals, Inc. Re: NDA #21-676, 21-873, 22-045. Yaz (drospirenone and ethinyl estradiol) Tablets. MACMIS ID # 16473. Warning Letter
Anonymous (1967) Risk of thromboembolic disease in women taking oral contraceptives. A preliminary communication to the Medical Research Council by a Subcommittee. Br Med J 2:355–359
Anonymous (1995) Effect of different progestagens in low oestrogen oral contraceptives on venous thromboembolic disease. World Health Organization collaborative study of cardiovascular disease and steroid hormone contraception. Lancet 346:1582–1588
Ashraf H (2002) UK high court dismisses risk of VTE in "pill" test case. Lancet 360:391
Berry DC, Raynor DK, Knapp P, Bersellini E (2002) Official warnings on thromboembolism risk with oral contraceptives fail to inform users adequately. Contraception 66:305–307
Bird ST, Delaney AC, Etmiman M, Brophy M, Hartzema AG (2013) Drospirenone and non-fatal venous thromboembolism: is there a risk difference by dosage of ethinyl-estradiol? J Thromb Haemost 11:1059–1068
Brynhildsen J (2014) Combined hormonal contraceptives: prescribing patterns, compliance, and benefits versus risks. Ther Adv Drug Saf 5:201–213
Child TJ, MacKenzie IZ, Rees M (1996) Terminations of pregnancy, not unplanned deliveries, increased as result of pill scare. BMJ 313:1005
de Bastos M, Stegeman BH, Rosendaal FR, Van Hylckama Vlieg A, Helmerhorst FM, Stijnen T, Dekkers OM (2014) Combined oral contraceptives: venous thrombosis. Cochrane Database Syst Rev (3):CD010813
de Vries CS, van den Berg PB, de Jong-van den Berg LT (1998) Oral contraceptive use before and after the latest pill scare in The Netherlands. Changes in oral contraceptive use and how users change. Contraception 57:247–249
Del Bono E, Francesconi M, Best NG (2011) Health information and health outcomes: an application of the regression discontinuity design to the 1995 UK contraceptive pill scare case, Institute for Social & Economic Research Working Paper Series 2011-16

Dhont M (2010) History of oral contraception. Eur J Contracept Reprod Health Care 15:S12–S18
Dinger J, Heinemann LAJ, Kuhl-Habich D (2007) The safety of a drospirenone-containing oral contraceptive: final results from the European Active Surveillance study on oral contraceptives based on 142,475 women-years of observation. Contraception 75:344–354
Dinger J, Assman A, Mohner S, Minh TD (2010) Risk of venous thromboembolism and the use of dienogest- and drospirenone-containing oral contraceptives: results from a German case-control study. J Fam Plann Reprod Health Care 36:123–129
Dinger J, Mohner S, Heinemann K (2016) Cardiovascular risks associated with the use of drospirenone-containing combined oral contraceptives. Contraception 93:378–385
Dukes MNG (2011) Side effects of drugs: third-generation oral contraceptives: time to look again? Side Effects of Drugs Annual 33:xli–xlvii
European Medicines Agency (2014) Benefits of combined hormonal contraceptives (CHCs) continue to outweigh risks
European Medicines Agency Pharmacovigilance Working Party (PhVWP) (2010) PhVWP discussions on safety concerns. YASMIN/YIRA (ethinylestradiol 30μg + drospirenone) – risk of venous thromboembolism (March 25, 2010 ed.)
European Medicines Agency Pharmacovigilance Working Party (PhVWP) (2011) Safety concerns. Ethinylestradiol + drospirenone-containing oral contraceptives (YASMIN, YASMINELLE and other products) – risk of venous thromboembolism
European Medicines Agency Pharmacovigilance Working Party (PhVWP) (2012) PhVWP Monthly report on safety concerns, guidelines and general matters. Ethinylestradiol + drospirenone-containing oral contraceptives (YASMIN, YASMINELLE and other products) – risk of venous thromboembolism
Farmer RD, Lawrenson RA, Thompson CR, Kennedy JG, Hambleton IR (1997) Population-based study of risk of venous thromboembolism associated with various oral contraceptives. Lancet 349:83–88
Flett G, Gurney E, McKessock L, Reid J (1998) Impact of the October 1995 pill scare in Grampian. Br J Fam Plann 24:18–20
Foran TM (2014) The newer contraceptive pills and venous thromboembolism risk. Med J Aust 200:376–377
Furedi A (1999) The public health implications of the 1995 'pill scare'. Hum Reprod Update 5:621–626
Gallo MF, Nanda K, Grimes DA, Lopez LM, Schulz KF (2011) 20 [micro]g versus >20 [micro] g estrogen combined oral contraceptives for contraception. Cochrane Database Syst Rev (4):CD003989
Geampana A (2016) Pregnancy is more dangerous than the pill: a critical analysis of professional responses to the Yaz/Yasmin controversy. Soc Sci Med 166:9–16
Greenhalgh T (1995) Making a scandal out of a scare – contraceptive pill scare. In: The times. UK
Gronich N, Lavi I, Rennert G (2011) Higher risk of venous thrombosis associated with drospirenone-containing oral contraceptives: a population-based cohort study. CMAJ 183:E1319–E1325
Haddad LB, Nour NM (2009) Unsafe abortion: unnecessary maternal mortality. Rev Obstet Gynecol 2:122–126
Han L, Jensen JT (2015) Does the progestogen used in combined hormonal contraception affect venous thrombosis risk? Obstet Gynecol Clin N Am 42:683
Hankin J (2003) Division of Drug Marketing, Advertising and Communications. US Food and Drug Administration. Letter to Nancy Konnerth, Berlex Laboratories. Re: NDA 21-098. Yasmin (drospirenone/ethinyl estradiol) Tablets, MACMIS ID#11730. July 10, 2003
Iversen OE, Nilsen ST (1996) The recent pill scare and number of legal abortions in Norway. Acta Obstet Gynecol Scand 75:690–691
Jick S (2015) Oral contraceptives and the risk of venous thromboembolism. In: Harrison-Woolrych M (ed) Medicines for women. Springer, Cham, pp 181–201
Jick S, Hernandez RK (2011) Risk of non-fatal venous thromboembolism in women using oral contraceptives containing drospirenone compared with women using oral contraceptives containing levonorgestrel: case-control study using United States claims data. BMJ 340:d2151

Jick H, Jick SS, Gurewich V, Myers MW, Vasilakis C (1995) Risk of idiopathic cardiovascular death and nonfatal venous thromboembolism in women using oral contraceptives with differing progestagen components. Lancet 346:1589–1593
Jick SS, Vasilakis C, Jick H (1998) Pregnancies and terminations after 1995 warning about third-generation oral contraceptives. Lancet 351:1404–1405
Jordan WM (1961) Pulmonary embolism. Lancet 2:1146
Kemmeren JM, Algra A, Grobbee DE (2001) Third generation oral contraceptives and risk of venous thrombosis: meta-analysis. Br Med J 323:131–U113
Kruvand M (2012) The pill at fifty: how The New York Times covered the birth control pill, 1960–2010. Am Journal 29:34–67
Lackie E, Fairchild A (2016) The birth control pill, thromboembolic disease, science and the media: a historical review of the relationship. Contraception 94:295–302
Laurance J (2012) Dramatic decline in teen pregnancies could be shortlived, campaigners fear. In: The independent. UK, 2012
Lewis MA (1999) The transnational study on oral contraceptives and the health of young women. Methods, results, new analyses and the healthy user effect. Hum Reprod Update 5:707–720
Lidegaard O, Lokkegaard E, Svendsen AL, Agger C (2009) Hormonal contraception and risk of venous thromboembolism: national follow-up study. Br Med J 339:b2890
Lidegaard O, Nielsen LH, Skovlund CW, Skjeldestad FE, Løkkegaard E (2011) Risk of venous thromboembolism from use of oral contraceptives containing different progestogens and oestrogen doses: Danish cohort study, 2001-9. BMJ 343:d6423
Loder E, Brizzell C, Godlee F (2015) Revisiting the commercial-academic interface in medical journals. BMJ 350:h2957
Lopez LM, Grimes DA, Gallo MF, Stockton LL, Schulz KF (2013) Skin patch and vaginal ring versus combined oral contraceptives for contraception. Cochrane Database Syst Rev (4):CD003552
Machado RB, Morimoto M, Santana N, Arruda LF, Bernardes CR, de Souza IM (2015) Effect of information on the perception of users and prospective users of combined oral contraceptives regarding the risk of venous thromboembolism. Gynecol Endocrinol 31:57–60
Martin RM, Hilton SR, Kerry SM (1997) The impact of the October 1995 'pill scare' on oral contraceptive use in the United Kingdom: analysis of a general practice automated database. Fam Pract 14:279–284
Martinez F, Ramirez I, Perez-Campos E, Latorre K, Lete I (2012) Venous and pulmonary thromboembolism and combined hormonal contraceptives. Systematic review and meta-analysis. Eu J Contracept Reprod Health Care 17:7–29
Milton C (1995) Clinics urge women not to panic – contraceptive 2011
Parkin L, Sharples K, Hernandez RK (2011) Risk of venous thromboembolism in users of oral contraceptives containing drospirenone or levonorgestrel: nested case-control study based on UK General Practice Research Database. BMJ 342:d2139
Pearce N (2008) Corporate influences on epidemiology. Int J Epidemiol 37:46–53
Pearce HM, Layton D, Wilton LV, Shakir SA (2005) Deep vein thrombosis and pulmonary embolism reported in the Prescription Event Monitoring Study of Yasmin. Br J Clin Pharmacol 60:98–102
Ramsay S (1996) UK "pill scare" led to abortion increase. Lancet 347:1109
Seaman B (1969) The doctor's case against the pill. Hunter House, Alameda
Seeger JD, Loughlin J, Eng PM, Clifford CR, Cutone J, Walker AM (2007) Risk of thromboembolism in women taking ethinylestradiol/drospirenone and other oral contraceptives. Obstet Gynecol 110:587–593
Shapiro S (2013) Combined hormonal contraceptives and the risk of venous and arterial thromboembolism and cardiovascular death: misuse of automated databases. J Fam Plann Reprod Health Care 39:89–96
Sidney S, Cheetham TC, Connell FA, Ouellet-Hellstrom R, Graham DJ, Davis D, Sorel M, Quesenberry CP Jr, Cooper WO (2013) Recent combined hormonal contraceptives (CHCs) and the risk of thromboembolism and other cardiovascular events in new users. Contraception 87:93–100

Skegg DCG (2000) Pitfalls of pharmacoepidemiology - oral contraceptive studies show a need for caution with databases. BMJ 321:1171–1172
Skjeldestad FE (1997) Increased number of induced abortions in Norway after media coverage of adverse vascular events from the use of third-generation oral contraceptives. Contraception 55:11–14
Society of Obstetricians and Gynaecologists of Canada (SOGC) (2013) Position Statement: hormonal contraception and the risks of venous thromboembolism
Spitzer WO (1997) The 1995 pill scare revisited: anatomy of a non-epidemic. Hum Reprod 12:2347–2357
Spitzer WO, Lewis MA, Heinemann LA, Thorogood M, MacRae KD (1996) Third generation oral contraceptives and risk of venous thromboembolic disorders: an international case-control study. Transnational Research Group on Oral Contraceptives and the Health of Young Women. BMJ 312:83–88
Suissa S, Spitzer WO, Rainville B, Cusson J, Lewis M, Heinemann L (2000) Recurrent use of newer oral contraceptives and the risk of venous thromboembolism. Hum Reprod 15: 817–821
Suissa S, Henry D, Caetano P, Dormuth CR, Ernst P, Hemmelgarn B, Lelorier J, Levy A, Martens PJ, Paterson JM, Platt RW, Sketris I, Teare G (2012) CNODES: the Canadian network for observational drug effect studies. Open Med 6:e134–e140
Toynbee P (1995) The pill is still a girl's best friend In: The independent. UK
Tricotel A, Collin C, Zureik M (2015) Impact of the sharp changes in the use of contraception in 2013 on the risk of pulmonary embolism in France. J Thromb Haemost 13:1576–1580
UK Committee on the Safety of Medicines (1995) Combined oral contraceptives and thromboembolism. London (Letter)
United Nations, Department of Economic and Social Affairs, Population Division (2015) Trends in contraceptive use worldwide 2015 (ST/ESA/SER.A/349)
US Food and Drug Administration (2012) FDA Drug Safety Communication: updated information about the risk of blood clots in women taking birth control pills containing drospirenone
van Hylckama Vlieg A, Helmerhorst FM, Vandenbroucke JP, Doggen CJ, Rosendaal FR (2009) The venous thrombotic risk of oral contraceptives, effects of oestrogen dose and progestogen type: results of the MEGA case-control study. BMJ 339:b2921
Veitch J (2001) Help me, there's a risk I'm going to die. In: The Scotsman, p. 4
Vinogradova Y, Coupland C, Hippisley-Cox J (2015) Use of combined oral contraceptives and risk of venous thromboembolism: nested case-control studies using the QResearch and CPRD databases. BMJ 350:h2135
Vlieg AV, Helmerhorst FM, Vandenbroucke JP, Doggen CJM, Rosendaal FR (2009) The venous thrombotic risk of oral contraceptives, effects of oestrogen dose and progestogen type: results of the MEGA case-control study. BMJ 339:b2921
World Health Organization (2017) WHO model list of essential medicines. 20th list. Geneva
World Health Organization Collaborative Study of Cardiovascular Disease and Steroid Hormone Contraception (1995) Venous thromboembolic disease and combined oral contraceptives: results of international multicentre case-control study. Lancet 346:1575–1582
Wu CQ, Grandi SM, Filion KB, Abenhaim HA, Joseph L, Eisenberg MJ (2013) Drospirenone-containing oral contraceptive pills and the risk of venous and arterial thrombosis: a systematic review. BJOG 120:801–811
Wu MH, Bartz D, Avorn J, Seeger JD (2016) Trends in direct-to-consumer advertising of prescription contraceptives. Contraception 93:398–405
Ziller M, Ziller V, Haas G, Rex J, Kostev K (2014) Risk of venous thrombosis in users of hormonal contraceptives in German gynaecological practices: a patient database analysis. Arch Gynecol Obstet 289:413–419

3 COX-2 Inhibitors: Communication of Accumulating Risk Evidence and a Product Withdrawal

Amy Rogers, Kerr Grieve, and Thomas M. MacDonald

Abstract

This chapter reflects on one of the biggest product withdrawals in pharmaceutical history, known as the "Vioxx story", and explores the discovery of cardiovascular risks with rofecoxib, the active substance in Vioxx®, and other COX-2 inhibitors, and the way that these risks were communicated to patients and healthcare professionals. It discusses specifically how evidence generation and communication are linked and how communication challenges arising from evidence accumulating over time demanded a need to frequently communicate to the public updated information. Examples from different countries and the impact on the World Health Organization's Essential Medicines List are presented. The chapter emphasises the link between the experiences of the Vioxx story and subsequent changes in the regulation of medicines in major jurisdictions, including legally mandated transparency of clinical studies. Ultimately, only with increased knowledge and communication about the safety of COX-2 inhibitors, patients can now be treated in the most effective and safe way.

A contribution from the author Sérgio Nishioka is included in this chapter as Appendix 3.1.

A. Rogers (✉) · K. Grieve · T. M. MacDonald
School of Medicine, Ninewells Hospital and Medical School, University of Dundee, Dundee, UK
e-mail: arogers@dundee.ac.uk

© Springer Nature Singapore Pte Ltd. 2020

P. Bahri (ed.), *Communicating about Risks and Safe Use of Medicines*,
https://doi.org/10.1007/978-981-15-3013-5_3

3.1 Situation: the Safety Concerns with COX-2 Inhibitors and Communication Challenges

When COX-2 selective anti-inflammatory agents were first introduced to the international market in 1999, they were seen by many as a new hope for the safe and effective treatment of chronic inflammatory conditions, such as rheumatoid arthritis or osteoarthritis (Feldman and McMahon 2000; Hawkey 1999; Lipsky 2001; Palmer 1999; Stuttaford 1999). A need for such a treatment option was increasingly apparent as data about gastrointestinal bleeding risks with older non-steroidal anti-inflammatory drugs (NSAIDs) accumulated (Hawkey 1990, 2000; Somerville et al. 1986).

The COX-2 inhibitors were designed to selectively target in the body the cyclooxygenase-2 enzyme (COX -2), an important facilitator in the production of prostaglandins, i.e., eicosanoid compounds that are critical mediators of pain and inflammation pathways. It was hoped that this selective action would be superior to older NSAIDs that act not only on cyclooxygenase -2, but also to inhibit cyclooxygenase-1 (COX-1). Although non-selective NSAIDs are beneficial anti-inflammatory and analgesic agents, through their inhibition of COX-2, the fact that they also act on COX-1 leads to greater risk of gastrointestinal bleeding because COX-1 activity is necessary for the production of prostaglandins with protective effects on the gastric mucosae.

This chapter explores and discusses the subsequent discovery of cardiovascular risks with the COX-2 inhibitors and the way that these risks were communicated to prescribers and patients. These substances remain effective tools in the control of chronic inflammatory conditions, but the shadow of the controversies around cardiovascular risks may mean that physicians and patients are reluctant to consider their use. Figure 3.1 lists some of the most commonly used non-steroidal anti-inflammatory agents that are discussed in this chapter.

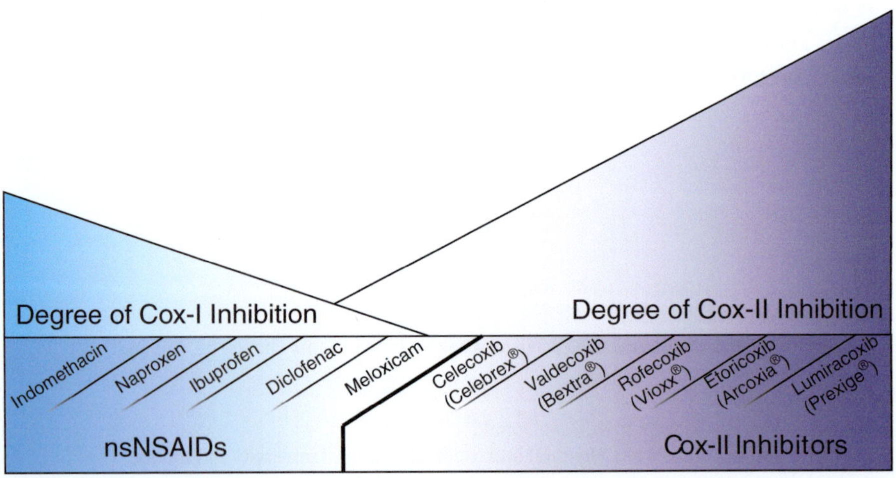

Fig. 3.1 Non-steroidal anti-inflammatory drugs and COX-2 selectivity (derived from Rao et al. 2008)

The Safety Concerns

Research into the pharmacological effects of COX-2 inhibitors suggested a plausible mechanism for promotion of blood clotting as early as 1999. COX-2 inhibitors had been demonstrated to have an unfavourable effect on the ratio of the eicosanoids, prostacyclin and thromboxane, which could potentially lead to promotion of thrombotic cardiovascular events (Bing and Lomnicka 2002; Krumholz et al. 2007). The Celecoxib Long-term Arthritis Safety Study (CLASS), comparing celecoxib with older NSAIDs for arthritis, had found beneficial reductions in gastrointestinal adverse effects without reporting any increase in cardiovascular events (Silverstein et al. 2000). However, concerns about the cardiovascular safety of COX-2 inhibitors began to be widely raised after the publication of the Vioxx Gastrointestinal Outcomes Research trial (VIGOR) in 2000. This study, by the manufacturer, compared rofecoxib (Vioxx®) against naproxen for the treatment of rheumatoid arthritis (Bombardier et al. 2000). The COX-2 inhibitor was associated with fewer gastrointestinal events, as anticipated. However, the authors reported a higher risk of myocardial infarction in the rofecoxib group despite similar overall mortality and efficacy (Bombardier et al. 2000). These early cardiovascular safety concerns led the US Food and Drug Administration (US FDA) to demand labelling changes for rofecoxib in the United States (US) in April 2002, urging caution in patients with a history of ischaemic heart disease and also stating that patients on anti-thrombo embolic medication such as acetylsalicylic acid (Aspirin®) should not discontinue anti-thrombo embolic medication (Yates and Merck and Co 2002). The European Medicines Agency (EMA, then called the European Agency for the Evaluation of Medicinal Products (EMEA)) completed its first review of the cardiovascular safety of all COX-2 inhibitors in November 2003 as part of a comprehensive safety review including also gastrointestinal, hypersensitivity and skin concerns. The EMA report concluded that the benefits of this class of medicines outweighed the risks but recommended caution in patients with a medical history of ischaemic heart disease or at high risk of gastrointestinal bleeding. Prescribers were reminded that COX-2 inhibitors should not be considered a substitute for acetylsalicylic acid for the secondary prevention of cardiovascular thrombo-embolic diseases. Changes to the product information across the European Union (EU) were demanded accordingly (European Medicines Agency 2004a).

In 2004, a trial aiming to support the hypothesis that COX-2 inhibitors may prevent colorectal tumours was halted early due to an excess of cardiovascular events in the active treatment group. This Adenomatous Polyp Prevention on Vioxx trial (APPROVe) followed up subjects treated with rofecoxib (Vioxx). While the active treatment group did suffer half the number of gastrointestinal adverse events relative to the placebo group, myocardial infarction risk was greatly increased with a reported relative risk of 5.0 (Baron et al. 2006). The manufacturer approached the US FDA in September 2004 and withdrew their product Vioxx from the market voluntarily on 30 September 2004 (Merck 2004; FDA US Food and Drug Administration 2004). This action by the manufacturer was not anticipated by regulators worldwide who issued press statements in reaction to the withdrawal, for example, in Asia, Australia, and Europe (IHS Global Insight Inc 2004; European Medicines Agency 2004b; Therapeutic Goods Administration 2004).

Another trial of a COX-2 inhibitor for prevention of bowel tumours, the Adenoma Prevention with Celecoxib trial (APC) published in March 2005, gave strength to calls for a new evaluation of possible COX-2 inhibitor class effects on cardiovascular risk. The APC investigators reported a dose-related increase in cardiovascular adverse events associated with celecoxib (Solomon et al. 2005).

The concerns about the cardiovascular safety of COX-2 inhibitors led to increased suspicions that the older non-selective NSAIDs may also be associated with risk of heart attack and stroke. Since 2005, the US FDA has mandated boxed warnings on the labels of all NSAIDs, warning of potential cardiovascular risks based upon data submitted for regulatory and new drug application purposes (Postmarket Drug Safety Information for Patients and Providers 2016). In 2006, the EMA reported that new data had highlighted a small increased risk in high dose non-selective NSAID use of long duration (European Medicines Agency 2006). As data continued to accumulate, including the research of the Safety of Non-Steroidal Anti-Inflammatory Drugs project (SOS) led by the ERASMUS University in Rotterdam, the EMA conducted an EU-wide review of the safety of NSAIDs in 2011/12 (European Commission 2015). This review suggested that diclofenac, a widely used non-selective NSAID, may carry the same increased cardiovascular risk as had been demonstrated in COX-2 inhibitors. A specific review of diclofenac followed at the request of the Medicines and Healthcare products Regulatory Agency (MHRA) of the United Kingdom (UK). The resulting EMA report advised that, in the EU, the product information of diclofenac should be strengthened similarly to that required for the remaining COX-2 inhibitors (European Medicines Agency 2013). The FDA ruled to strengthen the existing labelling of NSAIDs (except for acetylsalicylic acid) in July 2015 to highlight the now apparent cardiovascular risks associated with their use (FDA US Food and Drug Administration 2015).

It has been suggested that many of the adverse events seen in the original COX-2 inhibitors trials described above may have been due to the use of higher than usual doses. Observational studies have suggested that people using lower doses of rofecoxib and celecoxib are at no higher risk of serious heart disease than those taking other NSAIDs that are now considered to be safe (Ray et al. 2002, 2009).

What started as a new hope for chronic arthritis sufferers had developed from concerns about the safety of a single new medicine to suspicion over the safety profile of an entire product class with implications for prescribers and patients worldwide. Concerns around the withdrawal of rofecoxib and the subsequent re-examination of non-selective NSAIDs fed into discussions already underway between parties worldwide with an interest in improving safety (Tsintis and La Mache 2004).

The Communication Challenges

After the release of rofecoxib (Vioxx) to the market in 1999, heavy marketing and fears about the gastrointestinal risks of non-selective NSAIDs had resulted in approximately 80 million people worldwide having taken COX-2 inhibitors. In

England and Wales alone rofecoxib accounted for 2.1 million dispensed prescriptions in 2003 (Sukkar 2014). The abrupt withdrawal of Vioxx was one of the largest medicinal product withdrawals from the market with huge financial implications for its manufacturer. NSAIDs overall remain one of the most widely used categories of medication worldwide, both prescribed and over-the-counter (McGettigan and Henry 2013).

The associate director of the US FDA Office of Drug Safety at the time of the Vioxx withdrawal, David Graham, suggested that between 88,000 and 138,000 additional heart attacks and sudden cardiac deaths in the US might have been attributable to rofecoxib. Although disputed, the magnitude of these numbers implied a major public health concern. In contrast, the absolute risk of a person taking rofecoxib and therefore suffering a heart attack remained relatively small (Greener 2008).

It has been suggested that the withdrawal of the product and the litigation that followed led to a major loss of public confidence in not only pharmaceutical manufacturers but also in the regulatory framework that governs their actions. Questions were raised about the strength of marketing authorisation processes with suggestions that regulators were too close to manufacturers. Companies themselves have faced greater scrutiny after suggestions that the manufacturer should have acted sooner to withdraw rofecoxib from the market. Since news of the withdrawal broke in the global news media, there have been calls for greater transparency in trials and clearer requirements for post-authorisation surveillance of safety (Eichler et al. 2013; Goldacre et al. 2016).

The task of informing the public and healthcare professionals about the withdrawal of rofecoxib was in itself relatively straightforward. Communicating the subtler concept of absolute risk versus benefit for individual patients has proven more challenging. All medicines, by their nature, in taking effect on the body, have the potential to cause harmful side effects. It is essential that this potential risk is balanced against the potential benefits of effective treatments. Some commentators feel that the pendulum has swung too far in favour of minimising risk at the expense of patients' needs for effective treatments (Eichler et al. 2013). In minimising risks, access to potentially beneficial treatments may be restricted without giving patients the chance to choose how much risk they are personally willing to accept in pursuit of effective treatment.

The ideal anti-inflammatory agent would be 100% effective at relieving pain and improving function in 100% of people with no risk of adverse effects such as gastrointestinal bleeding, cardiovascular events or any other adverse reactions. In reality, each active substance and its effects in each patient will lie somewhere in between this ideal and the other extreme where the patient does not respond at all to the treatment but still experiences adverse reactions. The challenge for prescribers is, in the context of shared informed therapeutic decision-making with patients (see Chap. 16), to try and determine how risky a medicine is for a particular patient, and to allow that patient to choose whether they are willing to take the risk based upon their own values and priorities. Figure 3.2 illustrates the factors that affect each individual case.

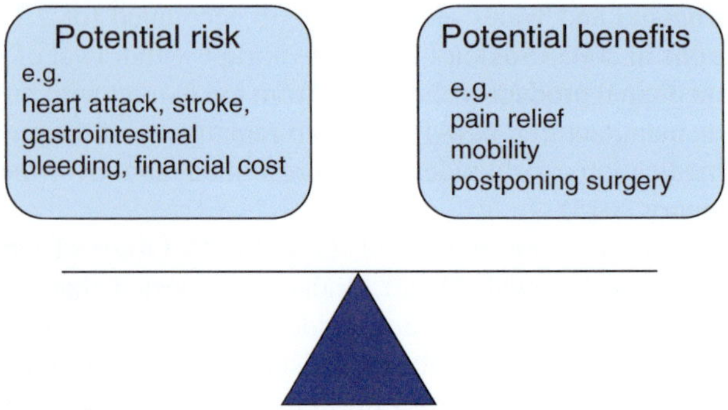

Fig. 3.2 Benefit–risk balance in therapeutic decision-making for individual patients

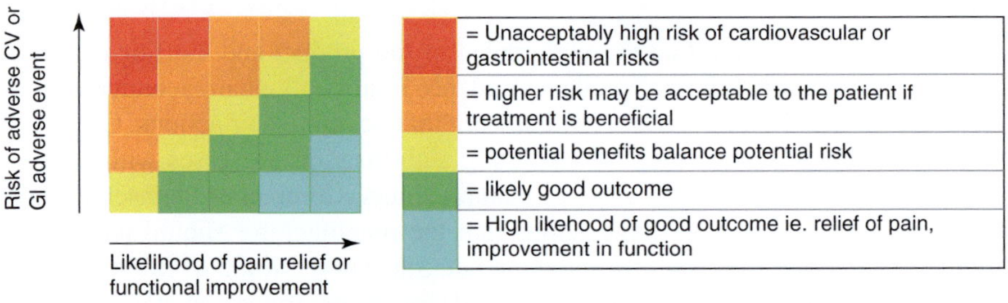

Fig. 3.3 Benefit–risk analysis in therapeutic decision-making for individual patients

Figure 3.3 shows a simplified representation of the risk–benefit analysis inherent in any such prescribing decision.

In the case of COX-2 inhibitors and other NSAIDs, many agents fall within the middle range where the ultimate decision of whether to prescribe needs to take individual patient preferences about potential risk and benefit into account. Gerd Gigerenzer, David Spiegelhalter and others have introduced and promoted the concept of risk literacy (Gigerenzer 2013; Spiegelhalter 2008; Spiegelhalter et al. 2011). They argue that in order to effectively communicate the complex interplay of risk and benefit, the audience needs to have an understanding of probability. Education of healthcare professionals and patients may be necessary before messages about risk and, given limited available evidence, uncertainty can be effectively communicated. Advances in information technology have meant that physicians in the UK can use internet-based risk calculators, such as the JBS3 calculator (for the estimation of cardiovascular risk) or the optiongrid.org (a generic tool), and patient information websites, such as patient.info, to facilitate conversations about risk. These resources use a combination of numerical, text and pictorial representations of risk that may be easier for patients, and doctors, to understand (Boon et al. 2014; Greenhalgh 2013; Joint British Societies for the Prevention of Cardiovascular Disease 2014; Option Grid 2015; Kenny and Newson 2016).

Further large scale safety research involving different patient groups will, hopefully, assist in more precisely estimating individual patient risks associated with NSAIDs. One concept that has been proposed as potentially useful in assisting decisions about which treatment is best for a risk literate patient is n-of-1 trials (Madhok and Fahey 2005). N-of-1 trials in clinical medicine are multiple, randomised, double blinded, crossover comparisons of alternative treatments conducted within a single patient. This experimental approach allows prescribers and patients to determine which treatment is most effective at controlling an individual's symptoms through structured trials of therapy, including placebos if appropriate, to clarify the benefit side of the risk–benefit equation.

Evidence to aid decision-making is accruing all the time. The Standard Care Versus Celecoxib Outcome Trial (SCOT), comparing cardiovascular and gastrointestinal outcomes for older arthritis patients with no history of cardiovascular disease, randomised participants to either celecoxib or a non-selective NSAID. The researchers found no significant difference in the cardiovascular event rate between the study arms. The low overall event rate in the study suggested that all such agents were reasonably safe with varying effectiveness and tolerability (MacDonald et al. 2016). The Prospective Randomized Evaluation of Celecoxib Integrated Safety Versus Ibuprofen Or Naproxen trial (PRECISION), published in November 2016, provided further information on the safety of these agents in patients with chronic arthritis and higher cardiovascular risk. Participants taking moderate doses of celecoxib in this study were not found to be at increased risk of cardiovascular events when compared to participants taking either naproxen or ibuprofen (Becker et al. 2009). Ultimately, truly informed prescribing decisions occur only when patient preference is combined with high quality safety and effectiveness data.

3.2 Events: the Communication Experiences

There are two main aspects of risk communication in the story about COX-2 inhibitors: the abrupt withdrawal of rofecoxib (Vioxx) from the market, and ongoing uncertainties about the cardiovascular risks of all NSAIDs. The following paragraphs will comment on the risk communication efforts in the UK. This necessarily concentrates on the main English language communications from the UK and US.

Communications regarding rofecoxib withdrawal in the UK required to be targeted at two main groups. Prescribers, who largely relied upon national prescribing guidance issued by authorities such as the MHRA and subsequent discussion in medical journals and magazines, were relatively easy to reach through these well-established channels. In contrast, the public needed to be informed promptly and without causing undue alarm. The press and broadcast media very quickly reported news of the withdrawal with reliance on the medical authorities to provide advice to their audiences (BBC 2004).

Prior to the withdrawal, UK newspaper coverage of rofecoxib was largely positive. Only close followers of the financial pages would have picked up on reports that manufacturers were not achieving the profits they had hoped for on the back of their new blockbuster arthritis drug, Vioxx, and the failure to launch its sister product Arcoxia® (etoricoxib) in the US (Kahn 2002). In 2002, The Times (London) reported that the EMA had been asked by the French authorities to investigate possible heart attack risks with rofecoxib. With some scepticism, the Times report concluded that "this result alone does not condemn the newer drug" (Hawkes 2002).

The abrupt withdrawal from the market of rofecoxib was reported by the UK press on 1 October 2004. This was a major story with front page coverage and numerous commentaries. Various agencies were called upon to advise readers, with reference to the Royal College of General Practitioners stating that there was "no cause for alarm, speak to a local pharmacist" and Arthritis Care, a charity, advising patients "not to panic" (BBC 2004). Although the coverage in the broadsheets was largely measured, some tabloid coverage appeared to be stoking public concern with prominent warnings of "DOUBLE risk of heart attacks" and "STOP giving it to patients" (Peake 2004). The UK health authorities braced themselves to deal with an onslaught of worried patients, issuing guidance through the MHRA to all prescribers and briefing the National Health Service (NHS) direct helpline (Lister 2004).

In October 2004, the newspapers The Times and The Independent (London) both reported on articles published in the medical press alleging failure of industry and regulators to conduct the necessary trials to ensure safety of new medicines. Regulators were accused of "astonishing complacency" as the US FDA was asserted to have suppressed unfavourable internal research (Graham 2004; Laurance 2004).

In December 2004, the press reported that the MHRA had issued interim guidance to prescribers advising that patients should be switched from COX-2 inhibitors after the APC trial was stopped early due to increased risk of heart attacks with Celebrex® (celecoxib) (Boseley 2004; Hall 2004).

A study conducted in the US following the later withdrawal of valdecoxib in 2005 found that several standard sources of information to prescribers took an average of 109.8 days to change their advice regarding the medication. This highlights the need for regulators to communicate directly with physicians to ensure timely change in prescribing behaviour. Information technology systems with automated alerts may be an efficient way of achieving this (Strayer et al. 2006).

The Vioxx withdrawal was a worldwide event and every country will have had its own unique communication challenges. Appendix 3.1 describes how matters were handled in Brazil as a further example.

The large scale regulatory changes and follow-up recommendations regarding the safety of all NSAIDs continued to be communicated efficiently through existing channels. Many physicians, however, feel that the real communication challenge lies in interactions between individual prescribers and patients as they make decisions about which treatments to choose amid continuing uncertainty about the risk that those treatments might pose to individuals.

3.3 Evaluation: Feedback, Outcomes and Lessons Learnt

Feedback

The communication of the immediate risk situation with rofecoxib was quickly and efficiently achieved through existing prescribing guidance channels. However, experience of the Vioxx withdrawal highlighted a desire by physicians and the general public for greater transparency and accountability surrounding new approvals of medicines and emerging safety concerns. Communicating issues of complex scientific uncertainty around class effects as more and more observational and interventional evidence has accumulated over time, has proven more challenging (European Medicines Agency 2014).

Outcomes

The final stage in risk communication is influencing behaviour. The complete withdrawal of rofecoxib left patients with no option but to stop this medication. This, of course, removed the potential harm, but there are other considerations. Faced with the removal of this treatment option and possible COX-2 inhibitors class effects, prescribers and patients had to choose whether to switch to another treatment with its own risks, or to remove analgesic treatment altogether.

An observational study from the Netherlands published in 2008 found that users of COX-2 inhibitors (including those not taking rofecoxib) were four times more likely to discontinue all prescribed analgesic medication compared with a similar group before the Vioxx withdrawal. This raises the suggestion that patients and prescribers may have feared a medicines class effect and that some patients may have been left undertreated. Those patients who did switch to an alternative analgesic largely moved to non-selective NSAIDs. 37% of rofecoxib users switched to a non-selective NSAID without additional gastro-protective medication, thus increasing their exposure to the risk of gastrointestinal bleeding. It was noted in this study that generalists such as family practitioners and internists were far more likely to avoid COX-2 inhibitors altogether when deciding on alternative treatment. Prescribing of opiates for chronic musculoskeletal pain also increased as such agents were used as alternatives to NSAIDs (Sukel et al. 2008).

Looking at the longer-term impact, a study published in 2013 found that diclofenac remained the most widely used NSAID despite evidence that it is associated with higher cardiovascular risks than other non-selective NSAIDs. In contrast, naproxen, thought to be one of the safest NSAIDs, claimed only a 10% market share across sampled countries. These findings were evident in high-, middle- and low-income countries. The authors suggested that although the absolute cardiovascular risk of diclofenac in many patients would be low, the use of this active substance in patients at higher risk may have contributed to over 14,000 excess cardiovascular deaths in China alone (McGettigan and Henry 2013). Since the publication of the paper, diclofenac has been removed from the World Health Organization Model List of Essential Medicines (EML). It is hoped that this will result in less risky prescribing patterns in low-income countries.

Recent prescription data from England demonstrated a reduction in diclofenac prescribing from 33% of prescribed NSAID items in January 2011 to just 9% in January 2015. Naproxen had a corresponding increase from 20% of items in 2011 to 55%, suggesting that the message has been getting through to prescribers and has resulted in behaviour change (EBM DataLab 2017).

Lessons Learnt
Communications with healthcare professionals, patients and the public need to be based upon robust evidence. A balance must be struck between the need for effective treatment choices and any potential risks of those treatments. Good quality and timely safety and effectiveness research will be essential in supplying the evidence required by those authorities that are responsible for protecting public health.

The relatively small absolute risk of cardiovascular adverse events found with rofecoxib meant that, unless a trial was specifically designed to assess cardiovascular safety, it would be unlikely to differentiate between commonly occurring events and those potentially caused by the study drug. Traditional phase III studies, powered to detect differences in primary effectiveness outcomes, cannot be relied upon to detect increases in already prevalent conditions, such as heart attacks. This highlights the need for improved methods of safety monitoring with an emphasis on post-authorisation surveillance and trials, which has led to an emerging role for regulatory authorities worldwide.

In response to criticism, regulators have made efforts to strengthen their frameworks for the conduct and reporting of clinical trials. The US Food and Drug Administration Amendments Act (FDAAA) of 2007 (FDA US Food and Drug Administration 2007), the EU Clinical Trials Directive of 2001 and now the EU Clinical Trials Regulation of 2014 (overwriting the Directive) (European Commission 2016) aim to promote safety of patients and strengthen the transparency of trial data. Clinical trials registers have been set up by the US National Institutes of Health (clinicaltrials.gov) and by the EMA (EudraCT). Regulators, at least those with stringent systems, now have legal powers to demand the conduct of post-authorisation safety studies and other risk management activities by manufacturers. This process of regulatory improvement is ongoing, with such developments as the European Network of Centres for Pharmacoepidemiology and Pharmacovigilance (ENCePP), a network established by the EMA for building independent research capacity to investigate safety and effectiveness of medicines, inviting voluntary participation of applicable centres (European Network of Centres for Pharmacoepidemiology and Pharmacovigilance (ENCEPP) 2020). Other endeavours such as opentrials.net and the Yale University Open Data Access project (YODA) have offered new ways to facilitate the sharing of trial data (Goldacre et al. 2016; Krumholz and Waldstreicher 2016).

It seems inevitable that medicinal product withdrawals will occur in the future as post-authorisation systems monitor medicines use in large, undifferentiated populations. The evolving assessment of risk requires that communication with patients and prescribers is done in a manner that promotes understanding of the inherent uncertainty in science, risk assessments and individual prescribing decisions, while maintaining confidence in medicines supply and regulatory rigour. Multidisciplinary methods to research and optimise communication are therefore needed (see Chap. 1). The developing story of COX-2 inhibitors and their safety profiles has undoubtedly impacted upon the current approach to pharmacovigilance and research. Ultimately, with better established knowledge and communication about the safety of these medicines, the COX-2 inhibitors can continue be effective agents for treating patients.

Conclusions

- Selective COX-2 inhibitors were marketed worldwide in the late 1990s and early 2000s as a safer alternative to older non-selective non-steroidal anti-inflammatory drugs (NSAIDs).
- Clinical trial data that emerged after marketing authorisation suggested that some COX-2 inhibitors might carry an increased risk of major cardiovascular events when compared with non-selective NSAIDs.
- The resulting abrupt withdrawal of the COX-2 inhibitor rofecoxib (Vioxx®) from sale by the marketing authorisation holder, i.e., the pharmaceutical company, in September 2004 necessitated a fast response in terms of assessment and communication from medicines regulators worldwide.
- The challenges of the "Vioxx story" have led to welcome change in medicines regulation and transparency alongside increasing awareness by healthcare professionals of the need to consider potential risks and benefits in the context of each individual patient.
- Medicines safety and its communication is a complex and evolving issue that should be discussed openly between companies, regulators, healthcare professionals and patients.

Appendix 3.1: Safety Evaluation and Communication About COX-2 Inhibitors—Experiences in Brazil at the Time of the Rofecoxib Withdrawal in 2004

Sérgio Nishioka

The withdrawal of rofecoxib (Vioxx®) from the US market in 2004 made its impact on clinical practice and on media headlines everywhere including in Brazil. As a consequence, the Brazilian medicines regulatory authority Anvisa decided to re-evaluate the safety of all COX-2 inhibitors already marketed in Brazil. By mid-February 2005 Anvisa's advisory committee CATEME had made general recommendations regarding the safety information in the package inserts in line with what other regulatory authorities were recommending at the time. A few remaining points were to be discussed in an ordinary meeting of that advisory committee scheduled for mid-April. Because it was felt to be an important issue, the local press was following up on this issue.

In early April 2005 the US Food and Drug Administration (US FDA) announced having requested the manufacturer Pfizer to voluntarily withdraw from the US market its COX-2 inhibitor valdecoxib (Bextra®). The European Medicines Agency and Health Canada took similar steps and Pfizer informed Anvisa accordingly. Anvisa decided to temporarily suspend the marketing of Bextra® in line with action taken by other authorities, but in Brazil there was an additional issue to deal with, different from elsewhere.

In 2003, the manufacturer Pharmacia, before its merger with Pfizer, had in its portfolio a COX-2 inhibitor, parecoxib, for parenteral use, which is a prodrug metabolised to valdecoxib. In Brazil only, perhaps because of the timing of registration, Pfizer registered parecoxib as Bextra IM/IV®, in order to support keeping patients who might have been prescribed parecoxib for perioperative pain control on oral valdecoxib thereafter, instead of switching to another analgesic. Parecoxib had been marketed in Europe and elsewhere under a different trade name, Dynastat®. Because both valdecoxib and parecoxib were marketed as Bextra® in Brazil, Anvisa decided that the temporary suspension of valdecoxib should also be applicable to parecoxib. Anvisa concluded that it would be difficult to communicate and make understandable to the public why one formulation of the same tradename would be kept on the market whereas the other would be withdrawn, even if only temporarily, considering that this would unnecessarily confuse the public. Five months later the evaluation was finalised; the marketing suspension of parecoxib was withdrawn while it remained valid for valdecoxib.

This is an example where a regulatory decision took into account the possible confusion through communication that might have been created on a very sensitive issue if only scientific rationales and actions by other regulatory authorities had been considered. The manufacturer in Brazil accepted this approach, and Anvisa, supported by CATEME, explained timely on its website every step taken. This facilitated the communication with the press and passed the image that CATEME had full control of the subject. During this time period, there was no major questioning by the Brazilian press of how Anvisa managed the case.

References

Baron JA, Sandler RS, Bresalier RS, Quan H, Riddell R, Lanas A, Bolognese JA, Oxenius B, Horgan K, Loftus S, Morton DG (2006) A randomized trial of rofecoxib for the chemoprevention of colorectal adenomas. Gastroenterology 131:1674–1682. https://doi.org/10.1053/j.gastro.2006.08.079

BBC (2004) Arthritis drug removed for safety. http://news.bbc.co.uk/1/hi/health/3704640.stm

Becker MC, Wang TH, Wisniewski L, Wolski K, Libby P, Luscher TF, Borer JS, Mascette AM, Husni ME, Solomon DH, Graham DY, Yeomans ND, Krum H, Ruschitzka F, Lincoff AM, Nissen SE (2009) Rationale, design, and governance of Prospective Randomized Evaluation of Celecoxib Integrated Safety versus Ibuprofen Or Naproxen (PRECISION), a cardiovascular end point trial of nonsteroidal antiinflammatory agents in patients with arthritis. Am Heart J 157:606–612. https://doi.org/10.1016/j.ahj.2008.12.014

Bing RJ, Lomnicka M (2002) Why do cyclo-oxygenase-2 inhibitors cause cardiovascular events? J Am Coll Cardiol 39:521–522. https://doi.org/10.1016/S0735-1097(01)01749-1

Bombardier C, Laine L, Reicin A, Shapiro D, Burgos-Vargas R, Davis B, Day R, Ferraz MB, Hawkey CJ, Hochberg MC, Kvien TK, Schnitzer TJ (2000) Comparison of upper gastrointestinal toxicity of rofecoxib and naproxen in patients with rheumatoid arthritis. VIGOR Study Group. N. Engl. J. Med. 343:1520–1528. https://doi.org/10.1056/nejm200011233432103

Boon N, Boyle R, Bradbury K, Buckley J, Connolly S, Craig S, Deanfield J, Doherty P, Feher M, Fox K, Goldsmith D, Grant P, Hingorani A, Hobbs R, Home P, Jackson S, Jennings C, Keenan J, Kirby M, Knapton M, Lovelidge L, Neely D, Pearson M, Potter J, Poulter N, Preiss D, Rees A, Sattar N, Simpson I, Sivers F, Spiegelhalter D, Stansby G, Stevens P, Taal M, Taylor C, Taylor PC, Weissberg P, Wheeler D, Wilding J, Williams B, Winocour P, Wood D (2014) Joint British Societies' consensus recommendations for the prevention of cardiovascular disease (JBS3). Heart 100:ii1–ii67. https://doi.org/10.1136/heartjnl-2014-305693

Boseley S (2004) Doctors told to stop using painkiller. The Guardian, 1–2

EBM DataLab (2017) OpenPrescribing.net, University of Oxford

Eichler HG, Bloechl-Daum B, Brasseur D, Breckenridge A, Leufkens H, Raine J, Salmonson T, Schneider CK, Rasi G (2013) The risks of risk aversion in drug regulation. Nat Rev Drug Discov 12:907–916. https://doi.org/10.1038/nrd4129

European Commission (2015) CORDIS: publications: final report—SOS (safety of non-steroidal anti-inflammatory drugs). http://cordis.europa.eu/publication/rcn/14115_en.html

European Commission (2016) Clinical trials—general information. http://ec.europa.eu/health/human-use/clinical-trials/information/index_en.htm#ct1

European Medicines Agency (2004a) Committee for Proprietary Medicinal Products (CPMP) opinion following an Article 31 referral for all medicinal products containing Celecoxib, Etoricoxib, Parecoxib, Rofecoxib or Valdecoxib. In: European Medicines Agency. https://www.ema.europa.eu/en/documents/referral/opinion-following-article-31-referral-all-medicinal-products-containing-celecoxib-etoricoxib_en-1.pdf. Accessed 4 Mar 2020

European Medicines Agency (2004b) Press release: EMEA statement following withdrawal of Vioxx (rofecoxib)

European Medicines Agency (2006) Public CHMP assessment report for medicinal products containing non-selective non steroidal anti-inflammatory drugs (NSAIDs). European Medicines Agency, London. http://www.ema.europa.eu

European Medicines Agency (2013) New safety advice for diclofenac. http://www.ema.europa.eu/docs/en_GB/document_library/Referrals_document/Diclofenac-containing_medicinal_products/European_Commission_final_decision/WC500155819.pdf

European Medicines Agency (2014) Benefit-risk communication to medicines users—How can regulators best meet the information needs of patients and healthcare professionals? Workshop report. http://www.ema.europa.eu/docs/en_GB/document_library/Report/2014/12/WC500178511.pdf

European Network of Centres for Pharmacoepidemiology and Pharmacovigilance (ENCEPP) (2020). http://www.encepp.eu

FDA US Food and Drug Administration (2004) Vioxx (rofecoxib) questions and answers. http://www.fda.gov/drugs/drugsafety/postmarketdrugsafetyinformationforpatientsandproviders/ucm106290.htm

FDA US Food and Drug Administration (2007) Regulatory information—full text of FDAAA law. www.fda.gov; http://www.fda.gov/RegulatoryInformation/Legislation/SignificantAmendmentstotheFDCAct/FoodandDrugAdministrationAmendmentsActof2007/FullTextofFDAAALaw/default.htm. Accessed 8 Nov 2016

FDA US Food and Drug Administration (2015) FDA strengthens warning that non-aspirin nonsteroidal anti-inflammatory drugs (NSAIDs) can cause heart attacks or strokes. US Food and Drug Administration. http://www.fda.gov/downloads/Drugs/DrugSafety/UCM453941.pdf

Feldman M, McMahon AT (2000) Do cyclooxygenase-2 inhibitors provide benefits similar to those of traditional nonsteroidal anti-inflammatory drugs, with less gastrointestinal toxicity? Ann Intern Med 132:134. https://doi.org/10.7326/0003-4819-132-2-200001180-00008

Gigerenzer G (2013) Risk literacy: Gerd Gigerenzer at TEDxZurich. https://www.youtube.com/watch?v=g4op2WNc1e4

Goldacre B, Gray J, Schmucker C, Goldacre B, O'Connor AB, Chan AW, Mathieu S, Boutron I, Moher D, Altman DG, Ravaud P, Chalmers I, Altman DG, Altman DG, Furberg CD, Grimshaw JM, Shanahan DR, Moja LP, Pfiffner PB, Oh J, Miller TA, Mandl KD, Wieseler B, Hartung DM, Boutron I, Dutton S, Ravaud P, Altman DG, Doshi P, Jefferson T, Mar C, Ip S, Jefferson T, Zarin DA, Tse T, Williams RJ, Califf RM, Ide NC, Huser V, Cimino JJ, Fecher B, Friesike S, Hebing M, Gray J, Davies TG (2016) OpenTrials: towards a collaborative open database of all available information on all clinical trials. Trials 17:164. https://doi.org/10.1186/s13063-016-1290-8

Graham D (2004) US officials' knew of Vioxx threat. The Times, 1–2

Greener M (2008) First do no harm. Improving drug safety through legislation and independent research. EMBO Rep 9:221–224. https://doi.org/10.1038/embor.2008.17

Greenhalgh T (2013) Option grids: an idea whose time has come? Br J Gen Pract 63:147–147. https://doi.org/10.3399/bjgp13X664315

Hall C (2004) Painkiller warning to arthritis sufferers. The Daily Telegraph, 22–23

Hawkes N (2002) Bestselling drugs face heart attack investigation. The Times, 4

Hawkey CJ (1990) Non-steroidal anti-inflammatory drugs and peptic ulcers. Brit Med J 300:278–284. http://www.ncbi.nlm.nih.gov/pubmed/2106956

Hawkey CJ (1999) COX-2 inhibitors. Lancet 353:307–314. https://doi.org/10.1016/S0140-6736(98)12154-2

Hawkey CJ (2000) Outcomes studies of drug induced ulcer complications: do we need them and how should they be done? Brit Med J 321:291–293. http://www.ncbi.nlm.nih.gov/pubmed/10915140

IHS Global Insight Inc (2004, October 13) Government of India to ban rofecoxib generics. Retrieved from Nexis Database. https://advance.lexis.com/api/permalink/39de5484-3b80-4825-aba2-f27c9f948a42/?context=1519360. Accessed 4 Mar 2020

Joint British Societies for the Prevention of Cardiovascular Disease (2014) JBS3 risk calculator. http://www.jbs3risk.com/

Kahn S (2002) City and business. The Express, 100

Kenny T, Newson L (2016) http://patient.info/health/absolute-risk-and-relative-risk

Krumholz HM, Waldstreicher J (2016) The Yale Open Data Access (YODA) project—a mechanism for data sharing. N Engl J Med 375:403–405. https://doi.org/10.1056/NEJMp1607342

Krumholz HM, Ross JS, Presler AH, Egilman DS (2007) What have we learnt from Vioxx? Brit Med J 334:120–123. https://doi.org/10.1136/bmj.39024.487720.68

Laurance J (2004) Drug giants "ignored dangers of painkiller in pursuit of profits" The Independent, 20

Lipsky PE (2001) Introduction. The role of COX-2-specific inhibitors in clinical practice. Am. J. Med. 110(Suppl 3A):1S–2S. https://www.ncbi.nlm.nih.gov/pubmed/11173042

Lister S (2004) Arthritis drugs check after Vioxx alert. The Times, 2

MacDonald TM, Hawkey CJ, Ford I, McMurray JJV, Scheiman JM, Hallas J, Findlay E, Grobbee DE, Hobbs FDR, Ralston SH, Reid DM, Walters MR, Webster J, Ruschitzka F, Ritchie

LD, Perez-Gutthann S, Connolly E, Greenlaw N, Wilson A, Wei L, Mackenzie IS (2016) Randomized trial of switching from prescribed non-selective non-steroidal anti-inflammatory drugs to prescribed celecoxib: the Standard care vs. Celecoxib Outcome Trial (SCOT). Eur Heart J. https://doi.org/10.1093/eurheartj/ehw387

Madhok V, Fahey T (2005) N-of-1 trials: an opportunity to tailor treatment in individual patients. Br J Gen Pract 55:171–172

McGettigan P, Henry D (2013) Use of non-steroidal anti-inflammatory drugs that elevate cardiovascular risk: an examination of sales and essential medicines lists in low-, middle-, and high-income countries. PLoS Med 10:e1001388. https://doi.org/10.1371/journal.pmed.1001388

Merck (2004) Press release: Merck announces voluntary worldwide withdrawal of VIOXX. http://www.pbm.va.gov/vacenterformedicationsafety/vioxx/DearHealthcareProfessional.pdf

Option Grid (2015). http://optiongrid.org/. Accessed 8 Nov 2016

Palmer J (1999) Family health: arthritis drug breakthrough. The Mirror, 38

Peake A (2004) Painkiller axed. The Sun

Postmarket Drug Safety Information for Patients and Providers (2016) COX-2 selective (includes Bextra, Celebrex, and Vioxx) and non-selective non-steroidal anti-inflammatory drugs (NSAIDs). http://www.fda.gov/Drugs/DrugSafety/PostmarketDrugSafetyInformationforPatientsandProviders/ucm429364.htm

Rao PNP, Knaus EE, Road TP, Jolla L (2008) Evolution of nonsteroidal anti-inflammatory cyclo-oxygenase (COX) inhibition and beyond drugs (NSAIDs). J Pharm Pharm Sci 11:81–110

Ray WA, Stein CM, Daugherty JR, Hall K, Arbogast PG, Griffin MR (2002) COX-2 selective non-steroidal anti-inflammatory drugs and risk of serious coronary heart disease. Lancet 360:1071–1073. https://doi.org/10.1016/S0140-6736(02)11131-7

Ray WA, Varas-Lorenzo C, Chung CP, Castellsague J, Murray KT, Stein CM, Daugherty JR, Arbogast PG, Garcia-Rodriguez LA (2009) Cardiovascular risks of nonsteroidal antiinflammatory drugs in patients after hospitalization for serious coronary heart disease. Circ Cardiovasc Qual Outcomes 2:155–163. https://doi.org/10.1161/CIRCOUTCOMES.108.805689

Silverstein FE, Faich G, Goldstein JL, Simon LS, Pincus T, Whelton A, Makuch R, Eisen G, Agrawal NM, Stenson WF, Burr AM, Zhao WW, Kent JD, Lefkowith JB, Verburg KM, Geis GS (2000) Gastrointestinal toxicity with celecoxib vs nonsteroidal anti-inflammatory drugs for osteoarthritis and rheumatoid arthritis: the CLASS study: a randomized controlled trial. Celecoxib long-term arthritis safety study. JAMA 284:1247–1255

Solomon SD, McMurray JJV, Pfeffer MA, Wittes J, Fowler R, Finn P, Anderson WF, Zauber A, Hawk E, Bertagnolli M (2005) Cardiovascular risk associated with celecoxib in a clinical trial for colorectal adenoma prevention. N Engl J Med 352:1071–1080. https://doi.org/10.1056/NEJMoa050405

Somerville K, Faulkner G, Langman M (1986) Non-steroidal anti-inflammatory drugs and bleeding peptic ulcer. Lancet 1:462–464. http://www.ncbi.nlm.nih.gov/pubmed/2869207

Spiegelhalter DJ (2008) Understanding uncertainty. Ann Fam Med 6:196–197. https://doi.org/10.1370/afm.848

Spiegelhalter D, Pearson M, Short I (2011) Visualizing uncertainty about the future. Science 333:1393–1400. https://doi.org/10.1126/science.1191181

Strayer SM, Slawson DC, Shaughnessy AF (2006) Disseminating drug prescribing information: the cox-2 inhibitors withdrawals. J Am Med Inform Assoc 13:396–398. https://doi.org/10.1197/jamia.M2045

Stuttaford T (1999) New drug gives hope to arthritis sufferers. The Times, 20. http://find.galegroup.com/ttda/infomark.do?&source=gale&prodId=TTDA&userGroupName=abe_ttda&tabID=T003&docPage=article&searchType=&docId=IF500952101&type=multipage&contentSet=LTO&version=1.0

Sukel MP, van der Linden MW, Chen C, Erkens JA, Herings RM (2008) Large-scale stopping and switching treatment with COX-2 inhibitors after the rofecoxib withdrawal. Pharmacoepidemiol Drug Saf 17:9–19. https://doi.org/10.1002/pds.1508

Sukkar E (2014) Still feeling the Vioxx pain. Pharm J. http://www.pharmaceutical-journal.com/news-and-analysis/features/still-feeling-the-vioxx-pain/20066485.article

Therapeutic Goods Administration (2004) Consumer level recall of arthritis drug. https://www.tga.gov.au/media-release/consumer-level-recall-arthritis-drug
Tsintis P, La Mache E (2004) CIOMS and ICH Initiatives in pharmacovigilance and risk management overview and implications. Drug Saf 27:509–517
Yates J, Merck & Co (2002) Important prescribing information. http://www.fda.gov/downloads/Safety/MedWatch/SafetyInformation/SafetyAlertsforHumanMedicalProducts/UCM171089.pdf

4 Isotretinoin: Communication for Preventing Birth Defects and Alerting of an Uncertain Risk of Suicide

Ineke Crijns

Abstract

This chapter discusses the succession of pregnancy prevention programmes (PPPs) for isotretinoin, a medicine effective against acne, but with high risks for birth defects and developmental disorders in the child when exposed during pregnancy. Strengthening of PPPs over time was considered necessary by regulators to increase the compliance with these programmes, but the communication for implementing "strict" PPPs in the healthcare system has been one of the most important challenges in the pharmaceutical field, due to its rejection by some opinion leaders among dermatologists and due to differences in cultures and expectations regarding sexual behaviour of women within and between countries. In addition, isotretinoin has been investigated for possible psychiatric adverse effects including suicidal behaviour, which caused media attention and even discussions in parliaments. Moreover, the chapter reflects on the inconclusive evidence to date in this respect and the associated needs for different regulatory action and handling of communication for isotretinoin and other retinoids. The best ways of how to communicate their risks and safe use recommendations will remain subject to discussion with a view to continuous improvement in every country of the world.

I. Crijns (✉)
Dutch Medicines Evaluation Board, Utrecht, The Netherlands
e-mail: hj.crijns@cbg-meb.nl

© Springer Nature Singapore Pte Ltd. 2020

P. Bahri (ed.), *Communicating about Risks and Safe Use of Medicines*,
https://doi.org/10.1007/978-981-15-3013-5_4

4.1 Situation: The Safety Concerns with Isotretinoin and Communication Challenges

Isotretinoin is an active substance highly effective for the treatment of severe forms of acne resistant to adequate courses of systemic antibiotics and topical therapy (Art 30 Referral Roaccutane 2003). Acne is a disease of the skin that may result in scars (Bhate and Williams 2013), and due to the acute and possibly life-long skin appearance, patients may experience reduced self-esteem, social phobia and suicidal thoughts and behaviour (Nguyen et al. 2016). The disease is the result of multiple factors taking place at the level of hair, hair follicle and sebaceous gland, and is an infectious and inflammatory process (Das and Reynolds 2014). Isotretinoin seems to have a mechanism to influence several factors of this process. It was first authorised in the United States (US) in 1982 as Accutane®. In member states of the European Union (EU), marketing authorisations were granted as of 1983.

4.1.1 The Safety Concerns

Over time, isotretinoin gave raise to some major safety concerns to manage, in particular congenital anomalies (birth defects) and developmental disorders in children exposed during pregnancy, psychiatric reactions and severe skin reactions. This chapter mainly reviews the communication around the teratogenic risk associated with pregnancy during isotretinoin use, but also highlights aspects of communication about concerns of depression and suicide.

Isotretinoin, or 13-cis-retinoic acid, is a vitamin A derivative. It is known since 1953 that retinoids can cause congenital anomalies in animals. Therefore, a contra-indication in pregnancy, a warning against becoming pregnant when using isotretinoin and the recommendation to monitor pregnancy exposures for their outcomes were already included in the initial product information for patients and healthcare professionals (Abroms et al. 2006). In 1983, one year after the initial marketing authorisation, first observations of human teratogenicity of isotretinoin were published (Rosa 1983). A range of severe congenital anomalies caused by isotretinoin were identified from case reports of teratogenic effects and prospective monitoring of exposed pregnancies, namely craniofacial, cardiac, thymic and central nervous system defects with a high frequency of 26% of exposed pregnancies (Lammer et al. 1985).

In the US, the manufacturer (or in legal terms: the marketing authorisation holder) was therefore requested to amend the product information by including a warning about the teratogenicity of isotretinoin in humans in bold font type. In addition, warning letters were sent to physicians, and red warning stickers were sent to pharmacies and wholesalers to be placed on the packages containing isotretinoin (Abroms et al. 2006). Because pregnancies during use of isotretinoin occurred despite these measures, requests for extending the risk minimisation measures further occurred several times during the product life cycle. From 1983 through 1988, the US Food and Drug Administration (US FDA) and the manufacturer strengthened the communication about the teratogenic risk. This included changes to the product information, repeated mailing of letters to healthcare professionals, articles in the US FDA's drug bulletin, distribution of specific patient information leaflets through prescribing physicians and press releases with background information for the general news media (Green 2002). However, there was evidence that despite these efforts isotretinoin continued to be used in the US by thousands of women of childbearing potential with less severe acne than what it was approved for (Bull 2000), possibly due to advertisement by the manufacturer (Green 2002), and the pregnancy rate was 3.4 per 1000 women using isotretinoin (Bull 2000). In 1988, the US FDA requested further actions from the manufacturer, such as educational materials and restrictions to the distribution of isotretinoin, and even proposed its removal from the market (Green 2002). This led to introducing the Pregnancy Prevention Program for Women on Accutane in the US in autumn 1988.

In the EU, the situation of granting marketing authorisation for isotretinoin was different in each member state, also due to their differences in the risk minimisation options available in each country. Since 1983, the product information of isotretinoin would contain strong warnings, and since 1988 a pregnancy prevention programme (PPP) was stated in the product information following the US. Based on the teratogenicity, isotretinoin did not even receive marketing authorisation in some member states but was made available only on named patient basis, for example, in Sweden (Crijns et al. 2011a). According to a British dermatologist, prescribers in Europe were overall more cautious because of the memory of the thalidomide tragedy in the early 1960s, which actually happened in Europe (Green 2002) (see Chaps. 1 and 15).

In 2002, the teratogenic risk of isotretinoin and the PPP was reviewed at EU level upon an arbitration request submitted by France to the Committee for Proprietary Medicinal Products (CPMP), the scientific committee of the European Agency for the Evaluation of Medicinal Products (EMEA) established in 1995 (now the European Medicines Agency (EMA)). The request mainly related to the PPP proposed for a generic product going, at the time, through the mutual recognition procedure (MRP), an EU procedure for national authorisations in more than one member state. Until then isotretinoin-containing products were authorised in member states through "purely" national procedures, i.e. without mutual recognition, which had resulted in differences in the PPPs between member states (Crijns et al. 2011a). The arbitration procedure was aimed at harmonising risk minimisation measures across the EU and resulted in a CPMP opinion, concluding that in view of the overall data isotretinoin for oral use may be granted a marketing authorisation through MRP, provided a strict PPP was implemented when prescribed to women of childbearing potential. This was disclosed to the public through the monthly report of the CPMP and directly to all manufactures in the EU.

Another safety concern for isotretinoin emerged in 2000/2001 with case reports of suspected adverse reactions such as anxiety, depression and suicidal behaviour. At the beginning of this century, retrospective cohort studies and case-control studies reported conflicting results in this respect and to date the evidence remains inconclusive (Jick et al. 2000; Wysowski et al. 2001). Regarding these adverse psychiatric events, questions have been raised in parliaments of the US, Ireland and other countries. These were triggered by suicides by adolescents and young adults using isotretinoin, which were also intensely discussed in news media (Ro/Accutane action group – news update 2002) and became subject of several lawsuits against the manufacturer of isotretinoin. The suspected psychiatric adverse reactions were addressed in the product information agreed through the above-mentioned arbitration review by the CPMP in 2002 (Art 30 Referral Roaccutane 2003).

The EU product information of 2002 also contained advice on how to avoid adverse reactions of the skin. However, the latest discussion at the EMA in relation to serious skin reactions resulted in an update of the product information and a direct healthcare professional communication (DHPC) in July 2010 (Isotretinoin and the risk of erythema multiforme 2010). The DHPC was implemented differently in each EU member state; for instance, in the Netherlands the DHPC was circulated to healthcare professionals in January 2011, while in the United Kingdom (UK) the DHPC was replaced by publishing the information in the national drug bulletin.

As the latest in the EU, on 7 July 2016, the UK submitted a so-called referral request to the Pharmacovigilance Risk Assessment Committee (PRAC), the EMA's scientific committee established in 2012 specifically for safety surveillance and risk management, asking for a review of current pregnancy prevention measures for all retinoid-containing medicines, to ensure that they are effective and appropriate. In addition, the PRAC will review the possible risk of psychiatric disorders such as depression, anxiety, psychotic disorders and suicidal behaviour with retinoids (Art 31 Referral Retinoid-containing medicines 2018).

The PRAC noted that despite the introduction of a PPP, cases of pregnancy during treatment with oral retinoids continued to be reported in the EU. As compliance with the PPP is crucial, the adequacy of the PPPs was reviewed to ensure that the available materials effectively encourage the implementation of the measures and the shared responsibility between patients, physicians and pharmacists to adhere to recommendations, and furthermore, that these measures are communicated consistently and effectively for these products. As the outcome of the referral, the PRAC imposed on the manufacturers specific studies to measure the effectiveness of the agreed changes to the PPP. In addition, the PRAC recommended amendments to the product information to reflect the teratogenic risk associated with the use and communication to healthcare professionals through a DHPC. Changes to the educational materials were recommended too, to ensure that healthcare professionals and patients are informed about the risks associated with oral retinoids in pregnant women and women of childbearing potential and on the measures necessary to minimise the risk. These measures include a patient reminder card, physician checklist/acknowledgement form and pharmacist checklist. Other elements of the PPP are to be considered and agreed at national level to account for the different healthcare systems in the member states of the EU. The PRAC has also recommended distributing the educational materials via electronic channels such as matrix bar codes and websites to make better use of the existing digital technology bearing in mind the young patient population.

Regarding psychiatric events, the PRAC recognised that the available data and the occurrence of these events have important limitations precluding the clear establishment of a causal association. The underlying risk of psychiatric disorders within the patient populations can be significant; however, it is advisable that patient taking oral retinoids is warned about the potential risks of psychiatric events.

4.1.2 The Communication Challenges

Isotretinoin is a medicine which posed very specific communication challenges, arising from the kind of risks to deal with and the patient population using isotretinoin. The teratogenicity can lead to serious adverse effects in the child and is a major concern, given that half of the patients are females (Nijsten et al. 2007), mostly in their reproductive years (Mitchell et al. 1995). Assessment and communication regarding the controversial causal association of depression and suicide with isotretinoin carries further challenges, on the one hand, because acne itself is associated with such psychiatric effects, and on the other hand, because of the inconclusive evidence, apart from the fact that depression and suicide are difficult topics to talk about anyway.

Also, isotretinoin came on the market before the digital era, when communication channels and tools were limited. Communication about the teratogenicity and the risk minimisation measures were in the beginning undertaken conservatively with the then available tools, i.e. DHPCs by paper mail or publications in national drug bulletins and scientific journals, and paper-based information for patients. With technical progress over time, the pregnancy prevention programmes could make increased use of internet-based tools with patient registration for individualised communication, new territory with its own challenges, such as data privacy. In fact, in the referral outcome of 2018, the PRAC specifically recommended, again, distribution of educational materials via electronic channels such as matrix bar codes and websites. The question remains however by the time of implementation, these channels are still the most appropriate ones. The digitalisation is moving forward with high speed, so one can hardly keep up-to-date with new technical tools and the media preferences, in particular of the younger patient group.

4.2 Events: The Communication Experiences

4.2.1 Risk of Birth Defects

There are several overviews on the actions taken by the US FDA and the manufacturer regarding the teratogenic risk of isotretinoin. A detailed chronology for isotretinoin in the US states that the manufacturer had circulated a number of DHPCs, two alone in 1983, due to pressure of the US FDA and the consumer rights advocacy group, Public Citizen (Green 2002). In addition, the manufacturer informed physicians through the Medical Director's Page in the widely read Journal of the American Medical Association (JAMA) in June 1984 (Fakour et al. 2014). In the previous year, the US FDA had also published their own article in the Lancet (Rosa 1983). Journalists participated in the debate by raising questions in major newspapers like the New York Times and the Washington Post (Green 2002).

The Pregnancy Prevention Program for Women on Accutane was introduced in the US in 1988, but as pregnancies during isotretinoin use still occurred, it was strengthened in 2002 with the name SMART for System to Manage Accutane Related Teratogenicity. This was extensively communicated by the US FDA and the manufacturer to healthcare professionals and patients (Woodcock 2002). This new PPP included yellow qualification stickers that should be put on the prescription. "Qualified" meant that a female patient had presented a negative pregnancy test each month, had signed an informed consent form, had agreed to use two effective forms of contraception or abstinence, and had been encouraged to join the follow-up survey to help monitor PPP performance. Prescribers could obtain these yellow stickers only after attesting to their cooperation with the programme. Pharmacists should only dispense upon presentation of a prescription with this yellow sticker for maximal 1 month and fill prescription within 7 days for the date of "qualification" (Shin et al. 2011). SMART and SMART-like PPPs had however limited success, as compliance with at least one method of contraception was low, only a very low increase was seen in the pregnancy testing rate and the number of pregnancies during use hardly declined (*note*: after patent expiration of Accutane in 2002, three marketing authorisations for generic formulations were granted by the US FDA with SMART-like PPPs (Memorandum on isotretinoin and pregnancy exposure 2004).

Upon request of the US FDA, the by then four manufacturers for isotretinoin therefore created the strengthened PPP called "iPLEDGE". This was implemented in 2006 and is the PPP still in place today. It requires that all stakeholders in the distribution chain and all patients receiving prescriptions—both male and female—register in a single database online or by telephone. Prior to prescribing, dispensing and receiving the medicine the prescriber and pharmacist have to enter information about the patient. Pharmacists are permitted to dispense only if this database shows that the prescriber and patient have complied with all requirements. For the prescriber the requirements are: annual renewal of their registration with iPLEDGE, confirmation of monthly counselling, specifying the two forms of contraception agreed with the patient and entering the test results of the monthly pregnancy tests. The patient should have monthly pregnancy test performed in certified laboratories, documented contraceptive counselling and present negative pregnancy results. Before and with the start of this programme there has been communication with the prescribers, pharmacists and wholesalers, to inform them that if they did not comply with the system, they were not allowed to prescribe/dispense isotretinoin (Abroms et al. 2006). This PPP led to several letters by dermatologists complaining about the burden and inflexibility of the new programme. Many were frustrated initially by technical glitches from the internet-based system coupled with inadequate telephone support. There have also been reports of patients experiencing difficulties in complying with the system's numerous requirements. Despite that iPLEDGE represents the most rigorous risk management programme in history for a widely prescribed medicine, the pregnancy rate decline is disappointing. To date, there is still resistance to iPLEDGE from dermatologists and other healthcare professionals (Pierson et al. 2015; Weinberg 2005).

Due to the relatively high pregnancy rate in the US compared to Europe, the US FDA took further measures to minimise the risk of pregnancy exposure of isotretinoin, and each amendment of the iPLEDGE PPP was communicated to prescribers, pharmacists and wholesalers and to patients. The media attention in the US continued too, as it can be expected for a teratogenic medicine evoking memories of the thalidomide tragedy. There have also been questions from representatives of the US parliament and the US FDA gave statements and testimonies to the US Congress regarding the teratogenicity (Green 2002).

At EU level, the outcome of the arbitration procedure for isotretinoin was published on the EMA website in the monthly report of the CPMP of April 2003 (Art 29 Referral Isotretinoin 2003), and physicians and pharmacists were also informed through DHPCs. The manufacturers were requested to provide PPPs compliant with the key elements stated in the European Commission decision of October 2003, finalised subsequent to the CPMP opinion. Patients were to be informed about the PPP by their treating physician, who should provide the patient with the contraception brochure and undertake the counselling.

This PPP was a strengthened version of the PPP introduced by the manufacturer in 1988 following the US. The PPPs implemented in EU member states since 2004 consist of patient counselling on the teratogenic risk and the use of preferably two effective contraceptive method(s) as of 1 month before starting treatment with isotretinoin, during the course of treatment and until at least 1 month after discontinuation of treatment. Two pregnancy tests have to be performed before the intended start of isotretinoin and require negative results for actual prescribing. Isotretinoin may be prescribed for maximum of 30 days and the prescription must be filled within 7 days. Pregnancy tests should be performed prior to each repeat prescription, which can only be written subject to a negative result, and a final pregnancy test has to be taken 1 month after discontinuation of treatment. The educational material consists of a physician's guide to prescribing isotretinoin, a checklist for prescribing to female patients, a patient information brochure, a brochure on contraception, an acknowledgement form for female patients and a pharmacist's guide to dispensing isotretinoin (Crijns et al. 2011a).

The referral to the PRAC triggered by the UK in 2016 for all retinoids resulted in recommendations of amendments to the product information, educational materials for healthcare professionals and patients, and the recommendation of communication to healthcare professionals through a DHPC. These amendments and communications were recommended to ensure healthcare professionals and patients are informed about the risks associated with oral retinoids (Art 31 Referral Retinoid-containing medicines 2018).

Isotretinoin is also subject to risk minimisation measures and communication elsewhere, and Australia and New Zealand are discussed here as further examples. The Australian marketing authorisation for isotretinoin requires the specialist prescriber to "ensure that the possibility of pregnancy has been excluded" before a woman can commence treatment and to advise her to avoid becoming pregnant during and 1 month after isotretinoin treatment. Women should receive the counselling and start effective contraception at least a month before beginning treatment (Australian Government, Department of Health 2005). In 2014, general practitioners (GPs) in Australia requested prescribing rights for isotretinoin especially in rural and remote areas to avoid undertreatment of patients with severe acne, and individual GPs may now be approved to prescribe it for patients without access to a specialist (The Royal Australian College of General Practitioners 2014). In view of the small number of publications in scientific journals, there seems to be less information from Australia, compared to the US and Europe, regarding the teratogenic risk minimisation measures on isotretinoin or the evaluation of these measures. The same applies for New Zealand. There, a review on isotretinoin was published in July 2015, stating that "medical authorities have tended to follow the UK, Europe and the US in the use of isotretinoin. This is because there are limits to the amount a small country can do in developing and researching a wide range of medicines" (Skelton 2016). This could explain the limited communication in the public domain found in this country and the fact that the New Zealand medicine data sheet of isotretinoin includes a contraindication and PPP that follows the EU (New Zealand Datasheet – Oratane 2016).

4.2.2 Risk of Psychiatric Effects

In the beginning of 2002, a 15-year-old pilot flew a small plane into a Florida skyscraper, with a suicidal intention. This adolescent had a prescription for isotretinoin and his last note made reference to his acne and the medication (Cosgrove-Mather 2016). It was discussed by the US media in detail whether the medication might have accounted for the boy's suicide. This media debate impacted also on other countries, and, for example, an action group in the UK issued a press statement on their meeting of the UK Medicines Control Agency, criticising what the group considered an inadequate warning on depression and suicide (Ro/Accutane action group – news update 2002). The mother of the boy filed a lawsuit against the manufacturer. In June 2002, the US FDA amended the labelling of isotretinoin with a warning of aggressive and/or violent behaviour in addition to the existing warning for depression and suicidal behaviour. This labelling amendment resulted in a US Congress hearing in December 2002 because of the suicide of the son of Congressman Stupak. Isotretinoin and suicide, as well as the related lawsuits, were frequently subject of news in the media at the time (Green 2002). Following the suicide of Stupak's son, the US FDA issued warning letters obliging the manufacturer to terminate advertisements aimed at minors (Bremner et al. 2012).

In fact, the possible risk of depression had already been included by the US FDA in the revised US product information ("labelling") in the mid-1980s (James 2016; Mitchell 2016). In 1996, the US FDA re-evaluated psychiatric effects because of emerging suicide cases reported for isotretinoin. This evaluation resulted in including suicidal ideation, suicide attempts, suicide, depression, psychosis and emotional instability in the product information, although causal association with isotretinoin was not established. The US FDA posted the conclusion on their website and issued a press release. In 1998, a comprehensive re-evaluation of the overall product information and risk management of isotretinoin was initiated, resulting in requests for studies from the manufacturers (FDA 2000) on interactions with hormones, a survey of isotretinoin use in women, a study on pregnancy occurrence and cumulative reviews of psychiatric cases and structured follow-up of suicide cases. The study on interactions with hormones did not show clinically relevant interactions. The survey on women using isotretinoin led to the strengthened PPP SMART.

While the possible causal association between isotretinoin and psychiatric effects remains to date inconclusive on the basis of all available evidence, a systematic review of 2012 presented evidence in support of a causal relationship (Bremner et al. 2012), which triggered a group of dermatologists and psychiatrists in Australia in 2013 to develop recommendations for safe prescribing of isotretinoin in adolescents. These aimed at increasing awareness in practitioners of both disciplines of the current evidence and the need for prompt recognition of symptoms and appropriate collaboration between dermatologists and mental health practitioners to ensure optimal patient care and safety (Rowe et al. 2014).

During the 2016–2018 EU referral, the PRAC recognised the limitations of the data relating to psychiatric events and considered it unlikely that this is a causal association between oral retinoids and these events. The current information in the product information following the 2003 referral was therefore considered to be still valid.

4.3 Evaluation: Feedback, Outcomes and Lessons Learnt

4.3.1 Feedback and Outcomes of Pregnancy Prevention Programmes

The following gives an overview of the worldwide research on the availability and effectiveness of PPPs for isotretinoin.

The effectiveness of the first PPP in the US, the Pregnancy Prevention Program for Women on Accutane, was evaluated over time, and so were the subsequent PPPs. At the beginning of 2008, the pregnancy rate declined from 3.11 per 1000 women of childbearing potential using isotretinoin under SMART to 2.67 under iPLEDGE (Marwick 1984). This was however not regarded to be a significant decrease of in utero exposure compared to the SMART programme. An overall conclusion is that DHCPs and warnings in the labelling are limited in effecting changes in healthcare professionals (Bremner et al. 2012).

Studies on the effectiveness of the PPPs in the EU were published in scientific journals (Crijns et al. 2011b; Isotretinoin and the effectiveness of the pregnancy prevention programme in Europe 2016) and despite announcements on public websites, received hardly media attention. For example, several surveys performed in the Netherlands showed that healthcare professionals and patients were informed about the PPP by different sources or did not receive any information at all (Crijns et al. 2013). Despite a certain level of knowledge of the PPP in the healthcare professionals, enforced by prescription alerts or pharmacy issuance system alerts, healthcare professionals and patients were not always compliant. It has also been shown that albeit a person is informed about the teratogenic risk and the PPP, he/she will decide differently in certain situations and not follow the imposed PPP. Situations such as where a holiday would overlap the 30 day prescription period, or a young religious patient is not sexually active, but also where the healthcare professional developed confidence in the patient being a responsible woman who will prevent a pregnancy in ways other than imposed by the PPP would be reason for non-compliance (Crijns et al. 2013).

In New Zealand, the pregnancy rate has been 7.3 per 1000 women aged 10–44 years using isotretinoin, i.e. more than twice the pregnancy rate during isotretinoin use by women of childbearing potential in the US before introduction of SMART (Bull 2000). Maybe that is due to the fact that there was less communication in this country for the reasons described above.

A survey performed in India showed that 10% of the participating isotretinoin-prescribing dermatologists had completed the documentation of pregnancy tests fully and provided the appropriate instructions, while 75% had only performed an initial pregnancy test with instructions but missed the follow-up with further counselling, and 15% had not performed a pregnancy test at all and only given instructions to the patient. The authors concluded that because the implementation of a PPP like iPLEDGE is practically difficult in India, mainly because of the absence of a fully functional pharmacovigilance system at national level and because it is a taboo to perform pregnancy tests for unmarried women. Therefore, a simpler and adapted risk minimisation programme needs to be developed to protect Indian females at risk, which needs to include a distinctive sensitive approach for unmarried women (Anwikar et al. 2010).

In Saudi Arabia an approach similar to the US PPP has been applied to isotretinoin, and a study investigating the compliance of dermatologists indicated that only 60% of the dermatologists had recommended pregnancy testing before treatment start, and only 16% requested monthly pregnancy tests. The pregnancy rate in isotretinoin-using women of childbearing potential was 8.8 per 1000 (n = 7), and 43% of the pregnancies were terminated. The authors concluded that the non-compliance of the dermatologists should be corrected, especially in countries with legal restrictions on pregnancy termination (AlGhamdi et al. 2011).

A longitudinal cohort study in Turkey showed no pregnancies in 57 female patients included in the study, but 81% of those were also not sexually active. This could indicate that there is good patient compliance with therapy and prohibitions. But, this may also be attributable to the young age and unmarried status of the patients using isotretinoin in communities favouring initiation of sexual activity late and within marriage. The low reportage of adverse pregnancy outcomes for isotretinoin in Turkey could therefore be due to the sociocultural profile of the female patients, strict adherence to contraceptive methods, and/or underreporting of teratogenic incidents due to lack of studies. Turkey has in place a controlled distribution programme for isotretinoin under the supervision of the Ministry of Health as well as other risk minimisation measures, including an informed consent form to be signed by female patients (Ozyurt and Kaptanoglu 2015).

A study performed in Iran concluded that besides the incorrectly prescribed dosages, the patients had not been adequately counselled about isotretinoin's teratogenicity and the severity of the possible birth defects. The study further reported that only 6.8% of the females of childbearing potential who receive isotretinoin and are sexually active (i.e. 25% of the women of childbearing potential receiving isotretinoin) use two effective methods of contraception (Entezari-Maleki et al. 2012). It should be noted that Iran has no PPP in place (correspondence with the author of (correspondence with the author of Entezari-Maleki et al. 2012)).

Likewise in the Republic of Korea, no PPP was available in 2012 when a study showed a high rate of terminated pregnancies occurring during isotretinoin use compared to terminations in women not using isotretinoin (Yook et al. 2012). In this country approximately 50% of all pregnancies are unplanned, as less than 30% of the sexually active population use contraception (Lim et al. 2016).

The outcome of a comparative review of pregnancy risk management programmes for isotretinoin across four continents, published in 2018, showed that because of the strictness of the programmes in the US and Europe, they are ineffective in reducing the risks of foetal exposure to isotretinoin when used alone (Kotvitwanichkanont and Driscoll 2018). The strict regulation would result in increased fear of teratogenic risks but did not translate in reducing the rate of isotretinoin-exposed pregnancies. The review concludes with recommending that education of effective contraception should be emphasised and the other requirements should be minimised to avoid undertreatment for acne in women of childbearing potential.

In addition to quantifying the effectiveness of PPPs and associated communications, it is also important to understand whether or not, and why, PPPs were accepted by those targeted.

In the US, protests were seen from healthcare professionals in form of open letters to scientific journals of medical, ethical (Cockerell and Thiboutot 2006) and legal focus (Doshi 2007), or journals like Medical Economics (Ortolon 2006) and medical specialist journal the Dermatologist (Darves 2016) with complaints about the restrictions imposed by iPLEDGE which could lead to disruption of treatment and create difficulties for prescribers, patients and pharmacists to obtain the registrations. Surveys performed in the Netherlands identified likewise critical notes on the PPP in place there. The PPPs were perceived by some as overly patronising and risk undertreating patients who are in need of isotretinoin but are not willing to consent to the PPP, e.g. to apply hormonal contraception as one necessary method of reliable contraception (Crijns et al. 2011b).

A literature review on publications on compliance on the PPP in Europe in 2011 was a reason for a group of dermatologists from Europe and the US to write a letter to the editor of the British Journal of Dermatology advocating for authorising isotretinoin with a more relaxed PPP because "it is the single most efficacious drug for acne and is sometimes the only effective treatment for patient with severe acne". They agreed that pregnancy exposure should be reduced as much as possible, but that a team of committee evaluating prescribing patterns and foetal exposure would be a valuable addition to the current system with the goal of improving patient access to treatment while avoiding use of isotretinoin during pregnancy (Thiboutot et al. 2012).

4.3.2 Feedback and Outcomes of Precautions Regarding Psychiatric Effects

Regarding the psychiatric effects, debates in newspapers and questions in parliaments (Ro/Accutane action group – news update 2002), especially raised by parents of patients with suicidal behaviour or committed suicides, indicate that some expect more information and restrictions in the product information of isotretinoin in this respect, and some think that perhaps isotretinoin should even be withdrawn from the market. This is a difficult debate; unfortunately there is scientific uncertainty, as the evidence to date is still inconclusive due to contradicting results of studies on the causal association of suicidal behaviour with isotretinoin, while there is evidence that successful treatment of acne can help patients to regain confidence over their appearance and free them of depression associated with the acne signs on their skin. For example, a Norwegian, cross-sectional, questionnaire-based study demonstrated the association of reported acne to increased risk of suicidal ideation, mental health problems and social impairment. Especially, an 80% higher level of suicidal ideation in adolescents with substantial acne was seen compared to those with no or little acne (Halvorsen et al. 2011). A study from Iran reported that isotretinoin improved the quality of life of patients treated for acne, *however the depression score increased* (Beck Depression Inventory (BDI)) in both male and female patients (Fakour et al. 2014). In contrast, the outcome of a study in India was that depression (Hamilton Rating Scale) decreased significantly in patients treated with isotretinoin and was not associated with an increased incidence of depression or suicidal behaviour (Gnanaraj et al. 2015). Because of the causal association between acne and psychiatric effects, it is difficult to investigate the risk of these effects with a treatment of acne, in individuals as well as at population level, a methodological issue called confounding in pharmacoepidemiology. This may explain the contradictory results of studies investigating psychiatric effects of isotretinoin in patients treated for acne, and the contradiction arising in scientific investigations poses a major communication challenge.

However, it is understandable that parents try to find out the reason why their child has committed suicide and speak about this in the media. This public debate presents an example of what is called "social risk amplification" (Kasperson et al. 1988), i.e. a situation where a public debate increases the perception of a risk. In 2005, a study was published which investigated the perception of patients on the association of isotretinoin with depression and suicide and showed that isotretinoin was perceived to be effective but dangerous and that depression and suicide were the most highly perceived risks (Magin et al. 2005), rather than the proven and severe teratogenicity. The study also reported that there was much media coverage in the US and Europe, but that in 2004 the issue was even discussed twice as much in Australian newspapers. In June 2005, the Therapeutic Goods Administration (TGA) reported on isotretinoin and suicide in their Australian Adverse Drug Reaction Bulletin.

4.3.3 Lessons Learnt

It seems that past experiences leave a mark on people and impact on how they handle certain risks in the future. Although the thalidomide tragedy is part of global knowledge in safety of medicines, in those countries where people had directly witnessed its risk of teratogenicity or personally met affected persons, the severe teratogenic risk of isotretinoin was handled in ways different from countries not having had that personal experience, as it was discussed in an article in the New York Times in April 1988 (Kolata 1985). Many dermatologists have expressed views that there is a need for an effective treatment of severe acne, and have complained that the restrictions imposed by regulatory authorities to prevent pregnancy during the use of isotretinoin oppose this medical need. It has become clear from these complaints and pressure of patients or their parents to be well informed of the risks that all patients and healthcare professionals must be involved in designing important risk minimisation measures, so that the measures are practical in the given healthcare and cultural environment and have a wide agreement and support for effective implementation. Multidisciplinary research is needed to understand the preferences of patients and healthcare professionals in relation to risk minimisation and communication for designing and evaluation measures (see Chap. 1). Also, risk minimisation measures will only be effective if they are communicated by using all available tools and channels, including the media most popular amongst patients and the general public use and increasingly the social media. Researching media preferences is therefore amongst the important areas of medicinal product risk communication research (see Chaps. 10 and 11).

Conclusions

- Isotretinoin has been authorised since 1982 as a medicinal product highly effective to treat severe forms of acne resistant to adequate courses of systemic antibiotics and topical therapy.
- Within a year after its marketing authorisation, cases of congenital anomalies and developmental disorders due to exposure to isotretinoin during pregnancy appeared, leading to imposing increasingly strict pregnancy prevention programmes (PPPs) by regulatory authorities in many, but not all countries.
- Countries, mainly in Europe and the US, monitor exposure and pregnancy outcomes of isotretinoin use during pregnancy, as use during pregnancy still occurs. The PPPs have been difficult to implement in healthcare, due to opposition by dermatologists who may perceive them as a burden and restriction to access to an effective treatment, as well as due to differences in cultures and expectations regarding sexual behaviour of women within and between countries.
- In the late 1990s, case reports of psychiatric adverse effects such as depression, suicidal behaviour and aggression lead to discussion in the media, and even parliaments.
- Investigations and studies aiming at clarifying whether isotretinoin can cause psychiatric effects have to date been inconclusive, and this uncertainty, together with the seriousness and sensitivity of the safety concern requires specific regulatory action and handling of communication.
- The best ways for communicating the risks and safe use advice for isotretinoin and other retinoids will remain subject to discussion with a view to continuous improvement in every country of the world.

Declarations The views expressed in this chapter are the author's personal views and may not be understood or quoted as being made on behalf of or reflecting the position of her employing organisation, i.e. the Dutch Medicines Evaluation Board, or the European Medicines Agency (EMA) or any of its committees or working parties, where she serves as an expert.

References

Abroms L, Maibach E, Lyon-Daniel K et al (2006) What is the best approach to reducing birth defects associated with isotretinoin? PLoS Med 3:1978–1983

AlGhamdi K, Khurram H, Asiri Y, Mandil A (2011) Dermatologists' level of compliance with the prescription guidelines of isotretinoin for females of childbearing potential. Int J Dermatol 50:1094–1098

Anwikar SR, Bandekar MS, Khopkar U, Kshirsagar NA (2010) Prescribing and dispensing of isotretinoin: a survey. Indian J Dermatol Venereol Leprol 76:412–413

Art 29 Referral Isotretinoin (2003) on EMA website. http://www.ema.europa.eu/ema/index.jsp?curl=pages/medicines/human/referrals/Isotretinoin/human_referral_000086.jsp&mid=WC0b01ac05805c516f

Art 30 Referral Roaccutane (2003) on EMA website. http://www.ema.europa.eu/ema/index.jsp?curl=pages/medicines/human/referrals/Roaccutane/human_referral_000085.jsp&mid=WC0b01ac05805c516f

Art 31 Referral Retinoid-containing medicines (2018) on EMA website. http://www.ema.europa.eu

Australian Government, Department of Health (2005) Safety information for health professionals: avoiding fetal abnormalities with isotretinoin. https://www.tga.gov.au/publication-issue/australian-adverse-drug-reactions-bulletin-vol-24-no-1#a2

Bhate K, Williams HC (2013) Epidemiology of acne vulgaris. Br J Dermatol 168:474–485

Bremner J, Shearer K, McCaffery P (2012) Retinoic acid and affective disorders: the evidence for an association. J Clin Psychiatry 73:37–50

Statement by Jonca Bull, MD, Deputy Office Director, Office of Drug Evaluation V, Center for Drug Evaluation and Research, US Food and Drug Administration, before the Committee of Government Reform, US House of Representatives on 5 December 2000

Cockerell CJ, Thiboutot DM (2006) iPLEDGE: a report from the front lines of dermatologic practice. AMA J Ethics 8:524–528

Cosgrove-Mather B (2016) Suicide pilot's mom blames Accutane. http://www.cbsnews.com/news/suicide-pilots-mom-blames-accutane/

Crijns I, Straus S, Luteijn M (2011a) Implementation of the harmonized EU isotretinoin pregnancy prevention programme: a questionnaire survey among European regulatory agencies. Drug Saf 36:27–32

Crijns H, Straus S, Gispen-de Wied C, de Jong-van den Berg L (2011b) Compliance with pregnancy prevention programmes of isotretinoin in Europe: a systematic review. Br J Dermatol 164:238–244

Crijns I, Mantel-Teeuwisse A, Bloemberg R et al (2013) Healthcare professionals surveys to investigate the implementation of the isotretinoin pregnancy prevention programme: a descriptive study. Expert Opin Drug Saf 12:29–38

Darves B (2016) Life after iPLEDGE. http://www.the-dermatologist.com/article/6137

Das S, Reynolds RV (2014) Recent advances in acne pathogenesis: implications for therapy. Am J Clin Dermatol 15:479–488

Doshi A (2007) The cost of clear skin: balancing the social and safety costs of iPLEDGE with the efficacy of Accutane (isotretinoin). Seton Hall Law Rev 37:625

Entezari-Maleki T, Hadjibabaie M, Dousti S et al (2012) Evaluation and monitoring of isotretinoin use in Iran. Arch Iran Med 15:409–412

Fakour Y, Noormohammadpour P, Ameri H et al (2014) The effect of isotretinoin (Roaccutane) therapy on depression and quality of life of patients with severe acne. Iran J Psychiatry 9:237–240

Dermatologic and Ophthalmic drugs advisory committee FDA, meeting 18-19 September 2000 – Briefing information – Accutane. http://www.fda.gov/ohrms/dockets/ac/00/backgrd/3639b1.htm
Gnanaraj P, Karthikeyan S, Narasimhan M, Rajagopalan V (2015) Decrease in "Hamilton Rating Scale for Depression" following isotretinoin therapy in acne: an open-label prospective study. Indian J Dermatol 60:461–464
Green J (2002) Babies, blemishes and FDA: a history of Accutane regulation in the United States. Harvard Law School. https://dash.harvard.edu/bitstream/handle/1/8963867/Green.html?sequence=2
Halvorsen J, Stern R, Dalgard F, Thoresen F, Bjertness E, Lien L (2011) Suicidal ideation, mental health problems, and social impairment are increased in adolescents with acne: a population-based study. J Invest Dermatol 131:363–370
Isotretinoin and the effectiveness of the pregnancy prevention programme in Europe (2016) www.encepp.eu/encepp/openAttachment/documents.otherDocument-0/4652
Isotretinoin and the risk of erythema multiforme. Final SPC and PL wording agreed by the PhVWP in June 2010. http://www.hma.eu/fileadmin/dateien/Human_Medicines/CMD_h_/Product_Information/PhVWP_Recommendations/Isotretinoin/CMDhPhVWP0212010_July10.pdf
James A (2016) The bitter pill - category: Accutane - Roche puts Accutane profits over lives of consumers. https://uniteforlife.wordpress.com/category/accutane/
Jick SS, Kremers HM, Vasilakis-Scaramozza C (2000) Isotretinoin use and risk of depression, psychotic symptoms, suicide, and attempted suicide. Arch Dermatol 136:1231–1236
Kasperson RE, Renn O, Slovic P, Brown HS, Emel J, Goble R et al (1988) The social amplification of risk: a conceptual framework. Risk Anal 8:177–187
Kolata G (1985) Europeans placed stiffer curbs on acne drug. New York Times 25:A1
Kotvitwanichkanont T, Driscoll T (2018) A comparative review of the isotretinoin pregnancy risk management programs across four continents. Int J Dermatol 57:1035–1046
Lammer E, Chen D, Hoar R et al (1985) Retinoic acid embryopathy. N Engl J Med 313: 837–841
Lim SH, Jang HI, Lee DY, Yoon BK, Choi DS (2016) Recent trends in contraceptive use among Korean adolescents: results from a nationwide survey from year 2013 to 2015. Obstet Gynecol Sci 59:519–524
Magin P, Adams J, Heading P et al (2005) Patients' perceptions of isotretinoin, depression and suicide: a qualitative study. Aust. Fam. Physician 34:795–797
Marwick C (1984) More cautionary labeling appears on isotretinoin. J Am Med Assoc 251:3208–3209
Memorandum on isotretinoin and pregnancy exposure (2004). http://www.fda.gov/ohrms/dockets/ac/04/briefing/4017B1-06a%20FDA%20Backgrounder-ODS%20Sec%20C%20Tab%203.pdf
Mitchell S. (2016) Congressional committee finds Accutane causes suicide. http://www.rense.com/general32/scu.htm
Mitchell A, Van Bennekom C, Louik C (1995) A pregnancy prevention program in women of childbearing age receiving isotretinoin. N Engl J Med 333:101–106
New Zealand Datasheet – Oratane (2016) http://www.medsafe.govt.nz/Profs/Datasheet/o/oratanecap.pdf
Nguyen CM, Beroukhim K, Danesh MJ, Babikian A, Koo J, Leon A (2016) The psychosocial impact of acne, vitiligo, and psoriasis: a review. Clin Cosmet Investig Dermatol 9:383–392
Nijsten T, Rombouts S, Lambert J (2007) Acne is prevalent but use of its treatments is infrequent among adolescents from the general population. J Eur Acad Dermatol Venereol 21:163–168
Ortolon K (2006) A pox on your practice: iPLEDGE program scars dermatologists. Tex Med 102:29–31
Ozyurt S, Kaptanoglu AS (2015) Systemic isotretinoin treatment and pregnancy: a longitudinal cohort study form Turkey. Eurasian J Med 47:179–183
Pierson JC, Ferris LK, Schwarz EB (2015) We pledge to change iPLEDGE. JAMA Dermatol 151:701–702
Ro/Accutane action group – news update (2002). http://www.accutaneaction.com/press/index.html
Rosa F (1983) Teratogenicity of isotretinoin. Lancet 2:513

Rowe C, Spelman L, Oziemski M et al (2014) Isotretinoin and mental health in adolescents: Australian consensus. Aust J Dermatol 55:162–167
Shin J, Cheetham T, Wong I et al (2011) The impact of the iPLEDGE program on isotretinoin fetal exposure in an integrated health care system. J Am Acad Dermatol 65:1117–1125
Skelton C (2016) Containing the impacts in New Zealand: acne and isotretinoin III. http://eveningreport.nz/2015/07/23/containing-the-impacts-in-nz-acne-and-isotretinoin-iii/
The Royal Australian College of General Practitioners (2014) GP prescribing rights for isotretinoin. http://www.racgp.org.au/yourracgp/news/reports/201405isotretinoin/
Thiboutot D, Gollnick H, Bettoli V et al (2012) Oral isotretinoin and pregnancy prevention programmes. Br J Dermatol 166:466–467
Weinberg JM (2005) iPLEDGE allegiance. Cutis 76:356
Woodcock J (2002) Concerns regarding Accutane (isotretinoin). www.fda.gov/NewsEvents/Testimony/ucm115126.htm
Wysowski DK, Pitts M, Beitz J (2001) An analysis of reports of depression and suicide in patients treated with isotretinoin. J Am Acad Dermatol 45:515–519
Yook JH, Han JY, Choi JS et al (2012) Pregnancy outcomes and factors associated with voluntary pregnancy termination in women who had been treated for acne with isotretinoin. Clin Toxicol 50:896–899

Pandemic Influenza Vaccines: Communication of Benefits, Risks, and Uncertainties

5

Glen J. Nowak, Emilie Karafillakis, and Heidi Larson

Abstract

Vaccines that would be recommended and offered in response to a novel influenza virus bring many communication challenges. This chapter identifies and describes some of the major issues that public health agencies and regulatory bodies, vaccine manufacturers, and healthcare professionals would face when it comes to pandemic influenza vaccines and immunisation recommendations. It does so by drawing upon experiences, findings, and outcomes from the H1N1 A influenza pandemic in 2009 that affected much of the world as well as lessons learnt from annual influenza prevention efforts. This chapter begins with challenges brought about by the uncertainties and complexities associated with influenza viruses and then highlights experiences from different countries with a focus on France as a relevant example, illustrating the similarities and differences that can affect pandemic influenza vaccine communication. The final section of the chapter reflects on some key communication-related research findings as well as lessons learnt that can help guide those doing vaccination-related communication responses and efforts in future influenza pandemics.

G. J. Nowak (✉)
Grady College of Journalism and Mass Communication, Grady College Center for Health and Risk Communication, Athens, GA, USA
e-mail: gnowak@uga.edu

E. Karafillakis
Vaccine Confidence Project™, Department of Epidemiology and Population Health, London School of Hygiene and Tropical Medicine, London, UK

H. Larson
Vaccine Confidence Project™, Department of Epidemiology and Population Health, London School of Hygiene and Tropical Medicine, London, UK

Department of Health Metrics Sciences, University of Washington, Seattle, WA, USA

© Springer Nature Singapore Pte Ltd. 2020

P. Bahri (ed.), *Communicating about Risks and Safe Use of Medicines*,
https://doi.org/10.1007/978-981-15-3013-5_5

5.1 Situation: Concerns About H1N1 A Pandemic Influenza and the Vaccines, and Communication Challenges

5.1.1 Influenza Viruses: A Continually Present Health Threat

According to the World Health Organization (WHO), every year, human influenza—commonly called "the flu"—rapidly spreads around the world in seasonal epidemics, resulting in an estimated three to five million cases of severe illness and up to 650,000 deaths linked to seasonal influenza (Iuliano et al. 2018). While it is certain that influenza is an annual health threat, each year there is much uncertainty regarding the severity, transmission, ultimate harm, and pandemic potential of the predominant circulating viruses. When WHO and other experts convene 6 months in advance of the Southern and Northern hemisphere flu seasons to review available data and make influenza vaccine strain selections, they do so aware that shifts and drifts in the viruses can greatly affect vaccine efficacy (e.g. substantially decrease it) and public health vaccination strategies (e.g. change in immunisation priorities). They also need to be continually mindful that novel influenza viruses can emerge, bringing with them the potential for a global pandemic as well as the need to quickly develop new vaccines.

5.1.2 The H1N1 A Influenza Pandemic in 2009

The 2009 H1N1 A influenza pandemic provides insights into how events can unfold after the recognition of a new influenza virus with pandemic potential (e.g. an influenza A virus). On 21 April 2009, the Centers for Disease Control and Prevention (CDC) in the United States (US) announced that it had identified a new H1N1 A influenza virus strain in two patients (CDC 2009). Shortly thereafter, public health agencies in Canada and Mexico announced they had determined the new virus had been widely circulating in Mexico and had caused much severe illness and many deaths. Following these reports, on 24 April 2009, WHO declared the outbreak a Public Health Emergency of International Concern (PHEIC) (Gerwin 2012). On 26 April, the US government declared the H1N1 A flu a public health emergency and soon after, similar declarations were made in other regions of the world (CDC 2009; Gerwin 2012; WHO 2009a). On 11 June, the outbreak reached a level that prompted WHO to declare a pandemic, with 74 countries reported being affected (Chan 2009). A year later, WHO reported that 214 countries and overseas territories or communities had laboratory confirmed cases of pandemic influenza, including over 18,156 laboratory-confirmed deaths from the virus (WHO 2010).

As is likely to be the case with pandemic influenza, the initial recognition of a novel influenza virus in April 2009 prompted swift and significant media, healthcare professional, public health and regulatory body, and public interest in influenza vaccines and influenza immunisation recommendations, including whether, when, and how new influenza vaccines would be tested, produced, distributed, and used. Shortly after identification of the new virus, a broad collaboration of international institutions, governments, public health authorities, scientists, and vaccine manufactures undertook a concerted effort to formulate, test, license, and produce a safe and effective pandemic influenza vaccine (Chan 2009; Abelin et al. 2011; EMA 2011). By September 2009, several manufacturers of inactivated and live attenuated influenza vaccines had completed vaccine development, received regulatory authorisation, and scaled up vaccine production (WHO 2009a; Abelin et al. 2011). By December 2009, over 30 vaccines had been licensed and more than 50 countries had formulated vaccination recommendations and started immunisation efforts (EMA 2010). Subsequently, the vaccine was administered and made available to millions of people, including the more than 40 million vaccinated in Europe and nearly 127 million doses distributed in the US by the end of March 2010 (Abelin et al. 2011; EMA 2010; CDC 2010a).

5.1.3 Communication Challenges

The 2009 H1N1 A influenza pandemic, along with experiences and findings gained every year from the use and promotion of annual vaccination against seasonal influenza, provides helpful insights into many of the major vaccine-related uncertainties and complexities that may arise or need to be addressed on the communication front (Bahri and Castillon Melero 2018; Nowak et al. 2015, 2017; Pistol and Steinu-Cercel 2013; Schmid et al. 2017; Walton and Seitz 2012; Wheelock et al. 2013). There are at least four communication challenges that public health agencies, regulatory bodies, vaccine manufacturers, and healthcare professionals need to be prepared for when it comes to communicating about pandemic influenza vaccines and vaccination to the public, patients and caregivers (e.g. parents who will need to make vaccination decisions for their children), and political leaders and policymakers. Each of these challenges greatly affect communication strategies, plans, and messaging, as well as the effects and effectiveness of influenza vaccine messages and materials. These challenges are as follows:

- *New influenza viruses with pandemic potential, as well as annual influenza vaccines that are not well matched with those found in seasonal influenza viruses, initially bring many hard-to-answer questions regarding the influenza disease, vaccines, and vaccination*: As the 2009 H1N1 A pandemic illustrates, in the aftermath of discovery of a new influenza virus, there will be much interest in predictions and projections, including whether the newly discovered virus will generate a pandemic (EMA 2011; Fisher et al. 2011). This will quickly be followed by much interest in whether, and how, the symptoms and illness caused by the pandemic influenza virus differs from that caused by circulating annual influenza viruses; how susceptible people are to infection with the newly discovered virus and whether some people (e.g. children, those 65 years old and older) are more susceptible to infection and/or more severe health outcomes; and how the virus is transmitted and how fast it is or may be spread. While regulatory bodies and public health agencies across the globe will be actively engaged in pandemic influenza vaccine development, immunisation efforts, and the monitoring of vaccine effectiveness and safety (EMA 2011; Fisher et al. 2011), questions and concerns regarding influenza disease, vaccines, and vaccination will likely vary by country. In some countries, for instance, the public and media may be very interested in vaccine efficacy, while in other countries the focus may be primarily on safety. It is also likely that concerns and issues beyond science will emerge, such as trust in the government officials who are recommending vaccination, and this will also vary by country. Cultural and country differences will add to the communication complexity (Poland 2010). However, high public and news media interest in whether and when vaccines will be available to protect people from the new virus should be expected, and initial questions in the public domain likely will include:

- How are the new flu vaccines being developed (e.g. what are the processes being used, will the pandemic vaccines be similar to annual vaccines in terms of composition and administration)?
- Who is sponsoring or funding the development of new vaccines (e.g. governments, industry, both)?
- How will vaccine safety and efficacy be evaluated or assessed, and which entities will do so?
- What is the timeline for vaccine development, testing, manufacturing, licensing, and distribution?
- What criteria will be used when determining whether to license a new flu vaccine, particularly those related to vaccine safety? and
- Who will be the priority sub-populations or groups for the initial vaccine doses, and what criteria were used to establish the priorities?

  In addition, influenza viruses, whether seasonal or pandemic, by their nature bring much uncertainty. Initial cases or outbreaks, for instance, by themselves are often not good indicators of future or additional cases; which communities or regions will experience cases or outbreaks; or the ultimate severity of an influenza pandemic.

- *There will be much demand for "risk" communication, but relatively limited understanding of the risk communication domain by non-experts*: The word "risk", for instance, encompasses many related yet distinct definitions, including (1) the likelihood or probability of the threat happening or occurring in general (e.g. an outbreak of pandemic flu in a community, country, or region); (2) the likelihood or susceptibility of a sub-population or individuals to a real or potential hazard or threat (e.g. contracting influenza, experiencing severe illness from influenza, or experiencing an adverse reaction to an influenza vaccine); (3) the outcome of threat or harm, such as the severity of harm or negative effects caused by a hazard or threat (e.g. it is often assumed that pandemic influenza viruses will cause more severe illness than annual influenza viruses); and (4) individuals' perceptions regarding the likelihood of personal exposure or of experiencing harm if exposed to the virus (e.g. in the case of seasonal influenza, many individuals believe their likelihood of contracting influenza is very small or that if they are infected, they will experience a "manageable" illness) (Nowak et al. 2015; Schmid et al. 2017). As such, pandemic vaccine and vaccination-related communications must acknowledge and address more than one type of risk. In addition, communication efforts, particularly the messages, must recognise that actual risk and perceived risk are two distinct concepts (see Chap. 7). Something can be an actual risk in the sense that it is known to cause harm and there is an estimation of likelihood or possibility. That, however, does not mean populations or individuals will perceive the hazard as a significant or personal health threat. As Peter M Sandman (2012) noted, "the most important truth in risk communication is the exceedingly low correlation between whether a risk is dangerous and whether it is upsetting. . . That is, the risks that kill people and the risks that upset people are completely unrelated. If you know a risk is dangerous, that tells you almost nothing about whether it is upsetting" (Sandman 2012).

- *Epidemiological information is essential for formulating vaccination priorities and recommendations but is often not enough for achieving high compliance with immunisation recommendations* (see Chap. 10): In the US, for instance, the estimated 2009 H1N1 A vaccination median immunisation rates at the end of a three-month concerted effort to achieve high vaccination coverage (i.e. late January 2010) was 23.9% among persons aged ≥6 months, 36.8% for children aged 6 months—17 years, and 20.1% for adults aged ≥18 years (CDC 2010b). It was also only 33.2% for persons in the US Advisory Committee on Immunization Practices (ACIP) initial priority groups (i.e. pregnant women, healthcare and emergency medical services personnel, children and young adults aged 6 months to 24 years, persons aged 25–64 years who had medical conditions that put them at higher risk for influenza-related complications, and persons who live with or provide care for infants aged <6 months) (CDC 2010b). In the UK, where H1N1 A vaccines were not available for large-scale use until the end of the second wave of infection in autumn 2009, vaccine uptake was also relatively low, including for two priority groups—children and healthcare workers (de Whalley and Pollard 2013).

As studies assessing annual influenza vaccination acceptance have found, campaigns and education efforts must go beyond simply providing information on vaccine safety and efficacy or increasing awareness of vaccination recommendations (Nowak et al. 2015; Schmid et al. 2017; Wheelock et al. 2013; MacDougall et al. 2015). It is not enough to simply provide factual and statistical information about disease incidence or vaccination benefits and risks in order foster "rational" decision-making (Bahri and Castillon Melero 2018; Bahri et al. 2019; Brewer et al. 2017; Simis et al. 2016). Rather, public health agencies and regulatory bodies must recognise that individuals, including parents of young children, often use subjective appraisals, perceived social norms, and heuristics (i.e. cognitive shortcuts) when making vaccination decisions (Wheelock et al. 2013; Simis et al. 2016; CDC 2018; Poland and Poland 2011), and that much medical-related decision-making is based on affect, feelings, and values (Brewer et al. 2017; Poland and Poland 2011; Lee et al. 2013). In the case of flu vaccination, for example, it has been found that risk perceptions measured in terms of feelings rather than in terms of cognitive probability judgments better predict adult vaccination (Sandman 2012; Weinstein et al. 2007) and that lack of confidence in flu vaccine is often based on doubts about its safety and effectiveness as well as lack of trust in health authorities (Schmid et al. 2017; Poland 2010; de Whalley and Pollard 2013).

- *Websites, social media, and other digital media, while widely used to transmit and exchange health-related information, bring significant additional challenges and communication resource demands*: As the 2009 H1N1 A pandemic and ongoing efforts related to annual influenza immunisation illustrate, public health agencies, and to a lesser extent government regulatory bodies, need to communicate about vaccines and vaccination recommendations through an array of channels, with websites, social media, and other digital media among the most visible and immediate. In addition, a wide array of digital are available, including texting, instant messaging (e.g. Twitter, Instagram, Snapchat), social networking sites, search engines, and internet-based content sites (e.g. YouTube). While digital media enable public health agencies and regulatory bodies to quickly post or disseminate content and materials that are completely within their control, and to do so when and how they choose, that does not mean those messages are reaching the needed people, being viewed or used by large numbers of people, or having significant impact on intentions and behaviours (Nowak et al. 2017; Brewer et al. 2017; Betsch et al. 2012).

  It is also the case that public health and regulatory body messages and content face enormous competition for attention. In 2018, each day an estimated 500 million tweets were sent and 4.75 billion pieces of content were shared (Desjardins 2018). It was also estimated that every 60 s, 187 million e-mails and 18 million text messages were sent, 4.3 million YouTube videos were watched, and 3.7 million Google search queries were done (Desjardins 2018). Widespread access and use of websites, social media, and other digital media mean that individuals can be reached with, or access, a plethora of information, misinformation, and disinformation, including "fake news", on any topic as well as select what to read and believe. Those opposed to vaccines use these channels to dissuade compliance with vaccination recommendations, and often do so without providing a scientific or medical basis for their assertions (e.g. they suggest those who would adhere should not trust government agencies) (Iuliano et al. 2018; Gerwin 2012). Given the volume and breadth of information disseminated via traditional news and novel digital media, public health and regulatory agencies should invest in listening and (media) monitoring capabilities or services. Knowing what information is being put forth enables detection of mis- and disinformation and guides the design of targeted communication responses. In addition, effectively using websites, social media, and other digital media often requires significant resources (e.g. programmers, content specialists), timely and rapid posting and responses, and high-quality production, which often are not available nor found in government agencies (e.g. most do not have adequate communication budgets and rapid review and message clearance processes) (Nowak et al. 2017). It is also the case that while many believe social media have much influence, relatively little is known about how social media affects vaccination-related beliefs and behaviours (Betsch et al. 2012).

5.2 Events: The Communication Experiences

The 2009 H1N1 A pandemic illustrated that novel influenza viruses will likely result in differences in responses as well as communication activities and needs. Related attitudes and intentions will differ across countries and cultures (Poland 2010). It was found, for instance, that in Hong Kong and Singapore, there was greater initial public support for government pandemic measures than in Western countries (Chor et al. 2009; Tan et al. 2010). Those high levels of support, however, did not prevent misconceptions and misunderstanding. In Hong Kong, where the public approved of government policies including the quarantining of hotel guests, large numbers of people avoided visiting crowded places, with many wrongly believing that this was a government recommendation. One assessment of the pandemic response in Asia thus concluded that "clear communication, updated scientific information and transparency on government decision-making were insufficient" (Fisher et al. 2011). Similarly, an assessment of response efforts in Europe found many countries reported a lack of public confidence in the pandemic recommendations from national authorities and that many healthcare professionals expressed lack of understanding of the benefits and risks of recommended pandemic vaccines (Hanquet et al. 2011). A comprehensive analysis of German press coverage of 2009 H1N1 A found high visibility throughout the pandemic but much variability in topics and messages, which was perceived as fostering the dissemination of incomplete, incorrect, and contradictory information to the public (Husemann and Fisher 2015).

5.2.1 The Influenza Pandemic in France: An Uncoordinated Response

France is one of the countries in the world with the lowest levels of public confidence in vaccines (Larson et al. 2016) and as such, can provide helpful insights into what may cause or contribute to low vaccine acceptance. In 2018, this was reflected by an extremely low uptake of human papillomavirus (HPV) vaccination as well as by the resurgence of devastating measles outbreaks, which highlighted insufficient uptake of measles vaccines. The roots of the low confidence can be traced back to a history of mistrust. One of the other major events that eroded public trust was the handling of the H1N1 A influenza pandemic in 2009. The French health authorities were criticised by news media, the public, and policy makers for the way they managed the response to the pandemic, including vaccine delivery and communication. Public mistrust led to a low uptake of the H1N1 A vaccine, with coverage ranging from 11.1% for the overall population, to 16.3% for individuals at risk of complications from flu infection and 30% for healthcare workers (Vaux et al. 2011). The unfolding events can be summarised as follows:

After the pandemic was declared, France purchased 94 million doses of the vaccine with the goal of vaccinating, free of charge, the entire French population (around 63.5 million inhabitants) (Schwarzinger et al. 2010a). While a similar decision was taken by other countries, it was seen as a particularly ambitious goal for France, where uptake of the seasonal flu vaccine is usually around 50% for targeted at-risk groups (e.g. those 65 years old and older) and less than 25% of the rest of the population (Schwarzinger et al. 2010b). During the influenza pandemic, communication campaigns targeted the wider French population, with few specific messages to individuals in targeted at-risk groups. However, as not enough vaccine was initially available for the entire population, it was given to different targeted groups in order of priority: (1) healthcare workers (including primary care doctors and nurses); (2) household contacts and caregivers of children under 6 months of age as well as other types of healthcare workers and individuals part of at-risk groups and aged between 6 months and 64 years; and (3) at-risk individuals over 65 years old. This phased strategy, which was implemented in concert with messages stressing the need for the entire population to be vaccinated, created confusion among the media and members of the public. The government was very quickly accused of over dramatising the pandemic, especially once it became clear that the disease was less severe than initially projected. The H1N1 A influenza pandemic was commonly referred by the French media as "grippette", or "little flu", in reference to the perceived low severity of the disease (Raude et al. 2010).

Public questioning of the rationale for mass vaccination, together with doubts about the safety of the new vaccine, led people to look for advice from their general practitioners (GPs). GPs are the traditional providers of vaccines in France, and as in many other European countries, they constitute one of the most trusted sources of medical information for the public (Bouder et al. 2015). However, GPs and paediatricians were deliberately not included in the national H1N1 A vaccination strategy to avoid overloading them in case of high demand (Vaux et al. 2011). During the pandemic, special vaccination centres were created in various public buildings throughout the country to avoid placing too much burden on GPs and hospitals. Some children were also vaccinated at schools, which is uncommon in France. This lack of engagement with typical vaccine providers created conflicts between GPs and health authorities and mistrust from the public. A study later found that French GPs had high acceptability of the vaccine, which shows that a more coordinated approach involving GPs could have helped increase public trust and vaccine acceptance (Schwarzinger et al. 2010a). The health authorities reversed the policy in January 2010 to authorise GPs to administer the pandemic vaccine, but this came too late, and followed months of debates and criticism of the vaccine on the media (Schwarzinger et al. 2010b).

As concerned parents and members of the public could not discuss the pandemic vaccine with their GPs, many sought information online or in the media. At the beginning of the pandemic, the government had a strong presence in the media, stressing the dangers of the pandemic by referring to daily reports of cases and fatalities. However, public perceptions soon began to change, and as the number of pandemic flu infections and severe cases decreased, concerns about pandemic flu vaccine safety started increasing. France was one of the countries where concerns about the safety of the pandemic vaccines were the strongest (Assemblée nationale 2010). Every day in the media, journalists, opinion leaders, and politicians issued concerns about the safety of a newly and rapidly developed vaccine, questioning the accelerated authorisation procedure for the vaccine and the motives of pharmaceutical companies (Schwarzinger et al. 2010b).

The adjuvants (used in the vaccine to enhance their efficacy) were also commonly debated, as they were considered unsafe, too novel, and insufficiently tested (Vaux et al. 2011). This could explain why concerns about adjuvants persist in France for any vaccine, more than in any other countries. Another characteristic of the French debates around the pandemic vaccine was the suggested correlation with the risk of Guillain-Barre syndrome (GBS), echoing the 1976 episode of GBS following administration of an earlier version of the H1N1 A vaccination in the United States (Pollack 2009). The GBS anxieties were also conveyed by some French nursing trade unions and contributed to low H1N1 A vaccination coverage among paramedical personnel (Tanguy et al. 2011). It is also likely that the nurses' reluctance to get vaccinated dissuaded some in the general public.

The 2009 H1N1 A influenza pandemic in France is often used as an example of an event that eroded public trust, with long-term effects on confidence in health authorities and vaccination. The challenge of communicating uncertainties around the vaccine and the disease led to confusing and sometimes conflicting messages from health authorities and created the perception of disagreement between experts. Communication was directed at the general population, using pre-existing communication mechanisms and failed to target at-risk groups or respond to concerns on digital and social media (Assemblée nationale 2010). The communication gap was quickly filled by negative public discourses, further exacerbated by a lack of consistent and coordinated messages from GPs and other traditional vaccine providers. While the government has drawn a long list of lessons learnt from the events (Assemblée nationale 2010), the long-term effects on public trust could prove to be extremely damaging in case of a future influenza pandemic. This was confirmed by a recent study, which showed that the events related to the 2009 H1N1 A influenza pandemic and the perceived responses from health authorities have had a dramatic impact on attitudes towards vaccination in general in France and has undermined public confidence in health authorities (Assemblée nationale 2010).

5.3 Evaluation: Feedback, Outcomes and Lessons Learnt

As has been shown, much has been learned from the 2009 H1N1 A pandemic, annual efforts designed to foster influenza vaccination, and research studies done to guide, inform, or evaluate influenza vaccine-related communications. Based on those experiences, findings, and research syntheses, learnings regarding how best to address the pandemic influenza-related communication challenges and complexities are specifically described in this section of the chapter.

5.3.1 Addressing Uncertainties and Complexities

Since influenza virus-related disease threats and risks involve uncertainties and complexities, core risk communication principles should be used to guide risk communication efforts and responses. This includes expressing empathy in response to public and sub-population fears and concerns, placing value on learning how members of target sub-populations perceive vaccine recommendations (including healthcare professionals), acknowledging uncertainties with regard to how events may play out, sharing dilemmas regarding public health recommendations and actions (e.g. those related to prioritising limited initial vaccine supplies), foreshadowing potential changes in recommendations and actions, recognising the influence of emotions and values in health decision-making, providing action steps, and setting appropriate expectations regarding public health and regulatory body actions (Bahri and Castillon Melero 2018; Nowak et al. 2017; Sandman 2012; CDC 2018; Lundgren and McMakin 2018; Topic Group 3 of the CIOMS Working Group on Vaccine Safety 2018).

5.3.2 Understanding Social and Behavioural Aspects

Effective influenza vaccine and vaccination-related communication requires more than providing information and seeking to increase awareness of public health recommendations and advice. As is being done with annual influenza vaccination communication efforts, behavioural and social science insights (see Chaps. 7 and 8), methods, and hence multidisciplinary research (see Chap. 1) should be used to inform communication strategies and messages. There is growing evidence that personal feelings, social networks, and social preferences positively and negatively influence vaccination acceptance (MacDougall et al. 2015; Brewer et al. 2017). Notably, a comprehensive review also found the most effective ways to increase vaccination compliance are ones that use reminders, defaults, sanctions, and incentives to change behaviour directly, rather than trying to change what people think or feel (Brewer et al. 2017).

5.3.3 Applying Communication Expertise

Public health and regulatory agencies, including WHO, the US CDC, the Council for International Organization of Medical Sciences (CIOMS), and others have developed resources to guide pandemic and annual influenza communication responses. They have also created vaccine safety-related communication resources. All of these resources are accessible (often in the internet) for guidance and use in developing and doing pandemic influenza-related communications. Examples include WHO's Pandemic Influenza Preparedness Risk Communication Framework (WHO 2018) and their guide for Vaccine Safety Events: Managing the Communications Response (WHO Europe 2013), the US CDC's Crisis and Emergency Communication Guide and supportive materials (CDC 2018), and the CIOMS Guide to Vaccine Safety Communications (Bahri et al. 2019).

5.3.4 Defining Clear Objectives and Appropriate Tools for Communication

It is necessary to know the specific communication purposes and objectives for the website, other digital media dissemination, and social media messages one plans to provide. Two questions that should be asked are: "What are we trying to achieve with our media tools and messages?" and "How will we know if we have been successful?" In the case of pandemic as well as annual influenza vaccination, the purposes and objectives should be focused on conveying the value, benefits, and safety of recommended vaccines. Consideration should also be given to how to use websites to provide guidance and information (e.g. pandemic influenza vaccine safety information) to healthcare professionals. Further, given the pervasiveness and reliance on digital and in particular social media by journalists, members of the public, and healthcare professionals, public health agencies need to have the ability, resources, and capabilities to use interactive, customised communication tools (Betsch et al. 2012).

5.3.5 Conducting Research for Planning, Monitoring, and Evaluating Communication

Audience and media research (see Chap. 10) as well as website, other digital, and in particular social media data and analytics, and social media research (see Chap. 11) should be used to both inform and evaluate content, messages, and communication strategies and materials (Bahri and Castillon Melero 2018; Nowak et al. 2017; Brewer et al. 2017; Betsch et al. 2012). In advance of a pandemic, public health agencies and regulatory bodies should undertake proactive efforts to gauge the effects and effectiveness of their communication efforts, and especially their websites, social media, and other digital media. During and after dissemination of information and interaction with the public, resources should be invested in assessing whether content is being accessed and understood, whether messages sent are reaching significant numbers of people in targeted audiences, and what information and misinformation is being sent, exchanged, and found on other digital and social media. These evaluation efforts will help in identifying information provision shortcomings and additional needs as well as guide efforts to address or counteract incorrect information (Lau et al. 2009; Peretti-Watel et al. 2013).

5.3.6 Global Considerations

While this chapter has primarily focused on US and EU approaches and lessons learnt from the 2009 H1N1 A influenza pandemic, many of the communication experiences and approaches have values across the globe. First, as multiple assessments of the effects and effectiveness of the pandemic response illustrated (Fisher et al. 2011; Poland 2010; de Whalley and Pollard 2013; Hanquet et al. 2011; Schwarzinger et al. 2010b), novel influenza viruses can quickly bring the need for rapid and extensive communication. Public health agencies and regulatory bodies will need to offer information, updates, and guidance in the face of much uncertainty, and likely much scepticism from healthcare professionals, the public, and individuals who may be at higher risk for medical complications. As such, most would benefit from gaining, practicing, and being able to quickly and effectively use risk communication principles and best practices. Second, the 2009 pandemic illustrated that while novel influenza viruses can pose a serious and significant health threat to many, that possibility by itself may not motivate healthcare professional or public acceptance of public health actions and recommendations. In 2009 and 2010, many countries found low public and priority group acceptance of H1N1 A vaccines, even among people who acknowledged the virus could cause serious illness. Healthcare professionals, who are often used as key sources of vaccination information, were of limited help because they had too little understanding of vaccination recommendations, priorities, and the safety of the vaccines. Thus, it would behove public health and regulatory bodies across the globe to assess how they communicate vaccine information, to more actively and systematically get input from healthcare professionals and the public (e.g. through use of communication, social and behavioural science research), and be prepared to actively engage with a wide range of partners (e.g. healthcare professionals, medical societies), media (e.g. journalists, websites), and affected groups (e.g. pregnant women, those with medical conditions that put them at higher risk of influenza complications) at the start of a potential influenza pandemic.

Conclusions

- The H1N1 A influenza pandemic in 2009 was declared a Public Health Emergency of International Concern (PHEIC) and public health emergency plans were evoked in many regions, with ultimately 214 countries affected by the pandemic and almost 20,000 laboratory-confirmed deaths worldwide.
- Vaccines against this novel pandemic influenza were produced in response, vaccination recommendations and priorities were established by public health advisory boards, and the safety of pandemic influenza vaccines were monitored in real time as they were distributed and used (WHO 2009b).
- Major challenges communication challenges arose from scientific uncertainties around the influenza disease, the vaccines, and vaccination recommendations. Additional challenges arose as a result of many public health officials and medical experts not having a strong understanding of how lay people perceive risk and make health-related decisions, inadequate application of risk communication expertise, and misinformation and disinformation disseminated on the internet and social media.
- As the example from France shows, trust in government officials, healthcare professional and public confidence in vaccines and vaccination recommendations, and early, meaningful involvement of healthcare professionals is essential in achieving acceptance and compliance with pandemic influenza vaccination recommendations. The absence of those elements fosters vaccine hesitancy and low uptake.
- Key lessons learnt from evaluating the communication efforts undertaken in response to the 2009 H1N1 A pandemic include the need to acknowledge and address uncertainties and complexities from the start, understand and utilise social, behavioural, and media science insights and methods, apply communication expertise early and throughout, define clear communication objectives, and use communication principles and research to guide strategies and messaging as well as to evaluate efforts.
- From a global perspective, the 2009 H1N1 A pandemic illustrated that public health agencies and regulatory bodies need to be able to quickly, effectively, and repeatedly communicate with healthcare professionals, journalists, the public, and those groups at higher risk of influenza complications; doing so will require expertise in risk communication as well as being able to obtain and use research data that can inform policy making and policy-related communication.

References

Abelin A, Colegate T, Gardner S, Hehmea N, Palache A (2011) Lessons from pandemic A (H1N1): the research-based vaccine industry's perspective. Vaccine 29(6):1135–1138

Assemblée nationale (2010) Rapport N2698 fait AU NOM DE LA COMMISSION D'ENQUÊTE sur la manière dont a été programmée, expliquée et gérée la campagne de vaccination contre la grippe A (H1N1). http://www.assemblee-nationale.fr/13/pdf/rap-enq/r2698.pdf

Bahri P, Castillon Melero M (2018) Listen to the public and fulfil their information interests: translating vaccine communication research findings into guidance for regulators. Br J Clin Pharmacol 84:1696–1705

Bahri P, Rägo L, CIOMS Working Group on Vaccine Safety (2019) CIOMS guide to vaccine safety communication: executive summary. Vaccine 37:401–408

Betsch C, Brewer NT, Brocard P, Davies P, Gaissmaier W et al (2012) Opportunities and challenges of Web 2.0 for vaccination decisions. Vaccine 30:3727–3733

Bouder F, Way D, Löfstedt R, Evensen D (2015) Transparency in Europe: a quantitative study. Risk Anal 35(7):1210–1229

Brewer NT, Chapman GB, Rothman AJ, Leask J, Kempe A (2017) Increasing vaccination: putting psychological science into action. Psychol Sci Public Interest 18(3):149–207

CDC (2009) Swine influenza A (H1N1) infection in two children – Southern California, March–April 2009. MMWR Morb Mortal Wkly Rep 58(15):400–402

CDC (2010a) Summary of 2009 monovalent H1N1 influenza vaccine data – vaccine adverse event reporting system. Data through 26 March 2010. http://vaers.hhs.gov/resources/2010H1N1Summary_Apr01.pdf

CDC (2010b) Interim results: state-specific influenza A (H1N1) 2009 monovalent vaccination coverage — United States, October 2009–January 2010. MMWR Morb Mortal Wkly Rep 59(12):363

CDC (2018) Crisis plus emergency risk communication manual. CDC, Atlanta. https://emergency.cdc.gov/cerc/manual/index.asp

Chan M (2009) World now at the start of 2009 influenza pandemic. World Health Organization press statement. http://www.who.int/mediacentre/news/statements/2009/h1n1_pandemic_phase6_20090611/en/

Chor JS, Ngai KL, Goggins WB, Wong MC, Wong SY, Lee N et al (2009) Willingness of Hong Kong healthcare workers to accept pre-pandemic influenza vaccination at different WHO alert levels: two questionnaire surveys. Br Med J 339:b3391

de Whalley PC, Pollard AJ (2013) Pandemic influenza A (H1N1) 2009 vaccination in children: a UK perspective. J Paediatr Child Health 49(3):E183–E188. https://doi.org/10.1111/jpc.12037

Desjardins J (2018) What happens in an internet minute in 2018? Visual Capitalist blog Posted on 14 May 2018. https://www.visualcapitalist.com/internet-minute-2018/

EMA (2010) 15th pandemic pharmacovigilance update. http://www.ema.europa.eu/pdfs/influenza/21323810en.pdf

EMA (2011) Pandemic report and lessons learned: outcome of the European Medicines Agency's activities during the 2009 (H1N1) flu pandemic. EMA, London

Fisher D, Hui DS, Gao Z, Lee C, Oh MD et al (2011) Pandemic response lessons from influenza H1N1 2009 in Asia. Respirology 16(6):876–882

Gerwin LE (2012) The challenge of providing the public with actionable information during a pandemic. J Law Med Ethics 40:630–654

Hanquet G, Van Damme P, Brasseur D, De Cuyper X, Gregor S, Holmberg M, Martin R, Molnár Z, Pompa MG, Snacken R, van der Sande M, Van Ranst M, Wirtz A, Neels P (2011) Lessons learnt from pandemic A (H1N1) 2009 influenza vaccination: highlights of a European workshop in Brussels (22 March 2010). Vaccine 10:370–377. (Epub 12 Nov 2010)

Husemann S, Fisher F (2015) Content analysis of press coverage during the H1N1 influenza pandemic in Germany 2009-2010. BMC Public Health 15:386. https://doi.org/10.1186/s12889-015-1742-1

Iuliano AD, Roguski KM, Chang HH, Muscatello DJ, Palekar R et al (2018) Estimates of global seasonal influenza-associated respiratory mortality: a modelling study. Lancet 391(10127):1285–1300. https://doi.org/10.1016/S0140-6736(17)33293-2

Larson HJ, de Figueiredo A, Xiahong Z, Schulz WS, Verger P, Johnston IG, Cook AR, Jones NS (2016) The state of vaccine confidence 2016: global insights through a 67-country survey. EBioMedicine 12:295–301

Lau JT, Griffiths S, Choi KC et al (2009) Widespread public misconception in the early phase of the H1N1 influenza pandemic. J Infect 59:122–127

Lee YK, Low WY, Ng CJ (2013) Exploring patient values in medical decision making: a qualitative study. PLoS One 8(11):e80051

Lundgren RE, McMakin AH (2018) Risk communication: a handbook for communicating environmental, safety, and health risks, 6th edn. Wiley, Hoboken

MacDougall DM, Halperin BA, MacKinnon-Cameron D et al (2015) The challenge of vaccinating adults: attitudes and beliefs of the Canadian public and healthcare providers. BMJ Open 5:e009062. https://doi.org/10.1136/bmjopen-2015-009062

Nowak GJ, Sheedy K, Bursey K, Smith TM, Basket M (2015) Promotion influenza vaccination: insights from a qualitative meta-analysis of 14 years of influenza-related communication research by the U.S. Centers for Disease Control and Prevention (CDC). Vaccine 33: 2741–2756

Nowak GJ, Shen AK, Schwartz JL (2017) Using campaigns to improve perceptions of the value of adult vaccination in the United States: health communication considerations and insights. Vaccine 35:5543–5550

Peretti-Watel P, Verger P, Raude J, Constant A, Gautier A, Jestin C, Beck F (2013) Dramatic change in public attitudes towards vaccination during the 2009 influenza A (H1N1) pandemic in France. Eur Secur 18(44):20623

Pistol A, Steinu-Cercel A (2013) Risk communication strategies used in the 2009 pandemic influenza A H1N1PDM. Public Health Manag 2(4):163–166

Poland CM (2010) The 2009-2010 influenza pandemic: effects on pandemic and seasonal vaccine uptake and lessons learned for seasonal vaccination campaigns. Vaccine 28S:D3–D13

Poland CM, Poland GA (2011) Vaccine education spectrum disorder: the importance of incorporating psychological and cognitive models into vaccine education. Vaccine 29:6145–6148

Pollack A (2009) Fear of a swine flu epidemic in 1976 offers some lessons, and concerns, today. New York Times [newspaper on the Internet]; Health. https://www.nytimes.com/2009/05/09/health/09vaccine.html

Raude J, Caille-Brillet AL, Setbon M (2010) The 2009 pandemic H1N1 influenza vaccination in France: who accepted to receive the vaccine and why? PLoS Curr 19:2

Sandman PM (2012) Responding to community outrage: strategies for effective risk communication. http://www.psandman.com/media/RespondingtoCommunityOutrage.pdf

Schmid P, Rauber D, Betsch C, Lidoit G, Denker ML (2017) Barriers of influenza vaccination intention and behavior – a systematic review of influenza vaccine hesitancy, 2005-2016. PLoS One 12:e0170550. https://doi.org/10.1371/journal.pone.0170550

Schwarzinger M, Verger P, Guerville MA, Aubry C, Rolland S, Obadia Y, Moatti JP (2010a) Positive attitudes of French general practitioners towards A/H1N1 influenza-pandemic vaccination: a missed opportunity to increase vaccination uptakes in the general public? Vaccine 28(15):2743–2748

Schwarzinger M, Flicoteaux R, Cortarenoda S, Obadia Y, Moatti JP (2010b) Low acceptability of A/H1N1 pandemic vaccination in French adult population: did public health policy fuel public dissonance? PLoS One 5(4):e10199

Simis MJ, Madden H, Cacciatore MA, Yeo SK (2016) The lure of rationality: why does the deficit model persist in science communication? Public Underst Sci 25(4):400–414

Tan WM, Chlebicka NL, Tan BH (2010) Attitudes of patients, visitors and healthcare workers at a tertiary hospital towards influenza A (H1N1) response measures. Ann Acad Med Singap 39:303–304

Tanguy M, Boyeau C, Pean S, Marijon E, Delhumeau A, Fanello S (2011) Acceptance of seasonal and pandemic a (H1N1) 2009 influenza vaccination by healthcare workers in a French teaching hospital. Vaccine 29(25):4190–4194

Topic Group 3 of the CIOMS Working Group on Vaccine Safety (2018) CIOMS guide to vaccine safety communication. Council for International Organizations of Medical Sciences (CIOMS), Genève

Vaux S, Van Cauteren D, Guthmann JP, Le Strat Y, Vaillant V, de Valk H, Lévy-Bruhl D (2011) Influenza vaccination coverage against seasonal and pandemic influenza and their determinants in France: a cross-sectional survey. BMC Public Health 11(1):30

Walton LR, Seitz HH (2012) Strategic use of YouTube during a national public health crisis: the CDC's response to the 2009 H1N1 flu epidemic. Case Stud Strateg Commun 1(3):25–37

Weinstein ND, Kwitel A, McCaul KD et al (2007) Risk perceptions: assessment and relationship to influenza vaccination. Health Psychol 26(2):146–151

Wheelock A, Thomson A, Sevdalis N (2013) Social and psychological factors underlying adult vaccination behavior: lessons from seasonal influenza vaccination in the US and the UK. Expert Rev Vaccines 12(8):1–9

WHO (2009a) Pandemic H1N1 2009 report of regional consultation on pandemic H1N1 2009 and strengthening country capacity for pandemic preparedness. Bangkok, Thailand, 9–11 July 2009

WHO (2009b) Statement from WHO global advisory committee on vaccine safety about the safety profile of pandemic influenza A (H1N1) 2009 vaccines. http://www.who.int/csr/resources/publications/swineflu/cp164_2009_1612_gacvs_h1n1_vaccine_safety.pdf

WHO (2010) Pandemic (H1N1) 2009 – weekly update 104. 11 June 2009. http://www.who.int/csr/don/2010_06_11/en/

WHO (2018) Pandemic influenza preparedness (PIP) risk communication. https://www.who.int/risk-communication/pandemic-influenza-preparedness/en/

WHO Europe (2013) Vaccine safety events: managing the communications response. http://www.euro.who.int/__data/assets/pdf_file/0007/187171/Vaccine-Safety-Events-managing-the-communications-response-final.pdf?ua=1

Part II

Tackling the Challenges: Methods for Medicinal Product Risk Communication Research

Ethical Frameworks

6

Ghislaine van Thiel

Abstract

Evidence about benefits and risks of medicines can guide the communication about risks and safe use of medicinal products—but not all the way. Ethical questions arise when science cannot produce conclusive answers to important questions or when there is a tension between scientific knowledge and other values, beliefs or perceptions. Examples are questions around new, inconclusive evidence about potential adverse effects of marketed medicines or regarding unintended effects of risk communication, such as shame, changes in therapy adherence or stigmatisation experienced by individuals using a certain medicine. Ensuring adequate and timely communication about risks and safe use of medicines therefore depends partly on ethical considerations, such as the duty of beneficence to patients and communities, the patient right to autonomy and collective responsibility. Health communication practices need to be based on a fair balance of relevant ethical norms and values. In this chapter, an ethical perspective on medicinal product risk communication will be introduced and four areas of ethical tension and the contexts of uncertainty and trust are discussed, which should be taken into account when planning or evaluating communication events.

G. van Thiel (✉)
Department of Medical Humanities, Julius Center for Health Sciences and Primary Care, University Medical Center Utrecht, Utrecht, Netherlands
e-mail: G.J.M.W.vanThiel@umcutrecht.nl

© Springer Nature Singapore Pte Ltd. 2020

P. Bahri (ed.), *Communicating about Risks and Safe Use of Medicines*,
https://doi.org/10.1007/978-981-15-3013-5_6

6.1 The Ethics Discipline: Scope, Theories and Principles

In recent years there have been a number of cases that are instructive to the challenges involved in communication of risks and safe use of medicines in the twenty-first century. One example is the human papillomavirus (HPV) vaccine scare, which had an important peak in Spain in February 2009 (see Fig. 6.1). This case clearly shows that in risk communication, facts are only part of the story. Interventions to overcome problems related to the risks and safety of medicines and the communications about it—especially vaccines—often take an approach of positioning a "rational", "expert" or "scientific" view as opposed to "irrational" view or fear of the general public. It is however questionable whether this dichotomy actually holds true and whether "shaming [the members of the public] into following expert advice" is an appropriate and sustainable strategy in health communication (Bergstresser 2015).

The questions that arise when science cannot produce conclusive answers to important questions or when there is a tension between scientific knowledge and other values, beliefs or perceptions are in part ethical in nature. This chapter starts out with a characterisation of the discipline of medical ethics. Subsequently, four areas of ethical tension in communicating risks and safe use of medicines are described:

1. the issue of the relation between autonomy and risk information;
2. the tension between attribution of individual responsibility and avoiding harm in risk communication;

On Friday, 6 February 2009, two girls from the Spanish province of Valencia were admitted to a hospital, shortly after having received the HPV vaccine Gardasil®. They were very agitated, and in both cases repeated and prolonged seizures and loss of consciousness were observed. Doctors became alarmed, as they diagnosed *Status Epilepticus* (SE) and decided to induce coma to put their brains to sleep. In a few days, this event escalated into a full-fledged controversy. The Valencia province's health authorities alerted the Spanish Ministry of Health without delay. Although staff members of the Spanish medicines agency were convinced that a safety issue with the vaccine was very unlikely, the provincial and central health authorities agreed to stop use of the batch. As soon as this was announced, the issue spread outside Spain. Italian authorities stopped the batch on 9 February, and the following day the marketing authorisation holder stopped use of the entire batch too. The mainstream press remained at first prudent about causal links. Soon, however, the same new soutlets suggested that profits had been put before safety.
Ten days after the "outbreak", the European Medicines Agency (EMA) issued a press release on the view of its Committee for Medicinal Products for Human Use (CHMP). This stated:
"Based on the current data, [CHMP] has concluded that the cases are unlikely to be related to vaccination with Gardasil and that the benefits of Gardasil continue to outweigh its risks. Therefore the Committee is recommending that vaccination with Gardasil should continue in accordance with national vaccination programmes in Member States."
In the same press release the CHMP also recommended an update of the product information of Gardasil, to reinforce information on syncope (fainting) as a side effect of vaccination with Gardasil.
The Spanish Health Directory General was in contact with the United States Centers for Disease Control (US CDC), which came up with likewise reassuring information. The Spanish authorities finally managed to put an end to the controversy by establishing an ad hoc committee of highly respected medical experts to look into the issue.
On 9 April 2009, this committee came to the conclusion –signed unanimously by its members –that this was an incident of "fictitious" and "hysterical" convulsions. In other words, there was no causal relationship with the vaccine other than purely "psychological" In the end, however, this crisis involved weeks of discussions, publications, papers, articles and heated television and radio coverage. A significant drop in vaccination was observed between February and April 2009, especially in the province of Valencia.

Fig. 6.1 The "Gardasil scare" (Löfstedt et al. 2011)

3. ethical aspects of knowledge governance; and
4. the value of trust in communication about risks and safe use of medicines.

Facts, norms and principles are described which together form an ethical perspective on each area of tension.

The chapter does not seek to resolve the ethical problems, since each would require extensive analysis and discussion, but intends instead to point out ways in which ethical analysis and debate could help the practice of medical product risk communication, its planning and evaluation and research overall move forward.

6.1.1 The Development of Bioethics

Ethics is concerned with questions about what *ought* to be done. To answer these questions, ethicists reflect on moral values and on rules and principles that reflect what human beings *ought* to do or what is *right* for them (Sidgwick 1962). Ethicists can employ a variety of methods for this reflection. The question of which methodology is the most appropriate is at the heart of a longstanding debate among scholars in the field (Anonymous 2007). Some authors argue that the disagreements regarding the primary method and standard of rigour are deeply problematic, while others have suggested that bioethics cannot be placed within the traditional framework of disciplines, instead considering it multidisciplinary (Adler and Zlotnik Shaul 2012; Ives et al. 2017). Notwithstanding the different methodological approaches, bioethics emerged as a discipline covering a relatively broad range of topics as well as methodologies. Its development during the twentieth century is generally seen as characterised by two "turns":

– the turn from abstract ethical theory to applied ethics; and
– the empirical turn.

6.1.1.1 From Philosophical Ethics to Applied Ethics

Towards the end of the twentieth century, the traditional philosophical approach of abstract theoretical argumentation about ethical issues was criticised as being too vague, contextless and inadequate to provide guidance in moral dilemmas that occur in the real world (Alvarez 2001). In the search for more adequate methods, two major approaches surfaced: casuistry and principlism.

Casuistry

In casuistry the answer to questions of good and right is sought in so-called paradigm cases: situations in which the right action is clear and agreed upon by virtually anyone familiar with the case and its particularities. From the perception of the correct actions in paradigm cases, we can proceed to more difficult cases by analogy. Difficult cases fall in between paradigms and the casuist must examine the circumstances of the case in detail to find which paradigm it most closely resembles (Kuczewski 1998). In this process, the focus is not on reasons, arguments and opinions. Instead, through a dialogical process, the case may be interpreted in a different way and new solutions to the moral problem may be found (Widdershoven et al. 2009).

Principlism

Principalists claim that certain principles can be considered as moral action guides. Beauchamp and Childress became famous for their so-called four-principles approach. They identified four principles for bioethics:

- respect for autonomy;
- nonmaleficence;
- beneficence; and
- justice.

These principles are always binding, but not absolutely binding. The principles create prima facie obligations. This means that each basic principle has weight, but when the connected duties conflict and we cannot fulfil all of them, no priority weighting or ranking should be applied a priori. To respect a patient's autonomy may infringe upon our duty to medically benefit him or her. In cases like these, we must balance the principles in conflict and determine which is weightier in the specific context. Which principle overrides in a case of conflict will depend on this context, which always has unique features (Beauchamp and Childress 2012).

6.1.1.2 The Empirical Turn

In the last decade of the twentieth century, bioethicists increasingly began to use empirical research methods from the social sciences for their research (Molewijk et al. 2004). This invited extensive discussion on the contributions and limitations of empirical information in ethics. In this—ongoing—debate a number of approaches for integrating empirical methods for advancing ethical research have been proposed.

In earlier research, we embraced John Rawls' model of *Reflective Equilibrium (RE)* as a method for justifying ethical judgements (van Thiel and van Delden 2010). The basic idea behind RE is that deciding on the right action in morally problematic cases requires an argumentative process in which a broad set of considerations is taken up. Adjustments are made to moral judgements, principles and theories to the point where a coherent view on the case is reached. The relevant considerations are then said to be in *reflective equilibrium.* The empirical elements in the model are morally relevant facts on the one hand (e.g. information on the level of public trust in an institution, facts on the incidence of euthanasia) and empirical information on moral intuitions of relevant actors on the other.

6.2 Provisions and Applications

The analysis of ethical issues in this chapter will be guided by the RE model. This implies that there will not be mainly elaboration of concepts or application of ethical theory. Instead, a description of morally relevant facts, ethical norms and principles relevant to the ethical aspects and tensions will be presented, to achieve a rich description of the issues with regard to medicinal product risk communication.

6.2.1 Risk Communication and the Ethical Principle of Respect for Autonomy

Communication about risks and safe use of medicines may be used to enhance the message recipients' autonomous choices by providing them with relevant information, or helping them to realise their genuine preferences. Fostering autonomy is generally seen as desirable and risk communication is a means to this end. Several aspects of risk communication may however render the message ineffective or even harmful, thereby failing its aim. More specifically, the following areas of tension have been pointed out:

6.2.1.1 Risk Literacy

First, risk communication should be aligned with the level of understanding of the target group(s). However, many people struggle with low risk literacy. Risk literacy refers to a person's ability to accurately evaluate and understand information about risk (Garcia-Retamero et al. 2015). A significant minority of the general population lacks the basic skills required to understand information about the risks and benefits of health-related behaviours and medical treatments (Galesic and Garcia-Retamero 2013; van Thiel and Stolk 2013). It is likely that among patients, limited risk literacy is more prevalent, because on average, the relative risk that patients with low numeracy suffer from chronic disease is roughly 40% greater than that of patients with high numeracy (Garcia-Retamero et al. 2015). Aside from errors in the understanding of the benefits and risks of treatment, people with low numerical skills typically overestimate the benefits of treatment (Fagerlin et al. 2007). A recent randomised controlled trial on the impact of changes in a medicines safety message on consumers' ability to understand and use the information, showed that a consumer's health literacy level was a key factor in respondents' level of understanding of the message that was studied (McCormack et al. 2016). Contrary to what many may believe, limited risk literacy may not only be a problem for patients. Problems with numeracy among healthcare staff have been repeatedly reported (Warburton 2010). It may apply not only to an estimated 30% of nurses, but also to physicians. In a study assessing numerical skills in a small sample of healthcare professionals (24 physicians, 4 nurses, 12 doctorate faculty and 5 medical students) the respondents were asked to answer 6 written questions, for example: "You have 5mg pills of warfarin and you take 7.5mg/d. If you have 9 pills left, would you have enough for 1 week?" 53% answered all 6 questions correctly (Estrada et al. 1999). This evidence shows that availability of accurate information is a necessary but insufficient prerequisite for autonomous decision-making. And although problems of health literacy are increasingly acknowledged, a ready solution is not at hand.

6.2.1.2 Psychological Reactance

Second, the phenomenon of so-called psychological reactance to health messages may limit their effectiveness and even invoke a counterproductive reaction. The theory of reactance suggests that when people feel threatened with a reduction of their freedom, they will become motivationally aroused. This arousal would be directed against any further loss of freedom and it would also be directed toward the

In the 1970s, an experimental evaluation of US broadcast warnings against certain medicines, such as "Using amphetamines and barbiturates can lead to serious trouble-if you're using them –stop now –before it's too late", found that there was a significant shift in a direction opposite to the one advocated in the messages. After repeated exposure to messages designed to engender or reinforce negative attitudes toward amphetamines/barbiturates, the targeted groups significantly shifted from generally negative attitudes to significantly less negative attitudes.

Another study on the effects of cigarette warning labels in the US, such as "SURGEON GENERAL'S WARNING: Quitting Smoking Now Greatly Reduces Serious Risks To Your Health", on actual smoking behaviour first measured adolescents' knowledge of the warning labels. Second, changes in adolescent smoking behaviour during the subsequent three months were monitored. The study revealed a paradoxical, significant increase in smoking from baseline to follow-up among those teenagers with greater knowledge of the warning labels on cigarette packages.

Fig. 6.2 Examples for warning statements and psychological reactance (Jones Ringold 2002)

re-establishment of whatever freedom had already been lost or threatened. This may cause a boomerang effect of health messages. In a comprehensive article on this effect, some illuminating examples are presented of research pointing towards the risk that health messages that are perceived as restricting autonomous choice are counterproductive (see Fig. 6.2) (Jones Ringold 2002).

A counterproductive effect has not only been reported with regard to reducing unhealthy behaviour. It has also been reported for campaigns concerning medicinal products, for example, promoting vaccines. A randomised trial testing the effectiveness of messages designed to reduce vaccine misperceptions and increase vaccination rates for the measles-mumps-rubella (MMR) vaccine (see Chap. 1) showed that the effectiveness of those messages may vary depending on pre-existing parental attitudes toward vaccines. For some parents, such messages may actually increase misperceptions or reduce vaccination intention (Nyhan et al. 2014). In addition to the failure to meet their goal, the use of risk communication messages that misrepresent statistics or use highly charged emotional appeals may fail to meet requirements of truthfulness and sincerity, as well as correctness and accuracy, which are not only scientific requirements but at a higher level ethical (Guttman and Salmon 2004). Considering the potential of reactance and other boomerang responses is important for successful risk communication. Communication strategies that are or may be perceived as reducing autonomy may be less likely to achieve the desired effect compared to messages that enhance autonomous decision-making.

Ensuring that critical health messages are aligned with the aim of respect for autonomy is an ethical imperative for public health agencies, organisations and professionals. The relationship between the norm of enhancing autonomy and the duty to inform is complex and failure to acknowledge this complexity could do more harm than good in risk communication about medicines.

6.2.2 Responsibility in Risk Communication and the Ethical Principles of Nonmaleficence, Beneficence and Justice

Next to the ethical imperative of respect for autonomy, the duties of beneficence and nonmaleficence are at the core of ethical practices in healthcare. The balance between optimising the benefits of better use of medicines and avoiding unintended potentially harmful consequences through risk communication relates to the attribution of personal responsibility for the safe use of medicines. Most people would argue that individual patients are at least partly responsible for the good use of medicines. They should not take medicines unnecessarily; and when they are prescribed to them, adherence and careful use can be reasonably expected. Adequate communication about the safe use of medicines is essential for enabling individuals to use them responsibly. In this way, risk communication promotes benefits and reduces risk of harm. Regardless of these positive effects, it has been argued that emphasising the individual's responsibility in health communication is ethically problematic because of its unintended harmful consequences.

Risk communication activities are generally viewed as benign interventions. Raising people's awareness of their own motivations, options and responsibility for safe use of medicines may be an effective way to attract the attention needed to promote the aims of risk communication. However, messages that make a strong causal link between a person's individual responsibility and their health can be ethically problematic for several reasons. First, this type of communication may fail to acknowledge that social factors affect individual behaviour. This may unduly locate the cause of risks within the individual instead of in social and environmental forces. In a review of the arguments regarding personal responsibility for health, it is pointed out that the idea of personal responsibility for risk avoidance is especially problematic in the case of people with low socioeconomic status (SES). A study among residents of a poverty neighbourhood in California showed a 40% excess mortality rate. Significant differences in mortality remained, even when smoking, diet, exercise and other traditional risk factors were controlled for. A frequently offered explanation for this phenomenon is that people at lower SES levels have less opportunity to control the circumstances and events that affect their lives, leading to a lower sense of "control over destiny" which, in turn, may translate into less healthy behaviours (Minkler 1999). Faulty attribution of responsibility may be harmful and unjust in the sense that it leads to "blaming the victim" (Marantz 1990). People who do not succeed in adopting healthy behaviours are pictured as irresponsible and weak and to blame for their health problems. This may invoke feelings of guilt and shame in people who feel they are not up to the task of following, for example, recommendations for the safe use of their medicines. A further ethically problematic consequence of blaming the victim is greater inequality because society is less willing to pay for the healthcare costs of certain groups of people, based on an overestimation of the role of individual responsibility on healthy behaviour (Guttman and Salmon 2004). Unjustified attribution of responsibility and the subsequent negative consequences constitute harm that should be avoided. A balance has to be sought between promoting responsible behaviour on the one hand and unduly blaming or punishing individuals on the other hand. Especially in healthcare, blame or guilt for health conditions is generally assigned limited weight in considering claims to healthcare. Physicians and other healthcare professionals have a duty to care for and respect patients regardless of their behaviour or guilt.

A specific form of risk communication about safe use of medicines is through decision support systems which can alert clinicians about inappropriate medications or harmful medication combinations. These alerts are designed with the aim to reduce the number of patient injuries due to medications. In a study of more than three million electronic prescriptions, in which 6.6% generated a safety alert, it was found that clinicians overrode almost 90% of high severity alerts of drug–drug interactions. The percentages for overriding moderate-severity and low-severity alerts were slightly higher with 92.7% and 92.9%, respectively (Isaac et al. 2009). An explanation for these percentages can be found in the phenomenon of alert fatigue. It occurs when the threshold for sending alerts to clinicians is set too low, and the warnings are not perceived as helpful for improving patient safety (Baker 2009). The problem of alert fatigue is that it can lead clinicians to override important warnings as well (Nyhan et al. 2014). The research on alert fatigue demonstrates that it is crucial to tailor communication strategies to the context and to monitor the beneficial as well as potential harmful effects that occur when in use.

Beyond the four bioethical principles that are relevant in general, more specific ethical norms are applicable in the context of medicinal product risk communication.

6.2.3 Knowledge Governance and the Duty to Inform in an Uncertain World

Uncertainties surrounding risks and safe use of pharmaceuticals could pertain to the quantity and quality of evidence, the risk-benefit profile or the effect of policy decisions on future risks. In a later report on ethical issues in studying the safety of approved medicines, the Institute of Medicine (IoM) in the USA stated that as a part of its public mission the US Food and Drug Administration (US FDA) should "help the public get the accurate, science-based information they need to use medicines and foods to improve their health." The IoM recommended that "modern tools for risk communication and public engagement should be used to ensure that all stakeholders—including physicians, other healthcare professionals, interested patients and their families and members of the public—understand the decision problem facing the agency, including what is known about the benefits and risks associated with the therapy in question and the pertinent uncertainties" (Institute of Medicine 2010).

In communication about safe use of medicines, these uncertainties create an ethical tension in the management and presentation of scientific uncertainty. This tension is caused between the duty of truthfulness about these uncertainties on the one hand and the expectation that scientific advisers will provide clear public guidance on the other. A normative analysis of strategies of dealing with this tension distinguishes between two extremes.

The first strategy is called concealment of uncertainty. It is grounded in the view that "the primary role of the scientific adviser is to feed scientific conclusions to the public, and that the adviser should act as an authority that settles matters once and for all" (Folker and Sandøe 2008). This strategy has been countered by appeals to autonomy and the right to be informed as an element thereof, and although it is hardly supported as a strategy, scientists involved in public debates may still feel that clear, unambiguous advice is expected from them. In addition, studies have found that it is difficult to break down expert/lay role expectations and to encourage collaboration between citizens and scientists as equals in policymaking (Goodwin and Honeycutt 2009). At the other end of the spectrum is the strategy to convey (all) scientific uncertainty. In light of the problematic paternalistic features of the first strategy, scientist could abandon the idea that the scientific expert should somehow act as a filter or mediator between science and the public. When communicating about science, this strategy involves the scientist *showing* the lay audience the evidence, as opposed to *telling* the lay audience the conclusion, implicitly asking them to trust the speaker and the conclusion he has drawn for his own reasons (Goodwin and Honeycutt 2009). The problem with the strategy to convey scientific uncertainty is that it will not serve the purpose of effectively informing public debate. The amount of scientific information and its inherent variety of uncertainties pose an impossible hurdle for scientists' effort to present an exhaustive account of all scientific uncertainties. Moreover, the public is in an inferior position when it comes to assessing scientific claims because of the complexity of underlying premises and reasoning. Therefore, selection is inevitable and scientists should provide the public with edited guidance within their domain of expertise. Relevant to the choice of communication between these extreme strategies is the phenomenon of social amplification. The term refers to the fact that communication of risk is not an isolated action, but instead evokes a wide range of psychological, social, institutional or political processes. In these interactive processes the perception of risk (severity) may be intensified or attenuated. Social amplification is hard to predict and control, especially in situations with high levels of uncertainty (Kasperson 2015). Social amplification may have negative effects on, for example, public consideration and communication of risk decisions. The problems of information overload as well as the risk of adverse effects of social amplification force to seek a balance between the two extremes. It has been argued that scientific advisers should be obligated to use their *best* judgement on what kinds of uncertainty it is necessary for the public to be informed about (Folker and Sandøe 2008). However, regardless of the value of the identification of relevant normative positions on the scientist's duty to inform the public on scientific uncertainty, the recommendation to use best judgement to select the information the public needs to assess scientific claims may not be sufficient to guide scientists in their role as expert advisors. This poses ethical dilemmas for scientists who engage as experts in public information campaigns or debates on risks and safe use of medicines.

6.2.4 Trust and Appeals Based on Scientific Expertise

Public trust in medicine, medicinal products and medical institutions is widely believed to be essential for the effectiveness of risk and safe use communication for medicines, vaccination campaigns, healthcare professional-patient relationships, care seeking, information disclosure and treatment adherence (Hall 2005). Therefore, the value of trust should be acknowledged and promoted. Currently, a lack of trust in information and claims based on scientific expertise is increasingly observed. In the pharmaceutical sector, safety controversies have diminished public trust in pharmaceutical companies and in medicines (Bauchner and Fontanarosa 2013).

In an analysis of one of the major controversies—about selective serotonin reuptake inhibitors (SSRIs) and suicidality (see Chap. 1)—we observed that trust in the ethical, professional and societal commitment of institutions is paramount to maintain and restore public trust in pharmaceutical companies and regulatory authorities. Patients tend to mediate or compensate their vulnerability by focusing on the competencies of these institutions. Thus, an important aspect of public trust is the reliance on the competence of companies, authorities and healthcare professionals to perform the tasks they are responsible for and expected to do. Risk communication may contribute to erosion of public trust when there is a strong focus on communicating risk while disregarding the role of credibility and public trust (Hernandez et al. 2014).

The gap between science and the public has been linked to a traditional style of regulation and communication about medicines, which has been called the consensual style. Characteristics of this way of governing the pharmaceutical sector are that (1) it was elitist in nature, made in consultation with a number of elite groups including heads of industry, senior regulators and trade representatives; and (2) it was practised in meetings behind closed doors (Löfstedt et al. 2011). In response to increased public distrust, regulators in many parts of Europe came to the conclusion that the consensual style of regulation was flawed and a new model was needed. Guidance on how experts can shape their engagement has recently been proposed, for example, by the Council of International Organizations of Medical Sciences (CIOMS) with regard to the role of regulatory authorities in vaccine safety communication. This guidance is based on a body of knowledge on effectiveness of communication strategies. It advocates finding ways forward in risk communication that go beyond the traditional approach of scientists merely trying to fill information gaps with the aim to enhance public perception and acceptance of risks. These include closing the monitoring of the public debate and creating meaningful participatory partnerships between the public, regulatory/public health authorities and international/global partners (Bahri and Rägo 2019). This approach aims to be more inclusive than exclusive, encouraging greater public and stakeholder participation in the policymaking process. Guidance can help actors in risk communication such as regulators to clarify their role and take specific responsibility that fits their role as part of a network of stakeholders in communication about safety of medicines.

6.2.5 Methodological Approaches in Ethics Research

Methods in ethics research involve investigations into concepts and basic principles that can guide responsible conduct. Section 6.1 comprises an outline of the main approaches in bioethics. Currently, many ethicists in bioethics apply a mixed method strategy: they combine conceptual and normative analysis with empirical research. In the model of normative-empirical reflective equilibrium, this combination is a key feature. Methods from the social sciences (see Chap. 8) are widely used to identify the empirical elements in the model (morally relevant facts and empirical information on moral intuitions of relevant actors). These involve quantitative research (e.g. prevalence study on the number of people who receive palliative sedation at the end of life), and qualitative methods such as interviews, focus groups and vignette studies (i.e. psychological and sociological experiments presenting participants with hypothetical situations) (e.g. into the moral intuitions or attitudes towards the use of human embryo's for research). Paramount for the soundness of ethical analysis is that the empirical information is interpreted in the light of normative principles and theories. Otherwise, bioethics would be no more than a series of naturalistic fallacies.

Methodology in normative bioethical analysis is informed by a significant body of literature on concepts and ethical theories relevant to healthcare issues (e.g. analysis of the concept of solidarity in healthcare and theories of autonomy and care). The methodology is philosophical and involves critical and reflective thinking.

6.3 Outlook: Relevance, Improvements and Future Potential

In the previous sections, ethical principles and areas of tension with regard to communications about risks and safe use of medicines were discussed. Based on literature from several disciplines (i.e. ethics, sociology, psychology) the ethical aspects of the practice are highlighted and illustrated. This discussion is limited by the current lack of a comprehensive approach which can inform a basic framework for addressing the ethical issues. A promising and thriving new area of ethical research could help overcome this limitation: *information ethics*.

6.3.1 Information Ethics

Initiated in the 1990s by Luciano Floridi—who developed the first ethical framework for dealing with the new challenges posed by information and communication technologies—information ethics is concerned with the conceptual nature and basic principles of information, including its ethical consequences (Floridi 2013). Floridi presents his framework of information ethics not as a perspective that overrides other ethical approaches but instead as additional and useful in guiding and evaluating the profound effects of information on the human condition, including among others the nature of communication, education, healthcare and social relations. An extensive presentation of concepts and theories in information ethics exceeds the scope of this chapter. Without the aim to do full justice to the framework of information ethics, a few characteristics which may be further specified for the context of communication about the safety of medicines can be pointed out. Essential to Floridi's view is that we all are part of a so-called *infosphere*. This is the whole informational environment constituted by all informational entities (human and non-human), their properties, interactions, processes and mutual relations. Non-human entities such as interfaces, machines, organisations, etc. form an engineered environment that is part of the infosphere. In the infosphere, the informational entities interact. The implication of this interaction is that we should no longer view informational entities as influences that affect and enter "our" human world. Instead we as human agents are *present* in the infosphere. The ethical obligations that come with this presence are focused on the effects of certain actions or arrangements on the status—or wellbeing—of informational entities (Floridi 2010). In further specifying these ethical duties it is essential to avoid corruption of the infosphere. Truthfulness is, for example, a necessary condition for information, and misinformation or disinformation constitute unethical acts (Vandekerckhove 2018). The ethics of information is an interesting new field of philosophical inquiry that can inform and complement bioethical thinking on issues related to the communication about risks and safe use of medicinal products. Information ethics emphasises the fundamental and significant value of information, rendering it worthy of autonomous philosophical investigation.

Together with more traditional approaches such as the four principles of bioethics and ethical considerations in the contexts of uncertainty and trust, information ethics can help design a multilayered approach to medicinal product risk communication research that integrates with medical humanities (see Chap. 1).

Conclusions

- Ethics is concerned with what ought to be done.
- In addressing ethical issues of communication, a mixed methods approach combining normative and empirical research is suitable.
- Ethical principles such as beneficence, nonmaleficence, autonomy and justice can serve as action guides in dealing with ethical tension around risk communication.
- Normative views on dealing with uncertainty and trust are relevant to the specific context of medicinal product risk communication.
- Information ethics is a new area of research that can further inform and enhance the debate on ethical issues in risk communication.

References

Adler D, Zlotnik Shaul R (2012) Disciplining bioethics: towards a standard of methodological rigor in bioethics research. Account Res 19(3):187–207

Alvarez AAA (2001) How rational should bioethics be? The value of empirical approaches. Bioethics 15:501–519

Anonymous (2007) The method in bioethics research. Kennedy Inst Ethics J 17:277–278

Bahri P, Rägo L (2019) CIOMS guide to vaccine safety communication: executive summary. Vaccine 37:401–408

Baker DE (2009) Medication alert fatigue: the potential for compromised patient safety. Hosp Pharm 449(6):460–462

Bauchner H, Fontanarosa PB (2013) Restoring confidence in the pharmaceutical industry. JAMA 309:607–609

Beauchamp TL, Childress JF (2012) Principles of biomedical ethics, vol 51, 7th revised edn. Oxford University Press, Oxford

Bergstresser SM (2015) Health communication, public mistrust, and the politics of "rationality". Am J Bioeth 15(4):57–59

Estrada C et al (1999) Health literacy and numeracy. JAMA 282(6):527

Fagerlin A, Ubel PA, Smith DM, Zikmund-Fisher BJ (2007) Making numbers matter: present and future research in risk communication. Am J Health Behav 31(Suppl 1): S47–S56

Floridi L (2010) Ethics after the information revolution. In: Floridi L (ed) The Cambridge handbook of information and computer ethics. Cambridge University Press, Cambridge, pp 3–19
Floridi L (2013) The ethics of information. Oxford University Press, Oxford
Folker AP, Sandøe P (2008) Leaping "out of the doubt" - nutrition advice: values at stake in communicating scientific uncertainty to the public. Health Care Anal 16:176–191
Galesic M, Garcia-Retamero R (2013) Using analogies to communicate information about health risks. Appl Cogn Psychol 27:33–42
Garcia-Retamero R, Andrade A, Sharit J, Ruiz JG (2015) Is patient's numeracy related to physical and mental health? Med Decis Mak 35:501–511
Goodwin J, Honeycutt L (2009) When science goes public: from technical arguments to appeals to authority. Stud Commun Sci 9(2):19–30
Guttman N, Salmon CT (2004) Guilt, fear, stigma and knowledge gaps: ethical issues in public health communication interventions. Bioethics 18(6):531–552
Hall MA (2005) The importance of trust for ethics, law, and public policy. Camb Q Healthc Ethics 14:156–167
Hernandez JF, van Thiel GJMW, Mantel-Teeuwisse AK, Raaijmakers JAM, Pieters T (2014) Restoring trust in the pharmaceutical sector on the basis of the SSRI case. Drug Discov Today 19:523–527
Institute of Medicine (2010) Ethical issues in studying the safety of approved drugs: a letter report. The National Academies Press, Washington, pp 3–6
Isaac T, Weissman JS, Davis RB, Massagli M, Cyrulik A, Sands DZ, Weingart SN (2009) Overrides of medication alerts in ambulatory care. Arch Intern Med 169(3):305–311
Ives J, Dunn M, Cribb A (2017) Theoretical perspectives: an introduction. In: Ives J, Dunn M, Cribb A (eds) Empirical bioethics. Theoretical and practical perspectives. Cambridge University Press, Cambridge, pp 3–16
Jones Ringold D (2002) Boomerang effects in response to public health interventions: some unintended consequences in the alcoholic beverage market. J Consum Policy 25:27–63
Kasperson RE (2015) Risk governance and the social amplification of risk: a commentary. In: Fra. Paleo U (ed) Risk governance. Springer, Dordrecht, pp 485–487
Kuczewski M (1998) Casuistry and principlism: the convergence of method in biomedical ethics. Theor Med Bioeth 19:509–524
Löfstedt R, Bouder F, Wardman J, Chakraborty S (2011) The changing nature of communication and regulation of risk in Europe. J Risk Res 14(4):409–429
Marantz PR (1990) Blaming the victim: the negative consequence of preventive medicine. Am J Public Health 80:1186–1187
McCormack L, Lefebvre RC, Bann C, Taylor O, Rausch P (2016) Consumer understanding, preferences, and responses to different versions of drug safety messages in the United States: a randomized controlled trial. Drug Saf 39:171–184
Minkler M (1999) Personal responsibility for health? A review of the arguments and the evidence at century's end. Health Educ Behav 26(1):121–140
Molewijk AC, Siggelbout A, Otten W, Dupuis H, Kievit J (2004) Empirical data and moral theory. A plea for integrated empirical ethics. Med Health Care Philos 7:71–79
Nyhan B, Reifler J, Richey S, Freed GL (2014) Effective messages in vaccine promotion: a randomized trial. Pediatrics 133(4):e835–e842
Sidgwick H (1962) The methods of ethics. Macmillan, London, p 1
van Thiel, GJMW, Stolk PS (2013) Patient and citizen involvement in priority setting for pharmaceutical innovation. Background paper for the WHO Priority Medicines for Europe and the World 2013 report. WHO, Geneva
van Thiel GJMW, van Delden JJM (2010) Reflective equilibrium as a normative empirical model. Ethical Perspect 17:183–202
Vandekerckhove W (2018) Whistleblowing and information ethics: facilitation, entropy, and ecopoiesis. J Bus Ethics 152:15–25
Warburton P (2010) Numeracy and patient safety: the need for regular staff assessment. Nurs Stand 24(27):42–44
Widdershoven G, Abma T, Molewijk B (2009) Empirical ethics as dialogical practice. Bioethics 23:236–248

The Cognitive and Behavioural Sciences

7

Sara Rubinelli, Nicola Diviani, and Maddalena Fiordelli

Abstract

This chapter focuses on the contribution of the cognitive and behavioural sciences to risk communication. First, it addresses the main theories that explain risk perception from a cognitive level and its impact at the behavioural level. Here, the main focus is on the shift from purely probabilistic accounts of risks to the heuristics and emotional and contextual factors that influence perceptions. Second, it reviews some of the main research methods used to study risk perceptions in the context of the safety of, and safe use of, medicines. Here, the main evidence from formative research and the evaluation of communication interventions are discussed. Third, it provides an overview of empirical cognitive and behavioural research by analytically presenting current evidence on risk communication in the field of medicine safety and appropriate usage. This chapter concludes by highlighting the steps necessary to implement successful risk communication in the field.

S. Rubinelli (✉) · N. Diviani
Department of Health Science and Medicine, University of Lucerne, Lucerne, Switzerland

Swiss Paraplegic Research, Nottwil, Switzerland
e-mail: sara.rubinelli@paraplegie.ch

M. Fiordelli
Faculty of Communication Sciences, Università della Svizzera italiana, Lugano, Switzerland

Swiss Paraplegic Research, Nottwil, Switzerland

© Springer Nature Singapore Pte Ltd. 2020

P. Bahri (ed.), *Communicating about Risks and Safe Use of Medicines*,
https://doi.org/10.1007/978-981-15-3013-5_7

7.1 The Disciplines of the Cognitive and Behavioural Sciences: Scope, Theories and Principles

If you're rational, you don't get to believe whatever you want to believe.
Michael Huemer

Risk and Risk Perception
As defined by Paek and Hove, "The concept of risk refers to the probability of experiencing harm or hazards" (Paek and Hove 2017). While a hazard refers to anything that can cause damage to people and the environment, the concept of probability refers to the percentage of possibilities that this damage will occur.

Risks are *perceived* by human beings. Risk perception is the subjective judgement that people make about risks and, specifically, about their characteristics and severity (Darker 2013). Risks perceptions are important determinants of health-related decisions, e.g. how to safely deal with medicines. They are more important than *actual* risks in predicting behaviour. Indeed, risks are always perceived (Shrader-Frechette 1991). Sometimes perceptions align with actual risks, but often they do not. Some perceptions may be more objective than others because they are firmly based on accurate data and statistics. However, exact understanding of risks is complex: it requires not only information about the nature of a risk, but also information on aspects including alternative options and the level of uncertainty regarding the available information (National Research Council 1989). Risk perceptions are thus key targets for interventions aimed at optimising health-related decision-making. Indeed, they are a main topic addressed by the field of study known as risk communication. Since its origin in the 1980s, risk communication significantly focused on how to best inform people about potential hazards (Pidgeon and Beattie 1998). Since then it has increasingly also focused on studying how communication can influence health-related decisions that involve risk evaluation, and in doing so, risk communication addresses risks perceptions in different dimensions.

Risk Perception and Communication
This chapter examines the study of risk perception as a relevant part of research into medicinal product risk communication by focusing on the main contributions made on this topic by the related cognitive sciences and behavioural sciences.

7.1.1 The Cognitive Science

By definition, the cognitive science aims to explain human intelligence and the mental processes underlying phenomena such as perception, reasoning, and communication. It embraces the frameworks and methods of the key disciplines including philosophy, psychology, neuroscience, linguistics, computer science, artificial intelligence, and anthropology (Thagard 1996).

As a starting point for the paragraphs that follow, it should be noted that, in recent decades, research in the cognitive and related sciences has disentangled a complexity behind the concept of risk perception. The focus has shifted from an interpretation of behaviour as purely rational to an understanding of behaviour as determined by more than the basic applications of the rules of logic and probability. In the context of decision-making regarding risks, it appears that actions do not simply result from an estimation of the nature of a hazard, the level of exposure, and the probability of being impacted.

Expected Utility Theory and Prospect Theory

Two main theories argued for the rationality of action, namely expected utility theory and prospect theory. For expected utility theory, which originates from the field of economics, decisions relating to risks or uncertain prospects are conceptualised as resulting from weighting the utilities of possible outcomes by the probability of their occurrence (von Neumann and Morgenstern 1944). According to this theory, decision-makers discharge lower utility. Prospect theory, developed by Daniel Kahneman and Amos Tversky, recognises that people do not make decisions by rigorously following the expected utility hypothesis (Kahneman and Tversky 1979). People seem to act within a framework of loss aversion and thus overestimate small probabilities when it is a matter of guarding against losses. Here, the way in which alternatives and options are presented make a difference to the evaluation. The authors specifically speak about the concept of framing. Generally, people prefer things that are framed as a sure gain over things that are framed as a probabilistic gain, and things that are framed as a probabilistic loss over things that are framed as a definite loss. Prospect theory was appreciated as a more descriptive theory of action compared to the normative nature of expected utility theory. However, it can also be considered too simplistic in nature—especially by critics in the field of psychology—to explain contexts where probabilities are unknown, and where one is operating under uncertainty.

Heuristics

It is Tversky and Kahneman who again, in their analysis of decision-making, enriched the description of risk perception by describing the concept of heuristics (Tversky and Kahneman 1974). They showed that people's evaluation under uncertainty can be driven by aspects that do not intrinsically relate to the uncertainty itself. By definition, heuristics are mental shortcuts that simplify thinking and reduce the cognitive burden of deep reflection. They can be useful in deciding how to act, but they can also lead to cognitive biases (that is, to errors in thinking that negatively impact risk perception and judgement generally) (Kahneman and Tversky 1972).

The list of most commonly used heuristics, and the possible resulting errors in (risk) judgement includes:

- *Representativeness*: This is based on evaluating the similarity of objects. People look at the degree to which two things resemble each other, or they compare one thing to their mental prototypes. Errors might occur when the comparison is not appropriate or when people miss or neglect information for the evaluation (Kahneman and Frederick 2002).
- *Availability heuristic*: This is applied when people evaluate something by relying on the closest examples or on what immediately comes to their mind. In doing so, judgments are made on the available information rather than on examining an issue in depth (Tversky and Kahneman 1973).

- *Anchoring and adjustment heuristic*: This describes cases where people rely heavily on a first piece of information (the "anchor"). In evaluating something they start from the anchor and make adjustments that are often insufficient to overcome the influence of the anchor (Tversky and Kahneman 1974).
- *Overconfidence*: This refers to a person's evaluation of the accuracy of his or her own thinking. People tend to consider their judgements to be more reliable than they actually are (Pallier et al. 2002).
- *Inconsistent intuition*: This refers to the tendency to overvalue intuition, even when this appears to be inconsistent with reality (Morrow 2009).
- *Belief perseverance*: This refers to the tendency to hold onto beliefs even when evidence contradicts them (Baumeister and Vohs 2007). Related to this heuristic, confirmation bias refers to people's predisposition towards searching for information that supports their points of views and beliefs (Nickerson 1998).

Overall, cognitive research on the determinants of risk perception shows that individuals often do not base their risk evaluation on probabilities and expected values, and that often, even when decisions are based on quantified values, they may apply biases.

Contextual and Fright Factors Influencing Risk Perception
In addition to this, the evidence shows that risk perception is also greatly influenced by other contextual factors. As explained by Ropeik (2012), the list of main contextual factors includes:

- *Trust*: People are less afraid of risks when they trust the sources of information about particular risks.
- *Origin*: People are more concerned about risks they perceive for other people than their own risks.
- *Imagination*: When a risk is not visible or difficult to understand, people tend to be more scared.
- *Familiarity*: New risks are considered more dangerous than familiar ones.
- *Fun factor*: Those risks that involve some form of fun or pleasure are perceived as less dangerous.

Some of the factors listed above can also be classified as fright factors. They refer to characteristics of risk communication that are known to raise particular concerns (Calman 2001). The list of additional fright factors includes: whether a risk is presented as inescapable, causing an irreversible damage, particularly challenging to small children, not well understood by science, and subject to contradictory statements.

Media Factors Influencing Risk Perception
As McCahrty, Brennan Boer, and Ritson further explained, risk perceptions are strongly influenced by the media (McCarthy et al. 2008). In particular, the list of impacting factors includes:

- *Media coverage*: The amount of attention that media give to something.
- *Media frames*: The perspectives and angles from which news is presented.

- *Media tones*: The attention to emotional aspects that can stimulate strong emotions.
- *Information sources*: The use of influencers and of people or institutions that can generate consensus or debate as sources.
- *Presentation formats*: Especially the use of verbal or numerical estimates.

Within these parameters, a special focus on the main role of affect and emotion in the evaluation of risks is placed within the so-called psychometric paradigm.

Psychometric Paradigm of Risk Perception
This paradigm decomposes risk perception into a set of psychological risk dimensions. Thus, Paul Slovic stressed the link between the perception of a benefit and of the derived pleasure of a risk and its tolerance (Slovic 2016). In addition, when people feel intense dread when they perceive a risk, they tend to evaluate it as more threatening.

Perception-to-Decision-Making Models
Overall, Vincent T Covello presented four models that explain risks from perception, to processing and decision-making that include cognitive and contextual factors (Covello et al. 2001). Cognitive aspects refer to intellectual functions that human beings utilise to deal with information, such as the use of knowledge, perceptions and beliefs, and the process of evaluation and memorization. Contextual factors are here intended as characteristics of the environment that can influence cognitive aspects (for instance, the source of information and its characteristics, and the way information that impact on human cognition is framed).

- *Risk perception model*: This assumes that risk perception is determined by a myriad of factors, some of which have been listed above. These also include personal stakes, ethical/moral values, and whether a risk has a human or a natural origin and fright factors.
- *Mental noise model*: This holds that when people are in a state of stress due to a perceived threat, their capacity for processing information is significantly impaired. When they are assisted in understanding risks, this processing improves.
- *Negative dominance model*: This focuses on the fact that when people are upset they tend to pay more attention to losses and negative information. It is thus important to counterbalance negative messages with solution-oriented ones.
- *Trust determination model*: The trust that people place on the communicator of risks is essential for the appraisal. Trust should be built well in advance because when people fear something or are upset, they tend not to trust authorities. The main factors that help build trust are honesty, expertise, and empathy.

Social Amplification of Risks
An important approach that clearly shows the complexity of risk appraisal is the conceptual framework of social amplification of risks, theorised by Roger Kasperson and colleagues (Kasperson et al. 1988).

This framework states that the perception of risk events is influenced by psychological, social, and cultural factors. A certain information system may amplify or weaken the information about a risk. Also, this information can be amplified by aspects including opinion leaders, activist organisations, scientists, and institutions.

Some risks may be experienced by individuals directly. Depending from this experience (for instance of a tragic car accident), people can amplify or attenuate risks. For many risks there is, however, no direct personal experience. Their perception can be influenced by factors including the quantity of media content and the phenomenon of "dramatisation".

In summary, the cognitive sciences clearly show that risk perception is influenced by complex and often unpredictable factors. The theoretical understanding of these factors, and their elaboration in the form of models and frameworks, is of great assistance in facilitating a communication of risks that minimises the possibility of misunderstanding and misappraisal. This understanding is also important for risk communication research.

7.1.2 The Behavioural Science

The behavioural science investigates human action, i.e. how people make decisions and how they interact with one another. They are based on knowledge from fields including psychology, the cognitive science, and social and cultural anthropology (Kerlinger 1979).

While the cognitive science explores risk perception in terms of its manifestation and determinants, the behavioural science has developed theories that show how risk perception can influence action. Some of these theories specifically focus on how to predict behaviour by highlighting several factors that determine it (risk perception is one of these factors). Some of the most popular theories in this field are presented below:

The Health Belief Model

The health belief model was developed by Godfrey H Hochbaum, Irwin M Rosenstock, and S Stephen Kegeles in the 1950s (Hochbaum et al. 1952). It shows that a behaviour results from:

- Perceived susceptibility, i.e. the perception of being at risk; people will not change behaviour if they do not perceive that they are at risk;
- Perceived severity, i.e. the perception of how serious the consequences of doing/not doing something are;
- Perceived benefits, i.e. the perceived positives of the change;
- Perceived barriers, i.e. the perceived difficulties and challenges of the change;
- Cues to action, i.e. anything external that might enhance a desire to make a change;
- Self-efficacy, i.e. the person's belief in his/her own ability to make a behaviour change.

Implementing this model, then, requires the facilitator(s) to:

- access who is at risk in the population;
- clearly present information to raise awareness, to understand the perceived severity, and to explain benefits and barriers; and to
- help overcome barriers and support self-efficacy through, for instance, skill development and the provision of external supportive tools.

The Protection Motivation Theory

According to the protection motivation theory of Ronald W Rogers, risk perception results from the interaction between the threat appraisal and the coping appraisal (Rogers 1983). The threat appraisal relates to perceived severity and the vulnerability, i.e. how people perceive their personal probability of the occurrence of something. The coping appraisal is based on self-efficacy and the perceived response efficacy, i.e. how people think that acting in a certain way will reduce a threat. Overall, according to the protection motivation theory, behavioural change depends on people's belief that a certain threat is severe and that acting in a certain way and having the perception of being able to act in a certain way will reduce that threat.

Extended Parallel Process Model

Similarly to the protection motivation theory, the extended parallel process model, developed by Kim Witte, focuses on the interaction between rational considerations and emotional reactions (Witte 1992). The motivation to act is determined by threat variables, i.e. perceived severity and perceived susceptibility, as well as by efficacy variables, i.e. self-efficacy and response efficacy.

Risk Perception Attitude Framework

The risk perception attitude framework, developed by Rajiv N Rimal and Kevin Real, explains behaviour as depending upon risk perception and efficacy beliefs (Rimal and Real 2003). This theory classifies people in four groups: responsive (with high risk perception and high self-efficacy); avoidance (with high risk perception and low self-efficacy); proactive (with low risk perception and high self-efficacy); and indifference (with low risk perception and low self-efficacy).

Theories of Risk Compensation and Homeostasis

Finally, the fact that people seem to become more careful when perceiving greater risk and less careful when they feel more protected is operationalised by the risk compensation theory. Linked to this theory is the theory of homeostasis, developed in the context of road safety by Gerald SJ Wilde, which presents the so-called target level of risk (Wilde 1982). People calculate risks by considering the expected benefits and costs both of the risky behaviour and of the safe behaviour.

As all these theories show, simply providing people with information about risks might not be sufficient to influence a behaviour. To plan a communication intervention, it is of key importance to carefully assess what people think about a certain risk, how they form this judgement, and how they relate to and address it. This understanding is also important for risk communication research.

7.2 Research Approaches and Methods

As outlined in the previous paragraphs, there is a multiplicity of factors potentially playing a role in medicine-related decisions, which consider their expected benefits and possible side effects. It is therefore of mainstream importance for those in charge of designing safety information materials (to be displayed, for instance, in patient information leaflets or on the packaging of medicines) to have a clear picture of how users perceive risks related to safety and safe use of medicines and to be familiar with evidence-based tools to effectively communicate them. This is where cognitive and behavioural sciences research comes into play. The underlying assumption here is that, the better consumers can evaluate and understand a risk (minimising the impact of false beliefs and cognitive biases in the process), the higher the chance they will follow the treatments as prescribed, with resulting increased safety. The purpose of the following paragraphs is to provide the reader with an overview of the research methods and approaches offered by the cognitive and behavioural sciences in order to support the understanding, preparing, and evaluating of communication processes and messages about the safety and safe use of medicines.

Measuring Risk Perception

Before starting with a description of the different research areas around communication of risks in the context of safety and safe use of medicines, a clarification is needed on how risk perception is measured. Unlike for other concepts of the cognitive and behavioural sciences, there is no universally accepted measure of risk perception. Studies around risk perception thus rely on a variety of self-reported measures, assessing different aspects of risk perception. Among the most commonly assessed aspects we find *perceived probability* (i.e. an estimation of the magnitude of the risk itself), *perceived likelihood* (i.e. beliefs about risk), and *perceived vulnerability* or *perceived susceptibility* (i.e. the extent to which one feels personally at risk). To assess perceived probability, individuals are usually asked to provide their estimate of a specific risk (e.g. "I think my chances of experiencing side-effects after taking this medication are…") and required to provide an answer on a verbal (e.g. from "very low" to "very high") or on a percentage scale. Beliefs about risk are usually assessed asking individual about the degree to which they agree with a series of statements (e.g. "I am sure I will experience side-effects after taking this medication"). Perceived vulnerability is usually assessed in a similar way, with the difference that the statements have a focus on the affective component (e.g. "I feel I am going to experience side-effects after taking this medication"). A study about different types of measures in the context of influenza vaccination showed that the measures of the affective type were the ones performing better in terms of predicting the behaviour (Weinstein et al. 2007).

In general, it is, according to Baruch Fischhoff, important to bear in mind that decision-making is the result of several different factors and usually happens in a complex environment (Fischhoff 1988). Let us think, for instance, to the decision about vaccinating against measles. An individual could correctly assess the risk of infection, but at the same time hold contrasting beliefs towards vaccinations in general (e.g. for religious motives) or might not have access to vaccines (e.g. for economical reasons) and, for these reasons, decide against vaccination. As a result, despite the "correct" risk perception, the behaviour is not optimal from a normative point of view. When planning a study in the field of risk perception, it is thus crucial that the choice of one or the other measure of risk perception, as well as the inclusion of potential confounders, is well thought through within the context and the objectives of the study.

A rapid review of recent empirical research about the communication of risks in the context of safety and safe use of medicines shows that research interest in this field mostly revolves around two distinct but strictly interrelated areas:

- *Formative research*: On the one hand, we have a stream of formative research, which focuses on examining the end users' perception and understanding of medicine safety information and their preferences in this context. Its results are crucial for the conceptualisation, development, and planning of evidence- and theory-based communication interventions, which are in turn the focus of the second research area.
- *Evaluative research*: The aim of this second research area is the evaluation of communication interventions to effectively communicate risks related to the safety and safe use of medicines. This has been done, for example, by examining whether and to what extent different tools can have an impact on understanding of risks, attitudes, and behaviour.

In the following section, we will discuss these two research areas in more detail, presenting a selective review of typical research questions, hypotheses, and methods of inquiry.

7.2.1 Methods for Formative Research: Literature Reviews, Qualitative Research Methods, and Surveys

Formative research in the context of safety and safe use of medicines essentially aims at answering basic questions about, for example, users' preferences for different types of safety-related information, their risk perception, and their ability to understand risk. It is also of interest to understand whether and how characteristics of the users (such as socio-demographics or risk tolerance) or of safety information itself are related to differences in risk perception. Research in this context has relied on a wide range of methods.

Literature Reviews

Systematic reviews of the scientific literature have commonly been used as a tool to identify gaps in research worth exploring in more detail and/or to build a solid evidence base for the intervention itself by summarising existing results. Over the years, several systematic reviews have been conducted on various topics within the field of communication about safety and safe use of medicines. These include studies on the role and effectiveness of written information available to patients about individual medicines (Raynor et al. 2007) or on the framing of treatment information comparing the effect of words versus numbers in communicating the probability of adverse effect to consumers (Büchter et al. 2014). Sometimes, generally when a specific aspect has only received scant attention in the field of medicines, the scope of the systematic reviews has been broadened to include literature from other fields of research. A review about pharmaceutical benefit-risk communication, for instance, included several tools that have been developed in the context of food safety and in the environmental/technological field (Way et al. 2017). Advice on how to build a search strategy and best conduct a systematic review is provided in (Higgins and Green 2008; Liberati et al. 2009). Although meta-analytic studies are recognised as the gold standard of evidence summaries, they have only rarely been conducted in this field, probably because of the relatively limited number of studies on each topic and of the heterogeneous nature of outcome measures used, which does not allow the calculation of pooled estimates (Sutton et al. 2000).

Qualitative Research Methods

Often, studies have used qualitative methodologies, for which principal research advice can be found in Chap. 8 dedicated to the social sciences. Qualitative studies in the area of the cognitive and behavioural sciences typically include users' perspective in order to get in-depth insights into preferences and perceptions about information on safety and safe use of medicines and into how the different ways of presenting information are perceived by the end users. They may also cover the processes involved in their evaluation of information for decision-making on, e.g. therapeutic options. Participants in these studies are usually presented with drug information leaflets or packages and asked to elaborate in a more or less structured way, either individually or in a group setting. Among other things, participants in interviews and focus groups have been asked to elaborate on the extent to which the safety information matches their needs, on whether the information is clear enough to enable them to make sense of the risk, on whether they would prefer the information to be presented in a different way, or on whether the safety information is enough for them to decide on the use of the medicines. As an example, in a study about the ramipril and clopidogrel, focus groups were used to explore consumers' perspectives, understanding, and treatment decision-making in response to written medicine information leaflets, containing information about side effect risks (Tong et al. 2015). Qualitative methods have also been used to capture the experts' perspective, as in a study where an expert consensus group of fourteen researchers from North America, Europe, and Australasia was given the task of identifying the main issues in risk communication to inform the development of a patient decision aid (Trevena et al. 2013).

The major advantages of using a qualitative methodology are its flexibility and the resulting increased richness of the data that can be obtained. Depending on the answers of the participants, the researcher can adapt his or her questions to get clarifications on specific aspects and thus gain a more in-depth understanding of the factors playing a role in the participants' perception. On the negative side, using a qualitative methodology it is not possible to reach generalisable conclusions about risk perception and its link with the use of different communication formats (Patton 2005).

Quantitative Research Methods, in Particular Surveys

This limitation can be at least partly overcome by using quantitative research methods. Large scale population surveys, for instance, have the major advantage of being able to provide researchers with generalisable information on preferences and perceptions and allow to quantitatively compare different risk communication formats. Surveys in this field have been conducted both among consumers and among experts. One context where consumers' perception about safety of medicines has often been examined through large scale surveys is that of childhood vaccinations. For instance, Chow and colleagues conducted a nationally representative online survey of Australian parents to determine associations between demographics and vaccination attitudes and behaviour (Chow et al. 2017). An example of surveys among experts is the one conducted among primary care clinicians by Finney-Rutten and colleagues to assess clinician knowledge, clinician barriers, and perceived parental barriers regarding HPV vaccination (Rutten et al. 2017). As mentioned before, the use of large scale surveys has a major advantage over qualitative methods in that it allows the researcher to obtain results that can be generalised, at least to a certain extent. On the other hand, the rigid structure of the questionnaires used in surveys limits the richness of the insights that can be gained, potentially hindering a holistic understanding of all the factors playing a role in safety-related perceptions and attitudes (Fowler 2013). General research advice on surveys is provided in Chap. 8 on the social sciences.

7.2.2 Methods for Evaluative Research: Randomised Controlled Trials

Research in the evaluation of different communication tools and interventions aims at answering more specific questions related to their effectiveness and strategies for information about safety and safe use of medicines. Typical tools or communication interventions in the context of safety and safe use of medicines include simple written information, effects tables, key benefits and risks summary tables, drug facts boxes, infographics, and warnings, and they have different uses. Written information has been used for changing both beliefs and behaviours. Effects tables, key benefits and risks summary tables, drug facts boxes, and infographics are commonly used for changing beliefs and attitudes, while warnings are usually aimed at changing behaviours. It is important to note that in recent years, more innovative approaches are under development, including those using digital media.

In contrast with what we observed in the case of research about risk perception and its determinants, the clear majority of evaluative studies have used quantitative approaches, particularly randomised controlled trials, where participants are randomly exposed to different versions of a tool to assess and compare their relative effects. The choice of an outcome measure depends on the specificity of the tool under investigation. According to Zipkin and colleagues, outcomes of interest in the field of risk communication from a cognitive-behavioural perspective can be grouped into three broad categories: cognitive (e.g. understanding or comprehension); affective (e.g. preferences for, or satisfaction with, information); and behavioural (i.e. actual or theoretical decision-making) (Zipkin et al. 2014). When assessing the impact of tools aiming at changing beliefs and attitudes or at improving understanding (such as drug facts boxes), outcomes measures are usually of the cognitive or affective type. As an example, Edwards and colleagues evaluated different risk presentation formats (numerical, graphical, and others) addressing the pros and cons of tight control versus usual treatment approaches for diabetes in a sample of people with diabetes and their carers. The two outcome measures of this randomised controlled trial were the degree of uncertainty and satisfaction with the information (Edwards et al. 2006). When evaluating the effectiveness of tools in changing behaviours, on the other hand, outcome measures are usually of the behavioural type. An example of a study of this type is a randomised controlled trial to evaluate the impact of an improved medication label. In this case the outcome measure was medication adherence (Shrank et al. 2009). One main limitation of research on the evaluation of tools is that it is often conducted in non-patient samples, thus limiting the validity of its results.

The research advice for experimental and quasi-experimental studies in Chap. 8 on the social sciences is applicable to cognitive and behavioural research.

7.3 Utility of Applied Methods for Researching Medicinal Product Risk Communication

As described in the previous section regarding methods, there are two main empirical research streams in the area of risk communication related to medicinal products within the cognitive and behavioural sciences. A first stream is formative research, which investigate users' preferences in terms of risk communication to inform the design and planning of communication tools and interventions, while a second stream investigates the effectiveness of the various tools and strategies on several outcomes. The multifaceted construct of risk perception, on the one hand, shapes the various outcomes of interest in these two areas, while the different methodologies allow for an attentive investigation of both the various approaches and the target groups. These combinations lead to the existence of a huge variety of studies which are hard to continuously monitor and appraise.

The purpose of this section is to provide an overall view of empirical cognitive and behavioural research by analytically presenting current evidence on risk communication in the field of safety and safe use of medicines. This demonstrates the best use and utility of the methods. This critical review has been developed in the form of a tabular presentation, organised by framing strategies (see below) and outcomes. For this purpose, the framework of cognitive, affective, and behavioural risk communication outcomes from Zipkin and colleagues (Zipkin et al. 2014) has been borrowed, which has been cited in the previous section. Table 7.1 hence highlights findings with potential to guide successful communication strategies while underscoring areas where there is paucity of research. As has already been pointed out in

Table 7.1 Utility of approaches and methods of the cognitive and behavioural sciences for medicinal product risk communication research in terms of the generated evidence

Framing strategy	Research method	Summary of generated evidence by communication outcomes
Negative versus positive framing	Randomised controlled trial, cross-sectional survey	*1. Cognitive* As shown in the field of genetic counselling, it is necessary to use both negative and positive framing in risk communication (Melas et al. 2012). The use of solely the negative or the positive framing of risk could lead to bias in the patients, therefore hindering their understanding. To allow patients to be autonomous in the decision-making process, facilitating understanding and avoiding biases generated by framing should be a primary concern for research and patient care (Edwards et al. 2002).
		2. Affective In relation to the presentation of pregnancy-related risks in genetic counselling, it has been shown that negative framing is perceived as more worrying than positive framing (Melas et al. 2012).
		3. Behavioural Positive framing increases the acceptance of therapies (Zipkin et al. 2014). This recent finding builds upon previous mixed evidence of positive versus negative framing effects on decision (Edwards et al. 2001). The biasing effect of positive and negative framing could also be cautiously exploited for behavioural interventions. However, ethical considerations are due.
Loss framing versus gain framing	Review of existing tools, literature review, meta-analysis, randomised controlled trial	*1. Cognitive* Few tools include information on both benefits and risks. Of those, many use frequencies to present a good outcome, and verbal descriptors or percentages to present adverse outcome (Flynn et al. 2013). Verbal descriptors lead to a bias of risk overestimation (see below: numerical representation versus verbal). Chronic patients have difficulties understanding materials mandated by the government, as these emphasise medication risks as opposed to benefits (Blalock 2017). The main problematic point remains the lack of a balanced presentation of benefits and risks for better patient understanding (Edwards et al. 2002).
		2. Affective Evidence is mixed or non-reported on affective outcomes. An experiment on breast self-examination comparing loss and gain framings showed a positive change in the attitude of the participants treated with the loss-frame messages (Edwards et al. 2001).
		3. Behavioural There is a greater effect of loss framing when compared to gain framing but a low effect significance. This is a clear pattern shown by older studies reviewed by Edwards and colleagues (Edwards et al. 2001) on detection and prevention behaviour. A more recent meta-analysis (Gallagher and Updegraff 2011) distinguished the effects of the two frames on different types of behaviour: loss-framed messages were not significantly more likely than gain-framed messages to promote detection behaviour but gain-framed messages were significantly more likely than loss-framed messages to promote prevention behaviour. This was found in the fields of skin cancer prevention, smoking cessation, and physical activity.

(continued)

Table 7.1 (continued)

Framing strategy	Research method	Summary of generated evidence by communication outcomes
Numerical and graphical representation versus only numerical	Focus group, interview, expert consensus, expert opinion, tool review, literature review, meta-analysis, survey, randomised controlled trial	*1. Cognitive* There is mixed evidence about the effectiveness of visual elements in risk representation. This probably derives from the fact that both numeracy and graph literacy skills play an important role in generating biases (Trevena et al. 2013; Hallgreen et al. 2016). Clear indications exist for the best way of developing graphical information, including: keeping information simple and focusing on essentials; choosing the best type of visual aid for the communication goal; depicting numerical information in addition to visual aids; effectively communicating through anticipation of user needs and skills; and scale validation studies to improve high-stakes interventions. (Garcia-Retamero and Cokely 2017). Graphical formats help understanding risk information, but different graphic formats suit different goals: i.e. bar graphs to compare several data points; line graphs to depict trends over time; distribution plot or forest plot to represent the statistical significance in the difference between alternatives; table to represent and present qualitative data, for example, text description, etc. (Hallgreen et al. 2016; Garcia-Retamero and Cokely 2017). In the USA, the drug facts box (a mix of visual and numerical information) is a positive example of risk communication, as it has shown particularly positive results in consumers' understanding of benefit data and of the whole content of the box itself (Way et al. 2017). As regards numerical information only, the presentation of numeric outcomes of decision is an important component and improves patient's accuracy of risk perception (Trevena et al. 2013). Also, evidence shows that to improve understanding it is important to express probabilities as event rates (percentages) or natural frequencies (numerator/denominator as whole numbers) (Zipkin et al. 2014).
		2. Affective Graphical representations, which complement and illustrate numerical representations, have the potential to catch and hold the attention of the audience (Lipkus 2007). However, no visual solution is absolutely superior to others for benefit-risk communication, as the most appropriate one highly depends on the targeted audience as well as on the information reported (Hallgreen et al. 2016).
		3. Behavioural In the USA, the drug facts box (mix of visual and numerical information) is a positive example of risk communication, as it showed positive results in patients' ability to make better and more informed choices regarding heartburn medicines (Way et al. 2017).

Table 7.1 (continued)

Framing strategy	Research method	Summary of generated evidence by communication outcomes
More data points versus less	Expert consensus, tools review, randomised controlled trial	*1. Cognitive* Tools for supporting decision-making should utilise evidence-based methods to present a balanced synopsis of probabilistic information on the full range of outcome states, suitable for different levels of health literacy (Flynn et al. 2013). This therefore shows the importance to present more statements that better depict the complexity of a risky event, rather than fewer.
		2. Affective As different strategies (visual, versus numerical, versus verbal) are suited for conveying different kind of information, and because people have different preferences regarding need and use of risk estimates (Büchter et al. 2014), it is advisable to use all the strategies to communicate more data points.
		3. Behavioural To make informed decisions, both patients and doctors are interested in having more data (i.e. longer-term outcomes) (Trevena et al. 2013). Having information that is more understandable to the patient is associated with a greater wariness to take treatments or tests (Edwards et al. 2002).
Numerical representation versus verbal	Randomised controlled trial, literature review	*1. Cognitive* Numerical information for risk representation is better understood when compared to verbal written information, even though it remains problematic for some people because of the intrinsic risk literacy issue. Both quantitative and verbal methods of communicating risk information have benefits and negative consequences associated with their use. Some studies show superiority of numerical presentation, but others show that semantic descriptors are easier to understand for people with lower literacy level (Young and Oppenheimer 2009). When verbal descriptors are used to communicate the frequencies of adverse effects in written health information (the ones indicated in the guidelines of the European Commission were tested, among others) lead to an overestimation of the probability of adverse effects if compared to numerical information. However, even people receiving numerical information overestimate the risk of adverse effect because people in general are poor in estimating risks (Büchter et al. 2014). Verbal information also results from interaction with healthcare professionals in support of written material. Verbal information from patient–physician encounters has been shown to be essential in complementing written material. On the other hand, pharmacists are not always effectively exploited as informational sources (Blalock 2017).
		2. Affective People tend to be more satisfied with numerical presentation of risk related information (Büchter et al. 2014).
		3. Behavioural People overestimate low risk events when given semantic descriptors, and their intention reflects this lack of calibration. The bias derived from verbal descriptors can discourage or encourage intentions to adhere to a prescribed behaviour, depending on whether the risks pertain to engaging or failing to engage in the stipulated behaviour (Young and Oppenheimer 2009). People seem to be more likely to take the drugs or continue taking them when they are presented numerical information (Büchter et al. 2014).

(continued)

Table 7.1 (continued)

Framing strategy	Research method	Summary of generated evidence by communication outcomes
Relative risk data versus absolute risk	Expert consensus, randomised controlled trial	*1. Cognitive* Expressing benefits and risks in absolute terms (such as absolute risk reduction) improves understanding of risk information. For the same reason, it is important to avoid expressing benefits as number needed to treat (Zipkin et al. 2014). Relative risk presentations tend to magnify risk perceptions and decrease understanding compared to absolute risk presentation (Trevena et al. 2013).
		2. Affective The evidence explored reports that in order to improve satisfaction it is essential to avoid the use of number needed to treat (Zipkin et al. 2014).
		3. Behavioural To have an effect on the acceptance of the intervention, it is important to realise that expressing numerical benefits as relative risk reduction has the greatest effect on decision-making (Zipkin et al. 2014; Edwards et al. 2002; McDowell et al. 2016). Adding baseline risks to both absolute risk reduction and relative risk reduction can equalise their effects on decision-making. (Zipkin et al. 2014).
Vivid portrayal of risk information versus abstract risk information	Literature review, expert consensus	*1. Cognitive* Few tools are prior tested by target groups. Therefore, they often do not respond to their needs (Flynn et al. 2013). Participatory design of information would ease the production of vivid portrayal.
		2. Affective No involvement of various stakeholders make the tools less acceptable for the consumers/patients (Flynn et al. 2013). To this extent, it is essential to involve the target audience in the production of information material.
		3. Behavioural Using narratives to present benefit and risk information may increase perceptions of risk severity, decrease the ability to accurately recall risk probabilities, and influence treatment choice. Narratives therefore: a) should be used with caution until research better clarifies their effects (positive and negative); and b) should be developed more cautiously when attempting to present unbiased information for informed decision-making than when attempting to be persuasive and to promote behaviour change (Trevena et al. 2013).
Lay terminology to present risk information versus usual medical terminology	Literature review, expert consensus, experiment	*1. Cognitive* Research on chronic conditions has shown a scarcity of evidence-based information presented in plain language, as well as programs designed to enhance patients' health literacy skills. Consequently, patients have limited knowledge of medication risks and benefits (Blalock 2017).
		2. Affective Few people read information leaflets, mostly because of the way they are structured and the complex terminology used. Patients suffering from chronic conditions reported that the written material about their treatment was not helpful (Way et al. 2017; Blalock 2017).
		3. Behavioural Insufficient evidence to support the effectiveness of both formats (Edwards et al. 2001; Moraes and Dal Pizzol 2018).

Table 7.1 (continued)

Framing strategy	Research method	Summary of generated evidence by communication outcomes
Manipulating base rate and "anchoring" points for frequencies	Randomised controlled trial	*1. Cognitive* As reported above, evidence shows that in order to improve understanding of risk information it is better to use a denominator of 1,000 participants for natural frequencies or as event rates (Zipkin et al. 2014). The judgement of an individual can be influenced more by altering the anchoring point, this is called the "base-rate neglect" bias (Edwards et al. 2001).
		2. Affective Studies related to this last category were scarce; moreover, the affective outcomes are often neglected.
		3. Behavioural Insufficient evidence to support the effectiveness of both formats.

the past by several authors, while there is attention on cognitive and behavioural outcomes, few studies assess affective outcomes. These are highly important when designing messages (Edwards et al. 2001). In light of current evidence, and as suggested by some of the scientists cited above and others, future research is needed to deepen understanding on the best way to communicate benefit and risk information in a balanced way (Blalock 2017). While it would be wise to consider borrowing successful visual strategies from other sectors (i.e. food safety) as well as other methods for developing tools such as the mental model approach (Way et al. 2017), it is also important to implement and test frameworks for risk-benefit communication which have been developed across the world (Pignatti et al. 2015).

Framing Strategies

The term "framing" describes how risks are presented, and nine framing strategies have inductively been derived by Edwards and colleagues (Edwards et al. 2001) in their review of risk communication interventions, namely:

1. *Negative versus positive framing*—presenting risk information in terms of negative consequences rather than positive terms;
2. *Loss framing versus gain framing*—presentation of the outcomes of an action in terms of disadvantages of not doing something versus the advantages of doing it;
3. *Numerical and graphical presentation versus numerical information only*—information presented in the form of numbers and graphs rather than only in the form of numbers;
4. *More data points versus fewer*—presentation of a great number of factual statements about a choice versus fewer statements;
5. *Numerical presentation of risk information versus verbal*—information quantitatively presented in the form of numbers versus information presented qualitatively with words;
6. *Relative risk versus absolute risk*—information is presented in terms of relative risk, which is the ratio between the probability of an outcome in an exposed

group to the probability of an outcome in an unexposed group compared to absolute risk (absolute risk is the probability that an event will occur and is usually presented as the ratio of the number of occurrences of an outcome in a group to the number of people in that group);
7. *Vivid portrayal of risk information* (by detailed or personalised vignettes) *versus abstract* (or general) *risk information*;
8. *Lay terminology to present risk information versus medical terminology*—information presented in simple terms compared to information presented only with clinical terms;
9. *Manipulating base rate* (absolute risk) *and "anchoring" points* (denominators) *for frequencies*—information presenting the efficacy of an action (i.e. medicine, treatment, or screening) in relative or absolute risk terms.

7.4 Outlook: Relevance, Improvements and Future Potential

Cognitive science considers beliefs as an integrative part of the cognitive process, and many behavioural theories (i.e. health belief model, theory of planned behaviour) either base their assumptions on or even include the belief concept into their models. A belief could explain why, when possessing the knowledge, we are still not able to take the right action, and it also explains why people with the same attitude toward an object yet differ in the extent of their behaviours (Ajzen and Fishbein 1972; Fishbein and Raven 1962). As shown above, communicating about risks with medicines so that people can form beliefs to facilitate appropriate decision-making by patients, healthcare professionals, and policy-makers in particular is not an easy task. There are many factors that, at both cognitive and behavioural level, can positively or negatively impact understanding and perception of these risks.

The evidence base for risk communication should be built around the topics of tailoring communication to different patient and consumer needs by moving beyond the "knowledge deficit model of communication" (Tong et al. 2015; Trevena et al. 2013). Science communication has historically been based on the paradigm that the public lacks adequate knowledge; therefore, the solution is to increase it by communicating factual expert knowledge. However, empirical evidence showed that the equation "expert thinking = laypeople thinking" is simply not working and when having more knowledge, laypeople do not necessarily make the expert-desired reasoning. The whole process is more complex, and people consider different factors (Hansen et al. 2003; Simis et al. 2016). As people have different preferences and needs with regard to presentation of risk estimates as well as different skills for interpreting information, various combinations of verbal, visual, and numerical formats could be implemented to best accommodate them. In order to implement this tailoring effort we still need to identify feasible solutions (Büchter et al. 2014). New communication strategies should be developed as a dynamic process and involve a range of actors from the outset, such as healthcare professionals, patients, and representatives from regulatory bodies (Karafillakis and Larson 2017). Another area that needs further exploration is the exploitation of potential of digital technologies (Trevena et al. 2013), which, we argue, would possibly facilitate this tailoring process. Table 7.1 also shows other important factors that need to be taken into account, such as health literacy and risk literacy. Those are important to consider as they can mediate the impact of different communication strategies. Health literacy has multiple accredited definitions, all broadly referring to the individual's ability to use (i.e. access, understand, process, and evaluate) health information and services (Sørensen et al. 2012). The concept of risk literacy can be considered as a context-specific health literacy related to the area of risk communication.

Overall, this chapter argues for the need to create communication interventions by coordinating key procedures that are well-established in the field of social marketing (Lee and Kotler 2011), the approach that aims to change or maintain an individual behaviour in his/her and the public benefit. Therefore, research from the cognitive and behavioural sciences should be used more for the key steps of planning and evaluating such interventions, including:

(1) to describe the background, purpose, and focus of the intervention;
(2) to define, segment, and characterise the audience (by focusing, for instance, on demographic data or on current behaviours, knowledge, and beliefs);
(3) to identify barriers and facilitators to decision-making (thus considering, for instance, misleading knowledge about a risk or existing incentives that can motivate people to act in certain ways);
(4) to create a message that it is clear, perceived to be relevant, engaging, and motivational, and is sensitive to possible cultural differences;
(5) to identify channels of communication (this step goes together with step 5 because the nature of the message is very much shaped by the type of channel that will be used deliver it, i.e. newspapers versus social media);
(6) to test and to refine the message (before being presented to the public, messages have to be tested with a sample of the target audience) (see Chap. 12 on design science for testing methods);
(7) to evaluate the impact of the message with the goal of establishing a correlation or even a proof of a causal relationship between the delivery of the message and specific outcomes (for instance, risk awareness or behaviour change).

For all this to happen, the engagement of stakeholders is essential, patients in particular (see Chap. 16). This can be achieved through co-design or participatory design (Sanders and Stappers 2008). These are processes where relevant stakeholders interact together with a moderator to work through the process of creation of, in this context, a strategy for risk communication and the messages it conveys. Here, it is important that representatives from all parties who have a significant interest in the outcome of a certain type of risk communication take part in the risk analysis and the risk communication planning. Last but not least, the multifaceted nature of risk perception and its complexity supports the need for healthcare institutions and organisations to dedicate financial, human, and technological resources to risk communication. For institutions and organisations to influence the public, it is essential that they go beyond a singular expertise in health and healthcare, and a framework supporting multidisciplinary research is required (see Chap. 1). A dialogue with experts from cognitive and behavioural sciences, health communication, and social marketing is the ideal basis for the delivery of successful risk communication.

Conclusions

- People's risk perceptions are more important than actual risks in determining behaviour, and as such are embedded in behavioural theories as one of the several different factors that predict behaviours.
- Risk perceptions are not formed by purely probabilistic evaluation and are greatly influenced by different factors including contextual, psychological, and emotional elements, as well as the media.
- Risk perceptions and evaluations of situations requiring decision-making are often driven by heuristics, which are mental shortcuts that can lead to cognitive biases.
- For planning a communication intervention, it is essential to go beyond the knowledge deficit model and determine the risk perceptions of the target groups in order to design appropriate messages for raising awareness and behaviour change.
- In order for healthcare institutions and organisations to adequately inform the public, motivate them for informed decision-making and facilitate behaviour change, it is essential that they go beyond a singular expertise in health and healthcare; a dialogue with experts from cognitive and behavioural sciences, health communication, and social marketing is the ideal basis for the delivery of successful risk communication.
- Overall, to successfully engage in risk communication, healthcare institutions and organisations need to engage with all relevant stakeholders in the field and have to invest in financial, human, and technological resources within a system underpinned by a suitable theoretical and empirical framework.

References

Ajzen I, Fishbein M (1972) Attitudes and normative beliefs as factors influencing behavioral intentions. J Pers Soc Psychol 21(1):1–9

Baumeister RF, Vohs KD (2007) Encyclopedia of social psychology. Sage, Thousand Oaks

Blalock SJ (2017) Medication risk communication in rheumatology: where are we and where do we go from here? Curr Rheumatol Rep 19:7

Büchter RB, Fechtelpeter D, Knelangen M, Ehrlich M, Waltering A (2014) Words or numbers? Communicating risk of adverse effects in written consumer health information: a systematic review and meta-analysis. BMC Med Inform Decis Mak 14:76

Calman K (2001) Issues of risk: this unique opportunity. Br J Gen Pract 51:47–51

Chow MYK, Danchin M, Willaby HW, Pemberton S, Leask J (2017) Parental attitudes, beliefs, behaviours and concerns towards childhood vaccinations in Australia: a national online survey. Aust Fam Physician 46:145

Covello VT, Peters RG, Wojtecki JG, Hyde RC (2001) Risk communication, the West Nile virus epidemic, and bioterrorism: responding to the communication challenges posed by the intentional or unintentional release of a pathogen in an urban setting. J Urban Health 78:382–391

Darker C (2013) Risk perception. In: Encyclopedia of behavioral medicine. Springer, New York, pp 1689–1691

Edwards A, Elwyn G, Covey J, Matthews E, Pill R (2001) Presenting risk information a review of the effects of framing and other manipulations on patient outcomes. J Health Commun 6:61–82

Edwards A, Elwyn G, Mulley A (2002) Explaining risks: turning numerical data into meaningful pictures. BMJ 324:827–830

Edwards A, Thomas R, Williams R, Ellner AL, Brown P, Elwyn G (2006) Presenting risk information to people with diabetes: evaluating effects and preferences for different formats by a web-based randomised controlled trial. Patient Educ Couns 63:336–349

Fischhoff B (1988) Judgment and decision making. In: Sternberg RJ, Smith EE (eds) The psychology of human thought. Cambridge University Press, New York, pp 153–187

Fishbein M, Raven BH (1962) The AB scales: an operational definition of belief and attitude. Hum Relat 15:35–44

Flynn D, Ford GA, Stobbart L, Rodgers H, Murtagh MJ, Thomson RG (2013) A review of decision support, risk communication and patient information tools for thrombolytic treatment in acute stroke: lessons for tool developers. BMC Health Serv Res 13:225

Fowler FJ Jr (2013) Survey research methods. Sage, Thousand Oaks

Gallagher KM, Updegraff JA (2011) Health message framing effects on attitudes, intentions, and behavior: a meta-analytic review. Ann Behav Med 43:101–116

Garcia-Retamero R, Cokely ET (2017) Designing visual aids that promote risk literacy: A systematic review of health research and evidence-based design heuristics. Hum Factors 59:582–627

Hallgreen CE, Mt-Isa S, Lieftucht A, Phillips LD, Hughes D, Talbot S, Asiimwe A, Downey G, Genov G, Hermann R (2016) Literature review of visual representation of the results of benefit–risk assessments of medicinal products. Pharmacoepidemiol Drug Saf 25:238–250

Hansen J, Holm L, Frewer L, Robinson P, Sandøe P (2003) Beyond the knowledge deficit: recent research into lay and expert attitudes to food risks. Appetite 41:111–121

Higgins JP, Green S (2008) Cochrane handbook for systematic reviews of interventions. Wiley Online Library, Chichester

Hochbaum G, Rosenstock I, Kegels S (1952) Health belief model. U S Public Health Service, Washington

Kahneman D, Frederick S (2002) Representativeness revisited: attribute substitution in intuitive judgment. In: Heuristics and biases: the psychology of intuitive judgment. Cambridge University Press, New York, pp 49–81

Kahneman D, Tversky A (1972) Subjective probability: a judgment of representativeness. In: The concept of probability in psychological experiments. Springer, Dordrecht, pp 25–48

Kahneman D, Tversky A (1979) Prospect theory: an analysis of decision under risk. Econometrics 47:263–291

Karafillakis E, Larson HJ (2017) The benefit of the doubt or doubts over benefits? A systematic literature review of perceived risks of vaccines in European populations. Vaccine 35: 4840–4850

Kasperson RE, Renn O, Slovic P, Brown HS, Emel J, Goble R, Kasperson JX, Ratick S (1988) The social amplification of risk: a conceptual framework. Risk Anal 8:177–187

Kerlinger FN (1979) Behavioral research: a conceptual approach. Holt, Rinehart and Winston, New York

Lee NR, Kotler P (2011) Social marketing: influencing behaviors for good. Sage, Thousand Oaks

Liberati A, Altman DG, Tetzlaff J, Mulrow C, Gøtzsche PC, Ioannidis JP, Clarke M, Devereaux PJ, Kleijnen J, Moher D (2009) The PRISMA statement for reporting systematic reviews and meta-analyses of studies that evaluate health care interventions: explanation and elaboration. PLoS Med 6:e1000100

Lipkus IM (2007) Numeric, verbal, and visual formats of conveying health risks: suggested best practices and future recommendations. Med Decis Making 27:696–713

McCarthy M, Brennan M, De Boer M, Ritson C (2008) Media risk communication–what was said by whom and how was it interpreted. J Risk Res 11:375–394
McDowell M, Rebitschek FG, Gigerenzer G, Wegwarth O (2016) A simple tool for communicating the benefits and harms of health interventions: a guide for creating a fact box. MDM Policy Pract 1:2381468316665365
Melas PA, Öhman SG, Juth N (2012) Information related to prenatal genetic counseling: interpretation by adolescents, effects on risk perception and ethical implications. J Genet Couns 21:536–546
Moraes CG, Dal Pizzol T d S (2018) Effect of different formats for information on side effects regarding medicine users' understanding: A randomized controlled trial. Patient Educ Couns 101:672–678
Morrow BH (2009) Risk behavior and risk communication: synthesis and expert interviews. Final Report for the NOAA Coastal Services Center 53.
National Research Council (1989) Understanding hazards and risks. In: Improving risk communication. National Academies Press (US), Washington
Nickerson RS (1998) Confirmation bias: a ubiquitous phenomenon in many guises. Rev Gen Psychol 2:175–220
Paek HJ, Hove T (2017) Risk perceptions and risk characteristics. In: Oxford research encyclopedia, communication. Oxford University Press, Oxford
Pallier G, Wilkinson R, Danthiir V, Kleitman S, Knezevic G, Stankov L, Roberts RD (2002) The role of individual differences in the accuracy of confidence judgments. J Gen Psychol 129:257–299
Patton MQ (2005) Qualitative research. Wiley Online Library
Pidgeon NF, Beattie J (1998) The psychology of risk and uncertainty. Blackwell Science, London
Pignatti F, Ashby D, Brass EP, Eichler H-G, Frey P, Hillege HL, Hori A, Levitan B, Liberti L, Löfstedt RE (2015) Structured frameworks to increase the transparency of the assessment of benefits and risks of medicines: current status and possible future directions. Clin Pharmacol Ther 98:522–533
Raynor DK, Blenkinsopp A, Knapp P, Grime J, Nicolson DJ, Pollock K, Dorer G, Gilbody S, Dickinson D, Maule AJ (2007) A systematic review of quantitative and qualitative research on the role and effectiveness of written information available to patients about individual medicines. Health Technol Assess 11(5):1–160
Rimal RN, Real K (2003) Perceived risk and efficacy beliefs as motivators of change: use of the risk perception attitude (RPA) framework to understand health behaviors. Hum Commun Res 29:370–399
Rogers RW (1983) Cognitive and psychological processes in fear appeals and attitude change: A revised theory of protection motivation. In: Cacioppo JT, Petty RE (eds) Social psychophysiology: a source book. Guilford Press, New York, pp 153–176
Ropeik D (2012) The perception gap: recognizing and managing the risks that arise when we get risk wrong. Food Chem Toxicol 50:1222–1225
Rutten LJF, Sauver JLS, Beebe TJ, Wilson PM, Jacobson DJ, Fan C, Breitkopf CR, Vadaparampil ST, Jacobson RM (2017) Clinician knowledge, clinician barriers, and perceived parental barriers regarding human papillomavirus vaccination: association with initiation and completion rates. Vaccine 35:164–169
Sanders EB-N, Stappers PJ (2008) Co-creation and the new landscapes of design. CoDesign 4:5–18. https://doi.org/10.1080/15710880701875068
Shrader-Frechette KS (1991) Risk and rationality: philosophical foundations for populist reforms. University of California Press, Berkeley
Shrank WH, Gleason PP, Canning C, Walters C, Heaton AH, Jan S, Patrick A, Brookhart MA, Schneeweiss S, Solomon DH (2009) Can improved prescription medication labeling influence adherence to chronic medications? An evaluation of the target pharmacy label. J Gen Intern Med 24:570–578
Simis MJ, Madden H, Cacciatore MA, Yeo SK (2016) The lure of rationality: why does the deficit model persist in science communication? Public Underst Sci 25:400–414

Slovic P (2016) The perception of risk. Routledge, Abingdon
Sørensen K, Van den Broucke S, Fullam J, Doyle G, Pelikan J, Slonska Z, Brand H (2012) Health literacy and public health: a systematic review and integration of definitions and models. BMC Public Health 12:80
Sutton AJ, Abrams KR, Jones DR, Jones DR, Sheldon TA, Song F (2000) Methods for meta-analysis in medical research. Wiley, Chichester
Thagard P (1996) Cognitive science. Johns Hopkins University, Irvine
Tong V, Raynor DK, Blalock SJ, Aslani P (2015) Consumer interpretation of ramipril and clopidogrel medication risk information–implications for risk communication strategies. Patient Prefer Adherence 9:983
Trevena LJ, Zikmund-Fisher BJ, Edwards A, Gaissmaier W, Galesic M, Han PK, King J, Lawson ML, Linder SK, Lipkus I (2013) Presenting quantitative information about decision outcomes: a risk communication primer for patient decision aid developers. BMC Med Inform Decis Mak 13:S7
Tversky A, Kahneman D (1973) Availability: a heuristic for judging frequency and probability. Cognit Psychol 5:207–232
Tversky A, Kahneman D (1974) Judgment under uncertainty: heuristics and biases. Science 185:1124–1131
von Neumann J, Morgenstern O (1944) Theory of games and economic behavior. Princeton University Press, Princeton
Way D, Blazsin H, Löfstedt R, Bouder F (2017) Pharmaceutical benefit–risk communication tools: a review of the literature. Drug Saf 40(1):1–22
Weinstein ND, Kwitel A, McCaul KD, Magnan RE, Gerrard M, Gibbons FX (2007) Risk perceptions: assessment and relationship to influenza vaccination. Health Psychol 26:146
Wilde GJ (1982) The theory of risk homeostasis: implications for safety and health. Risk Anal 2:209–225
Witte K (1992) Putting the fear back into fear appeals: the extended parallel process model. Commun Monogr 59:329–349
Young S, Oppenheimer DM (2009) Effect of communication strategy on personal risk perception and treatment adherence intentions. Psychol Health Med 14:430–442
Zipkin DA, Umscheid CA, Keating NL, Allen E, Aung K, Beyth R, Kaatz S, Mann DM, Sussman JB, Korenstein D (2014) Evidence-based risk communication: a systematic review. Ann Intern Med 161:270–280

The Social Sciences

8

Brian J. Taylor and S. Anne Moorhead

Abstract

Research methods commonly used in social sciences are appropriate for studies of how people deal with "risk" and for studies of risk communication. These approaches can be applied to understanding and appraising risk communications about medicines. This chapter reviews appropriateness and potential of social science research methods for this purpose, focusing on:

- qualitative studies (e.g. of experiences of a risk communication, or to create a theoretical conceptualisation or model of a risk communication);
- surveys for studying prevalence (e.g. of health behaviours or attitudes) and correlations (e.g. between communication types and health behaviours);
- (quasi-)experimental studies and intervention trials (for measuring effects of planned risk communication interventions); and
- mixed-method studies (combining features of the above designs).

The chapter explains the main features of these methods; discusses their strengths and limitations; considers examples; and makes suggestions for applying the methods effectively to improve the evidence base on risk communication about medicines. The chapter emphasises the distinctly different types of research question that are appropriate for each of these research designs.

B. J. Taylor (✉) · S. A. Moorhead
Ulster University, Newtownabbey, Northern Ireland, UK
e-mail: bj.taylor@ulster.ac.uk

© Springer Nature Singapore Pte Ltd. 2020

P. Bahri (ed.), *Communicating about Risks and Safe Use of Medicines*,
https://doi.org/10.1007/978-981-15-3013-5_8

8.1 The Discipline of the Social Sciences: Scope, Theories and Principles

It's like everything's a risk, everything's a danger.
I've always the belief, risk is not to be avoided; it is to be managed.
Well I think with medication they should, you know, tell you more about the side effects
Focus Group participants, cited in (Stevenson and Taylor 2016)

Communication about risks in life is an interaction between people—whether individuals, groups or organisations, and whether in government, research or commerce—and as such is a human process. Communication between people is a major focus of study in the social sciences. Appraising the quality of risk communication, and using research to understand and improve its effectiveness, requires a focus on the interaction and perceptual processes involved. This is a familiar type of social science research activity. As this book aims to develop multidisciplinary research, this chapter describes the methods offered by social sciences at a level which will be simple to some but novel to other, depending on the reader's background discipline. More details are provided in the indicated sources for the interested reader.

There is a broad international understanding that social science is the study of societies and the ways in which people behave, communicate and influence the world around them (see e.g. Economic and Social Research Council (2016), see also Wikipedia entry). The social sciences would commonly be regarded as including the domains of anthropology, archaeology, business studies, civics, communication studies, criminology, demography, development studies, economics, education, environmental studies, gerontology, human geography, international studies, law, library science, linguistics, management, marketing, organisational studies, political science, psychology, public administration, regional studies, social policy, social work, sociology and urban planning. Like the natural sciences, the social sciences seek to create an organised and systematic body of knowledge using scientific methods, and to develop practical applications. However the application of scientific methods to the study of people's attitudes, attributes, behaviour, beliefs, knowledge, opinions and reasoning presents particular challenges. It is generally harder than in the natural sciences to be precise, to achieve observations independent of the researcher, and to demonstrate causal links. The processes of theory informing empirical study and empirical study spurring development of theory exist in social sciences just as in the natural sciences (Taylor et al. 2015). The same research principles of replicability, testability, falsifiability and simplicity are used. Like the natural sciences, the social sciences encompass both pure and applied research. The practical applications of social sciences tend to have their focus on improving the way that societies and organisations operate (including in the provision of public services such as health), and in informing the knowledge and skills of professionals (including their communication and management of risk).

Developing and evaluating an intervention—including a psychosocial intervention such as a planned risk communication—requires a range of research methods suited to the stage of the process (Petticrew 2011), and a multidisciplinary approach can create synergy (see Chap. 1). In this chapter we discuss major research methods in the social sciences suited to stages of this process, each contributing appropriately to the type of research question (Petticrew et al. 2013a). In particular, the relevance of various research methods to risk communication about medicines is discussed, highlighting opportunities to develop these methods for future study. This chapter does not seek to describe, appraise or synthesise the findings of studies on risk communication about medicines. Types of risk communication interventions (Bahri 2010) are presented in Chap. 1. It is beyond the scope of this chapter to teach the knowledge and skills required to carry out the methods outlined, for which the interested reader is referred to sources at appropriate points.

8.1.1 Terminology

Risks of medicines include harm due to adverse reactions (commonly known as "side effects") with therapeutic use, and also harm due to misuse and abuse of a medicine (Mayall and Banerjee 2014 and see Chap. 1). Terminology regarding "risk" varies across and within social science disciplines, as well as differing from that common in other disciplines such as pharmacoepidemiology and pharmacovigilance (Council of the European Communities 1992; European Medicines Agency Benefit-risk Methodology Project Team 2011). In particular, theories and models for conceptualising risk derived from domains such as law (Carson and Bain 2008) or professional social work (Taylor 2012a, 2017a) may be internally consistent, but not in accord with terminology adopted by other professions or disciplines. This variable use of terminology needs to be considered in relation not only to the term "risk", but also to derivative phrases such as "risk management" (Taylor and Campbell 2011) or "risk minimisation". For example, the term "risk" may in itself be used on occasions in the social sciences to connote a balance between positive and negative outcomes (as in the everyday expression "taking a risk") rather than using the term "risk-benefit balance" used in pharmacovigilance to contrast risk as the chance of harm with the expected benefit (see European Union, Directive 2001/83/EC Art 1(28a) as amended). Interestingly, common usage of the term "risk" in social sciences, as in pharmacovigilance, does not usually restrict the term to being a synonym for "probability" or "likelihood" (of harm) as in many dictionary definitions. Thus the term "risk" is often used to encompass the concept of value, i.e. the seriousness of possible harm—as in pharmacovigilance phrases such as "identified risk" and "important identified risk" (European Medicines Agency 2017a)—in addition to referring to the concept of likelihood. A similar usage occurs in a range of health and social care professions (Stevenson et al. 2018). The terminology compiled for the good pharmacovigilance practices for the European Union (EU-GVP) (European Medicines Agency 2017a), which is largely based on or aligned with internationally agreed terms, is used in this chapter to ensure consistency within the book (see Chap. 1).

Terms relating to research in this chapter use terminology commonly accepted in the discourse of medicine, psychology and social sciences. For the purposes of this chapter we use the following definitions:

- *External Validity*: The extent to which the study findings may confidently be generalised to people and situations other than those studied.

- *Internal Validity*: The extent to which the measured effects of an intervention may be ascribed confidently to that intervention.
- *Reliability*: The consistency of research measures, primarily in terms of whether similar results are obtained if the study is repeated (Taylor et al. 2015).

Some jurisdictions, including the United Kingdom (UK), distinguish for the purposes of research governance between research, service evaluation, professional audit and uses of data for public health services (Health Research Authority 2016) (the term "research governance" includes both ethics and risks of the study). The distinction between research and evaluation depends primarily on whether the aim is generalisable new knowledge, which would then constitute research. In general terms a study of a risk communication intervention that is already designed and implemented as a "standard service" would be classified in the UK as evaluation (unless it involved experimental methods) or as a health and social care professional audit and not as research. The focus of this chapter is on the methods of research, some of which (particularly mixed methods) may be used within service evaluations (cf. European Medicines Agency 2017b, Appendix 1) as well as within research, rather than on governance categories. Our focus is on applying research methods to generate evidence for designing, planning, improving and evaluating communication interventions, including within evaluations after implementation (Australian Council for International Development 2016; European Medicines Agency 2017c).

8.1.2 Current Application of Social Science Methods for Medicinal Product Risk Communication Research: A Literature Review

Pharmaceutical regulators are requiring increased attention to risk minimisation, including risk communication (European Medicines Agency 2012, 2013; Food and Drug Administration 2005, 2007, 2009) in the context of concerns about the rigour of current research and evaluation (Bahri et al. 2017; Department of Health and Human Services. Office of Inspector General 2013; Dusetzina et al. 2012; Goedecke et al. 2018; Gridchyna et al. 2014; Mazzaglia et al. 2018; Smith and Morrato 2014). For the purpose of this chapter, a review of published research that used relevant social science methods on the general topic of risk communication regarding medicines was undertaken.

Using a thorough and systematic approach (Best et al. 2014; Centre for Reviews and Dissemination (CRD) 2009; McGinn et al. 2016; Taylor et al. 2003), the search included *Google Scholar* Web search engine and ten bibliographic databases: ASSIA; CINAHL; Communication Abstracts; Embase; Medline on Ovid; PsycINFO; PubMed; Scopus; and SCI and SSCI on Web of Science. The concept structure for the search was *risk AND communication AND medicines* (Stevenson and Taylor 2016; Bates et al. 2017; McFadden et al. 2012; Stevenson et al. 2016). The basic search formula (adapted for each database) involved 25 search terms as well as truncation variants. The search on bibliographic databases and the World Wide Web was supplemented by considering the references of included articles and recommendations by colleagues with expertise in the field. The search formula incorporated relevant terms from the Cochrane Review on personalised risk communication regarding screening tests (Edwards et al. 2013). As in the searches in that Cochrane Review, the terms "safety" and "warnings" (and their variants) were not included due to the high imprecision they would introduce. Hence some relevant research might not have been identified. As searching for diverse study designs was required (Petticrew et al. 2013b) it had to be accepted that the highest standard of sensitivity and precision was not achievable at the present time. As the aim was to retrieve examples to illustrate methodological issues, a totally exhaustive search strategy was not necessary even if it were possible.

The scope of the literature search was restricted to medicines in general. Searching for research on risk communication in relation to specific medicines (i.e. active substances and classes of medicines) was beyond our scope, although studies relating to specific medicines were included if retrieved by the generic search strategy. Editorials were excluded as were theoretical, opinion and policy papers. Articles on more general aspects of health and social care risk communication (including classic works such as Teigen, Brun (Taylor et al. 2015)) were excluded in order to maintain the focus on medicines, although it is recognised that such studies may have generalisable application.

The search, conducted in December 2015, retrieved 13 review articles (Butcher et al. 2014; Dodoo and Hugman 2012; Edwards et al. 2001; Lipkus and Hollands 1999; McComas 2006; Nelson et al. 2008; O'Connor et al. 2003; Reyna et al. 2009; Schmid et al. 2007; Visschers et al. 2009; West et al. 2013; Zipkin et al. 2014; Zolnierek and Dimatteo 2009), as well as the individual studies discussed below. Studies reviewed in these articles were considered against the criteria (above), for inclusion in the review conducted for this book. These reviews focused on synthesising findings rather than methodological aspects, which was the focus of our task. The overview of systematic reviews of interventions to improve safe and effective use of medicines in the Cochrane Library (Ryan et al. 2014) provides a useful framework for considering interventions and outcomes but was too broad in scope to be included.

Twenty-three relevant studies were retrieved (Andreas et al. 2010; Belcora et al. 2011; Berry et al. 2002; Brewer et al. 2009; Davis 2007; Davis et al. 2007; Gaissmaier et al. 2014; Han et al. 2014; Hutton et al. 2009; Ilic et al. 2012; Keller and Siegrist 2009; Kennedy et al. 2008; Kirkegaard et al. 2010; Langlois-Klassen et al. 2008; Längst et al. 2015; Makoul et al. 1995; Newman et al. 2009; Omedo et al. 2014; Reber et al. 2013; Schapira et al. 2006; Schwartz et al. 2009; Tong et al. 2015; Young and Oppenheimer 2006), originating from the United States (US), some European countries, Australia, Canada and one each on communication interventions in Kenya and Uganda. The retrieved studies were appraised using the appropriate tool from the suite in Taylor et al. (2015):

- QAT-S Quality Appraisal Tool—Survey Research
- QAT-Q Quality Appraisal Tool—Qualitative Research
- QAT-E Quality Appraisal Tool—(Quasi-)Experimental Research

Use of these appraisal tools facilitated a detailed understanding of the methods used in the studies. Each tool uses the same ten main headings, but the sub-headings are then tailored to the particular study design. Further discussion on the approach to study classification is in Sect. 8.2 and the approach to study appraisal in Sect. 8.3. However we are aware of the possible misuse of appraisal tools "if they convey the impression that one can simply add up scores so as to give a meaningful overall score of quality" (Taylor et al. 2015), and we did not use them for this purpose.

8.2 Research Approaches and Methods

This chapter outlines the relevance, limitations and opportunities of common social science research methods for the study of risk communication about medicines, presenting the following major research designs (Taylor et al. 2015):

- qualitative research for understanding experiences and perspectives, and for creating a theoretical conceptualisation or model;
- surveys to measure prevalence (e.g. of attitudes or behaviours) or correlations (e.g. between respondent characteristics and their behaviour);
- experimental and quasi-experimental studies—including intervention trials—measuring effects of a risk communication intervention; and,
- mixed-method studies using a composite of more than one of the basic designs above.

These research methods were chosen as the focus for this chapter because they are widely used in the social sciences and because they are less frequently used in pharmacoepidemiology (see Chap. 14). The title of this chapter and the focus on these methods does not imply that these methods are the only ones used within the social sciences, nor that these methods are not used outside social sciences. A distinction is sometimes drawn between experimental studies and those described as "observational" (Altman 1991), but for the present purpose this is unhelpful not least because of widely varying definitions of "observational". A more fine-grained categorisation is required (Bailar et al. 1986) to take account of, for example, study designs that use pre-post testing to measure the effect of the (risk communication) intervention but without a control group.

A key principle in creating knowledge is that the research design should be suited to the type of research question (Taylor et al. 2015). This can be considered in relation to the stages in the "Framework for Developing and Evaluating Complex Interventions" (2008) issued by the Medical Research Council (MRC) (Medical Research Council 2008) in the UK (Craig et al. 2008; Fischoff et al. 2011; Moore et al. 2015a, b). This framework poses various questions that need to be addressed in the process of creating and developing an intervention to the point of being ready for a randomised controlled trial of effectiveness. Such questions include understanding the prevalence of the problem (or issue) and factors that correlate with it; conceptualising (understanding, modelling) the need and intervention processes; designing the elements of the intervention (with engagement of appropriate stakeholders); estimating the intervention effect size; identifying or creating meaningful outcome measures and effective measurement tools; and considering feasibility and cost of implementation. These questions are then positioned in terms of a typical stage from conceptualisation through to a trial of the intervention. This chapter uses this framework to consider methods suited to various stages of the process of conceptualising through to creating and testing a risk communication intervention.

It is not possible in a brief chapter to provide guidance on how to carry out these types of research; there are many text-books for that purpose (Auspurg and Hinz 2014; Bickman and Rog 2008; Bland 2015; Bors 2018; Brewer 2000; Bryman 2016; Campbell et al. 2016; Charmaz 2014; Cresswell and Plano 2010; Engel and Schutt 2013; Gale et al. 2013; Gee 2005; Glaser and Strauss 1999; McColl et al. 2001; Ritchie and Lewis 2006; Smith et al. 2009). The focus here is to enable the reader to appreciate the main characteristics of the major types of research methods used in social sciences; to clarify the distinct purposes for which these social science research designs are appropriate; to help the reader to apply these appropriately to medicinal product risk communication research; and to develop an understanding of how research quality criteria might be applied properly to these designs.

8.2.1 Qualitative Research

Qualitative researchers study phenomena (including behaviours such as communication) in their natural settings, seeking to make sense of these in terms of the meanings that people attribute to them (Bryman 2016). This is in contrast to quantitative research which seeks to use numerical data to describe the world (surveys) or to measure the effects of a planned intervention (experimental and quasi-experimental studies). Qualitative research studies people and situations regarding their real-life experiences in their own words and concepts. It focuses on conceptual understandings of cognitive and social processes, and the social constructs (such as “cope with”, “purpose”, “risky”, “safety”, “self-image”, “trust”) through which people make sense of events and experiences (such as receipt of risk-communications). This “sense-making” is an essential part of the framework that people use to make decisions, such as about health and care in the context of risk (Taylor 2017a).

Essentially qualitative research analyses words or observed behaviours, and focuses on meanings and understandings. It is not suited to measuring distributions across populations or correlations. A common rationale for using qualitative research is that there is limited knowledge of the field and that exploratory research is required. Qualitative research can identify the language that people use, and gather useful data on people’s experiences of change processes, such as in response to receiving a risk communication. Qualitative studies are not suited to measuring the amount or effects of change. Qualitative research can be used to explore experiences of potential facilitators and barriers to change in response to a risk communication. Qualitative research is essentially inductive, i.e. it is concerned with creating, from data, new conceptualisations or understandings, which may be viewed as creating a theory. This contrasts with most quantitative research which is essentially deductive and concerned with testing the validity or applicability of an existing theory or related hypothesis. Qualitative studies may, however, lead to hypotheses which can be tested through deductive, quantitative research in a complementary, iterative process (Taylor et al. 2015).

In relation to risk communication about medicines, typical topics that might be explored through qualitative research are:

- the ways in which patients, clients and families conceptualise the risks, the risk communication process and risk management advice, including aspects such as emotion, motivation and trust;
- the ways that professionals conceptualise levels, likelihood or seriousness of "risk" and the issues they face in communicating about these to patients and clients; and,
- the ways in which numeric, verbal and visual communications are perceived and interpreted.

Qualitative data are typically gathered through semi-structured interviews or focus groups (see Table 8.1), but may be gathered also through observations, diaries or analysis of documents. One skill element in qualitative research where data is gathered directly from respondents is to tune-in to the context of the individuals so as to develop sufficient trust to elicit honest, in-depth responses. Context here might include socio-cultural norms; feelings (including such as fear, stigma or anticipated regret) that relate to the illness or the medicines; legal or organisational constraints; and abilities such as literacy and numeracy. As with interviews, the degree of specification of questions or prompts for discussion in focus groups may vary.

Table 8.1 Major data-gathering methods for qualitative research

Data-gathering method	Key features
Interview	An interviewer-guided discussion with an individual so as to elicit the interviewee's experience and understanding of the meaning of the topic being studied. Interviews are particularly appropriate if the topic might be embarrassing in group discussion, and are normally applied as "semi-structured" so as to prompt and facilitate responses without being too prescriptive or controlling. At the extreme of being tightly "structured", interviews might be used to gather data for a survey (see below)
Focus group	A facilitator-guided discussion with a group of people so as to elicit their experience and understanding of the meaning of the topic being studied. They are particularly appropriate if the synergy of discussion and sharing ideas is appropriate for developing a conceptual understanding of the topic. The degree of structuring through the "grand tour questions" may vary, and visual aids and other materials may also be used to prompt the discussion
Observation	May be used to study behaviours and communications, e.g. in the context of workflows, social rituals, information flows and customs. A template may be used to assist in ordering the data, but the focus is not on numeric data or measurement (see surveys) but on gaining a holistic understanding of the multiple facets of the situation or issue, in particular aspects that may be missed through pre-determined questions. Observation is common in ethnography, the systematic study of people and cultures

Analysis in qualitative studies focuses on the meaning of words that are spoken, recorded or written, and the meaning of behaviours that are observed (Campbell et al. 2016). Whilst the separation of what the study found from what the researchers' think it means is relatively straightforward in quantitative research, this distinction is not so straightforward in qualitative research (Greenhalgh 2014, p. 174). The strength of a qualitative design does not come from any attempt to "quantify" the qualitative data. Qualitative studies should use a clearly identified method, such as one of those in Table 8.2, each of which derives from a different epistemological approach to understanding knowledge (Spencer et al. 2003; Starks and Trinidad 2007).

The main quality feature of qualitative studies is external validity, that is, how true the data are to the real world, with an emphasis on natural settings (Kuper et al. 2008). The primary criterion for sampling in qualitative research is therefore that respondents should be "information rich" in relation to the topic of study (Taylor et al. 2015). Data gathering must relate to respondents' experience, and elicit some

Table 8.2 Selected major qualitative research designs

Data-gathering methods	Key features
Discourse analysis	• Focus on the way that language is used and the meanings attributed • Uses socio-historical context of speakers and dominant social rules • Data may be any mode of language, including written, oral and signed • May be called "documentary analysis" if data is from documents Further information: (Gee 2005)
Ethnography	• Focus on understanding shared meanings within a community • Data gathered through researcher immersion in the culture • Data gathering is primarily through observation • Ethics of immersing into and disengaging from a culture is a focus Further information: (Brewer 2000)
Framework analysis	• Focus on analysing data by individual cases as well as by themes • Data usually from focus groups or semi-structured interviews • Tabulation of data demonstrates its source Further information: (Gale et al. 2013)
Grounded theory	• Focus on generating theory grounded in real world experiences • Emphasises constant comparison of new with existing data • Data usually from focus groups or semi-structured interviews • Emerging findings may be used to inform subsequent data gathering • Concept of "saturation" of data as study progresses determines sample size Further information: (Charmaz 2014; Glaser and Strauss 1999)
Interpretative phenomenological analysis	• Focus on how a person makes sense of an emotional experience • Data usually from focus groups or semi-structured interviews • Can be used to refine or "test out" a theory in a new context • Twofold process of analysis, considering also the researcher's perspective Further information: (Smith et al. 2009)
Thematic (or narrative or content) analysis	• Focus on how people make sense of their experiences • Data usually from focus groups or semi-structured interviews • Simple basic method underpinning other approaches Further information: (Ritchie and Lewis 2006)

element of "the truth" despite factors (such as embarrassment at the illness or at the decision made in the face of risks) which might obscure reality. Because of the data-gathering methods required to obtain this type of data, it is rare in qualitative research for the researcher to be regarded as "objective". Rather, attention must be paid to reflection on the researcher's own background, role, attitudes and behaviour (e.g. during data gathering) so as to minimise bias from this source. This reflection might be carried out with a research supervisor, or through some group process associated with the research project.

Some measure of representativeness in sampling may be employed, but this is a secondary consideration in qualitative research as the purpose is not generalisability to a population but credibility in creating a theoretical understanding of the topic. This conceptualisation or model might then be tested through deductive research for the extent of its validity once hypotheses are developed. Such theoretical understandings from qualitative research inform the completion of the section "why the intervention might work" within the background section of a Cochrane Review (see, e.g. Akl et al. 2011). Qualitative methods may be used within mixed-method evaluations to gather illustrative material about people's "lived experience" of receiving the intervention. The in-depth qualitative analysis outlined here is appropriate to (generalisable) research, but a simpler approach may be taken to qualitative data within evaluations using thematic (narrative, content) analysis. Further detail on practical aspects of carrying out qualitative studies may be found in Campbell et al. (2016).

Theories, Concepts, Constructs and Models

The distinction between the terms "theory", "concepts", "construct" and "model" is not entirely clear-cut within the scientific community. A theory or model in social sciences is the creation of an abstract, simplified view of some aspect of the social world for a useful purpose. Within the social sciences it is perhaps most common to use the term "social construct" for a more static representation (e.g. stigma attributable to an illness) and the term "model" for dynamic systems (e.g. an understanding of the process of communicating about risks of medicines). The term "theory" might be most appropriate for a large-scale understanding with a number of constituent elements, and from which models are derived for particular applications, such as the "Theory of Planned Behaviour" to conceptualise an understanding of the cognitive processes of the recipient of the risk communication. Einstein's "Theory of Relativity" is an equivalent example in the natural sciences. The terms "concept" and "conceptualisation" are usually used more loosely, to describe an understanding that is recognised as partial and not yet formulated into a cohesive theory.

By "theory" in the context of risk communication about medicines we mean such things as our understanding of the sending or receiving of the risk communication messages (Granger et al. 2001); the way that the transfer of knowledge or emotion about the risk is understood (Taylor 2006a); conceptualisations of the sender, receiver, or method of the risk communication (Moorhead et al. 2013a); or models of the way that decisions are made as a result of the risk communication (Taylor 2017b). Qualitative research enables understanding of the need for, and the characteristics of, communication interventions and processes. Qualitative research can contribute to constructing or modifying a model of risk communication that "makes sense" in terms of the real world context, concepts and language of communicators and communication recipients as well as their relationships. This modelling has particular value at the early inductive stage of the research and development process, such as when a risk communication intervention is being first designed. It may also be useful later in the process when modifying the communication in the light of the experience. By comparison, a survey or experiment requires an appropriate understanding of the use of language, and concepts that are well developed and robust enough for the creation of meaningful measurement scales.

8.2.2 Survey Research

A survey is an investigation of the characteristics of a given population by collecting data from a sample of that population, and estimating the population characteristics through statistical analysis to detect patterns of relationship between variables (Bryman 2016). Surveys are cross-sectional, i.e. they provide a picture at a determined point in time. Surveys are suited to measuring the prevalence of characteristics in a population (for example, health literacy or computer literacy) and correlations amongst these characteristics (for example, the possibility that health literacy correlates with age or education). Surveys may identify barriers and facilitators of behavioural change, and may be used to measure constructs created through qualitative research. Surveys are not well-suited to measuring the effects of a planned intervention.

The data collection tool for a survey is commonly a questionnaire, i.e. a collection of questions administered to respondents. Questionnaires collect primarily quantitative data using closed questions (which may include scaled and multiple choice as well as dichotomous questions) but sometimes a few open questions are included to provide qualitative data with some simple form of qualitative analysis (see Sect. 8.2.1). The questionnaires may be provided in a printed or electronic format online. They may be completed either through self-completion by the respondents following distribution by the researchers (e.g. via email or post) or through a structured interview in person or via telephone. As a research design in social science and general epidemiology (Coggon et al. 2003), the term "cross-sectional survey" may be used also to include studies gathering data from a database (such as a patient and client database) relating to a point in time where the researcher completes the "questionnaire" on each person or event. Cohort studies, sometimes called "longitudinal surveys", studying data relating to more than one point in time in order to compare data at the time points are beyond the scope of this brief chapter, as are case-control and interrupted time series designs.

Regardless of method of administration, survey data are collected through use of standardised procedures, so that the same data are gathered on every event or responding participant. With the normal methods of administering a survey, questionnaire respondents have the opportunity to respond in a way and manner appropriate for them. The questionnaire used to gather the data needs to have a carefully constructed, structured format (Mayall and Banerjee 2014; Butcher et al. 2014). Depending on what is being analysed, the participants being surveyed may be representing themselves, or a group or organisation to which they belong.

The sampling process is an important element in the quality of surveys, so as to ensure representativeness and generalisability to the population of interest. "The sample survey has become a staple in the quiver of research design tools capable of enhancing our understanding of physical and social life" (Taylor and Zeller 2007, p. 33). There is a range of approaches to sampling for surveys, from convenience sampling at the least rigorous end of the spectrum to fully powered calculations for percentage effects for defined outcomes. The interested reader is referred to Bryman (2016) for further information on detail of sampling approaches.

The reliability of survey data depends on factors such as the following:

- clarity of definition of the population to which the survey is to be generalised;
- robustness of sampling method (ideally randomised) from the sampling frame;
- encouragement in wording so that respondents give accurate, honest answers;
- any data errors or bias due to missing responses to individual questions;
- the possibility of data error if response options are interpreted differently; and,
- limitations in self-perception, recall and those inherent in self-report studies generally.

There may be selection bias in that the respondents who choose to respond to a survey question may be different from those who chose not to respond. Data on non-respondents, if available, can be used to identify if responders and non-responders differ systematically in characteristics other than their choice over responding thus giving an indication of whether this is a source of error. In general, researchers assume that people with strongly-held views (in one direction or the other) are more likely to respond to surveys.

Some of the key benefits of surveys are:

- large-scale accessibility to individuals;
- opportunity for comparative studies across countries or regions;
- relatively easy administration;
- breadth of data types, e.g. attitudes, attributes, behaviour, beliefs, facts, opinions, values;
- convenience and anonymity for respondents;
- highly representative (if sampling and responding do not lead to selection bias);
- possibility to exclude observer subjectivity compared to qualitative studies;
- possibility of rapid data analysis and integration;
- testing for statistical significance and,
- cost effectiveness (cheap to administer).

In summary, surveys enable quick data collection from a large number of individuals from various population groups in a standardised format to enable generalisations.

Some of the key limitations of surveys are:

- inflexible in design compared to qualitative research;
- cannot collect additional data, only on the stated questions;
- cannot provide prompting for further information, especially with self-completion surveys;

- respondent concerns about presenting themselves in an unfavourable manner;
- may not be ideal for controversial issues if respondents are concerned about confidentiality;
- the possibility of inappropriate or misleading questions, or misinterpretation;
- they provide self-report data, and thus there may be over- or under- reporting and,
- excluding respondents whose literacy is limited or whose facility with the language of the questions is restricted.

The closed questions required for quantitative analysis in surveys (such as "yes-no" questions or scales) by their essence create lower external validity than qualitative research as the conceptualisation into categories is defined by the researcher, not the respondent.

Within social science research a survey is a common design, with a variety of purposes and methods of use. Within the area of risk communication in medicines, surveys can provide evidence on knowledge, attitude and behaviours of patients, regulators, service managers, health and social care professionals and sub-sections of these. The research topics may include their risk perceptions, interests, information sources, their media preferences, concerns and trust levels. This evidence can inform the preparation of communication interventions and the optimisation of risk management overall.

Surveys may be used within evaluations, such as to gather data across a representative sample of recipients of the intervention (European Medicines Agency (2017b), Appendix 1). A survey is essentially about measuring prevalence and correlation, but in its application to risk communication about medicines it might on occasion be viewed as a "proxy outcome" or "process measure" (Sobel 2016). For example the "reach" of communication material might be measured in terms of the prevalence of awareness of the message amongst the target recipient group, although studying attitudinal change would be stronger with a (quasi-)experimental design. A survey might demonstrate whether understanding of the message correlates with *intention* to act, although experimental and quasi-experimental designs (see Sect. 8.2.3) are more rigorous for measuring *actual* behavioural change than surveys if feasible. All research projects embody some consideration of efficiency or value-for-money (Taylor and Zeller 2007), and a survey may be sufficient for some purposes, making reasonable assumptions. Further detail on practical aspects of carrying out survey research may be found in Campbell et al. (2016), and further information on statistical analysis in Bors (2018).

8.2.3 Experimental and Quasi-Experimental Research

Experimental and quasi-experimental designs are quantitative, and are suited to providing insight into cause-and-effect and measuring the effect of a planned intervention, such as a risk communication intervention. Experimental and quasi-experimental studies are not suited to studying the "world as it is", but focus on limiting confounding ("real world") factors in order to avoid bias and better measure the effect of a planned intervention. Under this heading of experimental and quasi-experimental research we include not only trials of effectiveness of a planned risk communication intervention but also varieties of other experimental studies of the effects of particular elements of risk communication on respondents. These latter would include, for example, experimental studies on the use of particular words expressing likelihood (of harm) or verbal versus numeric presentations of data. This type of experimental studies may be within a (psychological) "laboratory" setting (for example, with students or members of the general public) or with professionals, patients and clients. For an experimental study, there is a comparison with an alternative situation such as non-receipt of the intervention or an alternative presentation format. In strict definitions of experimental research, the allocation of participants to receiving or not receiving the intervention must be within the control of the researcher. Naturally occurring situations, such as where one geographical region receives a particular risk communication and another does not, are generally called "natural experiments". For medicine risk communication these are less common, as once a product has been authorised for use in a jurisdiction, it may be required that all patients and health and social care professionals must receive the same information in the same format for equality. Comparisons between jurisdictions is an alternative natural experiment, although account needs to be taken of cultural differences. Studies of the effectiveness of an intervention may use pre- and post-intervention measures but without a control group (also occasionally called "before-and-after cross-sectional study": Goedecke et al. (2018), although the term "cross-sectional" in this context may be misleading). Pre-post studies are included here as "quasi-experimental" studies for simplicity of description as they have the same purpose as an experimental study, i.e. to measure effectiveness of a planned intervention, albeit with a weaker design for this purpose.

In the present context, typical questions that might be addressed through experimental or quasi-experimental research are measures of the effect on the knowledge, attitudes, perceptions, beliefs, emotions and behaviour of health and social care professionals, patients, clients or families caused by a planned and defined risk communication intervention about medicines (Gumucio 2011; Heins 1976). Experimental and quasi-experimental research focuses on measuring change and ascribing causality. These designs are not suited to understanding meanings (for which qualitative research is appropriate) nor for measuring prevalence or correlations within a population (such as identifying misunderstandings or misconceptions, and attributes that correlate with these) for which a survey design is appropriate.

Experimental and quasi-experimental studies measure whether a statistically significant difference exists between populations experiencing two or more different situations or conditions, such as before and after the intervention or in response to different risk communication elements. Scales to measure differences are created based on an appropriate theoretical framework, such as cognitive attributes (e.g. self-esteem), emotional state (e.g. anxiety), motivation (e.g. self-efficacy) or personality characteristics (e.g. trust, impulsivity). Many such constructs are relevant to the sending and receiving of risk communications. Detailed development work is required to create precise measures (Presser 2004). For reasons of efficiency and to enable comparison between study findings, studies may use existing scales. Validated tools are those that have had their properties of validity and reliability tested, and are thus particularly rigorous for their intended purpose. Whilst qualitative data may usefully be gathered during a trial of effectiveness as additional data, the purpose of the qualitative data would be to gather information about the experience of receiving the intervention or the experience of participating in the study, not to measure the effect of the intervention. The focus of experimental and quasi-experimental research is on internal validity, that is the extent to which the effect measured is attributable to the planned intervention. External validity, i.e. the extent to which the study results can be generalised to the "real world", is sacrificed by eliminating confounding factors so as to give greater confidence in attributing cause, and greater precision in measuring effects.

Where an intervention (such as a planned risk communication intervention) is being "done to" people in the framework of experimental or quasi-experimental research, there are stronger ethical issues to consider than when one is simply gathering data "from" or "about" people. The ethical principles developed for trials of complex health and social care interventions (Berry et al. 2002; Moore et al. 2015a; Greenhalgh 2014) should be considered in the context of a risk communication. For example, the development phase should include optimising the various components of the risk communication before a trial of the complete risk communication intervention. For general guidance on quality standards for studies of effectiveness of psychosocial interventions (such as risk communication), the Cochrane Collaboration Handbook (Higgins and Green 2011) is a good source. Further detail on practical aspects of carrying out experimental and quasi-experimental studies may be found in Engel and Schutt (2013) and further information on statistical analysis in Bland (2015) and Bors (2018).

8.2.4 Mixed-Methods Research

Mixed-methods research is a term that is employed usually to describe research that combines both quantitative and qualitative components (Bryman 2016). However the term may be used also to describe a study that combines different quantitative research methods or that combines different qualitative research approaches. Mixed-methods research may provide the in-depth and contextualised data of qualitative research coupled with the predictive power of quantitative research.

Mixed methods methodology takes advantage of using multiple ways to explore a research problem in a complementary way, and can overcome weaknesses inherent in a single study method. Mixed methods can be used to explore, explain and interpret a phenomenon, develop a theoretical perspective, or address a question at different levels. A mixed method study can be used to develop and test a new tool. They can therefore be useful when unexpected results arise from a prior study, and can position research in a transformative framework.

Mixed-methods research may be primarily qualitative or quantitative, and may use varied data collection techniques such as questionnaires, interviews or focus groups. It may involve continuing interpretation that can influence later stages in the research process (Cresswell and Plano 2010). A mixed methods approach may provide the opportunity for both depth (via a qualitative element) and breath (via a quantitative element). Limitations are that mixed-methods studies may be time consuming; designs may generate un-equal evidence; and they may pose challenges in deciding when to proceed in sequential designs. Common sequences are to use a qualitative study to provide the constructs, language and scale anchors for a subsequent quantitative study, or else to use a qualitative study after a quantitative study to explore meanings in the quantitative results or to make sense of outliers.

Within the domain of risk communication in medicines, mixed methods approaches can be useful to link theory with practice, for example providing a direct, normative link between paradigms, methods and types of data. Mixed methods are commonly used within evaluations to provide the richness of both qualitative and quantitative data: the quantitative data providing measures of key variables and the qualitative data "bringing alive" what may otherwise appear as dry statistical data. The challenge of mixed methods is in achieving rigour in the component methodological parts (to which the relevant criteria should be applied) without the whole project becoming unduly expensive and time consuming. The beauty of mixed methods is giving the reader "the statistics *and* the story", which is a balanced approach to convey study results. Further detail on practical aspects of carrying out mixed-method studies may be found in Cresswell and Plano (2010).

8.3 Utility of Applied Methods for Researching Medicinal Product Risk Communication

There are many challenges in defining criteria for designing and appraising research quality, and there are diverse opinions as to the optimal approach (Taylor et al. 2007). Notably the suite of tools in the (Critical Appraisal Skills Programme (CASP) 1998), which is well-known in the UK, contains no tool for surveys. The Bradford Hill criteria (Hill 1965) as applied in epidemiology (see Chap. 14) are useful to appraise diverse aspects of quality in studies of causality where experimental and quasi-experimental studies are not possible. For our purposes, any study with repeated measures that falls within the scope of this chapter (i.e. excluding cohort studies and interrupted time series) is being treated as quasi-experimental, and we apply to these designs widely accepted quality criteria for appraising studies of effectiveness.

Some people argue that certain criteria used to appraise quantitative research might be used for qualitative research, but that additional criteria are required also (Elliot et al. 1999). Some schemas to appraise qualitative research have been developed independently of any consideration of their relevance to quantitative research (Spencer et al. 2003; Santiago-Delefosse et al. 2016). Others propose that the same broad criteria may be used for quantitative and qualitative research, but that these must be applied appropriately. This last is the approach adopted here: using the same broad headings but applying them appropriately to each major type of research design. The tools in Taylor et al. (2015) are used to provide a framework of criteria for study design and appraisal for all study types (see summary in Table 8.3). These tools take account of the STROBE checklists for Strengthening the Reporting of Observational Studies in Epidemiology for quantitative research (von Elm et al. 2008) and encapsulate issues identified by Pluye et al. (2009) in appraising studies of diverse designs, including qualitative. These ten appraisal points (see box) can be

Table 8.3 General quality criteria for research design and appraisal (Taylor et al. 2015, adapted)

Major criteria for study design and appraisal	Sub-items
1. Is the rationale for the study adequately described?	• Does the study have a clearly formulated question, aims and objectives? • Was the question developed from a review of existing research and theory?
2. Is the study design appropriate?	• Is the design appropriate to the type of study question (for example, studying prevalence, correlation, effectiveness, real world experiences or theory-building)? • Is the design justified in relation to alternative study designs?
3. Are ethical issues adequately addressed?	• Was research ethics approval sought and obtained? • Has consultation with service users and practitioners been discussed? • Are informed consent and confidentiality discussed satisfactorily? • Are sponsorship and conflicts of interest considered?
4. Is the sampling strategy clearly defined and justified	• Have the characteristics of the sample been clearly described? • Is the sample suitable for the purpose?
5. Is the method for data collection appropriate?	• Is there an explicit and valid rationale for chosen method of administration? • Was the development or selection of the data collection tool appropriate? • Was the data collection tool piloted and lessons learnt noted?
6. Are the methods used for analysing data appropriate?	• Was the approach to data analysis clearly described and justified?
7. Are the research findings adequately presented?	• Are the findings presented in a manner that is clear and understandable? • Do the findings summarise fairly all the data gathered? • Is there discussion of any null, negative or contradictory outcomes?
8. Are the research findings credible?	• Do the findings address the research question? • Are limitations of the study discussed? • Are non-respondents, missing data or refusal to participate discussed?
9. Are the discussion and conclusions justified and appropriate?	• Are the findings discussed in the light of existing literature? • Are conclusions justified by the findings? • Have alternative explanations been explored and discounted?
10. To what extent are the findings of the study transferable to other settings?	• How different are the context and participants from your own setting? • How applicable are the findings to practice, policy or theoretical knowledge?

used when designing or reviewing research using these social sciences research methods for planning or evaluating risk communication interventions for medicines. It is recognised that appraisal scoring systems have limited use (Taylor et al. 2007, 2015). The criteria illustrated here assist in judging the extent to which the underlying research standards have been fulfilled rather than for a scoring system.

The basic principles underpinning each of these criteria are the same across study designs. However the operationalisation of these to a particular design needs attention to use of terminology. The term "validity" may refer to internal validity, i.e. how well a study measures or explores what it intends to explore. In experimental research (see Sect. 8.2.3) this is a key focus, and is used to refer to minimising confounding factors in the interests of demonstrating whether the planned intervention or experimental condition has a measurable effect. The term "validity" may be used also to refer to external validity, meaning how well the study corresponds to the reality of the real world. This is a key consideration in qualitative research (see Sect. 8.2.1) and surveys (see Sect. 8.2.2), but not in experimental studies which seek to eliminate external "real world" confounders in order to demonstrate internal validity. The generic term "credibility" is used here less precisely to refer to how believable the results of the study are. In relation to study designs common in pharmacoepidemiology and pharmacovigilance, this issue is addressed in the guide issued by the European Network of Centres for Pharmacoepidemiology and Pharmacovigilance (ENCePP) (2018) and Chap. 14. Across types of research, the term "credibility" includes issues such as how well the study addresses the research question; how well limitations are recognised and addressed; and whether data are available for inspection beyond the primary researchers. In qualitative research the concept of credibility includes also the richness of the information gathered, the perceived honesty of respondent data and whether the social constructs or models (see elsewhere for discussion of these) are plausible and coherent. In quantitative research the term "credibility" includes also the validity of measures used. In experimental studies, the term may include in addition the effectiveness of measures to eliminate confounding.

In this section the general criteria outlined above (see Table 8.3) for design and appraisal are applied in turn to qualitative, survey, (quasi-)experimental, and (more briefly) mixed-methods research. The general criteria are applied to the particular design with examples from the retrieved studies.

8.3.1 Qualitative Research

The general criteria for design and appraisal of research outlined in Table 8.2 are applied in this section to qualitative research using a structure adapted from Taylor et al. (2015). The criteria are illustrated with reference to the qualitative studies retrieved together with one mixed-methods study that had substantial enough qualitative part to merit consideration here.

1. *Is the rationale for the study adequately described?*

   Qualitative research is often appropriate where there is limited knowledge, but qualitative research may be framed or discussed in the context of existing research or theory. As a good example, Andreas et al. (2010, p. 1156) give context to their study along the lines of: "By viewing risk communication as a process of creating understanding, we can move beyond seeing information and choice merely as endpoints and begin to consider what other functions risk narratives might serve for patients…. Patients" narratives often serve as sense-making devices that organize ambiguous risk information and experiences'.

2. *Is the study design appropriate?*

   Qualitative research may seek to create a theoretical conceptualisation starting from a *tabula rasa*, or it may be positioned in relation to a theory that already exists in order to extend it or to test out its relevance in a new context. These aspects will influence the choice of approach (see Table 8.2). Amongst the studies reviewed, Newman et al. (2009) used elements of grounded theory, and one study (Omcdo et al. 2014) used the newly-developing framework analysis. In general, however, the use of robust qualitative designs is an area for development on this topic.
3. *Are ethical issues adequately addressed?*

   Issues of informed consent and confidentiality may be particularly an issue in qualitative research when exploring sensitive subjects, such as aspects of a person's health (Mooney-Somers and Olsen 2017). As an example, consider the issues of stigma and confidentiality in the study by Newman et al. (2009) which used focus groups in a study of HIV vaccine communication with people who were at high risk of this illness. Trusted interaction between researcher and respondent is required to explore topics in depth. Reflexivity on the part of the researcher is required to aid the reader in understanding the perspective of the researcher and possible associated bias. By "reflexivity" in the context of social research we mean the ability of the researcher to recognise the social forces that may influence their own perceptions and behaviours, such as in data gathering. On the topic of risk communication about medicines, important issues may be awareness of embarrassment regarding the illness or treatment and the responsibilities of health and social care professionals in their organisational context.
4. *Is the sampling strategy clearly defined and justified?*

   Data should be gathered from people who are "information-rich", that is who have experience of risk communication about medicines, whether as a patient, professional or in a management or regulatory role. Representativeness of the sample is a secondary consideration, but the researcher may seek people with diverse experiences of the topic, for example a range of ages of recipients of some risk communication, in order to build a more robust model. The important issue is that people are speaking from and about their own lived experience. Similarly the numbers who decline to participate is not such an issue in qualitative research as in a survey, as the purpose is distinctly different. Describing ("situating") the sample in terms of relevant characteristics is important so that the reader can relate the study to his or her own context.

   In terms of sample size, data saturation is now a well-established concept, and relates to the fact that as increasing qualitative data are gathered and analysed, the number of new themes reduces. Eventually no further major themes arise, given the breadth of the topic and the respondent type, and this is known as "saturation" (see Fig. 8.1, Morse 2015; Taylor and Donnelly 2006a). A more

> "A total of 11 focus groups were conducted with 76 participants (...). The focus group discussions were conducted until the data reached a point of theoretical saturation (...). Theoretical saturation of data was assessed at the conclusion of each focus group. Theoretical saturation was determined when the final focus group (from each of the respective PC and NPC groups) did not generate any further novel discussion points (...)."

Fig. 8.1 An example of reporting data saturation (from Ilic et al. 2012, p. 499, citations omitted)

refined determination of sample size in qualitative research is developing, which uses the concept of information power (Fugard and Potts 2015), embodying concepts such as expected population theme prevalence; number of desired instances of the theme; specificity of sample; quality of dialogue; and power of the study (Malterud 2001; Malterud et al. 2015).

5. *Is the method for data collection appropriate?*

   The data-gathering method should enable participants to communicate openly about their experiences. Skill is required to develop trust as well as to avoid leading questions. There should be an aide-mémoire on how to conduct the interviews or focus groups consistently, and this should be piloted. What has been learned from piloting and how this informed the data gathering should be noted in the paper. One criterion for using focus groups rather than individual interviews is that the group interaction may add to the richness of data, but that the topic is not too sensitive for honest discussion in this type of group. Diaries may be used to strengthen data reliability. Where more than one interviewer or focus group facilitator is used, attention should be paid to consistency (Blomgren et al. 2006).

6. *Are the methods used for analysing data appropriate?*

   Ilic et al. (2012) is a good example of clarity in method of data analysis, giving an effective description of their use of thematic analysis, coding and categorisation of focus group transcripts, thereby making the analysis process explicit and challengeable. Constant comparison of new data with existing data is a practical and sound method of analysis (Charmaz 2014). Theory may be used explicitly in data analysis, to assist in developing a new or refined conceptualisation. More novel approaches involve people similar to the research participants to assist in analysis (INVOLVE 2012, 2013; Stevenson and Taylor 2019; see also Chap. 16). An example of deriving theory from qualitative analysis is shown in Fig. 8.2.

7. *Are the research findings adequately presented?*

   Relevant characteristics of respondents should be reported in relation to each quotation used so that the reader can better understand the context of the comment. This also enables the reader to see the range of respondents quoted across the whole paper, and thus appraise the breadth of support for the conclusions drawn. As an example, Langlois-Klassen et al. (2008) helpfully quote a wide range of participants identified by age, gender and treatment. Demonstrating

> "Patients in focus groups appraised alternative information leaflets for medicines. The study draws out the following *social construct* to understand differing conceptualisations.
> 1. *"Glass half-empty consumers"* consider themselves as likely to experience the adverse effects mentioned in the leaflet; they perceived individual risk as higher than communicated risk.
> 2. *"Glass half-full consumers"* are generally confident that they will not experience the adverse effect(s) and perceive a favourable risk-benefit balance for themselves.
> 3. *"Middle-of-the-road consumers"* cannot ascertain their own likelihood of the adverse effect(s) from reading the information, but focus on individual risk rather than statistical risk and are inclined to trust in the prescribing doctor."

Fig. 8.2 An example of deriving theoretical constructs from qualitative analysis (from Tong et al. 2015)

the connection between the findings and the theoretical framework can present challenges. A good example is the study by Andreas et al. (2010), which helpfully explores one key theoretical concept for each of their research questions (such as burdens, responsibilities, adverse events, benefits of treatment), the findings being well-evidenced with respondent quotations.

8. *Are the research findings credible?*

   The main concept underpinning credibility in qualitative research is external validity, which depends on the richness of the information gathered, the perceived honesty of respondent data and whether the social constructs or models (see Sect. 8.2.1) are plausible and coherent with existing knowledge. Practical steps to enhance rigour include dual coding of data, sometimes by two researchers with a useful difference in perspective. In practice this leads to the creation of a refined document ("operational definitions of codes") by the end of the study listing the codes used, together with definitions of the scope of each and indications of how interface topics are coded. Another practical step to achieve rigour is to present findings to respondents or to people with expertise on the topic for comments on plausibility and coherence. These are known as "respondent validation" and "expert validation", respectively (Campbell et al. 2016). Use of these approaches to rigour in qualitative research is an area for development in this topic.

9. *Are the discussion and conclusions justified and appropriate?*

   Whilst there may (and perhaps, should) be development of a theoretical conceptualisation from the data in qualitative research, there is a line to be drawn to avoid over-extending the findings. In the best qualitative research one would expect a theoretical model to be derived from the qualitative data, and then the wider possible implications of the model discussed. As an example, Newman et al. (2009) presented to participants four mental models of how HIV vaccines work, and used findings from the study to develop a useful model.

10. *To what extent are the findings of the study transferable to other settings?*

    The concept of transferability in qualitative research relates primarily to theoretical generalisability, i.e. whether a conceptualisation or model is derived which has wider usefulness beyond the participants involved. This is different from the representational and inferential generalisability common in quantitative research (Ritchie and Lewis 2006). In the context of risk communication about medicines, the issue is the transferability of the model of risk communication across domains such as illness types, medicine types, cultures and legal jurisdictions. Despite the generic search terminology used for our review, retrieved studies typically confined their interest to a particular medicine, illness or setting, with limited exploration of the transferability of findings.

8.3.2 Survey Research

The general criteria for design and appraisal of research outlined in Table 8.3 are applied in this section to survey research using a structure adapted from Taylor et al.

(2015). The criteria are illustrated with reference to the surveys retrieved on risk communication about medicines.

1. *Is the rationale for the study adequately described?*

   The rationale for a survey might relate to measuring a construct developed through qualitative research or measuring the prevalence of some variable and its correlates derived from theory. As an example, Berry et al. (2002) set out to assess the general public's interpretation of the verbal descriptors for side effect frequency recommended for use in medicine information leaflets by a European Union guideline. They also examined the extent to which differences in interpretation affect people's perception of risk and their judgements of intention to comply with the prescribed treatment. Another example is the study by Gaissmaier et al. (2014), which conceptualised the information as being "complete", "transparent", "interpretable" or "persuasive" as a framework for the study.
2. *Is the study design appropriate?*

   It is important to be clear that a survey is an effective design for questions about prevalence or correlation of attributes, but not cause-and-effect of a planned intervention. An example of a survey measuring prevalence is illustrated in Fig. 8.3 and correlation Fig. 8.4. Other interesting and appropriate examples are the study by Davis (2007), which studied the prevalence of preferences for detailed risk information in media communications (see also Chap. 10), and the study by Brewer et al. (2009), where the correlation between estimates of recurrence risk and health literacy was measured.

   An example of measuring correlation in a survey (from Sanchez-Menegay and Stadler 1994) "Patients" expectations are fulfilled when they are expressed to physicians. There was no agreement between global or individual patient expectation and physician response (kappa ≤ 0.3). The physicians prescribed more medications than expected, and almost never discussed prevention or

"87% of the 1600 parents of young children (<6 years) in the sample regarded immunisation as extremely important. 173 (0.11%) respondents reported that they would not want any future child to have immunisation for varicella, with lower numbers opting out of other specific vaccines. Respondents indicated their perceptions of the severity of specific vaccine-preventable diseases, and their perception of the likelihood of infection. 84% indicated doctors as their main source of information about immunisation, with 18% indicating newspapers or magazines, and 12% books or journals, with lower numbers for other identified sources."

Fig. 8.3 An example of measuring prevalence in a survey (from Gellin et al. 2000)

"Patients' expectations are fulfilled when they are expressed to physicians. There was no agreement between global or individual patient expectation and physician response (kappa ≤ 0.3). The physicians prescribed more medications than expected, and almost never discussed prevention or prognosis. The characteristics of care were not different between the physicians who knew and those who did not know patient expectations."

Fig. 8.4 An example of measuring correlation in a survey (from Sanchez-Menegay and Stadler 1994)

prognosis. The characteristics of care were not different between the physicians who knew and those who did not know patient expectations."

3. *Are ethical issues adequately addressed?*

   Surveys are considered generally to be relatively low risk in ethical terms. The key ethical issues in surveys relate mainly to recruitment, consent, confidentiality and anonymity. Regarding recruitment and consent, people approached can readily decline to participate. Regarding confidentiality and anonymity similar considerations apply whether secondary data is used or whether data is gathered for the particular study.

4. *Is the sampling strategy clearly defined and justified?*

   The sampling in a survey needs to ensure that the respondents sampled provide data justifying conclusions generalisable to the target population from which the sample is drawn. The range of respondents in reviewed studies included adults (Gellin et al. 2000); women (Keller and Siegrist 2009); consecutive ambulatory patients (Sanchez-Menegay and Stadler 1994) and physicians (obstetricians and gynaecologists) (Gaissmaier et al. 2014). Researchers should make it clear how they came to invite a potential respondent. Sampling may vary from weak convenience sampling to calculations for sample size performed using G*Power software. Sample size required for significance is determined by effect size, measurement tool and the selected statistical significance criterion. Research methods literature suggests that at least 30 respondents as an absolute minimum are required for surveys to conduct statistical analysis (Bryman 2016). Most of the surveys reviewed had a reasonable sample size between 100 and 400. It is good practice to report the response rate of surveys, i.e. the percentage of those who were invited to complete the survey who actually complete and submit. Response rates in retrieved studies varied from 22% (Davis 2007; Kalet et al. 1994) to 72% (Gaissmaier et al. 2014). Response rates of 30–40% are typical for surveys of busy professionals (Taylor et al. 2018). The best practice guideline for surveys, especially e-surveys, is the CHERRIES statement which gives guidelines for sample selection and representative sampling (Eysenbach 2004).

5. *Is the method for data collection appropriate?*

   It is important that the mode of administration is suited to the respondents. An increasingly wide range of questionnaire administration methods is possible, with email and online surveys now complementing the time-honoured paper and telephone methods. Where more than one person gathers the data, attention to possible interviewer variability is required (Blomgren et al. 2006). Where cross-sectional data is gathered from existing databases, the question template is completed by the researcher. Validated scales promote reliability as well as validity of measures. This is a key area for development as there was little use of these in the reviewed studies. It is important that customised questionnaires are piloted to ensure that they are fit for purpose. The piloting—and the learning from it—should be reported, even if briefly.

6. *Are the methods used for analysing data appropriate?*

   In surveys, data are usually summarised (i.e. the number and percentages for each response option [variable] from each question) and then analysed using a statistical software package such as Excel, R, SAS, SPSS or Stata. These statistical packages calculate frequencies (e.g. number and percentages), descriptives (e.g. mean and standard deviation) and inferential statistics (significant differences using t-tests, ANOVA and relationships using correlations). A good study should comment on the possible impact of non-respondents and missing data on the validity of the statistical results.
7. *Are the research findings adequately presented?*

   A good study presentation is written bearing in mind the main readership, and with a sequence of findings that reads easily for them (Campbell et al. 2016). All tables and figures presenting survey data should be clear and standalone, and should support (not duplicate) material in the main text. Tables, graphs and bar-charts are generally regarded as clearer than pie charts. The best practice guideline for reporting results of surveys, especially e-surveys, is the Checklist for Reporting Results of Internet E-Surveys (CHERRIES Statement) (Eysenbach 2004).
8. *Are the research findings credible?*

   The key issue with credibility in surveys is validity and reliability of the data. Among the studies reviewed, validity and reliability were often limited due to lack of use of validated measurement tools and limited piloting of questionnaires. In communication research, it is common that a survey tool is developed for each research question. However, this means that due to lack of validated tools, limited comparison can be made between research projects. In some studies due to the low sample size and response rate, the generalisability of the results needs to be interpreted carefully in order not to overestimate the meaning. There was little use of powered sample size, limiting the credibility of results.
9. *Are the discussion and conclusions justified and appropriate?*

   Surveys can provide valid discussions and conclusions that can contribute to informing practice and policy guidelines. Amongst retrieved studies there were conclusions regarding: policy recommendations (Davis 2007); guidelines for industry (Leong et al. 2015) and enhancing patient care (Fry et al. 2007). Most studies reported limitations and recommendations for further research. A challenge for studies in this field is to put their research in a theoretical context and thereby link their results to the wider task of creating generalisable knowledge.
10. *To what extent are the findings of the study transferable to other settings?*

    Transferability (external validity) is stronger in surveys that include validated tools, which provide opportunities for comparison. It is important for surveys to be transferable and generalisable so the results can contribute to impact on enhancing risk communication in medicines among professionals, patients, regulators and industry. All of the reviewed surveys had potential for transferability in terms of practice and policy, but reporting of this could be clearer.

8.3.3 Experimental and Quasi-Experimental Research

The general criteria for design and appraisal of research outlined in Table 8.2 are applied in this section to experimental and quasi-experimental research intended to measure the effect of a planned medicine risk communication intervention using a structure adapted from Taylor et al. (2015). The criteria are illustrated with reference to the experimental and quasi-experimental studies retrieved on risk communication about medicines. This category includes both trials of the effectiveness of a planned, well-developed risk communication intervention about medicines, and (quasi-)experimental studies that might be viewed primarily as developing or optimising elements of risk communication, perhaps through (human) "laboratory" experiments. The gold standard for trials might be regarded as the level of rigour required to be included in a Cochrane Review. An example of an experimental study that is not a trial is shown in Figure 8.5.

An example of an experimental study that is not a trial (from Berry et al. 2002). Participants were presented with hypothetical but realistic vignettes about a visit to their general practitioner and being prescribed medication, participants being allocated at random to one of four experimental conditions. There were two between-subject factors (adverse reaction severity) and type of risk expression (percentage vs number out of 10,000), and one within-subject factor (frequency categories)."

1. *Is the rationale for the study adequately described?*

   The main focus for quality in experimental and quasi-experimental studies is on internal validity, that is, how well confounding factors are eliminated so that we can be confident (within a stated margin of error) that the observed effect is attributable to the risk communication intervention (or manipulation of a risk communication element). The feasibility, cost and operation of the planned intervention in the real world (external validity) are a secondary consideration in this type of study. The framework for developing interventions cited earlier (Medical Research Council 2008) provides a useful conceptualisation of key component parts required to justify the readiness of the state of knowledge on a topic to undertake an experimental study of effectiveness. Among reviewed papers, Han at al. (2014) articulated the study's question, aims and objectives reasonably clearly.
2. *Is the study design appropriate?*

   Study designs used in the retrieved studies included varieties of randomised trials; natural experiments; pre-post testing and various experimental and quasi-experimental manipulations. Explaining clearly the design of the study is particularly important for studies of effectiveness due to the complexity of possible

"Participants were presented with hypothetical but realistic vignettes about a visit to their general practitioner and being prescribed medication, participants being allocated at random to one of four experimental conditions. There were two between-subject factors (adverse reaction severity) and type of risk expression (percentage vs number out of 10,000), and one within-subject factor (frequency categories)."

Fig. 8.5 An example of an experimental study that is not a trial (from Berry et al. 2002)

designs and research issues. A full randomised controlled trial is often difficult in the field of communications because of the possibility of "contamination", i.e. where the difference in communication intervention between the groups to be compared cannot be fully controlled. For example in the case of doctor–patient communications, doctors in the control group might have informal contact with those in the experimental group and learn from them despite not receiving the intervention. Cluster-randomisation, with randomisation of groups (such as teams or medical practices) rather than individuals, is an obvious alternative to minimise this, although the power of the study will be reduced for a given number of participants. Measures to avoid contamination between trial groups should be indicated in a good study. Intervention fidelity, i.e. the extent to which those in the experimental group accurately received the risk communication under study (Taylor 2012b), is a key issue when an intervention becomes more complex. An example of a complex intervention studied in a trial is illustrated in Figure 8.6.

3. *Are ethical issues adequately addressed?*

   Ethical approval for studies of effectiveness has a distinct difference from qualitative research and surveys in that an intervention is being "provided for", or "done to", people rather than simply gathering data "about" them. A clear explanation of what is involved in the intervention is imperative, as is clarity about any sponsorship particularly by a manufacturer or provider of the risk communication (and sometimes also the associated medicine). A key issue is the potential negative emotional impact of the risk communication, particularly where the recipient has the illness for which the medicine is being considered.

4. *Is the sampling strategy clearly defined and justified?*

   Sufficient sample size for statistical significance is an essential element in demonstrating the effectiveness of an intervention or other experimental manipulation, and this is well rehearsed in the methods literature (Han et al. 2014; Bland 2015). A good study will compare intervention and control groups at the start to identify any major difference. If a study is randomised, concealment of allocation should be indicated as well as the method of randomisation so that the reader can appraise selection bias. The study report should state how many people declined to participate or dropped out, and comment on the understanding of reasons for this as well as explaining how this was addressed in analysis. Among

"The study illustrated risk communication as a complex intervention, the intervention comprising:
(1) feedback on the standardised patient encounter;
(2) academic detailing to review cancer screening guidelines;
(3) red flags for identifying low health-literacy patients;
(4) strategies for effective counselling; and
(5) a web-based tutorial of standardised patient comments and checklist items hyperlinked to reference materials.
Although the multiple diverse aspects of the intervention make it difficult to evaluate the effectiveness of any one part even with a satisfactory trial design, the intervention reflects the likely complexities of practice for more effective risk communication interventions."

Fig. 8.6 An example of a complex risk communication intervention subjected to a trial (from Price-Haywood et al. 2009)

reviewed studies, samples included professionals, patients and the public, although the limited number of studies for any one respondent group indicates the early stage of research on the topic, with little development yet of confirmatory studies with different samples of participants.

5. *Is the method for data collection appropriate?*

   For (quasi-)experimental studies it is important that data collection tools are sensitive, valid and reliable. These are crucial elements in the rigour of this type of study, and should be justified. In general one would expect the rigorous peer-review process required in funding applications and ethical approval of experimental studies to ensure that studies use effective data-gathering tools. This is particularly so in relation to trials given the high costs and the ethical issues in intervention studies. As an example of standardised scales, the Morisky Compliance Scale was to assess adherence to chosen treatment in the Kirkegaard et al. (2010) study. In the study by Han et al. (2014) standardised patients (actors) rated the students using a 5-item SP-Risk Communication Process tool; and students were observed by academic staff using the 13-item Risk Process Measure. This study had an interesting data collection feature in that the observed structured clinical examination of the medical students (involving communicating about risk) was video recorded, and these were independently evaluated by two faculty members.

6. *Are the methods used for analysing data appropriate?*

   For trials to measure the effect of a risk-communication intervention, the standards of the Cochrane Collaboration (Higgins and Green 2011) are an internationally accepted guide to risk of bias. Some important considerations are as follows:

   - allocation bias (allocation of participants to intervention and control groups);
   - attrition (the loss of participants during the experiment);
   - performance bias (systematic differences in the experience of the participants in the intervention and control groups other than the intervention being studied, including those due to participants behaviour being influenced by knowing whether they are in the intervention or control group).

   Cochrane guidelines suggest use of confidence intervals rather than p-values, and use of regression models to illustrate the influence of multiple factors (Vik 2014).

7. *Are the research findings adequately presented?*

   Avoiding reporting bias is particularly an issue for more complex study designs. The presentation should also include null or negative outcomes as these also may be a valuable contribution to knowledge. Amongst retrieved studies, the Schwartz et al. (2009) paper (on direct-to-consumer communication regarding two treatments and two preventive medicines) has an attractive presentation using box plots.

8. *Are the research findings credible?*

   In experimental studies, a participant may drop out or cross over from the intervention group to the control group. These are standard features of an experimental design and are generally well reported in higher-quality studies. Although experimental studies are designed to exclude the confounding effect of contemporaneous events, there would be merit in studies including some comment on the possible effects of the passage of time, where relevant, to the social context of the illness, risk message or medicine.

9. *Are the discussion and conclusions justified and appropriate?*

   Developing conclusions that extend beyond the evidence is particularly tempting if there is some status or commercial incentive to prove the effectiveness of a particular risk communication intervention. Structuring the discussion in relation to the findings assists with clarity. By detailing their discounting of alternative explanations, researchers can better justify the conclusions drawn. Linking to a theoretical conceptualisation may assist in meaningful discussion of findings. A theoretical model assists in relating study findings to wider conceptualisations and issues. Waters et al. (2006) is a good example, relating their treatment trade-off decisions (as a result of the risk communication) to "cognitive effort" theory. Han et al. (2014) used a three-stage model of shared decision making called "risk talk" (Elwyn et al. 2012) to frame how the risk communication interacts with the three decision tasks of:

   - choice talk;
   - option talk and,
   - decision talk.

Such theoretical conceptualisation helps subsequent studies to build on previous work.

10. *To what extent are the findings of the study transferable to other settings?*

    Transferability (external validity) is a particular challenge for experimental studies, because real world dimensions are deliberately limited so as to demonstrate more clearly the effects of the intervention itself (internal validity). Detail of the risk communication interventions was generally weak in retrieved studies, particularly the trials. Commercial gain may militate against detailed description, but understanding the intervention is essential for a paper to be meaningful to readers, regulators and researchers. There needs to be sufficient detail for the reader to reflect on how the findings may be applicable to their own context in relation to practice, policy or theory, and generalisable in general if knowledge on this topic is to develop optimally.

8.3.4 Mixed-Methods Research

The general criteria for design and appraisal of research outlined in Table 8.2 can be applied to mixed-methods research. Mixed methods studies can provide useful data both on the depth and breadth of risk communication in medicines. The study rationale should be provided, based on previous literature and the need or identified problem. A mixed method approach allows the different phases of the project to generate questions; test draft intervention and research materials; explain areas that are unfamiliar or not routinely studied and strengthen conclusions drawn across different phases of the study (e.g. Kennedy et al. 2008). The quality pointers for both quantitative and qualitative research outlined above apply as appropriate to component parts of studies using mixed methods.

8.4 Outlook: Relevance, Improvements and Potential

This section discusses the role and complementarity of methods for creating, developing and evaluating risk communication interventions about medicines (see Sects. 8.2 and 8.3), and then goes on to outline prospects for using the presented research methods for the study of risk communication about medicines. This section also comments briefly on developments in engaging patients, professionals and the public in these research designs, as well as the potential for progress through study synthesis and theoretical development.

8.4.1 Complementarity of Social Science Methods

The major research designs considered in this chapter are each important—and indeed, essential—for their contribution to the process of creating, developing and evaluating a psychosocial intervention such as risk communication about medicines (Medical Research Council 2008; Moore et al. 2015a, b). Diverse types of research questions require different—and complementary—research methods, as outlined here in their application to risk communication about medicines. A key message of this chapter in terms of the complementarity of research methods is perhaps captured in these words of Richard Feynman, Nobel laureate in physics:

> *I spent a few years trying to invent mathematical things that would permit me to solve the equations, but I didn't get anywhere, and then I decided that in order to do that I must first understand more or less how the answer probably looks. It's hard to explain this very well, but I had to get a qualitative idea of how the phenomenon works before I could get a good quantitative idea*
> (Feynman 1999, p. 18).

In addition to strengthening the research methods which are the focus of this chapter, social science expertise might contribute to the field of risk communication about medicines by:

- exploring different perceptions and conceptualisations of "risk" (Taylor and Donnelly 2006b);
- creating useful conceptualisations of the sender, receiver, content and method of the risk communication that aids transferable learning across studies (Moorhead et al. 2013b);
- linking the emotional uncertainty dimension of risk communication to the anxiety that may be experienced by the recipient, and human striving towards emotional equilibrium (Löwenstein et al. 2001);
- developing our understanding of the framing of risks in relation to the recipients' consequent decisions (Stevenson and Taylor 2016) and,
- connecting risk communication with the professional processes of judgement, decision making (including shared decision making), assessing and managing risk as part of holistic care planning by health and social care professionals (Taylor 2017a, 2012c; Taylor and Campbell 2011; Taylor and McKeown 2013).

The research methods common in social sciences have an essential contribution to the study and development of risk communication about medicines, complementing methods common in pharmacoepidemiology and other disciplines (multidisciplinarity) as presented in this book.

8.4.2 Prospects for Qualitative Research

Studies applying qualitative methods can provide an understanding of recipients' and communicators' experiences of risk communications and their related thought processes (Juanchich and Sirota 2013; Stevenson et al. 2019; Teigen and Brun 1999; Thomson et al. 2005; Young and Oppenheimer 2009). Qualitative studies are suited to creating theoretical conceptualisations or models of the risk communication processes. They have an essential place in creating a realistic and meaningful understanding of the real world upon which to build an effective risk communication intervention. Given the differences between people in understanding risk, it is important that future qualitative studies cover more diverse countries and cultural contexts so as to build theoretical understandings that are more generalisable.

There is much scope for improving the rigour of qualitative methods in relation to risk communication about medicines, as exemplified in Sect. 8.3 and also identified by others (Malterud 2001; Mays and Pope 2000). Although generic thematic (narrative, content) analysis is suitable for simpler studies, rigorous qualitative research should use more developed methods such as illustrated in Table 8.1. To build useful understandings of risk communication, the more developed and rigorous qualitative approaches such as grounded theory or interpretative phenomenological analysis will be required (see Sect. 8.3).

Although focus groups are likely to remain a major data-gathering tool, greater use could be made of individual interviews and diary methods, both written and digital, particularly where the participants are less articulate (Stevenson and Taylor 2019). The development of electronic media opens up the possibility of gaining insight into communication processes through monitoring the way that websites are used (see Chap. 11). Future qualitative research should attend to the sensitivity of the topic (the illness, the treatment and the communication message) in the data-gathering methods, and report more detail about piloting and what was learned from this. Well-established methods for enhancing rigour such as dual coding of data and respondent and expert validation could be used to good effect (Taylor et al. 2015). Researcher reflexivity is an essential component of qualitative research, and merits development in future studies on this topic.

Qualitative studies may help to shape new conceptualisations (Reyna and Adam 2003). For example, current models tend to think of a choice at a point in time, whereas the reality for patients in some situations may be that some anticipated benefits and risks are more immediate and others are long-term, and this may affect their response to the risk communication. Qualitative studies could clarify how recipients frame the decision (Bilgin and Brenner 2013; Peters 2008) regarding taking medication (or not) in response to the risk communication (Taylor et al. 2017). This may be in terms of decisions about the probability of benefit versus the probability of harm, rather than focusing only on the probability of harm. Or the reality may reflect a consideration of what symptoms to look out for, and "how I might manage those particular symptoms" rather than, or as well as, attention to likelihoods. As the research field develops, theoretical concepts might be tested out in a different context using interpretative phenomenological analysis to give greater generalisability. This might provide a rich theoretical conceptualisation across classes of medicines, and across organisational and cultural contexts (Reeves et al. 2008). Qualitative methods are also useful within mixed-methods studies and evaluations to build an understanding that includes both "statistics and story", which is often an effective research communication method!

8.4.3 Prospects for Survey Research

Surveys provide useful data on a range of issues, such as acceptability of communication modes. Surveys are suited to study prevalence, such as attitudes towards types of risk communication, and correlation, such as mode of communication with numeracy. The application of surveys in designing communication materials in user-centred manner is discussed in Chap. 12. Surveys are not well suited to measuring the effectiveness of a planned intervention or developing the initial conceptualisation of the topic. Sometimes the "reach" of a risk communication is measured with a survey. In terms of awareness, i.e. whether people are aware that a particular risk communication initiative has taken place, this might be regarded as a satisfactory design (Davis et al. 2006). However this is a weak design to measure effectiveness, for example in terms of change in perception or behaviour attributable to the intervention, as concurrent changes in the environment may have contributed to the observed change. An experimental or quasi-experimental design would be more appropriate.

There is a need to create and to use validated questionnaires to increase robustness and comparability of surveys. Piloting should be undertaken, and the amendments reported. Sample size calculations should be used to ensure representativeness to the population studied, and the response rate and details of non-respondents in terms of numbers and characteristics should be reported where possible. Approaches to ensure robust response rates should be used (McColl et al. 2001), although it has to be recognised that 30–40% is a typical response rate for busy professionals—and this is probably true also for busy members of the public! Surveys, and especially e-surveys, should follow the CHERRIES statement for reporting (Smith et al. 2018).

Survey methodology may be used within evaluations of established risk communication interventions, typically as part of a mixed-methods study. Where surveys are used for a purpose that could be considered as evaluation of an ongoing communication intervention (see Sect. 8.4.1; Sobel 2016) care needs to be taken to clarify that in effect these are measures of prevalence (e.g. that the communication has been received or prevalence of clinical knowledge at a point in time) or correlation (e.g. how clinical knowledge correlates with contextual characteristics or behaviour such as age of the prescriber or practice facilities). Surveys are not a strong design for measuring change in perceptions or behavioural change as a result of a risk communication intervention. Consideration of the distinct strengths of surveys compared to qualitative or experimental studies (as outlined above) assists in highlighting standards that are achievable and reasonable for the purposes of the study (European Medicines Agency 2017b).

With the development of the World Wide Web, there is now the potential for researchers to use web-based panels (see Chap. 11). Recruitment to surveys through website visitors has clear potential for the future. With the advent of "big data", there is potential for data mining using survey methodology (i.e. gathering data at a single point in time to study questions of prevalence and correlation) to generate predictive models, which have the potential to contribute to planning of communication interventions. If the dataset contains data on the same individuals at different points in time, then longitudinal (cohort) study methods (which are beyond the scope of this chapter and covered in Chap. 14) may be used.

8.4.4 Prospects for Experimental and Quasi-Experimental Research

Experimental and quasi-experimental methods are suited to measuring the effect of a planned risk communication intervention. Much preparatory work is required for a trial, so in general ethical approval and cost considerations ensure that these more complex designs are of a reasonable standard. However, by the time that risk communication interventions reach the stage of development of being ready for a (relatively more expensive) trial, there may be vested interests of public esteem or commercial gain at stake. Just as with medical interventions themselves, robust mechanisms may be required to ensure that scientific rigour and ethical principles are not jeopardised by such interests. Detail of the communication intervention and its causal mechanisms are required if knowledge in the field is to grow optimally (Smith et al. 2018; Mevissen et al. 2011). Greater use could be made of natural experiments where risk communication interventions are developed in one geographical area but not another. As attention is focused on more visual means of communicating risk (Taylor et al. 2018), particularly as facilitated by computers, there is likely to be increased need for more laboratory-type of experimental study, i.e. producing results with some generalisability but not necessarily representative of the final target population in every study. Researchers will also need to take cognizance of the fact that as psychosocial interventions, including risk communication interventions, become more effective the risk of harmful "side-effects" is likely to increase (Schüz et al. 2013).

Experimental studies other than trials often use varieties of factorial designs, presenting respondents with a series of vignettes for each of which they make a decision. As the general aim is to examine the response of groups (or "classes") of respondent, rather than to model the response of individuals, consideration should be given to using a wider range of factorial survey experimental designs (Auspurg and Hinz 2014; Killick and Taylor 2012; Taylor 2006b; Witry and Doucette 2015). In the factorial survey each respondent is presented with a unique randomised set of vignettes, each with randomised levels of the variables being studied. This randomised design enables efficient administration to a large sample, and has greater external validity than the more common factorial experiment as a larger number of variables, and more levels of variables, may be used (Taylor and Zeller 2007; Taylor 2006b). In these designs, respondents are forced to make trade-offs between factors, as in real-life responses to risk communications where decisions must be made about medicine use (or not) and the implications for everyday life. Natural frequencies have generally been found to be more readily understood than relative risks or odds-ratios (Galesic et al. 2009). One recently-developed tool for communicating risk using natural frequencies, the facts box (see Figure 8.7 for an example), provides a useful mechanism for developing and evaluating risk communication about medicines. As

"Numbers for children from 0 to 15 years of age with an acute middle ear infection who either received antibiotics or placebos over the course of 7 to 14 days.

	100 children who took a placebo	100 children who toook antibiotics
Benefits		
How many children experienced pain 4 to 7 days after the diagnosis?	24	18
How many children had conspicuous findings 2 to 4 weeks after the diagnosis that may indicate hearing problems?	48	40
How many children experienced a ruptured eardrum because of the infection?	5	2
Harms*		
How many children experienced adverse events (e.g., vomiting, diarrhea, or rash)?	20	27

The numbers in this fact box are rounded. They are based on 13 studies with 3,401 children.

*An overuse of antibiotics may lead to antibiotic resistance. Antibiotic resistance means that antibiotics lose their ability to kill bacteria or inhibit their growth. Acquired resistance, which occurs through genetic alterations to bacteria, isparticularly problematic because itreduces the effectiveness of antibiotic treatment.

Short summary: Pain, hearing problems, and a ruptured eardrum were less frequent for children who took antibiotics. However, antibiotics led to adverse events such as vomiting, diarrhea, and rashes.

Sources: [1] Venekamp et al. *Cochrane Database Syst Rev* 2015(6):CD000219. [2] BMG (ed.). 2015.

Last update: June 2016 www.harding-center.mpg.de/en/fact-boxes."

Fig. 8.7 An extract from a facts box (from Hinneburg and Ellermann 2016)

well as being a subject of study, such findings might also guide the presentation of study findings.

More attention is required to developing sensitive, valid and reliable measures for effective measurement of the effectiveness of risk communication as an aspect of risk management (European Medicines Agency 2017c). These measures need to correspond to the constructs of recipients of the risk communication. It needs to be recognised that the essence of experimental designs is to eliminate confounders. This may eliminate substantial numbers of real-life recipients, such as those with complex needs (including special communication needs) and those who are receiving multiple medications, thereby reducing external validity. As professional and vocational roles in relation to risk communication about medicines develop, it would be encouraging to see studies that focus on a wider range of health and social care staff groups in relation to their roles.

Future studies of effectiveness should pay more attention to the human (social and emotional) context of illness and treatment, and how communications relate to these. This will be particularly an issue for studies of risk communication regarding medicines for mental health conditions. Relevant dimensions should be considered as appropriate, such as the crisis context of illness and treatment; concerns about becoming addicted to the medication; and possible stigma of treatment (Taylor and Donnelly 2006a; Stevenson and Taylor 2017). Contextual information should demonstrate connection with the constructs of the public and professionals giving and receiving these communications as discussed above in relation to qualitative studies. Testing of product information or risk minimisation material with volunteer members of the public or patients prior to launch of a new medicinal product could use an experimental or quasi-experimental design for studying impact on knowledge, risk perception and attitude.

As more cohesive and complex risk communication interventions are developed (particularly in the context of more complex media opportunities, see Chap. 10), trials should aspire to the level of rigour required for inclusion in a Cochrane Review, perhaps for potential inclusion in a review of the *Cochrane Consumers and Communication Review Group* (http://cccrg.cochrane.org). Intervention fidelity will become more important as the risk communication interventions become more complex. The well-established "hierarchy of evidence" is a valuable framework for appraising the quality of studies designed to measure effectiveness (but not for the purposes appropriate to the other study designs discussed here) (Petticrew and Roberts 2003). Use of this as a reference standard could be developed more widely although a key issue is to improve researcher education so as to ensure that this evidence hierarchy is not mis-applied to studies designed to understand experiences and develop theory (appropriately qualitative) or prevalence and correlations (appropriately surveys), for which that framework is inappropriate (and misleading) for quality appraisal. Alternative quality frameworks are required for studies addressing such questions (Taylor et al. 2015).

Reporting of trials of risk communication about medicines requires improvement. Tools for this purpose include the recently-published RIMES Statement (Smith et al. 2018) (on reporting on trials of interventions to improve risk minimisation) as well as the CONSORT-SPI Statement (on reporting on trials of social and psychological interventions in general) (Montgomery et al. 2013). Improved reporting aligned to common standards will provide transparency; enable replication; facilitate synthesis across studies; and enhance usefulness in informing risk communication policy.

8.4.5 Prospects for Mixed-Methods Research

Mixed methods are useful to provide breadth as well as depth of data. However the different methods need to be interlinked and informed by each other. Mixed methods studies are often used for evaluations, but clear connection between study parts is required. Mixed methods are likely to be appropriate where both breadth and depth are required within the one study. The key for credibility of mixed-methods research is the clear linkage between the qualitative and quantitative methods, i.e. how does one method inform the other, as well as the importance and rigour of each method used in itself.

8.4.6 Involvement of Patients, Professionals and the Public

The involvement of patients, healthcare professionals and the general public in the processes of research is receiving increasing attention (Hanley et al. 2004, see also Chap. 16). The importance of their involvement is increasingly being recognised (INVOLVE 2012, 2013), and the social science methods should be further developed for their engagement as co-researchers in data gathering (Taylor et al. 2014), analysis (Stevenson and Taylor 2019) and dissemination. Giving greater attention to involvement of patients and the public in research will in itself doubtless lead to studies addressing more effectively the social and emotional context of illness, treatment and communication, as well as other benefits. The *Cochrane Consumers and Communication Review Group* (http://cccrg.cochrane.org) is a useful reference point, and it would be good to see more reviews of risk communication in the Cochrane Library.

8.4.7 Study Synthesis and Theoretical Development for Future Progress

As studies on the topic accumulate, the potential of, and challenge in, synthesising findings across studies become more apparent (Taylor et al. 2017; Gigerenzer and Edwards 2003; Wegwarth et al. 2011). Efforts at synthesis will highlight gaps in research, for example the lack of studies of professional-to-professional communication evident in the review underpinning this chapter (see Sect. 8.1.2). There are many challenges to evaluating complex interventions (Datta and Petticrew 2013; Raynor et al. 2013)—such as a risk communication—where there are complex human variables to consider. There is no space here to expand on the practicalities of (statistical) meta-analysis of experimental studies, meta-synthesis of qualitative data (using principles of qualitative research), and narrative review across study designs. The interested reader is referred to Taylor et al. (2015) and the *Cochrane Consumers and Communication Review Group* (http://cccrg.cochrane.org) for approaches to study synthesis.

It would be helpful to the creation of knowledge if studies were conceptualised as part of a research and development process from theoretical development through to post-implementation evaluation, passing through various stages (development, testing of component parts, evaluation, implementation) requiring as appropriate qualitative, survey and (quasi-)experimental studies along the journey. The guidance issued by the Medical Research Council in the UK (Medical Research Council 2008; see also Moore et al. 2015a) will be useful for this purpose, particularly now that the original guidance has been extended to include complex psychosocial interventions, such as risk communication. Even where interventions are well developed, process evaluation (where social science methods are valuable) in parallel to randomised trials is now recommended so as to develop an understanding of (as opposed to measurement of) causal mechanisms and their interaction with context (Moore et al. 2015b).

Developments in theoretical conceptualisation will assist in focusing the research question; selection of study design; analysis and interpretation of data; synthesis; and learning across studies. The review by Ryan et al. (2014) provides a useful taxonomy of intervention and outcome types which might inform syntheses and mechanisms through which the more pure (compared to applied) research on risk communication might be understood. Theoretical development may assist in facilitating reasoned learning from studies on health and social care risk communication generally, and from risk communication in more diverse fields such as climate change and financial instability (Hertwig and Erev 2009). As the cognitive and behavioural engagement in risk communications are studied in greater depth (see Chap. 7), it will be helpful to make more explicit the connection with theoretical and research developments in human judgement (Taylor 2017a), patient decision aids (Trevena et al. 2013) and shared decision making (Elwyn et al. 2012). The challenges of short timescales specified by regulators for communication to health care providers when a new safety concern has emerged give added urgency to the need to develop theoretical conceptualisations that span medicines and medicine types.

The connection between risk communication and decision making requires further exploration if risk communication about medicines is to develop beyond the need to fulfil legal requirements to avoid blame. There is a growing literature on the sociology, assessment, management and communication of risk, and—generally quite separately—a growing literature on informed choice, patient decision aids, professional judgement and shared decision making. The chasm between the literature on these two topics could be bridged by social science research methods (see Taylor et al. 2017, 2018; McDowell 2009), appropriately applied. There is great potential in increased collaboration between pharmacovigilance and social sciences so as to improve the study of risk communication about medicines and thus improve the service that professionals and organisations provide to patients, clients, families and the global public.

Conclusions

- The qualitative, survey and (quasi-)experimental methods commonly used in social sciences have much to contribute to the creation of generalisable knowledge to inform the development of risk communication approaches and to evaluate established risk communication interventions.
- The selection of research method must be suited to the type of question, and generally:
  - qualitative methods are suited to understanding perspectives in people's own words and creating a theoretical conceptualisation;
  - surveys are appropriate to studying prevalence (e.g. of attitudes towards types of risk communication or of ensuing behaviours) and correlation (e.g. risk perception in relation to illness severity);
  - experimental and quasi-experimental methods are suited to measuring the effect of a risk communication intervention or of some element or mode of this; and
  - mixed-methods studies combining survey and qualitative methods are particularly suited for evaluations of established risk communication interventions, combining breadth and depth.
- Qualitative studies have strengths in readily incorporating emotional and ethical as well as cognitive aspects of risk communication. Greater attention should be paid to standard methods for enhancing rigour, such as sampling to saturation, dual coding of data, and use of respondent and expert validation. Qualitative studies would be improved by being based on a specific robust paradigm such as grounded theory or interpretative phenomenological analysis.
- Surveys provide useful data on prevalence and correlation issues such as acceptability of communication modes in populations, whether of patients, health and social care professionals or the general public. There is a need to create and use more validated questionnaires to increase robustness and comparability of surveys.
- In experimental and quasi-experimental studies, more attention should be given to developing valid and reliable measures, and to ensuring that these correspond to the constructs of recipients and providers of the risk communication intervention. Effectiveness studies should demonstrate understanding of the human context of illness and treatment, and provide detail on the intervention studied. Trials should strive for the rigour required for inclusion in a Cochrane Review.
- Studies need clearer connection to a theoretical framework so as to build more effectively a cohesive conceptual understanding on risk communication about medicines. Theoretical development will assist in connecting risk communication with research and theory on judgement and decision making, including shared decision making with patients and clients.

- Guidance from regulatory bodies on research and evaluation of risk communication should be reviewed to ensure that methods specified are appropriate to the research questions, and that terminology is selected to be clearly understood by the range of interested researchers and other stakeholders.
- Journal editors and reviewers as well as researchers should note key recommendations in this chapter so as to improve the standard and reporting of studies using these designs.
- There is potential in increased collaboration between researchers in pharmacovigilance and social sciences so as to improve the study of risk communication about medicines and thus improve the service that professionals and organisations provide to patients, clients, families and the global public.

Acknowledgements The authors would like to acknowledge the support of Mrs. Joanne Knox and Miss Janice McQuilkin, Assistant Subject Librarians; Dr. Patricia Carlisle, Associate Lecturer; and Miss Mabel Stevenson, Research Assistant, all of Ulster University, Northern Ireland, who assisted with the literature review that underpins this chapter.

References[1]

Akl EA, Oxman AD, Herrin J, Vist GE, Terrenato I, Sperati F, Costiniuk C, Blank D, Schünemann H (2011) Using alternative statistical formats for presenting risks and risk reductions. Cochrane Database Syst Rev 3:CD006776. https://doi.org/10.1002/14651858.CD006776.pub2

Altman DG (1991) Practical statistics for medical research. Chapman and Hall, London

*Andreas DC, Abraham NS, Naik AD, Street RL Jr, Sharf BF (2010) Understanding risk communication through patient narratives about complex antithrombotic therapies. Qual Health Res 20(8):1155–1165. https://doi.org/10.1177/1049732310370154

Auspurg K, Hinz T (2014) Factorial survey experiments. Sage, London

Australian Council for International Development (2016) Principles and guidelines for ethical research and evaluation in development. ACFID, Canberra

Bahri P (2010) Public pharmacovigilance communication: a process calling for evidence-based, objective-driven strategies. Drug Saf 33(12):1065–1079. https://doi.org/10.2165/11539040-000000000-00000

Bahri P, Fogd J, Morales D, Kurz X, ADVANCE Consortium (2017) Application of real-time global media monitoring and 'derived questions' for enhancing communication by regulatory bodies: the case of human papillomavirus vaccines. BMC Med 15:91. https://doi.org/10.1186/s12916-017-0850-4

Bailar JC, Louis TA, Lavori PW, Polansky M (1986) A classification for biomedical research reports. N Engl J Med 311:1482–1487. https://doi.org/10.1056/NEJM198412063112305

Bates J, Best P, McQuilkin J, Taylor BJ (2017) Will web search engines replace bibliographic databases in the systematic identification of research? J Acad Libr 43(1):8–17. https://doi.org/10.1016/j.acalib.2016.11.003

[1] Studies included in the review are indicated by an asterisk (*).

*Belcora JK, Hutton DW, Moore DH, Siminoff LA (2011) Does use of the 'adjuvant!' Model influence use of adjuvant therapy through better risk communication? J Natl Compr Cancer Netw 9:707–712. https://doi.org/10.6004/jnccn.2011.0061

*Berry DC, Knapp PR, Raynor T (2002) Is 15 per cent very common? Informing people about the risks of medication side effects. Int J Pharm Pract 10:145–151. https://doi.org/10.1111/j.2042-7174.2002.tb00602.x

Best P, Taylor BJ, Manktelow R, McQuilkin J (2014) Systematically retrieving research in the digital age: case study on the topic of social networking sites and young people's mental health. J Inf Sci 40:346–356. https://doi.org/10.1177/0165551514521936

Bickman L, Rog DJ (eds) (2008) The sage handbook of applied social research methods, 2nd edn. Sage, Thousand Oaks

Bilgin B, Brenner L (2013) Context affects the interpretation of low but not high numerical probabilities: a hypothesis-testing account of subjective probability. Organ Behav Hum Decis Process 121:118–128. https://doi.org/10.1016/j.obhdp.2013.01.004

Bland M (2015) An introduction to medical statistics, 4th edn. Oxford University Press, Oxford

Blomgren KJ, Sundström A, Steineck G, Wilholm BE (2006) Interviewer variability: quality aspects in a case-control study. Eur J Epidemiol 21(4):267–277. https://doi.org/10.1007/s10654-006-0017-7

Bors D (2018) Data analysis for the social sciences: integrating theory and practice. Sage, London

Brewer J (2000) Ethnography. Open University, Buckingham

*Brewer NT, Tzeng JP, Lillie SE, Edwards AS, Peppercorn JM, Rimer BK (2009) Health literacy and cancer risk perception: implications for genomic risk communication. Med Decis Mak 29(2):157–166. https://doi.org/10.1177/0272989X08327111

Bryman A (2016) Social research methods, 5th edn. Oxford University Press, Oxford

Butcher RB, Fechtelpeter D, Knelangen M, Ehrlichg M, Waltering A (2014) Words or numbers? Communicating risk of adverse effects in written consumer health information: a systematic review and meta-analysis. BMC Med Inform Decis Mak 14:76–87. https://doi.org/10.1186/1472-6947-14-76

Campbell A, Taylor BJ, McGlade A (2016) Research design in social work: qualitative and quantitative methods. Sage, London

Carson D, Bain A (2008) Professional risk and working with people: decision-making in health, social care and criminal justice. Jessica Kingsley, London

Centre for Reviews and Dissemination (CRD) (2009) Systematic reviews: CRD's guidance for undertaking reviews in health care, 3rd edn. Centre for Reviews and Dissemination, University of York. www.york.ac.uk/crd/

Charmaz K (2014) Constructing grounded theory: a practical guide through qualitative analysis, 2nd edn. Sage, New York

Coggon D, Barker DJP, Rose G (2003) Epidemiology for the uninitiated, 5th edn. British Medical Journal, London

Council of the European Communities (1992) Council Directive 92/27/EEC of 31 March 1992 on the labelling of medicinal products for human use and on package leaflets. (Extended to the EEA by 21994D0628(01) SYN 231). Brussels: Official Journal

Craig P, Dieppe P, Macintyre S, Michie S, Nazareth I, Petticrew M (2008) Developing and evaluating complex interventions: the new Medical Research Council guidance. BMJ 337:a1655. https://doi.org/10.1136/bmj.a1655

Cresswell JW, Plano VL (2010) Designing and conducting mixed methods research, 2nd edn. Sage, London

Critical Appraisal Skills Programme (CASP) (1998) CASP checklists. Critical Appraisal Skills Programme, Oxford. http://www.casp-uk.net. Accessed 22 June 2017

Datta J, Petticrew M (2013) Challenges to evaluating complex interventions: a content analysis of published papers. BMC Public Health 13:568. https://doi.org/10.1186/1471-2458-13-568

*Davis JJ (2007) Consumers' preferences for the communication of risk information in drug advertising. Health Aff 26(3):863–870. https://doi.org/10.1377/hlthaff.26.3.863

∗Davis TC, Fredrickson DD, Kennen EM, Humiston SG, Arnold CL, Quinlin MS, Bocchini JA (2006) Vaccine risk/benefit communication: effect of an educational package for public health nurses. Health Educ Behav 33:787–801. https://doi.org/10.1111/j.0737-1209.2004.021305.x

∗Davis JJ, Cross E, Crowley J (2007) Pharmaceutical websites and the communication of risk. J Health Commun 12(1):29–39. https://doi.org/10.1080/10810730601091326

Department of Health and Human Services. Office of Inspector General (2013) FDA lacks comprehensive data to determine whether risk evaluation and mitigation strategies improve drug safety. Department of Health and Human Services, Office of Inspector General, Washington. https://oig.hhs.gov/oei/reports/oei-04-11-00510.pdf. Accessed 22 Jan 2018

Dodoo A, Hugman B (2012) Risk perception and communication in sub-Saharan Africa. Drug Saf 35(11):1041–1052. https://doi.org/10.2165/11636270-000000000-00000

Dusetzina SB, Higashi AS, Dorsey ER, Conti R, Huskamp HA, Zhu S, Garfield CF, Alexander GC (2012) Impact of FDA drug risk communications on healthcare utilization and health behaviors: a systematic review. Med Care 50(6):466–478. https://doi.org/10.1097/MLR.0b013e318245a160

Economic and Social Research Council (2016) What is social science? Economic and Social Research Council, London. http://www.esrc.ac.uk/about-us/what-is-social-science/

Edwards A, Elwyn G, Covey J, Matthews E, Pill R (2001) Presenting risk information a review of the effects of framing and other manipulations on patient outcomes. J Health Commun 6:61–82. https://doi.org/10.1080/10810730150501413

Edwards AGK, Naik G, Ahmed H, Elwyn GJ, Pickles T, Hood K, Playle R (2013) Personalised risk communication for informed decision making about taking screening tests. Cochrane Database Syst Rev 2:CD001865. https://doi.org/10.1002/14651858.CD001865.pub3

Elliot R, Fisher CT, Rennie DL (1999) Evolving guidelines for publication of qualitative research studies in psychology & related fields. Br J Clin Psychol. 38:215–219 [Erratum: Br J Clin Psychol. 2000;39:1:10]

Elwyn G, Frosch D, Thomson R, Joseph-Williams N, Lloyd A, Kinnersley P, Cording E, Tomson D, Dodd C, Rollnick S, Edwards A, Barry M (2012) Shared decision making: a model for clinical practice. J Gen Intern Med 27(10):1361–1367. https://doi.org/10.1007/s11606-012-2077-6

Engel RJ, Schutt RK (2013) The practice of research in social work, 3rd edn. Sage, Thousand Oaks

European Medicines Agency (2012) Guideline on good pharmacovigilance practices (GVP). Module V—risk management systems (rev 1). European Medicines Agency, London. http://www.ema.europa.eu/docs/en_GB/document_library/Scientific_guideline/2012/06/WC500129134.pdf. Accessed 24 Jan 2018

European Medicines Agency (2013) Guideline on good pharmacovigilance practices (GVP). Module XVI—risk minimisation measures: selection of tools and effectiveness indicators. European Medicines Agency, London. http://www.ema.europa.eu/docs/en_GB/document_library/Scientific_guideline/2013/06/WC500144010.pdf. Accessed 24 Jan 2018

European Medicines Agency (2017a) Guideline on good pharmacovigilance practices (GVP): annex I – definitions (rev 4). EMA/876333/2011 Rev 4∗. European Medicines Agency, London

European Medicines Agency (2017b) Guideline on good pharmacovigilance practices (GVP): module XVI: risk minimisation measures: selection of tools and effectiveness indicators (rev 2). European Medicines Agency, London

European Medicines Agency (2017c) Guideline on good pharmacovigilance practices (GVP): module VIII: post-authorisation safety studies (rev 3). [EMA/813938/2011 Rev 3∗]. European Medicines Agency, London 2017

European Medicines Agency Benefit-risk Methodology Project Team (2011) Work package 1 report: description of the current practice of benefit-risk assessment for centralised procedure products in the EU regulatory network: EMA/227124/2011. European Medicines Agency, London

European Network of Centres for Pharmacoepidemiology and Pharmacovigilance (ENCePP) (2018) Guide on methodological standards in pharmacoepidemiology (revision 7). EMA/95098/2010. European Medicines Agency, London

Eysenbach G (2004) Improving the quality of web surveys: the checklist for reporting results of internet e-surveys (CHERRIES). J Med Internet Res 6(3):e34. https://doi.org/10.2196/jmir.6.3.e34 [Erratum: J Med Internet Res. 2012; 14(1): e8. https://doi.org/10.2196/jmir.2042]

Feynman RP (1999) The pleasure of finding things out. Helix (Perseus), Cambridge

Fischoff B, Brewer NT, Downs JS (eds) (2011) Communicating risks and benefits: an evidence-based users' guide. Food and Drugs Administration, Silver Spring

Food and Drug Administration (2005) Guidance for industry: development and use of risk minimization action plans. Food and Drug Administration, Rockville. http://www.fda.gov/downloads/RegulatoryInformation/Guidances/UCM126830.pdf. Accessed 24 Jan 2018

Food and Drug Administration (2007) Food and Drug Administration Amendment Act of 2007. http://www.fda.gov/regulatoryinformation/legislation/federalfooddrugandcosmeticactfdcact/significantamendmentstothefdcact/foodanddrugadministrationamendmentsactof2007/default.htm. Accessed 24 Jan 2018

Food and Drug Administration (2009) Guidance for industry: format and content of proposed risk evaluation and mitigation strategies (REMS), REMS assessments, and proposed REMS modifications draft guidance 2009. Food and Drug Administration, Rockville. http://www.fda.gov/downloads/Drugs/Guidances/UCM184128.pdf. Accessed 22 Jan 2018

Fry RB, Ray MN, Cobaugh DJ, Weissman NW, Kiefe CI, Shewchuk RM, Saag KG, Curtis JR, Allison JJ (2007) Racial/ethnic disparities in patient-reported nonsteroidal antiinflammatory drug (NSAID) risk awareness, patient-doctor NSAID risk communication, and NSAID risk behavior. Arthritis Rheum 57(8):1539–1545. https://doi.org/10.1002/art.23084

Fugard AJB, Potts HWW (2015) Supporting thinking on sample sizes for thematic analyses: a quantitative tool. Int J Soc Res Methodol 18:669–684. https://doi.org/10.1080/13645579.2015.1005453

*Gaissmaier W, Anderson BL, Schulkin J (2014) How do physicians provide statistical information about antidepressants to hypothetical patients? Med Decis Mak 34:206–215. https://doi.org/10.1177/0272989X13501720

Gale NK, Heath G, Cameron E, Rashid S, Redwood S (2013) Using the framework method for the analysis of qualitative data in multi-disciplinary health research. BMC Med Res Methodol 13:117. https://doi.org/10.1186/1471-2288-13-117

Galesic M, Gigerenzer G, Straubinger N (2009) Natural frequencies help older adults and people with low numeracy to evaluate medical screening tests. Med Decis Mak 29:368–371. https://doi.org/10.1177/0272989X08329463

Gee JP (2005) An introduction to discourse analysis: theory and method. Routledge, London

Gellin BG, Maibach EW, Marcuse EK (2000) Do parents understand immunizations? A national telephone survey. Pediatrics 106(5):1097–1102. https://doi.org/10.1542/peds.106.5.109

Gigerenzer G, Edwards A (2003) Simple tools for understanding risks: from innumeracy to insight. BMJ 327(7417):741–744. https://doi.org/10.1136/bmj.327.7417.741

Glaser B, Strauss A (1999) The discovery of grounded theory: strategies for qualitative research. Aldine de Gruyter, New York

Goedecke T, Morales D, Pacurariu A, Kurz X (2018) Measuring the impact of medicines regulatory interventions: systematic review and methodological considerations. Br J Clin Pharmacol 84(3):419–433. https://doi.org/10.1111/bcp.13469

Granger MM, Fischhoff B, Bostrom A, Atman CJ (2001) Risk communication: a mental models approach. Cambridge University Press, Cambridge

Greenhalgh T (2014) How to read a paper: the basics of evidence-based medicine, 5th edn. Wiley and BMJ Books, Chichester

Gridchyna I, Cloutier AM, Nkeng L, Craig C, Frise S, Moride Y (2014) Methodological gaps in the assessment of risk minimization interventions: a systematic review. Pharmacoepidemiol Drug Saf 23(6):572–579. https://doi.org/10.1002/pds.3596

Gumucio S (2011) Data collection: quantitative methods: the KAP survey model (Knowledge, Attitude & Practices). Médecins du Monde, Paris

∗Han PKJ, Joekes K, Elwyn G, Mazor KM, Thomson R, Sedgwick P, Ibison J, Wong JB (2014) Development and evaluation of a risk communication curriculum for medical students. Patient Educ Couns 94:43–49. https://doi.org/10.1016/j.pec.2013.09.009

Hanley B, Bradburn J, Barnes M, Evans C, Goodare H, Kelson M, Kent A, Oliver S, Thomas S, Wallcraft J (2004) Involving the public in National Health Service, public health, and social care research: briefing notes for researchers. INVOLVE Support Unit, London

Health Research Authority (2016) Defining research. National Health Service, HRA, London

Heins H (1976) A KAP (knowledge-attitude-practice) approach to the regionalization of perinatal health. J Ark Med Soc 73(6):229–234

Hertwig R, Erev I (2009) The description-experience gap in risky choice. Trends Cogn Sci 13:517–523. https://doi.org/10.1016/j.tics.2009.09.004

Higgins JPT, Green S (eds) (2011) Cochrane Handbook for Systematic Reviews of Interventions, Version 5.1.0. The Cochrane Collaboration

Hill AB (1965) The environment and disease: association or causation? Proc R Soc Med 58(5):295–300

Hinneburg J, Ellermann C (2016) Antibiotics for acute middle ear infection in children: fact box. Harding Centre for Risk Literacy at the Max Planck Institute for Human Development, Berlin. https://www.harding-center.mpg.de/en/fact-boxes/use-of-antibiotics/acute-middle-ear-infection. Accessed 24 Jan 2018

∗Hutton DW, Belkora JK, Shachter RD, Moore DH (2009) Are patients getting the 'gist' in risk communication? Patient understanding of prognosis in breast cancer. J Cancer Educ 24:194–199. https://doi.org/10.1080/08858190902876452

∗Ilic D, Murphy K, Green S (2012) Risk communication and prostate cancer: identifying which summary statistics are best understood by men. Am J Mens Health 6(6):497–504. https://doi.org/10.1177/1557988312453616

INVOLVE (2012) Briefing notes for researchers: public involvement in NHS, public health and social care research. National Institute for Health Research, London

INVOLVE (2013) Exploring the impact of public involvement on the quality of research: examples. National Institute for Health Research, London

Juanchich M, Sirota M (2013) Do people really say it is "likely" when they believe it is only "possible"? Effect of politeness on risk communication. Q J Exp Psychol 66:1268–1275. https://doi.org/10.1080/17470218.2013.804582

Kalet A, Roberts JC, Fletcher R (1994) How do physicians talk with their patients about risks? J Gen Intern Med 9:402–404. https://doi.org/10.1007/BF02629523

∗Keller C, Siegrist M (2009) Effect of risk communication formats on risk perception depending on numeracy. Med Decis Mak 29(4):483–490. https://doi.org/10.1177/0272989X09333122

∗Kennedy A, Glasser J, Covello V, Gust D (2008) Development of vaccine risk communication messages using risk comparisons and mathematical modelling. J Health Commun 13:793–807. https://doi.org/10.1080/10810730802487463

Killick C, Taylor BJ (2012) Judgments of social care professionals on elder abuse referrals: a factorial survey. Br J Soc Work 42:814–832. https://doi.org/10.1093/bjsw/bcr109

∗Kirkegaard P, Edwards AGK, Hansen B, Hansen MD, Jensen MSA, Lauritzen T, Risoer MGB, Thomsen JL (2010) The RISAP-study: a complex intervention in risk communication and shared decision-making in general practice. BMC Fam Pract 11:70. https://doi.org/10.1186/1471-2296-11-70

Kuper A, Lingard L, Levinson W (2008) Critically appraising qualitative research. BMJ 337:a1035. https://doi.org/10.1136/bmj.a1035

∗Langlois-Klassen D, Kipp W, Rubaale T (2008) Who's talking? Communication between health providers and HIV-infected adults related to herbal medicine for AIDS treatment in western Uganda. Soc Sci Med 67(1):165–176. https://doi.org/10.1016/j.socscimed.2008.02.027

∗Längst G, Seidling HM, Stützle M, Ose D, Baudendistel I, Szecsenyi J, Wensing M, Mahler C (2015) Factors associated with medication information in diabetes care: differences in perceptions between patients and health care professionals. Patient Prefer Adherence 15:1431–1441. https://doi.org/10.2147/PPA.S88357

Leong J, Walker S, Salek S (2015) A practical approach to communicating benefit-risk decisions of medicines to stakeholders. Front Pharmacol 6:99. https://doi.org/10.3389/fphar.2015.00099

Lipkus IM, Hollands JG (1999) The visual communication of risk. J Natl Cancer Inst Monogr 25:149–163. https://doi.org/10.1093/oxfordjournals.jncimonographs.a024191

Löwenstein GF, Weber EY, Hsee CK, Welch N (2001) Risk as feelings. Psychol Bull 127(2):267–286. https://doi.org/10.1037/0033-2909.127.2.267

Makoul G, Arntson P, Schofield T (1995) Health promotion in primary care: physician-patient communication and decision making about prescription medications. Soc Sci Med 41(9):1241–1254. https://doi.org/10.1016/0277-9536(95)00061-B

Malterud K (2001) Qualitative research: standards, challenges and guidelines. Lancet 358:483–488. https://doi.org/10.1016/S0140-6736(01)05627-6

Malterud K, Siersma VD, Goassora AD (2015) Sample size in qualitative interview studies: guided by information power. Qual Health Res 26(13):1753–1760. https://doi.org/10.1177/1049732315617444

Mayall S, Banerjee AK (2014) Therapeutic risk management of medicines. Woodhead (Elsevier), Cambridge

Mays N, Pope C (2000) Qualitative research in health care: assessing quality in qualitative research. BMJ 320:50–52. https://doi.org/10.1136/bmj.320.7226.50

Mazzaglia G, Straus SMJ, Arlett P, da Silva D, Janssen H, Raine J, Alteri E (2018) Study design and evaluation of risk minimization measures: a review of studies submitted to the European Medicines Agency for cardiovascular, endocrinology, and metabolic drugs. Drug Saf 41(2):191–202. https://doi.org/10.1007/s40264-017-0604-4

McColl E, Jacoby A, Thomas L, Scoutter J, Bamford C, Steen N, Thomas R, Harvey E, Garratt A, Bond J (2001) Design and use of questionnaires: a review of best practice applicable to surveys of health service staff and patients. Health Technol Assess 5:31

McComas KA (2006) Defining moments in risk communication research: 1996–2005. J Health Commun 11(1):75–91. https://doi.org/10.1080/10810730500461091

McDowell M (2009) Making sense of numbers about health risks: the Facts Box (Chapter 19). In: Elwyn G, Edwards A, Thompson R (eds) Shared decision making in health care: achieving evidence-based patient choice, 2nd edn. Oxford University Press, Oxford, pp 123–128

McFadden P, Taylor BJ, Campbell A, McQuilkin J (2012) Systematically identifying relevant research: case study on child protection social workers' resilience. Res Soc Work Pract. 22:626–636. https://doi.org/10.1177/1049731512453209

McGinn AH, Taylor BJ, McColgan M, McQuilkin J (2016) Social work literature searching: current issues with databases and online search engines. Res Soc Work Pract 26(3):266–277. https://doi.org/10.1177/1049731514549423

Medical Research Council (2008) Developing and evaluating complex interventions. MRC, London. http://www.mrc.ac.uk/documents/pdf/complex-interventions-guidance/

Mevissen FDF, Ruiter RAC, Meertens RM, Zimbile F, Schaalma HP (2011) Justify your love: testing an online STI-risk communication intervention designed to promote condom use and STI-testing. Psychol Health 26:205–221. https://doi.org/10.1080/08870446.2011.531575

Montgomery P, Grant SP, Hopewell S, Macdonald G, Moher D, Michie S, Mayo-Wilson E (2013) Protocol for CONSORT-SPI: an extension for social and psychological interventions. Implement Sci 8(1):99. https://doi.org/10.1186/1748-5908-8-99

Mooney-Somers J, Olsen A (2017) Ethical review and qualitative research competence: guidance for reviewers and applicants. Res Ethics (3–4):128–138

Moore GF, Audrey S, Barker M, Bond L, Bonell C, Hardeman W, Moore L, O'Cathain A, Tinati T, Wight D, Baird J (2015a) Process evaluation of complex interventions: Medical Research Council guidance. BMJ 350:h1258. https://doi.org/10.1136/bmj.h1258

Moore GF, Audrey S, Barker M, Bond L, Bonell C, Hardeman W, Moore L, O'Cathain A, Tinati T, Wight D, Baird J (2015b) Process evaluation of complex interventions: a summary of Medical Research Council guidance. In: Richards DA, Hallberg IR (eds) Complex interventions in health: an overview of research methods. Routledge, Oxford, pp 222–231

Moorhead SA, Coates VE, Gallagher AM, Nolan G, Murphy K, Hazlett DE (2013a) Obesity communication among patients by health professionals: findings from the Weight Care Project. Health 5(8A3):100–109. https://doi.org/10.4236/health.2013.58A3015

Moorhead SA, Hazlett DE, Harrison L, Carroll JK, Irwin A, Hoving C (2013b) A new dimension of health care: systematic review of the uses, benefits, and limitations of social media for health communication. J Med Internet Res 15(4):e85. https://doi.org/10.2196/jmir.1933

Morse JM (2015) Data were saturated. Qual Health Res 25:587–588. https://doi.org/10.1177/1049732315576699

Nelson W, Reyna VF, Fagerlin A, Lipkus I, Peters E (2008) Clinical implications of numeracy: theory and practice. Ann Intern Med 35:261–274. https://doi.org/10.1007/s12160-008-9037-8

*Newman PA, Seiden DS, Roberts KJ, Kakinami L, Duan N (2009) A small dose of HIV? HIV vaccine mental models and risk communication. Health Educ Behav 36(2):321–333. https://doi.org/10.1177/1090198107305078

O'Connor AM, Legare F, Stacey D (2003) Risk communication in practice: the contribution of decision aids. BMJ 327(7417):736–740. https://doi.org/10.1136/bmj.327.7417.736

*Omedo M, Ogutu M, Awiti A, Musuva R, Muchiri G, Montgomery SP, Secor WE, Miwinzi P (2014) The effect of a health communication campaign on compliance with mass drug administration for schistosomiasis control in Western Kenya: The SCORE Project. Am J Trop Med Hyg 91(5):982. https://doi.org/10.4269/ajtmh.14-0136

Peters E (2008) Numeracy and the perception and communication of risk. Ann N Y Acad Sci 1128:1–7. https://doi.org/10.1196/annals.1399.001

Petticrew M (2011) When are complex interventions 'complex'? When are simple interventions 'simple'? Eur J Pub Health 21:397–398. https://doi.org/10.1093/eurpub/ckr084

Petticrew M, Roberts H (2003) Evidence, hierarchies, and typologies: horses for courses. J Epidemiol Community Health 57:527–529. https://doi.org/10.1136/jech.57.7.527

Petticrew M, Rehfuess E, Noyes J, Higgins JPT, Mayhew A, Pantoha T, Shemilt I, Sowden A (2013a) Synthesising evidence on complex interventions: how meta-analytic, qualitative and mixed-methods approaches can contribute. J Clin Epidemiol 66:1230–1243. https://doi.org/10.1016/j.jclinepi.2013.06.005

Petticrew M, Anderson L, Elder R, Grimshaw J, Hopkins D, Hahn R, Krause L, Kristjansson E, Mercer S, Sipe T, Tugwell P, Ueffing E, Waters E, Welch V (2013b) Complex interventions and their implications for systematic reviews: a pragmatic approach. J Clin Epidemiol 66:1209–1214. https://doi.org/10.1016/j.jclinepi.2013.06.004

Pluye P, Gagnon MP, Griffiths F, Johnson-Lafleur J (2009) A scoring system for appraising mixed methods research, and concomitantly appraising qualitative, quantitative and mixed methods primary studies in mixed studies reviews. Int J Nurs Stud 46(4):529–546. https://doi.org/10.1016/j.ijnurstu.2009.01.009

Presser S (ed) (2004) Methods for testing and evaluating survey questionnaires. Wiley, Hoboken

Price-Haywood EG, Roth KG, Shelby K, Cooper LA (2009) Cancer risk communication with low health literacy patients: a continuing medical education program. J Gen Intern Med 25(Suppl 2):126–129. https://doi.org/10.1007/s11606-009-1211-6

Raynor DK, de Veene P, Bryant D (2013) The effectiveness of the Summary of Product Characteristics (SmPC) and recommendations for improvement. Ther Innov Regul Sci 48:255–265. https://doi.org/10.1177/2168479013501311

*Reber KC, Wieringa JE, Piening S, De Graeff PA,Haaijer-Ruskamp F, Mol PGM, Straus SMJM, Raine JM (2013) When direct health-care professional communications have an impact on inappropriate and unsafe use of medicines. Clin Pharmacol Ther 93(4):360–365. https://doi.org/10.1038/clpt.2012.262

Reeves S, Albert M, Kuper A, Hodges BD (2008) Qualitative research: why use theories in qualitative research? BMJ 337(7226):631–634. https://doi.org/10.1136/bmj.a949

Reyna VF, Adam MB (2003) Fuzzy-trace theory, risk communication and product labelling in sexually transmitted diseases. Risk Anal 23:325–342. https://doi.org/10.1111/1539-6924.00332

Reyna VF, Nelson WL, Han PK, Dieckmann NF (2009) How numeracy influences risk comprehension and medical decision making. Psychol Bull 135:943–973. https://doi.org/10.1037/a0017327

Ritchie J, Lewis J (2006) Qualitative research practice: a guide for social science students and researchers. Sage, London

Ryan R, Santesso N, Lowe D, Hill S, Grimshaw J, Prictor M, Kaufman C, Cowie G, Taylor M (2014) Interventions to improve safe and effective medicines use by consumers: an overview of systematic reviews. Cochrane Database Syst Rev 4:CD007768. https://doi.org/10.1002/14651858.CD007768.pub3

Sanchez-Menegay C, Stadler H (1994) Do physicians take into account patients' expectations? J Gen Intern Med 9(7):404–406

Santiago-Delefosse M, Gavin A, Bruchez C, Roux P, Stephen SL (2016) Quality of qualitative research in the health sciences: analysis of the common criteria present in 58 assessment guidelines by expert users. Soc Sci Med 148:142–151. https://doi.org/10.1016/j.socscimed.2015.11.007

*Schapira MM, Nattinger AB, McAuliffe TL (2006) The influence of graphic format on breast cancer risk communication. J Health Commun 11(6):569–582. https://doi.org/10.1080/10810730600829916

Schmid EF, Smith DA, Ryder SW (2007) Communicating the risks and benefits of medicines. Drug Discov Today 12:355–364. https://doi.org/10.1016/j.drudis.2007.03.003

Schüz N, Schüz B, Eid M (2013) When risk communication backfires: randomised controlled trial on self-affirmation and reactance to personalised risk feedback in high-risk individuals. Health Psychol 32:561–570. https://doi.org/10.1037/a0029887

Schwartz LM, Woloshin S, Welch HG (2009) Using a drug facts box to communicate drug benefits and harms. Ann Intern Med 150:516–527. https://doi.org/10.7326/0003-4819-150-8-200904210-00106

Smith MY, Morrato E (2014) Advancing the field of pharmaceutical risk minimization through application of implementation science best practices. Drug Saf 37(7):569–580. https://doi.org/10.1007/s40264-014-0197-0

Smith JA, Flowers P, Larkin M (2009) Interpretative phenomenological analysis: theory, method and research. Sage, London

Smith MY, Russell A, Bahri P, Mol PGM, Frise S, Freeman E, Morrato EH (2018) The RIMES statement: a checklist to assess the quality of studies evaluating risk minimization programs for medicinal products. Drug Saf 41:389–401. https://doi.org/10.1007/s40264-017-0619-x

Sobel R (2016) Evaluating the effectiveness of additional risk minimisation measures via surveys in Europe: challenges and recommendations. Bethesda, International Society for Pharmacoepidemiology

Spencer L, Ritchie J, Lewis J, Dillon L (2003) Quality in qualitative evaluation: a framework for assessing research evidence. Cabinet Office, London

Starks H, Trinidad SB (2007) Choose your method: a comparison of phenomenology, discourse analysis, and grounded theory. Qual Health Res 17:1372–1380. https://doi.org/10.1177/1049732307307031

Stevenson M, Taylor BJ (2016) Risk communication in dementia care: family perspectives. J Risk Res 21(6):692–709. https://doi.org/10.1080/13669877.2016.1235604

Stevenson M, Taylor BJ (2017) Risk communication in dementia care: professional perspectives on consequences, likelihood, words and numbers. Br J Soc Work 47(7):1940–1958. https://doi.org/10.1093/bjsw/bcw161

Stevenson M, Taylor BJ (2019 Feb) Involving individuals with dementia as co-researchers in analysis of findings from a qualitative study. Dementia (London) 18(2):701–712. https://doi.org/10.1177/1471301217690904

Stevenson M, Taylor BJ, Knox J (2016) Risk in dementia care: searching for the evidence. Health Risk Soc 18(1–2):4–20. https://doi.org/10.1080/13698575.2015.1119256

Stevenson M, McDowell ME, Taylor BJ (2018) Concepts for communication about risk in dementia care: a review of the literature. Dementia (London) 17(3):359–390. https://doi.org/10.1177/1471301216647542

Stevenson M, Savage B, Taylor BJ (2019) Perception and communication of risk in decision making by persons with a dementia. Dementia (London) 18:1108–1127. https://doi.org/10.1177/1471301217704119

Taylor BJ (2006a) Risk management paradigms in health and social services for professional decision making on the long-term care of older people. Br J Soc Work. 36:1411–1429. https://doi.org/10.1093/bjsw/bch406

Taylor BJ (2006b) Factorial surveys: using vignettes to study professional judgement. Br J Soc Work 36:1187–1207. https://doi.org/10.1093/bjsw/bch345

Taylor BJ (2012a) Developing an integrated assessment tool for the health and social care of older people. Br J Soc Work 42:1293–1314. https://doi.org/10.1093/bjsw/bcr133

Taylor BJ (2012b) Intervention research (Chapter 27). In: Gray M, Midgley J, Webb S (eds) Social work handbook. Sage, New York, pp 424–439

Taylor BJ (2012c) Models for professional judgement in social work. Eur J Soc Work 15:546–562. https://doi.org/10.1080/13691457.2012.702310

Taylor BJ (2017a) Decision making, assessment and risk in social work, 3rd edn. Sage, London

Taylor BJ (2017b) Heuristics in professional judgement: a psycho-social rationality model. Br J Soc Work 47(4):1043–1060. https://doi.org/10.1093/bjsw/bcw084

Taylor BJ, Campbell B (2011) Quality, risk and governance: social workers' perspectives. Int J Leadership Public Services 7:256–272. https://doi.org/10.1108/17479881111194152

Taylor BJ, Donnelly M (2006a) Professional perspectives on decision making about the long-term care of older people. Br J Soc Work 36:807–826. https://doi.org/10.1093/bjsw/bch322

Taylor BJ, Donnelly M (2006b) Risks to home care workers: professional perspectives. Health Risk Soc 8:239–256. https://doi.org/10.1080/13698570600871695

Taylor BJ, McKeown C (2013) Assessing and managing risk with people with physical disabilities: development of a safety checklist. Health Risk Soc 15:162–175. https://doi.org/10.1080/13698575.2013.764973

Taylor BJ, Zeller RA (2007) Getting robust and valid data on decision policies: the factorial survey. Irish J Psychol 28(1–2):27–42. https://doi.org/10.1080/03033910.2007.10446246

Taylor BJ, Dempster M, Donnelly M (2003) Hidden gems: systematically searching electronic databases for research publications for social work and social care. Br J Soc Work 33:423–439. https://doi.org/10.1093/bjsw/33.4.423

Taylor BJ, Dempster M, Donnelly M (2007) Grading gems: appraising the quality of research for social work and social care. Br J Soc Work 37:335–354. https://doi.org/10.1093/bjsw/bch361

Taylor BJ, Killick C, O'Brien M, Begley E, Carter-Anand J (2014) Older people's conceptualisation of elder abuse and neglect. J Elder Abuse Negl 26(3):223–243. https://doi.org/10.1080/08946566.2013.795881

Taylor BJ, Killick C, McGlade A (2015) Understanding and using research in social work. Sage, London

Taylor BJ, Killick C, Bertotti T, Enosh G, Gautschi J, Hietamäki J, Sicora A, Whittaker A (2017) European Social Work Research Association SIG to study decisions, assessment and risk. J Evid Inf Soc Work 15(1):82–94. https://doi.org/10.1080/23761407.2017.1394244

Taylor BJ, Stevenson M, McDowell M (2018) Communicating risk in dementia care: survey of health and social care professionals. Health Soc Care Community 26(2):e291–e303. https://doi.org/10.1111/hsc.12519

Teigen KH, Brun W (1999) The directionality of verbal probability expressions: effects on decisions, predictions and probabilistic reasoning. Organ Behav Hum Decis Process 80:155–190. https://doi.org/10.1006/obhd.1999.2857

Thomson R, Edwards A, Grey J (2005) Risk communication in the clinical consultation. Clin Med 5:465–469

*Tong V, Raynor DK, Blalock SJ, Aslani P (2015) Consumer interpretation of ramipril and clopidogrel medication risk information: implications for risk communication strategies. Patient Prefer Adherence 9:983–988. https://doi.org/10.2147/PPA.S86414

Trevena LJ, Zikmund-Fisher BJ, Edwards A, Gaissmaier W, Galesic M, Han PKJ, King J, Lawson ML, Linder SK, Lipkus I, Ozanne E, Peters E, Timmermans D, Woloshin S (2013) Presenting quantitative information about decision outcomes: a risk communication primer for patient decision aid developers. BMC Med Inform Decis Mak 13(Suppl 2):S7. https://doi.org/10.1186/1472-6947-13-S2-S7

Vik P (2014) Regression, ANOVA and the general linear model: a statistics primer. Sage, Thousand Oaks

Visschers VH, Meertens RM, Passchier WW, De Vries NN (2009) Probability information in risk communication: a review of the research literature. Risk Anal 29:267–287. https://doi.org/10.1111/j.1539-6924.2008.01137.x

von Elm E, Altman DG, Egger M, Pocock SJ, Gøtzsche PC, Vandenbroucke JP, STROBE Initiative (2008) The Strengthening the Reporting of Observational Studies in Epidemiology (STROBE) statement: guidelines for reporting observational studies. J Clin Epidemiol 61(4):344–349. https://doi.org/10.1371/journal.pmed.0040297

Waters EA, Weinstein ND, Colditz GA, Emmons K (2006) Formats for improving risk communication in medical tradeoff decisions. J Health Commun 11:167–182. https://doi.org/10.1080/10810730500526695

Wegwarth O, Gaissmaier W, Gigerenzer G (2011) Deceiving numbers: survival rates and their impact on doctors' risk communication. Med Decis Mak 31(3):386–394. https://doi.org/10.1177/0272989X10391469

West SL, Squiers LB, Mccormack L, Southwell BG, Brouwer ES, Ashok M, Lux L, Boudewyns V, O'Donoghue A, Sullivan HW (2013) Communicating quantitative risks and benefits in promotional prescription drug labeling or print advertising. Pharmacoepidemiol Drug Saf 22:447–458. https://doi.org/10.1002/pds.3416

Witry MJ, Doucette WR (2015) Factors influencing community pharmacists' likelihood to ask medication monitoring questions: a factorial survey. Res Soc Adm Pharm 11:639–650. https://doi.org/10.1016/j.sapharm.2014.11.007

∗Young SD, Oppenheimer DM (2006) Different methods of presenting risk information and their influence on medication compliance intentions: results of three studies. Clin Ther 28:129–139. https://doi.org/10.1016/j.clinthera.2006.01.013

∗Young S, Oppenheimer DM (2009) Effect of communication strategy on personal risk perception and treatment adherence intentions. Psychol Health Med 14(4):430–442. https://doi.org/10.1080/13548500902890103

Zipkin DMA, Umscheid CA, Keating NL, Allen E, Aung K, Beyth R, Kaatz S, Mann DM, Sussman JB, Korenstein D, Schardt C, Nagi A, Sloane R, Feldstein DA (2014) Evidence-based risk communication: a systematic review. Ann Intern Med 161:270–280. https://doi.org/10.7326/M14-0295

Zolnierek KB, Dimatteo MR (2009) Physician communication and patient adherence to treatment: a meta-analysis. Med Care 47:826–834. https://doi.org/10.1097/MLR.0b013e31819a5acc

Rhetoric and Science and Technology Studies

9

Mathias Møllebæk

Abstract

The safety of medicines is increasingly becoming an issue of public concern, and calls for more transparency and public involvement abound. However, the notion of "public" is inherently ambiguous and loaded with values and normative expectations, which may have significant consequences for communicators involved with medicines safety. This chapter illustrates how methods and insights from two disciplines, rhetoric and science and technology studies (STS), can elucidate issues related to the publicity of medicines safety communication. In the first of two case studies a rhetorical analysis of a public hearing is presented and subsequently related to existing discussions of public hearings in STS scholarship. In the second case study an STS-driven analysis of a medicines safety controversy in the media is presented, and afterwards rhetorical insights are leveraged to discuss the meaning and implications of the controversy in medicines safety communication.

M. Møllebæk (✉)
University of Copenhagen, Copenhagen, Denmark
e-mail: mathias.moellebaek@sund.ku.dk

© Springer Nature Singapore Pte Ltd. 2020

P. Bahri (ed.), *Communicating about Risks and Safe Use of Medicines*,
https://doi.org/10.1007/978-981-15-3013-5_9

9.1 The Disciplines of Rhetoric and Science and Technology Studies: Scope, Theories and Principles

9.1.1 The Public and Medicines Safety

In the last days of September 2017, a French online petition demanding the reintroduction of a then-retired formulation of levothyroxine, i.e. Levothyrox®, indicated for an underactive thyroid gland, or hypothyroidism, reached an astonishing 300,000 signatures after only 3 months (Pétition 2017). The marketing of the new formulation, Euthyrox®, had resulted in a surge of adverse events reports reaching more than 9000 in short time (Melville 2017). In protest marches in front of the French National Assembly in Paris and multiple appearances in news shows patients demanded that manufacturers and authorities re-issue the old formulation, even though the French regulatory agency affirmed the safety of the new one.

Simultaneously, on 26 September 2017, the European Medicines Agency (EMA) in London convened its first-ever public hearing. The medicine in question, valproate, was and still is indicated for epilepsy and bipolar disorder, but bears significant risks of congenital malformations for children born to mothers taking this medicine. When the unresolved risk management of valproate triggered the public hearing, patients and mothers, and an affected daughter, took the stand and testified to their experiences with valproate, and together with patient advocacy representatives presented knowledge on the ineffectiveness of the risk minimisation activities mandatory at the time. At the receiving end of the testimonies were EMA's Pharmacovigilance and Risk Assessment Committee (PRAC), who ultimately would decide on what to do next with valproate, based on scientific evidence and the perspectives brought forth by the public voices.

The two events testify to the ways in which medicines safety is increasingly becoming a matter of public attention and concern. Like in other areas of health technology, medicines risk communication is no longer a matter of conveying technical facts to non-experts (Fischhoff 2014; Council of Canadian Academies 2015). Rather, the complexity of risks combined with the increased expectations of transparency and public involvement in risk management raise the need to critically examine how current medicines safety communication mediate the relation between scientific expertise and the public. In juxtaposition, the two events above shed light on very different aspects of this issue. In both situations members of the public and regulatory authorities communicated knowledge, opinions, and experiences. However, despite their proximity in time, these two events differ radically as communication situations. Does a *public* protest about medicine safety and *public* hearing on medicines safety refer to the same public? Which of these two events give the most true representation of the public? Do protesters who march the streets of Paris by their own volition speak more authentically and authoritatively as "the public" than those who have formally applied to and were then accepted to a public hearing hosted by an official authority? Peering into the question of what we mean by the term "the public" is important, if nothing else, because references to the public are ubiquitous. Regulators of medicines deal with *public* administration in order advise on *public* policy which then protects *public* health, as well as provide *public* information and increasingly engage with the *public*. These vastly different fields of knowledge are underpinned by various assumptions of what a public is and how to relate to it through communication.

The purpose of this chapter is to present methods and concepts that facilitate critical inquiry into the communication between medicines safety professionals and the public. Specifically, the chapter provides tools for understanding the potentially problematic assumptions about publics that undergird encounters between regulatory authorities and the public. On the basis of current research in rhetoric and science and technology studies (STS), the chapter shows that the ways in which medicines safety professionals communicate with the public are not always beneficial to the aims they attempt to achieve.

This chapter first provides a methodological overview of rhetoric and STS. Key concepts from these disciplines are then applied and discussed in various ways in two case studies. This is to illustrate how rhetoric and STS can equally offer hands-on methods for analysing as well as providing perspectives on such analytical insights. The case studies reflect two important communicative encounters that regulators and other professionals may have with the public: controversies about the safety of a medicine discussed in public spaces, and public hearings on a medicine where participants representing the public are formally heard by scientific experts. Although varying in scale, safety controversies are a recurring phenomenon and central to how medicines have been regulated historically and how regulators and industry are perceived by citizens (Carpenter 2010). Public hearings, on the other hand, comprise a relatively new way of relating to the public and one that is driven by certain ideals about the proper relation between citizens and the regulating state. The case studies also investigate whether such ideals can be supportive or obstructive to the communication of medicines safety. The chapter then proceeds with a discussion of the potential value, use and perspectives of an approach to communication informed by rhetoric and STS research. Suggestions for future research conclude the chapter.

9.1.2 Rhetoric

The term "rhetoric" is often associated with empty speech or manipulation in everyday discourse. As an area of communication research, however, rhetorical scholarship provides critical and practical insights into how language and other symbolic systems are used to perform actions. Whereas communication research may refer to many forms of studies on informational or symbolic exchange between humans and/or machines, rhetoric is the study and practice of how humans use language and other symbols to influence each other and reach agreement in order to coordinate social action (Hauser 2002). This complements research into language and discourse performed by linguists (see Chap. 1). Many rhetorical scholars identify as critics and examine how power is distributed and contested by means of language in order to evaluate public discourse against norms of liberal democracy. A central concern within rhetorical research, then, is how language and argumentation accomplishes or disappoints democratic ideals of modern liberal society.

9.1.3 Science and Technology Studies (STS)

Scholars in science and technology studies (STS) investigate how society and politics influence scientific research and technological innovation and, conversely, how science and technology affect society, politics and culture. As such, STS, like communication research to which rhetoric belongs, is part of the social sciences. Extending Thomas Kuhn's influential *The Structure of Scientific Revolutions* from 1962, STS generally assigns fundamental importance to the historical, political or institutional context in which science and technology are developed, regulated and used. This entails that concepts from social sciences, such as deliberative democracy from political science, are not separated from the analysis of science and technology but rather become analytical lenses and ethical principles through which science and technology are to be conceived and evaluated. STS studies of medicines have in recent years been referred to as part of a wider field of social studies in the pharmaceutical field, dubbed "pharmaceutical studies" (as opposed to "pharmaceutical sciences") (Sismondo and Greene 2015).

9.2 Research Approaches and Methods

9.2.1 Overview of Methodology in Rhetoric

The majority of rhetorical studies are textual analyses of publicly disseminated texts, speeches or visuals. Here, textual analysis refers to the systematic reading of textual objects with a view towards deeper meanings (Brummett 2010). However, the use of methods from the social sciences is increasing (McKinnon 2016), and quantitative content analysis and qualitative methods, like ethnography, interviews and focus groups (see Chap. 8), have become more integrated in rhetorical studies. Furthermore, rhetorical theory and methods are increasingly finding use in health and medical contexts (Meloncon and Scott 2017). Very broadly construed, rhetorical analysis follows three kinds of approaches:

1. a *close reading-approach* which puts focus on a selected text of political or social importance in order to understand its meaning and to assess its wider implications; this approach largely follows inductive, case study logic (Brummett 2010);
2. a *critical rhetoric-approach* which focuses on a socially or politically important phenomenon that is not contained in a single text but rather observable across multiple texts; this approach generally follows deductive reasoning and is often informed by broader social theory, such as class, disability or gender (Mckerrow 1989); and
3. a *conceptually oriented approach* in which a socially and politically salient research question is examined through the simultaneous examination of a relevant theoretical concept (e.g. "consensus") and a relevant empirical text (e.g. a public hearing transcript); this approach follows abductive reasoning, which refers to a back and forth reflective oscillation between the object of study and the chosen theoretical concept (Jasinski 2001a).

Relevant concepts for rhetorical analysis include (for a comprehensive list of concepts see Jasinski 2001b) the following:

- *Framing* is the rhetorical act of making some aspects of reality more accessible and salient than others. As a metaphor for framing a picture, a rhetorical frame "induce[s] us to filter our perceptions of the world in particular ways, essentially making some aspects of our multidimensional reality more noticeable than other aspects" (Kuypers 2009). Importantly, framing is a precondition for communication because no one can perceive every aspect of reality at once. In other words, it is impossible *not* to frame information when communicating. The important question, then, is the meaning and implications of the chosen frame.
- *Second persona* is the implied audience of a speech or a text (Black 1970). Whereas the first persona describes the "I" in a text, that is, how the author comes across in the text, the second persona describes the implied "you" in the text, that is, how the audience is implicitly described in the text. The second persona is an indicator of how the communicator seeks to influence his audience's behaviours and beliefs.
- *Antithesis* is a rhetorical figure that places terms in opposition to achieve a contrastive effect. Antitheses have been found to have a significant argumentative function in the sciences where commonly accepted pairs of opposition are used to promote a scientific argument (Fahnestock 1999). Some terms can be opposed through negation (e.g. "rational" versus "*ir*rational"), while others can be constructed and become commonplace over time (e.g. "anecdote" versus "evidence"). Part of their argumentative function is the implicit suggestion of the binary pair as exhaustive alternatives.

This chapter illustrates in Sect. 9.2.3.1 how framing, second persona and antithesis can be used to analyse a public hearing on medicines safety. This relies on Teston et al.'s rhetorical-qualitative analysis of the 581-page transcription of a public hearing at the United States Food and Drug Administration (US FDA) (Teston et al. 2014). While their study differs in purpose and methods, their analysis and conclusions provide an instructive background and resource for the purpose of introducing the methodology of this chapter. Teston et al. employ a grounded theory approach (Glaser and Strauss 1967) (see Chap. 8) with rhetorical argumentation concepts (Toulmin 2003) to examine how the public voices were incorporated in the hearing.

9.2.2 Overview of Methodology in STS

The methodological suite of STS reflects its interdisciplinary history and wide array of topics. While many STS researchers have preference for ethnography and/or document research, a wide assortment of empirical social science methods (see Chap. 8) is employed for STS-related purposes.

Actor-network theory To mention one particular approach, actor-network theory (ANT) has been a very influential theoretical and methodological resource in the last three decades in STS (Sismondo 2010). Rather than a theory in the sense of a coherent framework with predictive and explanatory capabilities, ANT is a theory in the sense of a repository of terms and "methodological reflexes" (Mol 2010) which supports the exploration of interaction of the natural, observable world and the social, experienced world. A central tenet in ANT is that the social and natural world exists in continuously changing network of relations between actors which may equally be human subjects, organisations, institutions or material objects and technologies. The term "network" in this field is different from the technical definition of network in, e.g. engineering where "network" describes a final and stabilised relation of nodes of which some are more crucial to the network's functionality than others (Latour 1996). In ANT, the term "network" captures a fundamental view on the world rather than a technical object. In this view, any object of scientific inquiry is the outcome of the ongoing interaction of multiple components (Callon 1987). Aligned with a constructivist tradition of social sciences, one key insight is that the fundamental categories whereby science and society are typically understood (e.g. "nature" and "culture") are not eternal truths but rather outcomes of a network of relations. In other words, the dividing line between "nature" and "culture" is continuously maintained, disputed and altered by a cast of actors. ANT-inspired empirical research typically investigates the ways in which networks emerge, change and disintegrate.

Some relevant concepts from STS research include the following (for more see Sismondo 2010; Jasanoff et al. 1995):

- *Risk colonisation theory* refers to the dynamic between the management of risks in society (societal risks) and the management of "threats to regulatory organisations and/or the legitimacy of rules and methods of regulation" (Rothstein et al. 2006) (institutional risks). The regulation of societal risks gives rise to institutional risks because the inevitable limitations of regulation may be exposed in light of increasing expectations of accountability and transparency.
- *Public deficit model* refers to a set of assumptions (rather than a model) about communication as a mediating factor between science and society. It posits that the communication of scientific facts to the general public is problematic because the public lacks general understanding of science, and, consequently, that the mission for science communicators is to infuse the public with scientific knowledge and thereby enfranchise it (Irwin and Wynne 1996; Wynne 2016). STS scholars have generally seen the wide use of the model as a central problem in science-society relations (Jasanoff 2012). It can be compared to problem and critique of paternalism in clinical medicine.
- *Regulatory capture* refers to a situation in which a regulating institution advances or is perceived to advance the interests of the regulated industry instead of the public interests it was intended to serve. Although regulatory capture is used across disciplines like economics and law, STS scholars examining pharmaceuticals have mostly used the concept to describe the implications of scientific biases in the regulation of medicines (Abraham 2002).

The case study in Sect. 9.2.3.3 exemplifies how ANT, risk colonisation, public deficit model and regulatory capture can be used in an STS analysis. It relies on Dew and Gardner's ANT-informed analysis of a public controversy in New Zealand (Dew et al. 2017), as it is, like Teston et al., an instructive resource to this chapter's introduction of STS.

9.2.3 Two Case Studies

Rather than explore the two recent events sketched in Sect. 9.1.1, the case studies rely on existing research on similar, earlier incidents. A public hearing on bevacizumab initiated by the US FDA sheds light on the qualities of public participation in the regulation of medicines (Teston et al. 2014; Teston 2017). As for the public protests, prior to any protest in France over the reformulation of Levothyrox, the New Zealand public protested vigorously about an almost identical issue in 2008. Existing research on the development of the case in the media and the medical merits of the protests (Dew et al. 2017; Faasse et al. 2010; Gardner and Dew 2011) constitute useful stepping stones for a discussion of the communicative aspects.

9.2.3.1 The US FDA Public Hearing on Avastin: A Rhetorical Analysis

On 28 and 29 June 2011, the US FDA convened a public hearing about a recent recommendation to revoke a breast cancer indication for Avastin®, a medicine containing the active substance bevacizumab and authorised for the treatment of various types of cancer. The announcement to revoke the indication 7 months prior had caused worry among breast cancer patients using the product, because they were likely to lose insurance funding for the expensive treatment without an approved indication. In response patients, physicians, and cancer patient organisations lobbied their political representatives in Congress. At the same time, the manufacturer filed an appeal against the recommendation from the FDA's Oncologic Drugs Advisory Committee (ODAC) to revoke the indication. The roster of participants at the hearing included patients, physicians, researchers, patients organisation representatives and representatives from the manufacturer. Over the two days each participant presented their views to a panel of jurors appointed by the ODAC, consisting of one patient representative, five representatives from the oncological research community and one representative from the pharmaceuticals industry who did not have a vote. The hearing revolved around four questions posed by the ODAC to the participants:

> "1. Do the AVADO and RIBBON 1 trials [fail to] verify the clinical benefit of Avastin for the breast cancer indication for which it was approved?
>
> 2[a]. Does the available evidence on Avastin demonstrate that the drug has not been shown to be effective for the breast cancer indication for which it was approved?
>
> 2[b]. Does the available evidence on Avastin demonstrate that the drug has not been shown to be safe for the breast cancer indication for which it was approved and that Avastin has not been shown to present a clinical benefit that justifies the risks associated with use of the product for this indication?

> 3. If the Commissioner agrees with the grounds for withdrawal set out in Issue 1, Issue 2[a] or Issue 2[b], should the FDA nevertheless continue the approval of the breast cancer indication while the sponsor designs and conducts additional studies intended to verify the drug's clinical benefit? (Petryna 2009)"

Put simply, the official point of contention in the hearing was whether the medicinal product showed "significant clinical benefit" to keep its indication for breast cancer. The four key questions helped frame the hearing so as to keep it focused, similar to a meeting agenda. Following the concept of rhetorical frames, however, such framing questions inevitably feature some perspectives over others and thereby implicitly assign certain roles to participants.

This raises the first research question for analysing the public hearing: How is the public involved? Or posed through the concept of the second persona, how are the public participants implicitly described in the frame that the four questions establish in the beginning of the hearing? Judging from the four questions posed by the ODAC, the role of the non-researching public is hard to establish. Each question implicitly presumes the participants' expertise in assessing the veracity of the evidence provided for clinical benefit, efficacy and risks for the breast cancer indication. Extending this observation in a rhetorical analysis of the entire hearing, Teston et al. (Teston et al. 2014) argue that the premises securing the relevance of citizen contributions were not reached at any point in the hearing because the discussion centred on whether the medicine was assessed clinically beneficial enough, as suggested by the four questions. Moreover, the discussion specifically revolved around the methodological question of which endpoints could constitute such evidence. According to Teston et al., this essentially meant that citizen testimonies "could be bracketed off as merely anecdotal" (Teston et al. 2014). In other words, due to the dissensus about clinical benefit among scientific representatives, the public perspectives articulated by patient and patient group advocates fell short of the actual focus of discussion.

Adding a second research question about how the hearing is framed, it would be relevant to investigate how the discussion at the hearing actually unfolded: How did the representatives of the public participate? Teston et al. concluded that the inclusion of diverse participants across numerous expert and lay perspectives did not ensure that "all included parties were able to participate equally in the debate" (Teston et al. 2014). For example, they found that even though participants representing the public (such as breast cancer survivors and their friends and family members) made up 21 of the 47 participants, they accounted for only about 7% of utterances made throughout the hearing. As the design of the public hearing revolved around inclusive dialogue, this inequality resulted from the fact that patients, their representatives and family members were at no point asked any specific questions, and none of the questions they asked were answered.

A third research question about the evaluation of expert and lay contributions needs to be examined too: Can the difference between expertise and public participants that the ODAC initial framing establishes be traced in other parts of the hearing? Closely related to the differentiation between scientific expertise and public perspective in the framing created through the ODAC questions, an antithesis between data and anecdote was observable throughout the hearing. This antithesis became particularly clear in the voting section of the hearing: "The research evidence does not demonstrate a clinical benefit. And even though we have anecdotal information, we don't show any improvement in quality of life or in overall survival" (Dr. Natalie Compagni-Portis, ODAC, Teston et al. 2014), and: "I was once taught that the plural of anecdote is not data. So we each have one story of somebody who felt better while responding, but if the facts don't support that, then that's not something that we can rely on" (Dr. Mikkael Skeers, ODAC, Teston et al. 2014). From a biomedical perspective the differentiation between the constitution and reliability of data versus anecdote is crucial and perhaps represents the utmost scientific concern in medical and pharmaceutical research. However, in the context of a public hearing which explicitly seeks to expand the perspective of the communication beyond the biomedical domain, the data/anecdote antithesis in principle and practice hinders the potential for a positive estimation of patient perspectives presented in the hearing.

What, then, counts as public participation? If the deliberation in the public hearing is primarily a scientific one between dissenting experts, where does that leave the invited public? At what stage and by what kind of input are citizens imagined to contribute to decision-making? How does this process help to assuage the public distrust in scientific governance and regulation? These are the questions which arise from the above rhetorical analysis of the public hearing as a communication encounter.

9.2.3.2 The US FDA Public Hearing on Avastin: STS Perspectives

STS scholars have examined the efforts to engage the public in technological and scientific matters extensively, and this proves helpful when discussing a public hearing. The problem with many efforts to engage the public, according to, for example, Wynne (Wynne 2016), is the predominant perception in scientific institutions and authorities that the public is inherently external to the work of science and technological regulation. A fixed and passive externality, a public is imagined to lack knowledge about science, and in response scientific actors should aspire to educate the public and assist in making decisions more rationally. Hence, the public deficit model prevails (Irwin and Wynne 1996).

Although policy makers and representatives from scientific institutions have attempted to move their communication beyond the assumptions underlying the public deficit model, it has proved difficult. For example, Hagendijk (Hagendijk 2004) notes that the intention to incorporate the critique of the public deficit model in the European Commission's paper "Science, Society and Citizen in Europe" (European Commission 2000) resulted in two competing voices throughout the vision described by the European Commission. According to Hagendijk, "The dominant voice is the inclusive voice, assuring the reader that citizens' concerns should be taken seriously, and ought not to be treated in a condescending way. In contrast with this, however, a more "scientistic" voice argues that the public can only contribute properly if it is adequately educated and instructed." (Hagendijk 2004).

From the literature on public engagement in STS, we can identify two modes of reasoning behind having public hearings. The "input reason" holds that public engagement such as hearings may contribute with perspectives informed by values, experiences and real-life characteristics. In this line of thinking, patients, healthcare professionals and patient advocate representatives are expected to bring knowledge to the process of decision-making, which balances the strict scientific rationales driving regulatory decisions. Secondly, the "remedial reason" holds that the public increasingly lacks trust in scientific authority and in the government institutions that regulate by applying scientific principles and evidence. Public hearing as one modality of public engagement is a remedy to this lack of public trust. However, hearings may become problematic at the intersections of these two modes of reasoning, raising the following questions: Are public engagements, which provide input for decision-making, beneficial to public trust? And vice versa, can efforts to assuage public trust produce relevant input for decision-makers?

The Avastin hearing clearly exemplifies the intention to engage the public in a matter of scientific regulation, thus ostensibly taking us further than the public deficit model. Yet, as presented in Teston et al. (2014), the framing of the hearing performed by the ODAC questions, the participation of non-researchers and the assessment of their contributions in the voting section suggest that the implicitly described public (that is, the second persona) fall between both the input reason and the remedial reason for arranging public hearings. Perhaps most clearly in the data/anecdote antithesis, the hearing did probably not provide new and useful input from non-researchers on the defined questions, nor is it likely to have improved the public trust through the inclusion of citizens' perspectives, as they "could be bracketed off" (Teston et al. 2014). As the frame of the deliberation created by the ODAC questions corresponds to the scientific approach of affirming efficacy and clinical benefit and of higher evidence strength of "data over anecdote", public contributions, such as patients' experiences with medicines or healthcare professionals' experiences with patient care, are destined to miss the scientific threshold set in the structure of the deliberations.

9.2.3.3 The New Zealand Controversy Over Eltroxin: An STS Analysis

In July 2007, the New Zealand Medicines and Medical Devices Safety Authority (MedSafe) approved the introduction of a new formulation of levothyroxine, Eltroxin®, a prescription-only medicine for low function of the thyroid gland (hypothyroidism), produced by a German manufacturer. A year later, as the new formulation replaced the old one, patients began reporting a range of adverse events, such as joint and muscle pain, skin rash, weight gain and visual disturbances. According to Dew and Gardner (Dew et al. 2017), what eventually turned into a two-month long controversy in the public domain in 2008, started when a user of Eltroxin talked about suspected adverse reactions in a radio show. This story was picked up by regional newspapers in the New Southland region, including one particular article in which a local pharmacist, Allen Campbell, accused the manufacturer and regulators of attempting to suppress the story.

After three weeks of increasing news coverage in multiple regional media outlets MedSafe issued a press release confirming the safety profile and prescription advice and cited "poor patient compliance" as the probable cause of the reports of suspected adverse reactions (MedSafe 2008a). The press release did not halt the public attention, however. A patient support group had formed and was cited in a news story as suggesting that Eltroxin users could shift to a named alternative product to avoid adverse reactions (MedSafe 2008b). After the MedSafe announcement and the support group statements circulated in five regional newspapers, two members of parliament (MPs), Jackie Blue and Sue Kedgley, each issued press releases in which they criticised the authorities and sympathised with the patients who felt disregarded.

On 11 September 2008, the New Zealand Ministry of Health distributed a press release which (1) confirmed an ongoing subsidisation approval process of medicines alternative to Eltroxin; (2) affirmed that the safety profile of Eltroxin was satisfactory; and (3) repudiated unverified claims that Eltroxin was manufactured in India or using "genetic engineering" (MedSafe 2008b).

In the end, on 23 October 2008, MedSafe approved two additional levothyroxine products, giving worried users alternatives (MedSafe 2008c).

Why Focus on Social Aspects and Relations?

While an STS analysis allows us to reach a more comprehensive understanding of the Eltroxin case as a social phenomenon, taking up a controversy over medicines safety requires some justification first.

As with the Avastin case, a discussion of the communication in this series of events is easily reduced to a discussion of being "scientifically right" with regards to the statistical basis for patients' claims about side effects with little attention to the social nature of the events. Indeed, in the *British Medical Journal* one team of researchers argued that the Eltroxin case was a quintessential health scare (Faasse et al. 2010, 2012) in which unwarranted claims about a medicinal product's safety were unjustly amplified through media outlets triggering a chain reaction which eventually led to regulatory intervention. Based on the bioequivalence studies of the old and the new formulation presented by the New Zealand authorities, the authors concluded that it was "unlikely that the constitution of the medication itself was responsible for the large increase in reported adverse reactions" (Faasse et al. 2010). Rather, they argued, the spike in reporting of suspected adverse reactions was more likely due to "external factors" such as public distrust in authorities, critiques of authorities by politicians and accusations from a local pharmacist, as well as the emotional distress of hypothyroidism patients resulting from incorrectly perceived adverse reactions.

Health scares and controversies about medicines safety are often considered anomalies when they, in fact, recur so often and are well-described in scientific literature that they should be considered an integral part of public health and risk communication. From a biomedical perspective, strict evaluation of the correctness and validity of the claims made by patients and healthcare professionals are doubtlessly important. From a communication perspective, however, such focus fails to account for the complexity of a health scare as a social phenomenon that significantly shapes the public's attitude towards scientific and governmental authorities.

While Faase et al. (2010) rightly argue that multiple factors were at play in the Eltroxin case (as will be described below), their distinction between internal and external factors is inhibitive to understanding the inherent social nature of medicines safety controversy.

An analysis informed by STS approaches allows us to shed light on social and public aspects of the Eltroxin case. Based on ANT and corresponding mapping of technical controversies (Berker et al. 2011), the following analysis identifies the communication positions of the main actors in the public controversy based on the synthesised narrative account in the beginning of Sect. 9.2.3.3 (see Dew et al. 2017; Gardner and Dew 2011, for more elaborate accounts). The first step is to identify the actors, assess their similarities and differences in the controversy and arrange them accordingly. The second step is to describe the actions and the relations they form based on the first step.

Actor-Network Analysis: Mapping Actors and Relations

Figure 9.1 lists the cast of actors in the controversy. They can all be described as actors because some action related to the controversy originates from them or is conferred on them. In principle this means that the roster of actors can be infinite, so it remains a methodological choice how to scope the range of the network to suit the research question.

To get a more comprehensive overview of the actors and their relations, a diagrammatic representation can be helpful. Figure 9.2 is a simple network diagram of

Fig. 9.1 Actors in the New Zealand controversy over Eltroxin

- The national regulatory body MedSafe
- The manufacturer of Eltroxin
- The patient on radio talking about suspected adverse reactions
- Regional news papers
- Allan Campbell, pharmacist
- Patient support group
- Member of parliament (MP) Jackie Blue
- Member of parliament (MP) Sue Kedgley
- The New Zealand Ministry of Health

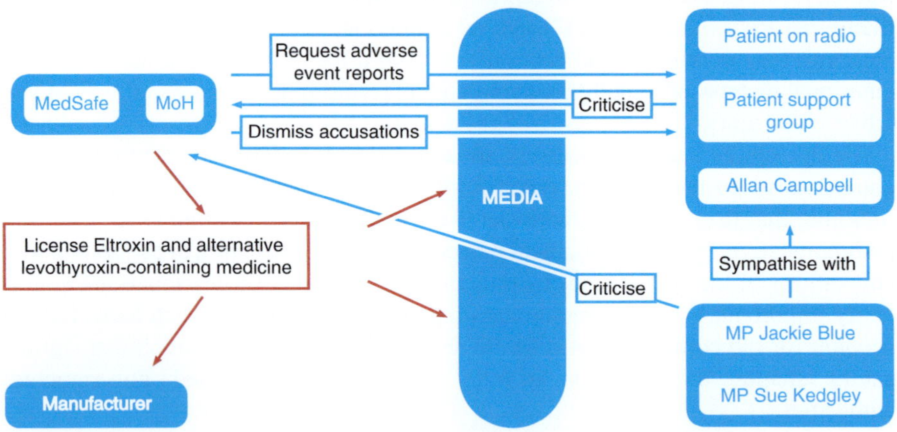

Fig. 9.2 Network diagram of actors in the New Zealand controversy over Eltroxin

the actors listed in Figure 9.1. Importantly, it is not an objective representation of the network or the controversy. Rather, it is the outcome a series of analytical steps guided by ANT: identifying, assessing and arranging actors in their relations. Identifying an actor and plotting it on the map attributes equal significance to all actors. This meets the research need for representing the actors as unassumingly as possible. For example, one would normally expect different degrees of influence from national health authorities as opposed to private individuals, but the map helps to equalise these and provides a basis for a STS analysis that is as unassuming as possible. All actors (except the media and the manufacturer, as will be explained later) are arranged in clusters (marked by dotted lines) according to the similarities and differences of their communication position in the controversy. This highlights how some actors align, while others oppose each other. Importantly, the actors' positions here reflect the network of relations in which the Eltroxin public controversy emerged. Positions do not reflect other networks of relations in which these actors may be involved.

The map consists of three clusters of actors and two individual actors, the media and the manufacturer of Eltroxin. The cluster in the top-left corner consists of the two public authorities who were involved in the public controversy, MedSafe and the Ministry of Health. While the two government organisations have different legal mandates, different responsibilities for public health and carry out different functions in the management of risks of medicinal products, they take similar positions in the controversy where these differences are less significant. They both emerged as actors who to the public hold a double responsibility for public safety with regards to medicines and for market oversight and regulation. The double responsibility and the direct regulatory association with manufacturers prime the potential for the regulatory capture critique, which we will explore rhetorically below. As the blue lines pointing away from the cluster indicate, the authorities actively dismissed the public critique raised by patients and simultaneously requested adverse events reports from patients. These two activities point to a potential risk colonisation dynamic of institutional and societal risk. While a comprehensive risk colonisation analysis is beyond the scope here, it should be noted that the public critique of the authorities cluster is an institutional risk to the legitimacy of the methods and rules of regulation, and the adverse events reporting is a measure to manage the risks to members of society. Managing institutional risks and societal risks at the same time are known to produce a difficult tension in the responsibility and interests of authorities which could "sensitise regulators to take account of societal risks in different ways" (Rothstein et al. 2006).

The cluster in the top-right corner encompasses patient voices. Again, while there are notable differences between casual remarks from a patient on the radio and the organised patient group with regular meetings and official mission statement (and even further to an individual pharmacist), the similarity of the cluster is the position they take in the controversy. What defines this cluster of actors is the collective criticism of the authorities and the lack of formal power to intervene in the situation. The actors in this cluster emerged as representatives of the public who the authorities are meant to protect, and they voiced different kinds of criticism of the authorities' handling of the situation. Furthermore, they garnered sympathy from MPs who do have some degree of formal power to intervene but more relevantly can gather and direct media attention as way of support and sympathy.

The cluster on the bottom-right consists of the two MPs. They represent different political parties and probably have different political views on other issues, yet their beliefs and statements in the Eltroxin controversy are aligned in the sympathy for the patient cluster and the critique of the authorities. Although the MPs most probably had a significantly and democratically important impact on the development of the controversy by augmenting it to a national level of attention, it is important to note that they emerged relatively late in the controversy. The two MPs did not emerge as actors until the controversy was established in the regional media, and, as I will discuss below, the MPs could have an electoral interest in making themselves heard in this controversy in addition to the support of the patients. Methodologically, the late emergence of this cluster points to the limitations of the actor mapping and the strength of the narrative account the beginning of Sect. 9.2.3.3. While the map provides overview that cuts across every stage of the controversy, the narrative provides a chronology that describes how it unfolds over time as a process with multiple stage. This complementarity may give important nuance.

Two actors are not placed within clusters. The manufacturer of Eltroxin plays a passive role in the controversy given the accusation of regulatory capture. The manufacturer is the object of critique but does not respond publicly. The media is not clustered with other actors either because it had an important double function as both an arena and actor. Instead, media are placed centrally in the diagram because it had a connective and infrastructural function to other actors allowing relations between them to form. However, the media were also an actor in and of itself. In general, media outlets are not neutral conduits of facts and statements. Newspaper editors have editorial trajectories informed by their readership and commercial and public interest. Moreover, journalists select sources and propagate some frames over others, even though they principally aim to balance divergent perspectives on a newsworthy event. Media analysis can further elucidate such processes (see Chap. 10).

9.2.3.4 The New Zealand Controversy over Eltroxin: Rhetorical Perspectives

The actor-network diagram provides an overview of relations between actors in the public controversy around Eltroxin. The arrows signify the actions taken by actors as described in the narrative account. Two types of actions are observed: Blue arrows describe actions that are communicative in nature, whereas the red arrows describe regulatory actions. As the majority of actions in this controversy are communicative and mediated, rhetorical concepts can further the analysis. In particular, the communication of Ministry of Health and the critiques raised by Allan Campbell and the MPs deserve further rhetorical consideration.

First, New Zealand's Ministry of Health chose in their press release regarding the potential approval of an alternative brand of levothyroxine to announce that Eltroxin "…is not manufactured in India" and that "its manufacture does not involve any genetic engineering" (MedSafe 2008b). These two points are outlandish in the context of the rest of the press release, and none of the claims were made in news outlets reporting the Eltroxin case, according to Dew et al. (Dew et al. 2017), so the nature and origin of these claims are unknown. While these points were undoubtedly intended to reassure the public of the quality of the product, responding directly to such unspecified and undocumented claims may risk equivocating publicised patient experiences with speculation and rumours, effectively rendering the public less "rationally minded" and possibly even seeding doubts on topics where there were none before. Or readers who are already critical of the authorities' handling of the Eltroxin case may perceive the Ministry of Health's attempt to discredit claims as "straw man argumentation", in which the authorities misrepresent claims made by the public in order to respond to it in a superior way.

Second, Allan Campbell and MPs Jackie Blue and Sue Kedgley repeatedly criticised authorities for the management of the controversy. But by which standards should the criticism be evaluated? Allen Campbell was quoted for saying that the manufacturer and New Zealand regulators colluded to suppress the story and that "the Government should face up and fund an alternative brand until the whole mess can be cleared up" (Dew et al. 2017). Aligned with Campbell, Blue sympathised with the patient public by stating that "the problem is definitely real. The people we have been talking to are not neurotic…" (Dew et al. 2017), effectively insinuating that patients who reported adverse events were deemed "neurotic" by authorities. Lastly, MP Sue Kedgley stated in a press release that "It's time for MedSafe to tell the drug manufacturer that the new formulation is not acceptable for many New Zealanders and that they should provide an alternative drug".

While all three critiques are charged against the authorities, they differ in their substance and should therefore be evaluated by different standards. Whereas Blue charged authorities in an ethical register with stigmatising patients, Kedgley argued that MedSafe was too lenient with the manufacturer and neglected public safety. Most forcefully, Campbell expressed the regulatory capture critique (a critique identified primarily in STS). Most probably, his critique gained influence by his vocation as a community pharmacist whose professional training grants him expertise within pharmaceuticals. On the other hand, keeping in mind that a collusion was not observed at any point, healthcare professionals, including pharmacists, are expected to have a higher standard of their claims about medicines than non-professionals when raising such accusations in public. While less explicit than Campbell's, Blue and Kegdley's critiques are more important because they are MPs and wield significant agenda-setting powers in national debate. With the Eltroxin controversy unfolding less than 4 months before the national parliament election, suspicion of political and self-serving motivations behind siding with patient population does not seem unwarranted. In any circumstance, recent experience has shown that ill-guided interventions by public figures in controversies around medicines can have detrimental effects (e.g. vaccine scepticism (Gottlieb 2016)), so any involvement by elected politicians in similar emergent controversies should be made with a view towards the risk of distorting and inhibiting the public deliberation of medicines issues.

In sum, the STS analysis inspired by ANT has provided an overview of actors, actions and relations involved in the Eltroxin controversy. Significantly, the diagram showed that citizens and elected politicians aligned in their communicative actions and in their opposition to health authorities. Rhetorical perspectives further suggested standards by which the actors' communicative actions should be evaluated.

9.3 Utility of Applied Methods for Researching Medicinal Product Risk Communication

Even though rhetorical scholars have only begun to systematically engage with medicines and health issues within the last two decades (Reed 2016; Segal 2005), recent such studies reveal the utility and value of rhetorical engagement with issues of medicines communication (Teston et al. 2014; Graham and Herndl 2011; Graham et al. 2018; Segal 2018). Like the case study provided in this chapter, this research highlights the need for closer examination and evaluation of the communication processes by which the public is involved in formal dialogues about medicines and risk. In contrast to rhetoric, STS scholars have a longer history with research in medicines and risks. This research has produced novel insights into the industrial outsourcing of pharmaceutical research (Petryna 2009), mobilisation of social protest against the regulation of medicines (Epstein 1996) and the "pharmaceuticalization" of everyday life (Williams et al. 2011; see Sismondo and Greene 2015, for an overview). However, few STS scholars have directly related their conclusions to medicines communication. As the second case study in this chapter has illustrated, the use of STS methods and concepts provide important resources for understanding the crucial role of communication in the mediation of science-society relations. Chap. 1 provides a comprehensive overview of how STS, rhetoric and other disciplines introduced in this chapter may contribute to a multilayered analysis of medicinal product risk communication.

9.4 Outlook: Relevance, Improvements and Future Potential

In combination, rhetoric and STS can equip medicine communicators with more nuanced conceptual understandings and reflection on the concepts that are put to work—more or less consciously—in medicinal product risk communication. In particular, scholars across vaccine communication (Hausman et al. 2017) and public hearings on medicines (Teston et al. 2014) have argued from empirical evidence that a stronger understanding of the emotional, sociological and political intricacies of medicinal product risk communication would most probably help communicators realise aspirations of a more connected, responsible and viable understanding between authorities and the variety of publics they engage. More research and derived recommendations guiding this engagement is needed.

Conclusions

- Medicines risk communication is increasingly becoming an object of public attention and concern.
- Concepts from interpretive social sciences are needed to understand, evaluate and improve current communication in public and political contexts.
- Rhetoric enables textual analysis of how issues are framed, how publics are included and how contrastive rhetoric may exacerbate gaps between publics and scientific counterparts.
- Science and technology studies (STS) enables critical analysis of risk management, science-society relations and relations between actors in controversies.

References

Abraham J (2002) The pharmaceutical industry as a political player. Lancet 360(9344):1498–1502

Berker T, Callon M, Lascoumes P, Barthe Y (2011) Acting in an uncertain world: an essay on technical democracy. MIT, Cambridge

Black E (1970) The second persona. Q J Speech 56(2):109–119

Brummett B (2010) Techniques of close reading. SAGE, Thousand Oaks, p 137

Callon M (1987) Society in the making: the study of technology as a tool for sociological analysis. In: The social construction of technological systems: new directions in the sociology and history of technology. MIT, Cambridge, pp 83–103

Carpenter D (2010) Reputation and power. In: Organizational image and pharmaceutical regulation at the FDA. Princeton University Press, Princeton, p 802

Council of Canadian Academies (2015) Health product risk communication: is the message getting through? Council of Canadian Academies, Ottawa

Dew K, Gardner J, Morrato EH, Norris P, Chamberlain K, Hodgetts D et al (2017) Public engagement and the role of the media in post-marketing drug safety: the case of Eltroxin® (levothyroxine) in New Zealand. Crit Public Health 1596:1–14

Epstein S (1996) Impure science: AIDS, activism, and the politics of knowledge. University of California Press, Berkeley, p 466

European Commission (2000) Science, society and citizen in Europe, vol 1. Commission of the European Communities, Brussels

Faasse K, Cundy T, Petrie KJ (2010) Thyroxine: anatomy of a health scare. BMJ 339(7736):20–21

Faasse K, Gamble G, Cundy T, Petrie KJ (2012) Impact of television coverage on the number and type of symptoms reported during a health scare: a retrospective pre-post observational study. BMJ 2(4):e001607

Fahnestock J (1999) Rhetorical figures in science. Oxford University Press, Oxford, p 234

Fischhoff B (2014) Four answers to four questions (about risk communication). J Risk Res 17(10):1265–1267

Gardner J, Dew K (2011) The Eltroxin controversy: Risk and how actors construct their world. Health Risk Soc 13(5):397–411

Glaser BG, Strauss AL (1967) The discovery of grounded theory: strategies for qualitative research. Aldine, Chicago, p 271

Gottlieb SD (2016) Vaccine resistances reconsidered: Vaccine skeptics and the Jenny McCarthy effect. BioSocieties 11(2):152–174

Graham SS, Herndl CG (2011) Talking off-label: the role of stasis in transforming the discursive formation of pain science. Rhetor Soc Q 41(2):145–167

Graham SS, Kessler MM, Kim S-Y, Ahn S, Card D (2018) Assessing perspectivalism in patient participation: an evaluation of FDA patient and consumer representative programs. Rhetor Heal Med 1(1):58–89

Hagendijk RP (2004) The public understanding of science and public participation in regulated worlds. Minerva 42:41–59
Hauser GA (2002) Introduction to rhetorical theory. Waveland Press, Mountain View, p 303
Hausman BL, Dannenberg CJ, Marmagas WJ, Harriman K (2017) Immunity, modernity, and the biopolitics of vaccination resistance. Configurations 25(3):279–300
Irwin A, Wynne B (eds) (1996) Misunderstanding science? Cambridge University Press, Cambridge
Jasanoff S (2012) Science and public reason. Routledge, New York, p 306
Jasanoff S, Markle G, Peterson J, Pinch T (1995) Handbook of science and technology studies. SAGE, Thousand Oaks
Jasinski J (2001a) The status of theory and method in rhetorical criticism. West J Commun. 65(3):249–270
Jasinski J (2001b) Sourcebook on rhetoric: key concepts in contemporary rhetorical studies. SAGE, Thousand Oaks, p 641
Kuypers JA (2009) "Framing analysis" How to conduct a framing study. In: Rhetorical criticism: perspectives in action. Lexington, Lanham, pp 181–203. Available from: https://www.researchgate.net/publication/318926032_Framing_Analysis_How_to_Conduct_a_Framing_Study
Latour B (1996) On actor-network theory: A few clarifications. Soz Welt. 47:369–381
Mckerrow RE (1989) Critical rhetoric: theory and praxis. Commun Monogr. 56(2):91–111
McKinnon SL (2016) In: Sara L, Asen R, Chávez KR, Howard RG (eds) Text + field: innovations in rhetorical method. Pennsylvania State University Press, University Park, PA, p 231
MedSafe (2008a) Eltroxin formulation change—monitor patients and adjust dosing if necessary. Available from: http://www.medsafe.govt.nz/hot/alerts/Eltroxin.asp. Accessed Jun 26
MedSafe (2008b) Eltroxin: further information. Available from: http://www.medsafe.govt.nz/hot/media/media2008.asp#11Sept. Accessed Sept 11
MedSafe (2008c) MedSafe approves two additional levothyroxine products. Available from: http://www.medsafe.govt.nz/hot/media/media2008.asp#23Oct. Accessed Oct 23
Meloncon LK, Scott JB (2017) Methodologies for the rhetoric of health and medicine. Routledge, New York
Melville NA (2017) Side effects Skyrocket in France with levothyroxine reformulation. Medscape.com. Available from: https://www.medscape.com/viewarticle/886900. Accessed Oct 11
Mol A (2010) Actor-network theory: sensitive terms and enduring tensions. Kölner Zeitschrift für Soziologie und Sozialpsychologie Sonderh 50:253–269
Pétition (2017) Contre le nouveau Levothyrox dangereux pour les patients! Available from: https://www.mesopinions.com/petition/sante/contre-nouveau-levothyrox-dangereux-patients/31185
Petryna A (2009) When experiments travel: Clinical trials and the global search for human subjects. Princeton University Press, Princeton, pp 1–258
Reed AR (2016) Building on bibliography: toward useful categorization of research in rhetorics of health and medicine. J Tech Writ Commun 48(2):1–24
Rothstein H, Huber M, Gaskell G (2006) A theory of risk colonization: the spiralling regulatory logics of societal and institutional risk. Econ Soc. 35(1):91–112
Segal JZ (2005) Health and rhetoric of medicine. In: SAGE handbook of rhetorical studies. SAGE, Thousand Oaks
Segal JZ (2018) Sex, drugs, and rhetoric: the case of flibanserin for 'female sexual dysfunction. Soc Stud Sci. 48(4):459–482
Sismondo S (2010) An introduction to science and technology studies. Wiley, New York, p 244
Sismondo S, Greene JA (2015) The Pharmaceutical Studies Reader. Wiley, Malden, p 296
Teston C (2017) Bodies in flux: scientific methods for negotiating medical uncertainty. University of Chicago Press, Chicago
Teston CB, Graham SS, Baldwinson R, Li A, Swift J (2014) Public voices in pharmaceutical deliberations: negotiating "clinical benefit" in the FDA's Avastin hearing. J Med Humanit 35(2):149–170
Toulmin SE (2003) The uses of argument. Cambridge University Press, Cambridge, p 247
Williams SJ, Martin P, Gabe J (2011) The pharmaceuticalisation of society? A framework for analysis. Sociol Health Illn. 33(5):710–725
Wynne B (2016) Ghosts of the machine: publics, meanings and social science in a time of expert dogma and denial. In: Chilvers J, Kearnes M (eds) Remaking participation: science, environment and emergent publics. Routledge, New York

Media Science and Practice

10

Glen J. Nowak and Michael A. Cacciatore

Abstract

Given their influence and visibility, understanding how news media cover topics involving medicines and how they provide information to their target audiences is essential when it comes to medicinal product risk communication research. While information about health and medicine are found in entertainment and social media, this chapter introduces media science with a focus, albeit not exclusively, on journalist-based news media. It presents an overview of relevant theories as well as methods that academics, government agencies, professional societies and pharmaceutical companies can use to understand communication flows in the media and their potential effects. Particularly, it reviews in more depth, the methodological aspects of content analyses as well as discusses research approaches, including those involving journalists, which could be used to guide or strengthen medicinal product risk communication. Media science-based research can inform the preparations of communication strategies and materials; and studying what is actually happening in the news media is relevant to establishing communication models and evaluating communication interventions in a rapidly changing media landscape.

G. J. Nowak (✉) · M. A. Cacciatore
Grady College of Journalism and Mass Communication, Grady College Center for Health and Risk Communication, Athens, GA, USA
e-mail: gnowak@uga.edu

© Springer Nature Singapore Pte Ltd. 2020

P. Bahri (ed.), *Communicating about Risks and Safe Use of Medicines*,
https://doi.org/10.1007/978-981-15-3013-5_10

10.1 The Discipline of Media Science and Practice: Scope, Theories and Principles

People around the world get much information about medicines, including vaccines, from a wide array of media. Every day, news stories, websites, advertising and education campaigns, social media posts, and entertainment programmes provide information about the availability, benefits, and risks of medicinal products to the general public, current and prospective patients, and healthcare professionals. With so much health information available from so many sources, it is quite challenging for patients and healthcare professionals to discern valid and relevant information from unreliable information, and for government agencies, pharmaceutical companies, and others to use journalist or news media-based communication as a channel to provide information on the effective and safe use of medicines. The communication about combined hormonal contraceptives (see Chap. 2), rofecoxib (see Chap. 3), and measles-mumps-rubella (MMR) vaccines (see Chap. 1) are recent prominent examples in this respect. Much behaviour and social science research indicates that it is rarely the case that simply providing more information, highlighting statistics and data, or refuting misinformation will improve consumers' perceptions and knowledge or influence their intentions and behaviours with respect to medicinal products (Larson 2016; Nyhan et al. 2014; Reyna 2008). Rather, efforts to improve public, patient, healthcare professional, and journalists' perceptions and knowledge, and appropriate patient use behaviours or acceptance of medicinal products require a strong understanding of media science and best practices (Nowak et al. 2015). Such efforts also require a willingness to make the necessary time and resources investments for conducting research or applying research findings and derived best practices (Nowak et al. 2015; Bahri 2010; Nowak et al. 2017).

The media environment for the companies that provide medicinal products, including vaccines, and the government agencies and healthcare professional societies that offer recommendations and advice regarding the use of those products, is usually complex, dynamic, and challenging. Countries also vary when it comes to the laws and regulations that affect what can be communicated and how. As of 2018, the United States (US) and New Zealand, for example, are the only countries that allow direct-to-consumer advertising for prescription medicines in the media. However, regardless of where one is in the world, information on the benefits, risks, and safe use of medicinal products is most effectively transmitted to the public, patients, and healthcare professionals when guided by research and best practices from communication science, of which media science is a major sub-discipline. As such, this chapter's primary focus is on journalist or news media science and practice considerations, particularly those related to objectives, strategy, research, and evaluation.

Therefore, this chapter (1) provides an overview of theories and principles related to news media interests or journalists' coverage of medicinal products; (2) describes research methods and findings related to identifying the news media and information preferences of audiences; (3) gives directions and examples for how to assess or gauge the impact of news media efforts and content on target audiences and public opinion; and (4) offers guidance and recommendations for improving and using news media-related research to provide information about medicinal products to public and healthcare professional audiences. A distinguishing characteristic of journalist or news media communication channels is that the placement, presentation, tone, and final content of news stories and articles are determined by third parties, such as the journalists and their editors, rather than a purchase of media time or space (e.g. advertising) that ensures when, where, and how the information will appear. As such, trust is a key component; journalists must trust the people and organisations providing them information, and the people and organisations must trust that journalists will use or convey the information in a fair, accurate, and appropriate manner.

10.1.1 Terminology

It is important to first recognise the words "media" and "science" have multiple meanings, and their definitions have implications when it comes to doing medicinal product benefit–risk communication as well as undertaking research to inform or evaluate such communication efforts.

The Term "Media"

For instance, at its broadest, the term "media" can refer to the wide array of communication channels available or used to disseminate materials, information, and messages. This would encompass everything from mass media (e.g. television, radio, national newspapers, general interest magazines) to targeted media (e.g. local or community-based television, radio, newspapers, special interest magazines) to websites (e.g. news organisation sites, advocacy group sites) to social media (e.g. Twitter, Facebook) to place-based media (e.g. billboards, interactive content made available on tablet computers, or leaflets placed in physician offices or clinics), and include entertainment and educational media along with news media. More narrowly, the term media can be used to primarily refer to news media outlets and sources; that is, television, radio, print, websites, and other channels where news articles, stories, and content primarily independently produced by journalists and reporters (i.e. a journalist who gathers information from multiple sources and does own research in this respect) is made available. News-related definitions of media typically mean primary control of information, including its use and dissemination, lies with news organisations and external parties such as publishers, journalists, and editors rather than with the entity producing or providing the medicinal product or service or an organisation putting forward recommendations regarding its use.

For government agencies, healthcare professional organisations, and companies that manufacture and provide medicinal products, the domain of news media strategies and tactics encompasses media advocacy and outreach, media news or press releases and advisories that seek to achieve or "earn" journalist attention, donated media (e.g. public service announcements), entertainment-education efforts where health information is embedded in entertainment programming or shows, issues management, public affairs, and news media response (e.g. responding to news media inquiries) (duPre 2017; Hicks and Nichols 2017). "Earned media" refers to medical product attention or mentions in news media stories as well as positive reviews, reposts, or recommendations within news stories that were "earned" by successful proactive outreach to journalists and news media content writers, typically done by appealing to or piquing their interest in a product, recommendation, or new development (Parvanta et al. 2018). Oftentimes, public relations firms are hired for their expertise in undertaking such efforts.

The Term "Science"

Similarly, definitions of the word "science" vary in terms of breadth and scope. In the health and medical fields, the term refers to objective, systematic, and theory-based approaches to studying phenomena and discovering results that will be generalisable across populations, time, and places. Experimental designs, randomised control trials, and dose–response approaches are common research methods.

The Term "Media Science"

Communication and media science, systematic, and theory-based, but given the varied, complex, and dynamic nature of media, audiences, and messages, randomised control trials and dose–response approaches are often not used or possible and generalisability is typically context and/or audience dependent. In addition, much media practice, especially those related to news media, is informed or assessed using interviews and focus groups with audience or potential audience members, qualitative and quantitative content analyses, and judgments regarding actual or potential media and message exposure. As a result, it is important to recognise that "media science" has important differences from health and medical science in terms of assumptions, methods, and generalisability. Much learning in the media world is based on qualitative research, surveys that measure global knowledge or beliefs regarding a health issue or medicinal product, and experience and judgments regarding the effects and effectiveness of media content. It also emanates from media and public relations practitioner experiences and case studies that have yielded many helpful insights into "best" or "effective" practices.

Given these definitions, this chapter highlights and describes news media-related research findings, examples, and methods that academics, government agencies, professional medical or health societies, and companies who provide medicinal products can use to inform their preparations of communications on benefits, risks, and appropriate use information to the general public, journalists, targeted sub-populations (e.g. the patients who currently use them), and healthcare professionals. News media outreach and advocacy, news media content (e.g. stories, articles), and education/information campaigns that involve earned or donated media time and space are the communication channels and tools of primary interest. In recent years, much has been learned from academic studies and professional practice regarding how news media channels inform, educate, and persuade people, including healthcare professionals, about the benefits, risks, and use of medicinal products.

10.1.2 Theories

As public relations practice illustrates, news media and public service or information campaigns have been, and can be, used to convey health and medical information in a variety of ways and with a wide range of results (Nowak et al. 2015; Schiavo 2014). Given the multidisciplinary nature of public and media relations, many theories and communication frameworks have guided news media planning, research, and evaluation (Parvanta et al. 2018; Schiavo 2014; Lattimore et al. 2012), including:

Systems Theory

Systems theory focuses on the communication structure that guides an organisation in achieving its organisational goals. According to this theory, every organisation is part of a system with three components: the organisation, its publics, and its goals. Organisations with open systems use news media, primarily through public relations efforts, to engage with key stakeholders, such as government agencies, customers, and non-governmental organisations and advocacy groups as well as journalists. When it comes to communicating about medicinal products through the news media, systems theory highlights the need for organisations to understand the media environment (e.g. who are the key media outlets and journalists), develop sound relationships with key stakeholders and news media that are most influential, and recognise that success often involves knowing and accounting for the relationship needs of the major parties. For example, news media and journalists not only need information about medicinal products, they usually favour information related to new developments and need to be able to present the information as part of audience-relevant and interesting stories.

Situational Theory

Situational theory states that not all stakeholders or people in stakeholder groups are equally interested in or likely to communicate with an organisation. Instead, organisations using public relations or media outreach can more effectively manage communications by identifying where specific publics or people are with respect to the topic or issue (e.g. actively engaged and seeking information versus passive receivers of information). Situational theory is used when organisations identify stakeholder and/or news media awareness, perceptions/beliefs, and level of involvement or interest in an issue as integral to developing a communications strategy or effort. In the case of medicinal products, this theory highlights the need for research that identifies the likely interest and knowledge levels of various news media outlets, journalists, and media audiences and whether or how differences affect their questions and concerns regarding medicines or medicine-related recommendations. Those who are highly interested in or sceptical about a medicinal product typically want and need greater information about benefits, risks, and appropriate use while communication efforts directed at those for whom the product is relevant but who are currently less involved, will need information that will pique their interest.

Diffusion Theory, Also Called Diffusion of Innovation Theory
Diffusion theory focuses on how people process and accept new ideas, practices, or offerings, such as a new vaccine or therapeutic. It posits that people accept a new recommendation, product, or service, particularly one that is distinct from those presently available, only after going through five discrete steps: awareness (e.g. exposure to a message or information about the new offering); interest (e.g. they pay attention to the message or information); evaluation (e.g. they consider the message or information and use it to assess the usefulness or relevance of the new offering); trial (e.g. they discuss the new offering with others or try a sample); and adoption (e.g. they act or behave accordingly). The theory also identifies and defines five subgroups of people, based on their willingness to accept and adopt innovations: innovators, early adopters, early majority, late majority, and laggards. Early adopters usually decide faster than those in other groups to adopt new ideas, practices, or offerings, and thus can serve as role models and endorsers. News media stories and content are often especially helpful in creating awareness and interest that can facilitate trial by others. Journalists are also often interested in doing stories on people who try new products, including medicinal products, for stories that describe an individual's experiences. Further, news stories highlighting early adopters and their experiences can surface questions and concerns that journalists and others will likely ask as the product or recommendation increases in visibility; and facilitate or inhibit adoption by others (e.g. through endorsements or critiques).

Social Learning Theory
Social learning theory posits that people learn and maintain behaviours, beliefs, and attitudes by observing others, including how those others process and respond to information in the media. Albert Bandura, the social psychologist who developed social learning theory in the 1960s and 1970s, noted that people are more likely to adopt beliefs and behaviours if they notice others are getting positive attention or recognition (Bandura 1977; 1986), both of which can happen with media attention and coverage. Conversely, negative news media attention and stories can discourage or inhibit adoption or maintenance of a belief or behaviour. Social learning theory can be especially relevant when it comes to new health recommendations or new medicinal products, with endorsements and use by prominent or similar others often helpful in fostering adoption and appropriate use.

Agenda Setting Theory
Agenda setting theory recognises that news and other media have the ability to influence the importance of a topic or item on the public or targeted audience's "agenda"; that is, whether and how much individuals pay attention to it and make it a priority. In the case of medicinal products, new treatments or vaccines will likely attract more healthcare professional and prospective patient interest if the disease or condition involved is one that has significant public awareness and media attention. Agenda setting theory also brings forth the notion that while the news media often are unsuccessful in terms of telling people what to think, they are frequently successful in telling them what to think and talk *about, including what issues and*

concerns are important. In the case of health and medicine, media attention and coverage can influence whether people think about the need, benefits, and safety of new or recommended medicines and vaccines as well as what they believe about the disease, health condition involved (e.g. do they believe people like themselves are susceptible), and the benefits and risks involved.

Framing Theory

Framing theory puts the focus on *how the* news media *package and present information to the public or targeted audiences (e.g. prospective patients and healthcare professionals).* According to this theory, how journalists and the news media select and present information and material (i.e. the "frames" used) affects the meaning and interpretation by media audiences; that is, it intentionally or indirectly seeks to influence how they think about the issue. In some cases, media outlets and journalists purposely use framing to influence interpretation and beliefs, while in other cases, the frame that is used is the one deemed most appropriate. By emphasising one angle over another or mentioning some interpretations and ignoring others (e.g. through the sources quoted and the quotes used), media stories can encourage or discourage certain interpretations (e.g. whether a medicinal product is safe or not). The media frames can arise from conscious decisions by journalists and editors regarding what information to include and emphasise, from the metaphors and examples used in a media story, from a media outlet or journalist's preference or bias for science-based or "natural" medicine, or from the culture in which the news media operate (e.g. cultures grounded in individualism will favour different frames than cultures grounded in collectivism). Also numerical frames (e.g. either focusing on the minority or majority of experiencing or not an event) can be highly influential on the formation of preferences.

10.1.3 Principles of Communication Through the Media

There are a number of professional experience and evidence-based principles that increase the likelihood of effectiveness and success in using news media to communicate and convey information about medicinal products to the general public, the individuals who are using the product or are potential users, or healthcare professionals, such as those would be recommending a medicine or vaccine or answering questions about it. These are important to understand for media and communication research, as they affect decisions regarding research goals and objectives, formulation of hypotheses, research designs and methods, and expectations regarding whether one's media-related efforts are likely to have discernible effects or impact. Primary among these are:

- *Identify the goal or purpose for seeking or responding to news media attention related to a medicinal product.* To effectively do communication research, one needs to know what outcomes are being sought so that appropriate measures of message framing, information content, and outcomes are used. This is essential for communication research designed to inform communication campaigns and messaging as well as communication research designed to assess or evaluate communication outcomes. There are many possible media communication goals or purposes. They include increasing awareness or visibility for a new or forthcoming medicinal product; increasing understanding of a safe use recommendation among potential users, healthcare professionals, or journalists; creating or altering frames of how journalists, the general public, or others think about a medicinal product or use recommendation; informing journalists, current or prospective users, and/or healthcare professionals about a product's benefits, risks, and/or appropriate use; influencing perceptions and mitigating safety-related concerns, including by providing context; and fostering appropriate product use.

- *Newsworthiness and audience relevance matter.* Information provided to journalists and news media outlets usually has to meet their inclusion criteria before they will further consider or use it as the basis of a story or as part of a story. Their criteria favour information that is new, unique, or relatively unusual, would be of interest or relevance to many in the media outlet's audience, and timely. In addition, most news media package and present information in the form of stories, with the most desirable stories being ones that involve conflict, controversy, confrontation, unexpected or breakthrough developments, and human interest. Proactive use of these criteria increases the likelihood of attracting journalist or news media interest to doing a story related to or involving a medicinal product. If media interest emanates independent of an organisation's efforts, these criteria can help in preparing for journalist interviews and preparing for the story, particularly in cases where the news media focus encompasses disagreement among health and science experts. In many countries, it is often the case that news media and journalists believe it is their job duty and mandate (e.g. as the fourth component of democracy) to question the claims of authorities, including healthcare professionals and public health/regulatory agencies, give visibility to those with concerns or different perspectives about medicines, or report on the conflicts and controversy more so than the benefits of a medicinal product, even when a consensus exists that the benefits far outweigh the risks.
- *There are many ways to seek news media attention, but message content primarily determines success.* Government agencies, professional health and medical organisations, and companies that provide medicinal products often have many tools for communicating with news media and the public. These include press/media releases, opinion-editorial columns ("op-eds"), letters-to-the media, video news releases, public service announcements, podcasts, online news websites, and direct outreach to individual journalists. Often, success, as measured in terms of journalist, media, or public interest and use, is contingent upon having content that is relevant, timely, interesting, and addresses important health and medical issues or questions. Media news releases, for instance, need helpful quotes that convey key points in relatively short, understandable, and interesting ways. Research can be used to identify the types of content or message framing that would most interest news media as well to evaluate whether news media

stories included the content and frames put forward by medicinal product companies or government agencies (e.g. in press releases or interviews).

- *News media outreach and engagement are important but have notable limitations.* When developing communicating plans for medicinal products, it is often necessary to assess and supplement news media-related efforts because news media and journalists may not see or use a media release (e.g. do a news story); some topics and products may be of greater interest to media outlets and journalists; information provided to news media may not be used or may be placed into a different context; and news media and journalists often use information from other sources, including to present divergent views (Lundgren and McMakin 2013; Rickard et al. 2013; US Food and Drug Administration 2011).

10.2 Research Approaches and Methods

10.2.1 Categories of Media Science Communication Research

Three major categories of research are important to media communication: formative research, message and material testing research, and evaluative research.

Formative Research

Formative research occurs first and is concerned with building an in-depth understanding of the problem or issue that needs addressing, setting the stage for a successful communication or media strategy, and guiding the development of news media plans and messages (e.g. by learning what information healthcare professionals or targeted audiences are most interested in knowing more about). Formative research can be used to inform decisions regarding which news media outlets or journalists to focus on, how to frame and present messages, and which questions or concerns to place a priority on when developing materials for healthcare professionals, prospective patients, or media interviews (Wilcox et al. 2015). During the formative research stage, a major focus is on better understanding the targeted audiences, including their current knowledge and beliefs about a disease or medical condition, their attitudes and beliefs toward the medicinal product or product use recommendation, how they make decisions regarding medicinal products, the communication channels they trust and use for health information, and how they perceive the benefits and risks associated with a medical condition and related medicinal products.

In the formative communication stage, the research team might also need to understand the legislative or policy environment they will be communicating within (see Chap. 15) as well as the competitive landscape for the product or service. This may mean that formative research, such as in-depth interviews or focus groups (see Chap. 8), may need to involve policymakers or key stakeholders as participants, as well as consumers. It may also involve reviewing articles published in both academic and non-academic professional publications (e.g. print or internet-based magazines or newsletters which provide stories, ideas, products, or services to people in a specific industry or type of business, such as *Pharmacy Today*) for insights, including relevant research findings. Regardless of who the participants represent, formative research needs to surface information and insights that can help medicinal product companies, government agencies, or public health officials more effectively communicate the value, benefits, risks, and appropriate usage of a medical product to (1) the healthcare professionals involved in recommending and administering it; (2) the people or patients who would benefit from using it; and (3) news media and journalists who may do stories.

Materials and Message Testing Research

Once the initial communication materials, including media messages, have been drafted, researchers move into the testing phase of research. As the name suggests, this phase focuses on materials testing for the messages and communication materials that have emerged from earlier formative research. This might include the testing of specific "frames" or ways of presenting information to different target audiences. Often, testing research is done to gauge whether it would be more effective to use a positive frame (e.g. an emphasis on the benefits gained from product use) or a negative frame (e.g. the harm caused by a health condition). Qualitative research is generally privileged at this stage, with focus groups offering a particularly attractive option for researchers. Other options are available, however, including survey questionnaires, one-on-one personal interviews, and experiments (Nicols 2017). The testing phase typically focuses on four key attributes related to the message or materials that have been developed (Nicols 2017):

- *Clarity*: The first is a focus on clarity and calls to action. Regardless of the methodology employed (focus groups, surveys, experiments, interviews, etc.), participants at this stage are asked to evaluate the overall clarity of the messages being communicated. In doing so they may be asked how well they understood the information, to identify any problematic ideas or terminology in the materials, to identify, in their own words, the primary messages of the materials, or to describe what next steps they believe the materials are asking them to take (Lewis et al. 2016). The goal here is on increasing the likelihood the materials will be adequately understood by most members of the targeted audiences as well as journalists who may receive them as part of their information gathering and reporting efforts.
- *Appeal*: Next is a focus on the appeal of the messages (Nicols 2017). Here the research is focused on understanding respondents' sentiments as they relate to the information and major messages. Key questions include: Is the information personally relevant and appealing? Does the tone and information fill them with hope or despair? Do the messages produce feelings of powerlessness, control, or self-efficacy? Do the messages come across as believable and relatable? Would they want to continue viewing or otherwise interacting with the content?
- *Relevance*: Similarly, researchers must determine the personal relevance of their materials for those in the targeted audiences, including news media. To do so, they might ask participants whether and how the messages got their attention or what might be done to ensure this information would stand out in a crowded information environment. Respondents might also be asked about words or phrases that

should be added (or omitted) from the message to help it better speak to them on a personal level (Nicols 2017). Researchers must be careful about crafting messages that are too broad or narrow at this stage and should always be cognizant of how the information will be received by targeted audiences. In the case of journalists, for instance, would the information be considered newsworthy?

- *Formation of intent*: Finally, researchers should evaluate the potential behavioural outcomes on those receiving the messages. The focus here encompasses outcomes such as self-efficacy (e.g. perceived ability to do) and ease of compliance with the message's call to action. Respondents should be asked about any possible barriers to compliance, including what can be done to overcome such barriers. Likelihood scales for better understanding audience compliance might be especially effective for tapping into behavioural intent. A major challenge here, however, is that much formative communication research, particularly that involving message or material testing or related to behavioural intention, generally cannot be done with journalists, editors, or other key news media members who make decisions about news stories and content. Journalists and news media members usually do not and cannot participate because of organisational policies or professional standards and practices (Association of Health Care Journalists 2018). Most journalists and news media members purposely seek to be independent, and maintain independence, from companies and agencies seeking their attention, including those involved with medicinal products.

Chap. 12 on design science discusses testing methods further.

Evaluative Research
Once a communication effort, such as a media campaign to launch a new medicinal product, has run its course, evaluative research can be used to assess outcomes and effectiveness. Such research efforts seek to collect information that can be used to determine if key communication objectives were met and might also be used to improve future communication efforts. Evaluative research is generally concerned with two key areas of focus: process measures (a.k.a., measures of potential exposure to information) and outcome measures (a.k.a., measures of knowledge, awareness, attitudes, and actions) (Nicols 2017).

Evaluation of Exposure to Information
Measures of potential media exposure are easiest to collect (Wilcox et al. 2015). These might focus on broad indicators of news media success, such as whether the information appeared in news media stories, how many and which news media outlets carried stories about the medicinal product, the number of people reached by the media outlets in which the information appeared, or the number of visitors to a news media website where the information appeared. These assessments may also involve content analysing all the media coverage or selected stories to identify the tone, frames, and content used. For instance, trained coders may be asked to analyse the stories or articles that appeared in key media outlets (e.g. major newspapers or blogs) to determine what percentage of the overall content was favourable, unfavourable, or neutral in tone toward the organisation, the product, or service.

Online tools have emerged as particularly important for studying news in the internet as well as identifying and understanding social media impacts of news media stories. These tools track metrics like click-through rates (e.g. how many people used the website link included in a tweet or press release), page visits, top traffic sources, engagement duration (e.g. how long audience members spent on specific pages), activity ratios (e.g. the proportion of active to passive members on your web or Facebook pages), the virality of content and conversion rates (e.g. turning visitors who went to a webpage into consumers of a product or service). Organisations can also track increases in Twitter followers or Facebook friends, as well as the number of "likes", "retweets", or "shares" that different posts received (Wilcox et al. 2015).

While social media and audience reach/exposure metrics are helpful for getting a sense of how many people may have seen a story or specific types of information or what appeared in media stories, they generally fail to provide information into audience responses to a news media story or the messages found in news stories. Mere exposure to a news media story does not equate to individuals' reading or viewing the story nor does it mean that those who read or viewed the story gave much thought or consideration to the information. Measures of reach, exposure, or media content also do not provide any information related to attitudes, beliefs, or intentions among audiences. For instance, even a flattering blog post or news article about a pharmaceutical company or medicinal product might generate sceptical or negative reactions among many of those who saw it, resulting in distrust of the information and a net negative change in attitude toward the company or product.

Evaluation of Communication Impact

The second type of evaluative research thus aims to go beyond measures of reach and exposure and obtain information about effects (e.g. what happened?) and effectiveness (e.g. did what we want to happen occur?). These types of media studies use methods and measures to discern impact on outcomes such as awareness, knowledge gain, shifts in attitudes, and ultimately, behaviour (or future behavioural intentions) (Nicols 2017). Unlike with process measures, evaluative research seeks to obtain information on whether and how audiences processed the information that was communicated rather than speculating on such impacts. However, given the volume and dynamic nature of news media stories, it is often very difficult to identify and discern the effects of specific news media content on readers or viewers. If one can assume that large numbers of people will be exposed to, and thus potentially be aware of, news media content related to a medicinal product, pre-post surveys can be used to compare the knowledge and attitudes of those who recall exposure versus those who do not.

10.2.2 Overview of Methods

Media science applies a range of methods, many emanating from the broader social sciences, to which communication and media science belongs. As noted, the principle research methods used in media science are focus groups and interviews; surveys; experiments; and news media content analysis.

While most of these methods are presented in detail and with references to further methodological guidance in Chap. 8 dedicated to the social sciences, the next section of this chapter describes and exemplifies their application and utility for the specific objectives of media research. In addition, as the news media contribute to generating public knowledge and sentiments, methods for analysing public sentiments are also relevant to studying the effects of the media, and this is also reflected in Chap. 11 on social media research. The cited studies that follow in this chapter on media science and practice have been chosen as recent examples of how a given research methodology has been employed in the published international research focusing on medicinal product risk communication. It is, of course, impossible to have a full knowledge of how these methodologies are being employed by private organisations like pharmaceutical companies, for instance, but references to the published research provide a reasonable proxy for how private organisations are likely exploring similar issues. We discuss methodologies in approximate chronological order, beginning with those methods most often employed in the early formative and testing phases of research before ending with those more commonly associated with evaluative approaches.

10.3 Utility of Applied Methods for Researching Medicinal Product Risk Communication

10.3.1 Focus Group and Interview Studies

Focus groups and interviews are qualitative research methods and especially well-suited for both formative and testing research. Both can be quickly and inexpensively conducted, provided the organisation has access to key stakeholders and members of targeted audiences. In the case of media research, focus group discussions with members of targeted patient audiences can provide insights into current knowledge and beliefs regarding the medicinal product or product category, while one-on-one interviews with healthcare professionals are often used to identify their beliefs and communication needs. Both methods allow for a detailed understanding of audience thoughts, with focus groups allowing for such an understanding in a social setting where participants can respond to the thoughts of others in the room. The discussion can provide an expanded understanding of how audiences might view messages (Wimmer and Dominick 2011). The nature of these data collection methods also means that the interviewer or moderator can ask follow-up questions to clarify participant comments or to explore further topics and issues arising from participant comments but not previously known to be significant (Wimmer and Dominick 2011).

At the same time, the information learned from interviews and focus groups is not generalisable to a larger population, in part because the methods typically rely upon very small convenience samples of respondents. Each also brings the need for skill in conducting interviews and guiding discussions. For example, it can be difficult to create an environment where participants feel comfortable sharing their thoughts. Shyness or a reluctance to express a minority viewpoint is oftentimes compounded in social settings (Wimmer and Dominick 2011). Extroverts might also monopolise the conversation in a focus group setting, reducing the researcher's ability to gain the perspective of all participants. A skilled and trained moderator or interviewer is therefore a necessity (Wimmer and Dominick 2011).

It is likely that companies and the firms they hire to implement marketing and communication campaigns for medicines and pharmaceuticals have learned much about the effects and effectiveness of their media efforts and news stories through interviews and focus groups. However, such entities do not generally make their research findings public. However, academics are often involved in formative communication studies. One recent study in the US, for example, used focus group discussions to gain insights into how mothers and caregivers who were hesitant about recommended childhood vaccinations would respond to short educational videos and infographics designed to show the benefits of vaccines were significantly greater than the risks (Mendel-Van Alstyne et al. 2017). After viewing, participants were asked how understandable and appealing the materials were, and whether the key messages made them more positive and confident about childhood vaccinations. The authors found evidence that videos were better received than infographics, and that most participants found the creative attempts to explain the value of vaccines worthwhile. In addition, the study indicated some materials resonated better with some participants than others, suggesting a portfolio of vaccine information materials would likely be needed rather than a single video or infographic.

Researchers in the Netherlands examined whether media use resulted in patients being more active communicators with their doctors during medical consultations, and whether differences existed between native Dutch and Turkish-Dutch patients (Schinkel et al. 2015). In addition, the study assessed the relationship between patient participation and communication outcomes. A total of 191 patients participated in the study, which involved pre- and post-consultation questionnaires assessing their information seeking as well as the recording and content analysis of 120 patient-general practitioner (GP) consultation. Native Dutch patients were less likely to have consulted traditional media sources (e.g. books, newspapers, magazines, radio, TV) and participated to a greater extent during the consultations (e.g. asked more questions) than Turkish-Dutch patients of similar educational levels. The Turkish-Dutch patients used a wider variety of media in their search for health information and used these sources more frequently than native Dutch patients.

10.3.2 Surveys

Surveys, when properly designed and administered, can overcome the generalisability issues that limit the value of interviews and focus group research (Wimmer and Dominick 2011; Babbie 2007; Frey et al. 2000), making them potentially useful for all phases of research, particularly the formative and evaluative phases. In the formative phase, a well-designed and administered survey to a random selected sample of respondents in a target population can yield valuable insights for what information needs to be conveyed and how messages should be presented to the broader population. However, high-quality surveys can be expensive to implement. Careful attention must be paid to the wording of items and the order of response options as even seemingly minor changes in these areas can impact how audiences respond to a given question (Moy et al. 2001). Similarly, different survey methods (e.g. in-person, telephone, online) carry with them their own set of advantages and disadvantages with regards to issues like response rates, costs, the honesty of respondents, and the timeliness of the data collection. While there are differences across formats, surveys using random probability samples can be expensive to administer, with costs typically in the tens of thousands of US dollars (Wimmer and Dominick 2011; Babbie 2007; Frey et al. 2000) Further, the key advantage of generalisability is lost when non-probability samples—that is, samples where not every member of the population has a non-zero, known, and equal chance of being selected into the study—are utilised. Thus, the selection of respondents is critical and oftentimes requires outsourcing work to major public opinion or polling firms.

Surveys are also a research method that has been successfully used to learn more about how journalists consider and cover health-related topics, though much of this research involves US media. In one of the largest such studies, 468 reporters and editors representing 463 local and national broadcast and print media outlets in the US were surveyed to learn more about their educational and demographic backgrounds and how they initiate, prioritise, and develop health and medical news stories (Viswanath et al. 2008). They found 70% had a bachelor's degree and 19% had a master's degree, but only 8% were life science majors in college. The three primary sources of initial ideas for health and medical stories were "a person with whom the reporter is frequently in contact with", press conferences and press releases, and newswire items. The primary factors that determined whether an idea would become a story were potential for public impact, new information or development, supervisor/editor interest, and ability to provide a human angle. With respect to the latter, a 2013 study used a survey to gain insights into how journalists select the people and case examples used in medical news stories (Hinnant et al. 2013). They found reporters often sought and highlighted interesting, likeable people who were perceived to be similar to those in the media outlet's audience, with most journalists seeing inclusion of such sources as adding a needed human element that medical experts and government officials could not provide.

10.3.3 Experiments

Experiments can be particularly helpful at the testing and evaluative stages of research. Experiments are well-suited for assessing the effects and effectiveness of different variations in the wording, content, or creative presentation of a message or piece of communication. Attitudes and beliefs toward a medicinal product can be assessed before participants are randomly assigned to a message condition. Once the participants receive their assigned message they can be asked again to indicate their attitude and beliefs toward the product of interest. Researchers can then compare before and after responses to see whether message exposure changed attitudes or whether one presentation performed better than the rest. The condition or conditions producing the most favourable change in attitudes can then be selected for broader use. With advances in technology, messaging experiments can now be easily done using most online survey platforms, including those provided by Qualtrics, YouGov, GfK Knowledge Networks, and the National Opinion Research Center. The key advantage of experiments is control—specifically the ability to pinpoint the message or communication as the cause of any change in attitude by controlling for other confounding factors; however, most experiments rely on non-probability samples, making generalisability difficult (Wimmer and Dominick 2011; Babbie 2007; Frey et al. 2000).

Message testing experiments are particularly popular in health communication research. For example, experiments with United Kingdom (UK) participants were utilised to investigate the impacts of more or less personalised styles of information presentation when prescribing medicines. The study found that more personalised methods of information delivery were associated with higher reported satisfaction with the information and lower reported concerns about the likelihood of side effects or other risks to health (Berry et al. 2003). Researchers in Australia have developed a general framework for message design and testing that can be used to systematically guide the development and evaluation of persuasive health-related messages, including to inform media strategies (Lewis et al. 2016). The framework—the Step Approach to Message Design and Testing (SatMDT)—was developed to guide road safety health promotion efforts but is based on persuasion and health theories that have guided many health media and advertising campaigns.

From an outcomes perspective, an evaluative approach to message testing was, for example, taken concerning the issue of vaccinations (Nyhan et al. 2014). Looking at US parents' intentions to vaccinate children against measles-mumps-rubella (MMR), this study randomly assigned parents to receive one of four possible communication interventions that were currently being used to educate parents about MMR vaccine benefits and risks. Overall, the findings from the study were disheartening, with none of the educational materials increasing parents' intentions to vaccinate a child in the future. Some of the interventions even backfired in that they reduced parents' vaccination intention. The study does, however, illustrate that messaging success is not guaranteed and that message testing can also help identify messages or materials that may produce negative effects, including those designed to address safety fears or concerns.

10.3.4 Content Analyses

Content analysis is a common method for examining media coverage and public sentiment, particularly during the evaluative phase of research. Further, as the methodology is not dependent on direct interaction with members of the public, content analyses and media tracking have emerged as cost-effective proxies for public opinion. This approach can be as simple as compiling clippings of product mentions from major newspapers or magazines or it can be more sophisticated. For example, an analysis of the tone of conversation will require the creation of a codebook for identifying relevant content and for defining the key categories of interest. These categories might be arrived at inductively based on a close reading of media content, or deductively based on a broader theoretical understanding of the topic. Then, coders will need to be identified and trained to ensure they classify content in the appropriate categories of interest and to make certain the validity of the findings (for an overview of the content analysis methodology, see Krippendorff 2013). Depending on the outlets and timeline of interest, tools like LexisNexis may need to be purchased to gain access to content.

Traditional content analysis approaches are best suited for traditional media outlets, like newspapers, magazines, radio, and television. The sheer volume of content online makes human coding through traditional content analysis techniques difficult at best, and impossible for high media coverage events or products (Su et al. 2017). Many academic studies have used content analyses involving traditional news media outlets to examine how vaccines, particularly perceptions of benefits, risk, and safety are conveyed. One such study content analysed 1147 US newspaper stories involving mention of immunisation safety topics or issues from 1995 to 2005 (Hussain et al. 2011). The findings included most were news articles (81%) rather than editorials or opinion pieces, typically they were 500 words or less in length, and 72% were written because of a policy/programme or announcement about vaccines. Vaccine-safety concerns and vaccine policy were the most frequent topics, with the main topic in 20% of the stories being vaccines are safe. More recently, a number of media content analyses have examined Human Papillomavirus (HPV) vaccine and immunisation recommendation news stories, for example, in the US, the UK, and worldwide (Bahri et al. 2017; Casciotti et al. 2014; Hilton et al. 2010). Findings included that most news articles were prompted by research/scientific advancement or immunisation policy actions, a large percentage of the stories highlighted HPV vaccine benefits, many stories highlighted conflicts and controversies regarding the vaccine or a vaccination recommendation (e.g. the vaccine would foster earlier sexual initiation), and personal testimonies were frequently used to convey messages.

10.4 Outlook: Relevance, Improvements and Future Potential

10.4.1 Future Research Contributions from the Media Science and Journalists

The news media landscape across the globe will likely continue to be dynamic and varied. As such, there are many needs and opportunities for additional studies that can inform, evaluate, and guide medicinal product information provision through news media channels. First, given the potential impact news media can have in generating initial interest and perceptions regarding medicinal products, particularly new offerings, further studies with journalists and editors are needed to gain insights into current practices and perspectives. As more news content moves online, and frequently encompasses greater use of video and graphics, it will be important to learn whether and how their story preferences and medicinal product content needs are affected. In addition, as medicine becomes more individualised and tailored, does this affect how journalists and editors report and write about the benefits, risks, and safety of medicinal products. Second, given the significant differences that exist across the globe with respect to news media outlets, journalist background, and news media independence from government, more studies are needed in a wider variety of places. At present, much of the published research involves high income countries, with relatively little known about low- and middle-income countries and how media in those places report and present medicinal benefit, risk, and safety information.

10.4.2 Medicinal Product Risk Communication Research in a Rapidly Changing Media Landscape

The Internet

With the growth of Web 2.0 technologies, companies like Crimson Hexagon and Radian6 have become popular for the so-called social media listening. These platforms offer medicinal product organisations and government health agencies the ability to track social media discussions about products, the organisations who manufacture and market them, and health recommendations, including assessments of the tone of online postings and conversation, levels of audience engagement, key influencers, and the timeline of postings and discussions. These platforms generally work by conducting a census of all content that researchers identify via a keyword search. Companies like Crimson Hexagon and Radian6 work with social media companies to ensure complete access to publicly available content (Su et al. 2017). Many, if not most public relations and advertising firms employ some form of social media listening and analytics for their clients. Methods using social media as a data source for medicinal product risk communication are covered in greater depth in the next Chap. 11.

Virtual and Augmented Realities

In addition to advances in social media, the technologies of virtual and augmented realities are emerging as promising areas of research for communication and media science scholars, including those working in areas of health and medicines. The promise of being able to engage audiences by exposing them to simulated scenarios involving illnesses or diseases without physical exposure to any actual or "real world" danger is viewed as an exciting frontier for health and medicinal communication. Such technologies could also be used to help journalists better understand how vaccines and therapeutics work or how their safety was established. While there remains much to learn in these spaces, the early evidence suggests that there is great promise in providing medical and health-related information to individuals via virtual and augmented realities, with more immersive environments often associated with greater retention of message information, better understanding of key concepts, and a stronger likelihood of following prescribed behaviours. It will be interesting to see how fully and with what strategies health and medicinal product organisations and government health agencies embrace these new communication technologies.

Conclusions

- Medicines and vaccines are subject to reports in the news media, like print, television, radio, and internet-based media, and in some jurisdictions are also advertised by manufacturers in such media; as such the news media are an important source of information to the public, patients, people who should or may benefit from using a medicinal product, and healthcare professionals.
- Media science-based research makes an essential contribution to medicinal product risk communication, in particular, for informing news media communication strategies, optimising interactions with journalists and news media outlets, and evaluating the outcomes of news media stories and content.
- Relevant theories underpinning media science-based research come primarily from the literatures in communication, psychology, and sociology. These include systems theory, situational theory, diffusion theory, social learning theory, agenda setting theory, and framing theory.
- Methods applied include both qualitative and quantitative approaches, ranging from one-on-one interviews to large scale tracking of traditional and social media content and product mentions. While the published literature remains a rich source for understanding the effectiveness of communication, data is not frequently shared by private organisations.
- Future work on the communication of medicinal product risk information is likely to focus heavily on the information that can be gleaned from social media discussions as well as traditional news media analyses.
- Future research related to medicinal product risk information would benefit from additional studies involving journalists, including those in a broader array of countries, as well as assessing the potential value of virtual and augmented realities as methods for providing benefit, risk, and safety information to different audiences.

References

Association of Health Care Journalists (2018) Statement of principles of the Association of Health Care Journalists. https://healthjournalism.org/secondarypage-details.php?id=56. Accessed 6 July 2018

Babbie E (2007) The practice of social research, 11th edn. Thomson Wadsworth, Belmont, CA

Bahri P (2010) Public pharmacovigilance communication: a process calling for evidence-based objective driven strategies. Drug Saf 33(12):1065–1079

Bahri P, Fogd J, Morales D, Kurz X, ADVANCE Consortium (2017) Application of real-time global media monitoring and 'derived questions' for enhancing communication by regulatory bodies: the case of human papillomavirus vaccines. BMC Med 15:91

Bandura A (1977) Self-efficacy: toward a unifying theory of behavioral change. Psychol Rev 84:191–215

Bandura A (1986) Social foundations of thought and action: a social cognitive theory. Prentice-Hall, Upper Saddle River

Berry DC, Michas IC, Bersellini E (2003) Communicating information about medication: the benefits of making it personal. Psychol Health 18(1):127–139

Casciotti DM, Smith KC, Klassen AC (2014) Topics associated with conflict in print news coverage of the HPV vaccine during 2005 to 2009. Hum Vaccin Immunother 10(12):3466–3474

duPre A (2017) Communicating about health: current issues and perspectives, 5th edn. Oxford University Press, New York

Frey LR, Botan CH, Kreps GL (2000) Investigating communication: an introduction to research methods, 2nd edn. Allyn & Bacon, Needham Heights

Hicks NJ, Nichols CM (2017) Health industry communication: new media, new methods, new message, 2nd edn. Jones & Bartlett Learning, Burlington

Hilton S, Hunt K, Langan M, Bedford H, Petticrew M (2010) Newsprint media representations of the introduction of the HPV vaccination programme for cervical cancer in the U.K. (2005–2008). Soc Sci Med 70(6):942–950

Hinnant A, Len-Rios ME, Young R (2013) Journalistic use of exemplars to humanize health news. Journal Stud 14(4):539–554

Hussain H, Omer SB, Manganello JA, Kromm EE et al (2011) Immunization safety in US print media. Pediatrics 127:S100–S106

Krippendorff K (2013) Content analysis: an introduction to its methodology, 3rd edn. Sage, Thousand Oaks

Larson HJ (2016) Vaccine trust and the limits of information. Science 353(6305):1207–1208

Lattimore D, Baskin O, Heiman S, Toth E (2012) Public relations: the profession and the practice, 4th edn. McGraw-Hill Education, Columbus

Lewis I, Watson B, White KM (2016) The Step approach to Message Design and Testing (SatMDT): a conceptual framework to guide the development and evaluation of persuasive health messages. Accid Anal Prev 97:309–314

Lundgren RE, McMakin AH (2013) Risk communication: a handbook for communicating environmental, safety, and health risks, 5th edn. Wiley, Hoboken

Mendel-Van Alstyne JA, Nowak GJ, Aikin AL (2017) What is 'confidence' and what could affect it? A qualitative study of mothers who are hesitant about vaccines. Vaccine. https://doi.org/10.1016/j.vaccine.2017.09.007

Moy P, Scheufele DA, Eveland WP, McLeod JM (2001) Support for the death penalty and rehabilitation: question order or communication effect? J Appl Soc Psychol 31(11):2230–2255

Nicols CM (2017) The communication planning process. In: Hicks NJ, Nicols CM (eds) Health industry communication: new media, new methods, new message, 2nd edn. Jones & Bartlett Learning, Burlington, pp 53–86

Nowak GJ, Gellin BG, NE MD, Butler R, SAGE Working Group on Vaccine Hesitancy (2015) Addressing vaccine hesitancy: the potential value of commercial and social marketing principles and practices. Vaccine 33:4204–4211

Nowak GJ, Shen AK, Schwartz JL (2017) Using campaigns to improve perceptions of the value of adult vaccination in the United States: health communication considerations and insights. Vaccine 35:5543–5550

Nyhan B, Reifler J, Richey S, Freed GL (2014) Effective messages in vaccine promotion: a randomized trial. Pediatrics 133(4):1–8

Parvanta CF, Nelson DE, Harner RN (2018) Public health communication: critical tools and strategies. Jones & Bartlett Learning, Burlington

Reyna VF (2008) A theory of medical decision making and health: fuzzy trace theory. Med Decis Mak 28(6):850–865

Rickard LN, McComas KA, Clarke CE, Stedman RC, Decker DJ (2013) Exploring risk attenuation and crisis communication after a plague death in Grand Canyon. J Risk Res 16(2):145–167

Schiavo R (2014) Health communication: from theory to practice, 2nd edn. Jossey-Bass, San Francisco

Schinkel S, Van Weert JCM, Kester JAM, Smit EG, Schouten BC (2015) Does media use result in more active communicators? Differences between native Dutch and Turkish-Dutch patients in information-seeking behavior and participation during consultations with general practitioners. J Health Commun 20:910–919

Su LY-F, Cacciatore MA, Liang X, Brossard D, Scheufele DA, Xenos MA (2017) Analyzing public sentiments online: a new content analysis tool combining human- and computer-based coding. Inf Commun Soc 20(3):406–427. https://doi.org/10.1080/1369118X.2016.1182197

US Food and Drug Administration (2011) Communicating risks and benefits: an evidence-based user's guide. FDA, Washington, D.C. http://www.fda.gov/ScienceResearch/SpecialTopics/RiskCommunication/default.htm

Viswanath K, Blake KD, Meissner HI, Saiontz NG et al (2008) Occupational practices and the making of health news: a national survey of U.S. health and medical science journalists. J Health Commun 13:759–777

Wilcox DL, Cameron GT, Reber BH (2015) Public relations: strategies and tactics, 11th edn. Pearson, New York

Wimmer RD, Dominick JR (2011) Mass media research: an introduction. Wadsworth, Boston

Social Media Research

11

Nabarun Dasgupta, Carly Winokur, and Carrie Pierce

Abstract

The use of the social media by people around the globe is widespread. This chapter discusses the contribution which social media research can offer to pharmacovigilance and medicinal product risk communication research. While the use of the social media itself and the development of social media strategies are important topics for research, this chapter focusses on the methods of social media listening and crowdsourcing of information, and provides examples of their utility. It highlights opportunities, limitations, challenges as well as ethical and legal aspects that need to be addressed for future research.

N. Dasgupta (✉)
Eshelman School of Pharmacy and Injury Prevention Research Center,
University of North Carolina, Chapel Hill, NC, USA
e-mail: nab@unc.edu

C. Winokur · C. Pierce
Booz Allen Hamilton, McLean, VA, USA

© Springer Nature Singapore Pte Ltd. 2020

P. Bahri (ed.), *Communicating about Risks and Safe Use of Medicines*,
https://doi.org/10.1007/978-981-15-3013-5_11

11.1 The Discipline of Social Media Research: Scope, Theories and Principles

11.1.1 An Introduction to Social Media Research

The internet has had widespread uptake around the globe and offers opportunities and challenges for risk communication in safety of medicines. In 2015, there were 3.2 billion (International Telecommunication Union (ICU) 2015) internet users worldwide; 63% were from low- and middle-income countries (International Telecommunication Union (ICU) 2015). Even in least-developed countries, a significant number of people access the internet regularly, especially from handheld devices operating over cellular data networks. The internet is used for disseminating and accessing information via websites, electronic mail, purchasing goods, and engaging via social media. In 2015, nearly two-thirds of adults (65%) in the United States (US) used a social networking site. While the majority of these individuals were aged between 18 and 29, 35% of adults aged 65 and older were using social media (Perrin 2015).

11.1.1.1 Social Media Listening

Billions of people interacting with the internet, or being "online", on a daily basis generate traces of important information that can be aggregated and analysed for research purposes. The process of using social media to understand how consumers discuss specific topics in online spaces is known as social media listening (Powell et al. 2015). Typically, social media listening is a passive process for the social media users and has been used for commercial purposes, like marketing and retail. However, a large amount of daily discussions in social media pertains to health information and diseases, as well as biomedical and medical products that address these conditions (medicines, devices, vitamins, supplements, etc.) (Powell et al. 2015). Many of these health-related discussions are generated by patients, comprising a large corpus of free-text narratives that can be leveraged for health-specific research (Powell et al. 2015).

11.1.1.2 Crowdsourcing of Information

Crowdsourcing of information, on the other hand, is generally an active process whereby online participants are solicited for specific information. It may be defined as the systematic effort to collect information from a wide audience, particularly through online tools that can provide mutual benefits to participants and activity sponsors (Bahk et al. 2015).

In practice, both active and passive processes may be used within a single research project. For example, social media listening may be used to form hypotheses, which are then tested using crowdsourced data. Conversely, social media listening can be used post hoc to contextualise and make sense of unexpected crowdsourced information, such as jargon and acronyms.

Information from patients is traditionally captured through qualitative research or surveys, usually with a series of standardised questions (see Chap. 8). However, listening to the patient voice in this structured way may limit the scope of patients' responses and their willingness to discuss sensitive topics. In contrast, unstructured discussions acquired from online forums—particularly those dedicated to discussions regarding a specific therapeutic area or treatment—could provide a wealth of patient information that typically is not captured in traditional studies due to hearing directly from the patient. Metadata derived from posts and user account profiles can provide a more complete picture for research-related applications than relying solely on a single post, and has the possible benefit of painting a more comprehensive view of a patient's life than just based on a cross-sectional survey response.

The body of literature on digital health is expanding rapidly (Rothman et al. 2015). While the use of the social media and the development of social media strategies are important topics for research, in this chapter we narrow the focus. Our aim is to describe how to apply emerging tools of social media research—a new discipline under formation—to the post-authorisation safety surveillance of medicinal products and pharmacovigilance overall. This additionally includes the application to medicinal product risk communication research in particular, including for the purpose of planning and evaluation of communication interventions.

11.1.2 Pharmacovigilance, Risk Communication and the Social Media

Pharmacovigilance monitors a medicinal product to identify and assess adverse events that may occur in patients. Adverse events causally associated with a medicine (i.e. adverse reactions) pose a patient and public health problem. However, both rare and late reactions are difficult to uncover through clinical trials during the development process of a medicine because trials typically include a couple of thousand patients at maximum and are relatively short in duration compared to long-term medicines use in real life. For this reason, safety surveillance after product approval by the regulatory body and during use in healthcare is of critical importance to safeguarding the availability and development of pharmaceutical medicines. Legal obligations for pharmaceutical manufacturers and established practices during this post-authorisation phase refer to characterising, preventing, and minimising risks related to medicinal products. Fundamental to these pharmacovigilance processes are continuous exchange and (re)assessment of risk information. Many organisations currently use a combination of automated and manual processes to perform necessary pharmacovigilance duties, including with traditional individual case safety reports, i.e. reports of an adverse reaction suspected in a patient, that are submitted as the so-called spontaneous reports through national reporting systems. Harms related to medication errors or product quality concerns may also be reported depending on national definitions and requirements. Reports can be submitted via telephone, paper, email, fax, online forms, and mobile apps. Nowadays evidence from observational studies, in addition to spontaneous reports, is very important for further investigating safety concerns or proactively monitoring a medicine at the population level.

More recently, regulatory authorities and other stakeholders have recognised the importance of capturing the patient voice and data contribution for pharmacovigilance. As such, regulatory authorities in many countries recommend to patients to report adverse events they suspect with their medicines, and recommend testing of risk communication for patient comprehension, even asking for patient input on proposed risk minimisation/communication plans and strategies (Snipes 2015). In general, the patient voice has been established as an important addition to a variety of medical research initiatives (Smith and Benattia 2016). Patient-reported outcomes are now accepted in clinical trials, and there is a renewed focus on patient-reported outcomes derived from unstructured data in other types of research, such as comparative effectiveness (Peacock 2014).

Starting in 2011, questions about the future of social media and pharmacovigilance were raised by senior figures in the field (Edwards and Lindquist 2011). With the rise of social media usage, there is potential for social media to be incorporated into effective pharmacovigilance (PatientsLikeMe 2019), including risk communication, by manufacturers, regulators, and others involved. Social media can be perceived as a new data source to inform pharmacovigilance and risk communication. Nevertheless, the volume and concerns about tenuous causality give rise to legitimate concerns about muddling data from social media with vetted data from carefully honed pharmacovigilance information systems. Yet, the processes in place globally for pharmacovigilance information processing offer a potential framework for dealing with social media data. This will require a careful balance of human and machine tasks, tempered by vastly different concepts of privacy and collaboration.

This chapter provides an overview of how social media research may be used to augment current medicines safety surveillance and risk communication practices through case studies, discussion of its potential opportunities for benefits and limitations, ethical and legal concerns, as well as practical lessons learnt and future outlook. This includes a synopsis of the current public debate on the usefulness of social media research in pharmacovigilance, underpinned by examples. Many high-quality reviews of existing applications have been published recently (Rees et al. 2018; Convertino et al. 2018; Tricco et al. 2018; Wong et al. 2018; Demner-Fushman and Elhadad 2016; Golder et al. 2015; Lardon et al. 2015; Sloane et al. 2015; Sarker et al. 2015) and should be consulted for more in-depth discussion of topics like the merits of particular data sources and computational methods.

11.2 Research Approaches and Methods

11.2.1 Selection of Social Media Sites

For clinical trials and epidemiological studies, site selection is central to investigating causal inference from observed associations. Similarly, a wide variety of social media platforms currently exist, and each may be used primarily by a different population; therefore, one social media site may be more appropriate for a specific research purpose than another. Permissions associated with a specific site might only allow for use of certain information. Additionally, each site's users may have a unique demographic profile that could change over time. For research projects that are interested in specific, well-defined topics or events, Twitter might be useful due to the hashtag (#) feature, which groups posts into a folder system; hashtags are a means of organising content in social media, akin to folders in traditional computer operating systems or electronic mail (Grajaless et al. 2014), but limited by length of content. Researchers specifically have been able to utilise Twitter to connect with patients or potential patients about a variety of health topics. However, for privacy reasons, healthcare professionals and patients should be cautious about what content they publicly share (Grajaless et al. 2014). Closed social media platforms such as a site for patients of a clinical practice allows patients to be actively involved in their care coordination, track their clinical progress, and have greater access to their physicians (Grajaless et al. 2014). While this is beneficial to the patient, this information is often unavailable for research projects. Alternatively, online patient communities offer a theoretically more secure healthcare forum for patients to communicate with one another. These sites are more likely to partner with stakeholders who are interested in using online patient narratives in research that will directly benefit the patients who originally generated the data; however, a site's terms of use may require organisations to pay or to follow certain guidelines to access the raw data, with varying standard of informing or obtaining consent from patients.

11.2.2 Study Designs

Studies using social media data often default to cross-sectional epidemiologic designs because they are straightforward to conduct. Metadata about the user account (such as patient gender and location) that accompanies an individual message posted to a site may be used to define prospective cohorts, bringing such research more in line with other epidemiological study designs. For example, if a medicine safety communication intervention is targeted to a high risk subset of patients (say, women of reproductive age actively seeking to become pregnant that should avoid a suspected teratogenic medicine), then individuals with the underlying disease condition who meet the high risk criteria could be identified in social media from post histories and metadata. This subset of patients could be enrolled in a prospective cohort to evaluate message penetration (say, by seeing if these individuals repost warning materials generated from the information campaign).

11.2.3 Social Media Listening

Early initiators (Knezevic et al. 2011; Bian et al. 2012; Wu et al. 2013; Chary et al. 2013; Abou Taam et al. 2014) presented technical modalities when social media surfaced as an untapped data source for pharmacovigilance. The general approach to social media listening remains the same, even as new tools are developed:

- First, data are generated by users of a social media site, usually a general-purpose social network or a disease-specific patient forum.
- Second, with permission from site administrators, unformatted text and metadata on user characteristics are transferred to servers held by the analyst.
- Third, text is standardised and formatted for machine processing, including removal of verbatim multiplicate copies (e.g. reposts or forwards) (Sharpe 2014), perhaps with steps to preserve anonymity of social media users.

- Then, an automated or semi-automated process is conducted to isolate the name of the medicine and the description of the suspected adverse reaction or another medicine-related problem, often with the use of purpose-built or existing publicly available medical semantic language tools. Machine learning tools are usually required to separate the indication for using the medicinal product from the suspected adverse reaction, as well as the removal of spam, advertisements, etc.
- A further step of manual review is often executed, with vastly different amounts of human effort involved. The most intensive individual case reviews are conducted by pharmacovigilance experts, and more commonly cursory review is completed by entry-level analysts.
- Finally, quantitative descriptive statistics are generated through summarisation, including comparisons to traditional sources of pharmacovigilance data, leading either to a publication for disseminating the evidence or to support internal decision-making, such as for risk management at a pharmaceutical company.

Social media listening to patient and other relevant various communities can be performed manually or through automated tools that filter and/or classify information acquired from social media. It is most commonly performed through a mixed method process of automatic tools coupled with manual review or curation (Tufts Center for the Study of Drug Development 2014). Automated data processes typically employ normalisation (i.e. organising data so that there is no redundancy, and ensuring related items are stored together), text-matching, and natural language processing techniques to collect and filter data, enabling researchers to amass a larger, more complete database (Sharpe 2014). Best analytical practices will likely require a hybrid approach leveraging automated and manual processes to contextualise the data. Manual work may be needed to develop taxonomies for translating colloquial phrases from social media into standardised medicine and medical condition concepts. Human curation is crucial for validating and improving outputs from machine learning tools for data classification. In essence, machine learning tools are excellent at replicating tasks that humans perform well through applying consistency. On the other hand, machine learning stumbles on tasks where discretion is involved, such as when humans disagree on classifications, highlighting the importance of human curation.

There are specific challenges with using data from social media listening in pharmacovigilance that have been well addressed in the scientific literature: determining which posts deserve manual review (Comfort et al. 2018; Alvaro et al. 2015), vernacular patient language (i.e. the language commonly spoken in the respective region as mother tongue) (Sharpe 2014; Jiang et al. 2018a; Emadzadeh et al. 2018; Cocos et al. 2017; Carbonell et al. 2015), 3326 misspellings of medicine and disease names (Bian et al. 2012; Carbonell et al. 2015), drawbacks to manual annotation of training a corpus (Jiang et al. 2018b; Gupta et al. 2018; Liu et al. 2018; Nikfarjam et al. 2015), and separating side effects from indications or benefits within a post (Liu and Wang 2018; Abdellaoui et al. 2017; Eshleman and Singh 2016; Liu et al. 2016; Sarker et al. 2016; Segura-Bedmar et al. 2015). Other issues being addressed by creative computer science include: dealing with constantly evolving internet slang and visual elements of text (e.g. emoticons, emoji), geolocation of social media posts, maintenance costs of complex dynamic visualisation displays of real-time data, the burn-out from demands of human curation, purposefully misleading information disseminated by malicious actors using automated methods (e.g. bots), the ability to perform retrospective analyses on historical data, and the ability to remove personally identifiable information (PII) (Tufts Center for the Study of Drug Development 2014).

Social media listening can be used for a number of research purposes, including understanding aspects of medicines use and risks, or simply understanding what kind of information patients are asking for. It can also be used to understand audiences of risk communication, their characteristics, communication needs, and preferences more comprehensively for communication planning. Following a communication intervention, social media listening can be used to evaluate its impact.

11.2.4 Understanding Aspects of Medicines Use and Risks

Social media listening, or monitoring, involves two-way communication, where organisations engage in disseminating messages and also in listening to populations. For pharmacovigilance, insights may be obtained to serve risk assessment and provide for the contextualisation of risk—for example, what it means to patients—in communication materials.

More specifically, healthcare professionals generally underutilise voluntary spontaneous reporting systems of adverse reactions of medicines, due to bandwidth constraints precluding them from having time to submit reports. Patients and informal caregivers may be unaware of the importance or mechanisms by which to report adverse reactions. Additionally, some national authorities may be wary of becoming inundated with reports of minor side effects, as it could distract them from paying attention to more serious problems. Further limitations of spontaneous reporting—regardless of whether it is voluntary or mandatory—include significant underreporting of events, incomplete data quality for clinical evaluation, a lack of geographic diversity (most reports are from the US and Europe), persistent reporting of known adverse reactions, duplicate reports, and unspecified causal links (Sarker et al. 2015). Spontaneous reporting has been described as efficient for rare and very serious events. However, the sizeable limitations leave information gaps among regulatory agencies, healthcare professionals, stakeholders, and patients. While social media cannot fill all gaps and overcome all problems, there may be certain areas in which social media content can complement what is collected via traditional systems.

Two case studies (see Figs. 11.1 and 11.2) provide a methodological introduction and exemplify how social media listening can support understanding aspects of medicines use and risks. These examples demonstrate that social media data can provide the context of real world use of medicines, help identify safety concerns and risk factors, and offer additional information not typically captured by existing reporting systems, such as benefits or lack of efficacy. These two case

Description: A pharmaceutical company was interested in exploring the use of a social media monitoring platform to unlock the potential of Twitter and Facebook discussions for safety surveillance. They contracted a third party, Epidemico, to further develop Epidemico's MedWatcher Social that had been created with support from the US Food and Drug Administration. MedWatcher Social is a unique social media monitoring tool that was designed to complement safety surveillance by providing real-time access to publicly available, online patient discussions about medicinal products. The project's goal was to characterise social media as a data source and to determine whether these discussions could provide real world contextualisation of medicines use to safety reviewers.
Start date: October 2012
End date: October 2014
Data source: Facebook and Twitter
Number of events captured: 22,091,787
Number of events reviewed for analysis: 15,490

Methods overview: MedWatcher Social was designed to separate patient discussions in social media from 'noise' (i.e. irrelevant data and signals) and prepare social media data for medicine safety analysis via four distinct components: filtering, translation, de-identification and supplementation. In the filtering step, a Bayesian probabilistic model developed through statistical machine learning computation was applied to each social media post to determine its relevance to medicines safety and to remove spam. Next, natural language processing (NLP) was utilised to translate symptom descriptions into standardised medical terminology (Medical Dictionary for Regulatory Activities (MedDRA) (http://www.meddra.org)) using a proprietary vernacular-to-regulatory language dictionary (Falzon D et al (2016) Digital health for the End TB Strategy: developing priority products and making them work. Eur Respir J 26(48):29–45). Third, data were de-identified using text and pattern matching methods to remove all person-identifying information (PII). Finally, the resulting data were compared to data from traditional spontaneous data sources.

Challenges: Social media is a relatively new data source, which few organisations leverage and incorporate into different pharmacovigilance strategies –if at all. The volatility of publicly available social media data vendors exacerbates this challenge. There has been a lack of regulatory guidance on whether or how to implement digital listening tools for pharmacovigilance, leaving many industry stakeholders unclear how to proceed with social media data that may describe adverse reactions. Finally, the structure or public visibility of social media platforms may prevent patients from describing their events in detail. For example, some social media posts may not provide as much information as reports from other sources due to character count limitations. It may be tempting for some organisations to follow up with patients to obtain more information. However, obtaining contact information or devising a protocol that supports this activity can be both ethically and technically difficult. In order to protect patient privacy and make the data research-ready, the social media posts in this use case were de-identified. No attempt was made to follow up with patients.

Results: 6,441,679 proto-adverse events were captured between October 2012 and October 2014 from Twitter and 15,650,108 events from Facebook, representing 702 and 946 individual Preferred Terms (PTs) from MedDRA, respectively. The five most commonly discussed PTs were 'Pain', 'Altered state of consciousness', 'Headache', 'Malaise' and 'Drug ineffective'. Among the medicinal products that were studied in this analysis, diphenhydramine, influenza vaccines, dextroamphetamine, codeine and morphine were most commonly associated with an event. Additionally, it was determined that 26% of posts included discussions regarding medicinal product benefits such as efficacy or unexpected positive outcomes.

Key points: Social media listening is an important tool to be used in conjunction with traditional post-authorisation safety surveillance methods. When effectively acquired and filtered, social media data can provide the context of real world use of medicines, help identify related safety concerns and offer additional information not typically captured in existing reporting systems, such as benefit or lack of efficacy discussions. Given the aforementioned challenges involved in social media listening activities and the novelty of this data source, understanding the full potential of social media listening will require collaboration among all stakeholders.

Fig. 11.1 Case study 1 on social media listening for routine post-authorisation safety surveillance of medicines (Powell et al. 2015)

studies provide interesting parallels and contrasts. Case study 1 (see Fig. 11.1) was conducted using Facebook and Twitter data by a large pharmaceutical company with considerable reliance on manual review and an annotated training corpus. Case study 2 (see Fig. 11.2) comes from an academic group that used consumer-generated product reviews from Amazon online marketplace in a highly automated manner. Both approaches revealed new insights into the safety of the substances and patient perceptions of them. A third case study 3 (see Fig. 11.3) describes how online news and social media could be used to understand infectious disease outbreaks and support safety surveillance of anti-infectives as well patients in making healthy choices.

Description: Nutritional, or dietary, supplements are a diverse set of products used by consumers often without medical supervision, including vitamins, weight loss aids and muscle builders. They are regulated differently from bone fide medicines and hence may lack safety and efficacy studies and have less stringent reporting requirements than medicines. Data on safety concerns of dietary supplements are also hampered by a lack of standardised coding schemes. Accordingly, these are types of substances that might benefit from social media monitoring to fill knowledge gaps. Also, dietary supplements are often taken in conjunction with medicines and not disclosed to the treating physician.
Data source: Amazon.com product reviews from consumers
Number of posts: approximately 40,000 reviews mentioning 2,708 dietary supplements

Methods overview: Data were harvested from Amazon.com using a custom-built automated computer script that accesses, downloads and simplifies each costumer review ("scraper" or "crawler"). The authors used a fully automated variant of an existing computer algorithm called Latent Dirichlet Allocation (LDA). This modeling method relied on external data from the open source SIDER (Side Effect Resource (sideeffects.embl.de)) (Eshleman R, Singh R (2016) Leveraging graph topology and semantic context for pharmacovigilance through twitter-streams. BMC Bioinformatics 17(Suppl 13):335. Accessible at:https://bmcbioinformatics.biomedcentral.com/articles/10.1186/s12859-016-1220-5 Liu J, Zhao S, Zhang X (2016) An ensemble method for extracting adverse drug events from social media. Artif Intell Med 70:62–76. Accessible at: ttps://linkinghub.elsevier.com/retrieve/pii/S0933-3657(15)30037-3) to compile a structured dictionary of adverse reactions known from medications. An empirical adverse reaction risk score for each product was calculated based on internal variance in the data. The LDA algorithm was validated against an existing annotated corpus of Tweets as well as human review of final results.

Results: Clusters of words associated with each type of dietary supplement emerged from the LDA algorithm. For example, in a weight loss pill, jitteriness and headaches clustered together as well as palpitations and high blood pressure, offering a sense of internal validity. The adverse reaction risk scores that were generated were placed in three tiers. Human expert comparisons to these scores revealed general concordance, with the greatest empirical concern for products promising to disrupt metabolism (e.g. weight loss), including specific products known to have substantial side effects requiring medical attention. On the other end of the spectrum, some dietary supplements were of low real world concern (e.g. saffron tea for sleep) but scored in the intermediate range of the adverse reaction risk score because numerous trivial reactions generated a higher score than one serious adverse reaction. The authors point out that this limitation, as well limitations arising from distinguishing between indication-versus-side effect and fake-versus-real reviews, could be addressed using other data processing tools in a composite fashion.

Key points: Fully automated data processing approaches can yield rapid results when mining large datasets of unstructured text. As each new tool is published to address each emergent data integrity concern, automated methods will require regular upkeep to ensure that these features are included in future versions.

Fig. 11.2 Case study 2 on social media listening by analysing consumer reviews on an online marketplace for identifying potentially unsafe nutritional supplements (Sullivan et al. 2016)

11.2.5 Understanding Audiences of Risk Communication and Their Information Needs

Since various social media platforms are used by large proportions of the general population, they can provide stakeholders with access to more diverse and comprehensive patient cohorts than those used in traditional studies (Rothman et al. 2015). Integration of traditional data sources with alternatives such as social media, partnered with rapid buy-in from key stakeholders may allow regulators, pharmaceutical industry, academia, and healthcare professionals to better understand the patient communities they serve. This in turn enables patients' first-hand experiences to improve the care they receive (Smart Patients, Inc 2015). To leverage this effectively, methods are needed to filter out noise and distil insights from patients (Larkin 2014). A 2015 analysis of vaccine sentiments in Twitter users in the US performed illustrates the application of social media listening to better understand audiences to develop strategies and communication intervention to address their concerns. The analysis showed which themes and terms were more prevalent in positive, neutral, and negative sentiment networks. This approach could guide which messages and words to use for reaching and improving vaccine confidence in the respective populations. Methodologically, the study was performed through coding, creation of semantic networks, and their analysis (Kang et al. 2017).

Description: How can social listening help stakeholders grasp the prevalence of and experience with infectious disease and anti-infectives was the question of this research project. The World Health Organization (WHO) developed the End TB Strategy in 2014 in response to the worldwide tuberculosis (TB) epidemic. As part of this initiative, the WHO established the Global Task Force on Digital Health for TB in April 2015, specifically to develop digital health innovations in global efforts to improve TB care and prevention. By developing and effectively applying digital health products on a large scale, the task force aims to meet the needs of TB patients, their caregivers, innovators, funders, policy-makers, advocacy groups and affected communities (Abou Taam M, Rossard C, Cantaloube L, Bouscaren N, Roche G, Pochard L, Montastruc F,Herxheimer A, Montastruc JL, Bagheri H (2014) Analysis of patients' narratives posted on social media websites on benfluorex's (Mediator®) withdrawal in France. J Clin Pharm Ther. 39:53–55. Accessible at: https://onlinelibrary.wiley.com/doi/abs/10.1111/jcpt.12103). Previous digital health innovations (also known as electronic health (eHealth) and mobile health (mHealth)) have attempted to implement interventions that could be used in both affluent and resource-constrained settings to meet the needs of a TB intervention, such as patient care, surveillance, program management, advocacy, staff development and the engagement of civil society. Many previous efforts in this space lacked scale, end-user ownership and population-level impact. The WHO wished to improve this situation by exploring other options, such as online surveillance, to meet the critical needs of a TB intervention.
Date range: 2016
Data source: Over 200, 000 sources including news, eyewitness reports, expert-curated discussions, validated official reports and social media

Methods overview: HealthMap (www.healthmap.org) at the Boston Children's Hospital is an organisation utilising formal and informal online sources for global disease outbreak monitoring. HealthMap leverages data that have been automatically aggregated from over 200,000 online sources including news, eyewitness reports, expert-curated discussions, validated official reports and social media. HealthMap employs machine learning and natural language processing (NLP) to tag, filter, analyse and visualise infectious disease outbreak alerts that are reviewed manually by public health experts. An interactive geospatial dashboard displays information that facilitates real-time analysis.

Challenge: Implementing a functional TB public health surveillance system has remained challenging in many countries over the years for a variety of reasons: inaccurate reporting and/or underreporting of TB cases, inconsistent case definitions and reporting parameters, little buy-in for reporting from healthcare professionals, lack of coordination between different surveillance information sources, poor quality data, limited resources in many health systems, technology barriers and an inadequate number of healthcare workers with the required knowledge, skills, time, resources, pay, training and support. TB medicines safety monitoring is considered to be even less-developed from general disease surveillance; this is due to a variety of factors: many countries lack a functional medicines safety monitoring framework (and have weak health systems), a lack of support for routine monitoring of toxicity and product quality defects, and inadequate follow-up of newly available and repurposed medicines.

Results: A basic yet effective digital tool that could overcome the challenges and collect, and also consolidate, disease surveillance and medicines safety data would be beneficial for country stakeholders, so they could access relevant information on an ongoing, real-time basis and act upon it as required. Social listening using online news and social media monitoring could therefore be applied, and HealthMap that is currently available in several different languages and ready for immediate use could fulfil the needs of the TB strategy. In addition, patients could be granted access to the data and be empowered to make choices to prevent TB spread, treat TB with anti-infectives and discuss concerns or alternative treatment options with their healthcare professionals.

Key points: Stakeholders overseeing public health interventions need to remain aware of initiative effectiveness and programmatic circumstances including feasibility, time to implementation, resource use, benefits, and support structure. Digital health interventions should include robust monitoring and follow-up capabilities, and a notification system to improve patient care. Digital health, specifically via the methods proposed above, has the potential to help address major components of the End TB Strategy by tapping into pre-existing data and technology that amplifies the patient voice. Digital health can overcome several barriers, access vulnerable populations and allow cross-border partnerships and rapid translation of information to necessary stakeholders. Social listening and online surveillance have the ability to combat many of traditional surveillance's shortcomings and should be considered as an additional tool to end TB.

Fig. 11.3 Case study 3 on surveillance of disease outbreaks and safety of anti-infectives through social listening based on news media and social media monitoring

11.2.6 Crowdsourcing of Information

Social media cannot fill all gaps and overcome all problems seen with traditional data sources used for pharmacovigilance. Nonetheless, there may be certain areas in which social media content can complement what traditional systems collect, such as data directly from patients. Traditional systems for spontaneous reporting of suspected adverse reactions are burdensome and time-consuming for healthcare professionals and patients, for whom reporting is mostly voluntary. Patients completing reports through traditional channels can take up to an hour. As a result, only 2% of reports received by the US Food and Drug Administration (US FDA) are reported by patients directly, i.e. not by or via a healthcare professional. Online and mobile tools have been developed to address barriers to reports, streamline the reporting process, and make them more user-friendly. Additional tools have been developed to perform digital disease detection in the form of online surveillance and social media listening, allowing for a more complete, accurate picture of medicinal product—adverse event pairs (Bahk et al. 2015). These tools' hallmark is the ability to support a concept known as crowdsourcing.

Crowdsourcing tools enable stakeholders to directly engage with a patient community. Patient community outreach can be successful if conducted through social media platforms where community groups may pre-exist. These communities may look different depending on the networking site. For example, Facebook hosts pages or member groups that can be set up by any member to provide a space for dedicated discussion according to a patient population, interest group, or disease area (Bahk et al. 2015). A Twitter-based community would be organised by hashtags that identify different patient populations or concepts that are aggregated by a folder system to be easily identified through a simple query (Grajaless et al. 2014). For example, Twitter users may use the hashtag #teamnosleep to self-identify themselves as insomniacs. Social media patient communities typically openly discuss experiences with their disease(s) and/or treatment(s) that include conversations about adverse events and benefits of medicines, news in scientific journals, and official communications, such regulatory guidelines, label changes, and product recalls. Organisations can access these group members by contacting the group administrator(s) for permission to engage with members and discuss the benefits of utilising an online crowdsourcing tool (Bahk et al. 2015). Administrators may encourage the group to participate in the crowdsourcing. This could include utilising social media to share information about potential adverse reactions of a medicine among a specific patient group (Bahk et al. 2015). This method of patient engagement is illustrated in the motivation-incentive-activation-behaviour (MIAB) concept. In the MIAB concept, motivation is the reason for patient interest, and incentive is what leads the patient to act. Activation is the set of factors that lead to the patient's actual participation, and behaviour is the activity of interest and outcome—in this case, submitting a suspected adverse reaction report (Bahk et al. 2015). It has been proven that patients are more likely to engage in activities that reduce their own burden or that provide some benefit in exchange for some equal level of effort (Bahk et al. 2015). A proven history of patient buy-in to social listening and to other digital tools for pharmacovigilance may encourage patients to participate in crowdsourcing activities. This can be seen as a more active form of two-way communication, which has implications for traditional communication efforts as well as offering opportunities.

11.3 Utility of Applied Methods for Researching Medicinal Product Risk Communication

11.3.1 Opportunities of Social Media Research

"Fast", "cost-effective", "large-scale", "transparent", "patient-generated", "real-time" and "general usefulness" are all phrases commonly used to describe the strengths of social media listening and crowdsourcing.

Social media listening is often available prospectively and in real time, allowing stakeholders to quickly grasp disease prevalence and other epidemiological insights, the impact of a medical intervention, (like a medicine), health topics, and questions of interest to medicine users. Pharmaceutical companies often use such listening alongside launches of new medicines or post-authorisation studies to gather information on how the patient population is responding to treatments. It has also been used to determine where to host a study or launch a new product or intervention due to previously unknown medical need and patient demand (Larkin 2014). Just as importantly, medicinal risk communication may benefit from social media mining, in monitoring and evaluations of communication interventions, or even in the planning phase of communication. Reliance on online health forums for medical advice could be risky to patients; they could be misinformed by each other, improperly self-diagnose, or inappropriately use a medication. Hence, it could be beneficial to capture complex topics and confusing messages. These insights can be used to inform healthcare professional communications to patients, for example. Social media listening enables capturing a large amount of unsolicited, patient-generated data that are available publicly or with permission. End users are provided with the resulting data either in verbatim form or in aggregate, via datasets, summary reports, or visualisations. Since the population of social media users is pre-existing, this method is thought to be cost-effective for the potential amount of data and information gathered from these sources (O'Connor et al. 2014). To collect, clean, analyse, and visualise the same volume of data from other sources would take years, and the timely actionable insight provided would be limited due to the time required to disseminate results (Donahue 2012).

As patients become more knowledgeable about their medical conditions, their articulation of first-hand experiences and perspectives contribute to a valuable data source that can improve the care they receive (Smart Patients, Inc 2015). The widespread use of social media platforms provides communication researchers and practitioners with the ability to understand and design communication interventions for populations that would otherwise be hard-to-reach audiences. The use of new technology and the rapid uptake of social media will provide for better responses to the patient communities they serve.

Many patients report a lack of trust in healthcare professionals, preferring to share information with fellow patients and caregivers (Peacock 2015). Since some diseases, specifically rare diseases or those with social stigma, are associated with an isolating experience that can span several geographical areas, many individuals look to social media to communicate with their peers (Peacock 2015). These patient forums offer anonymity and privacy that may result in patients providing unfiltered data that are more readily available than data from traditional sources. This content can be incredibly beneficial to organisations leveraging social media listening as a research tool: these conversations are unsolicited, and often unfiltered and unabashed. Online discussions among patients about medicines often extend to wider aspects of use, such as off-label use (i.e. use with a medical purpose not in accordance with the terms of the marketing authorisation), as well as issues with product quality, formulation, handling and disposal, sensitive or stigmatised topics, and reluctance to adhere to treatment due to troublesome adverse reactions.

Crowdsourcing offers the opportunity to specifically solicit information on medicines' use behaviours, risk knowledge and perceptions, communication needs, and preferences as well as feedback on communication events.

Finally, information from patient populations may reflect preconceived notions of shared beliefs due to community mentality, which should be considered in research projects. A carefully planned social listening campaign that accounts for nuances of social media data and potential biases gleans insights from a diverse range of global patient populations.

11.3.2 Limitations of Social Media Research

While social media data may be readily available in unprecedented volumes, these data represent unsolicited responses, often making it challenging to understanding its quantity or quality. Once personal identifiers are removed from social media data, it is impossible—and ethically challenging—to verify a reported adverse event by following up with a social media user. Additionally, it is difficult to validate the information until data from traditional sources are available for a comparison analysis. Despite the exuberance generated by the potential of social media mining, in practice there has been a vigorous and necessary debate about the practical application of social media mining for pharmacovigilance. In fact, multiple recent, sophisticated, large-scale efforts and systematic reviews have concluded that routine use of social media for pharmacovigilance underperforms pharmacovigilance data collection systems, including industry-dominated traditional reports of suspected adverse reactions submitted to national authorities (Rees et al. 2018; Convertino et al. 2018; Caster et al. 2018; Kheloufi et al. 2017; Pierce et al. 2017). Others have acknowledged these limitations and noted that social media may fill niche knowledge gaps in medicine safety or may require the use of more sophisticated computing tools (Lardon et al. 2018; Bousquet et al. 2018; Anderson et al. 2017). In most cases of serious adverse reactions identified by regulatory authorities, vigilant physician reporters were the most consistent and earliest source of information on new safety signals, compared to social media.

The authors of the largest evaluation to date (Caster et al. 2018) identified key limitations. In their evaluation, they analysed more than two million Twitter, Facebook, and patient forum posts, using an automated Bayesian classifier and purpose-built patient vernacular dictionary to assign risk scores to posts. Two reference datasets of known positive and negative controls were used for comparison. In addition, a major global database of adverse reactions (i.e. VigiBase) was used in head-to-head comparisons with social media. The analysis calculated traditional pharmacovigilance reporting disproportionality ratios for each medicine in social media and compared them against controls. The results were extensive and decisive: "This study investigated the potential usefulness of social media as a broad-based stand-alone data source for statistical signal detection in pharmacovigilance. Our results provide very little evidence in favour of social media in this respect: in neither of the two complementary reference sets, containing validated safety signals and label changes, respectively, did standard disproportionality analysis yield any predictive ability in a large dataset of combined Facebook and Twitter posts… [M]anual assessment of Facebook and Twitter posts underlying 25 early signals of disproportionality showed that only 40% of posts contained the correct drug and the correct event as an adverse experience, and for only three of those 25 signals did the posts strengthen the belief in a causal association" (Caster et al. 2018). The authors offered some possible explanations. First, some medications may have very little discussion in social media channels. Second, identifying rare events in social media may be difficult if the specific colloquial terms are not detected, and the underlying algorithm to detect adverse reactions may have limited detection ability for the types of very rare events of interest to safety reviewers. Third, there is possible bias when comparing social media results to established reference or validation datasets of known signals. Relatively few reference datasets are in public scientific literature, and the nature of the comparison can vary greatly. Fourth, using statistical aberration detection methods originally optimised for traditional pharmacovigilance systems may not be appropriate for social media-based applications (Caster et al. 2018).

In relation to medicinal product risk communication research, like many other data sources, social media data have inherent biases that must be considered when interpreting results. Biases specific to social media data result from each social media network having its own user demographic profile, making it difficult to generalise findings to a larger population of patients who may not fit this profile. This could, for example, influence the provision of useful data pertaining to medicines most commonly used by specific populations, like older or paediatric patients. In addition, certain brands or types of medicinal products may be represented differentially in the social media; thus, an organisation ought to consider determining how often products are discussed online prior to launching a social media research project. Another bias dimension of using unstructured text is literacy bias. Individuals with limited written language skills will only be represented in the data if someone else posts about their experiences for them. The use of emoji and voice-to-text tools may be able to mitigate some of this bias.

For some products, such as medicines against the human immunodeficiency virus (HIV) and acquired immune deficiency syndrome (AIDS), or hepatitis B, individuals may not be willing to communicate publicly about their treatment experiences due to stigmas associated with their diseases and concerns about being identifiable. This could result in bias due to large self-selection or incomplete information sharing. Honest conversations are more likely to be found on specific patient forums as opposed to on public social media sites. Moreover, if patients suspect that they are being monitored, they may go elsewhere to post comments about their disease or treatment regimen, posing a risk to social listening projects.

There is another issue to consider. The need to improve health outcomes, increase safety and safe use of medicines and manage risk are major drivers behind collecting patient data. Communication practitioners and researchers should note that as more data have been collected, concerns about privacy have grown beyond patient privacy. Notably, one of the biggest lessons learnt from using social media for pharmacovigilance is that patients will talk. While this may seem to many like a treasure trove of information, there is major concern that patients will become unblinded when social media is used alongside clinical trials (Lipset 2014). This occurred during a 2009 clinical trial when a patient discovered that she had been placed on the study product (as opposed to placebo or comparator) (Lipset 2014). This realisation led to more individuals seeking online patient communities to share symptoms and compare notes about pill formulations and taste to try to determine which treatment they were receiving. Many patients do not understand the consequences of these interactions, which could end a clinical trial early, and delay or even prevent a new treatment from becoming available to other afflicted patients. This underscores the importance of clinical trial subjects understanding that their social media discussions may compromise randomisation and be an inherent threat to validity in clinical trials. Such discussions among clinical trial participants should be discouraged or sequestered while the clinical trial is underway. Social media monitoring for such discussions could therefore be useful to proactively understand this threat to clinical trial validity.

11.3.3 Ethical and Legal Aspects

Regulatory guidelines and best practices are slowly emerging regarding when and which organisations have the legal responsibility for mining patient narratives through social media listening (Lengsavath et al. 2017). The regulatory dimensions are addressed as part of the WEB-RADR project (web-radr.eu) (Ghosh and Lewis 2015) and by a few authors (Sloane et al. 2015; Lengsavath et al. 2017; Naik et al. 2015). Despite the ambiguity and evolving regulatory environment, major pharmaceutical companies have executed social media listening projects in recent years (Powell et al. 2015; Comfort et al. 2018; Caster et al. 2018). Currently, the most evident disadvantage to using social media for research relating to medicinal product safety and communication is the lack of regulatory guidance and best practices regarding the use of social media data.

Social media listening also poses ethical and privacy concerns, especially within private online communities (Stergiopoulos 2014). To meet moral obligation, many organisations will only listen in and/or engage with patients on public social media platforms once they have announced their affiliation and presence to the patient(s) (Stergiopoulos 2014). In addition, ethical and privacy regulations are distinct across different geographic regions. Hence, organisations that wish to engage in social media listening must be cognisant of these differences to avoid or address privacy breaches in a timely manner (Stergiopoulos 2014). Due to the speed at which information travels on social media, a researcher may benefit from considering issues that may arise from inappropriately using social media (Stergiopoulos 2014).

Pharmaceutical manufacturers must also consider, as part of their protocol, how to conduct social media listening activities in a way that addresses liability and compliance, meeting regulatory requirements. Legally required reporting of suspected adverse reactions necessitates patient information. This poses a challenge in social media listening, as there is limited ability to confirm that individuals are using their true identity when posting on social media sites, or to approach them if they are obviously using an alias name. When monitoring social media alongside clinical trials, this challenge becomes more complicated, as there is often no way of confirming a patient's participation in a specific clinical trial (Thompson 2014). Furthermore, even if a person can be confirmed as a trial participant, there would be no way of confirming in which arm of the trial a participant is participating, which treatment(s) that participant is receiving, or if any adverse event reported in social media has already been recorded and dealt with appropriately (Barry 2014). It is therefore highly recommended that legal and compliance departments review the use of any social media for recruitment or use alongside a clinical trial, prior to the start of social media listening activities (Dizon et al. 2012). This practice could also be subject to institutional review board (IRB) approval and require compliance with national privacy laws (Dizon et al. 2012). Alternatively, the rules and requirements for surveillance campaigns and observational studies are often less scrutinising. Therefore, it is important to determine the feasibility of using social media for a specific project prior to committing resources.

When considering the use of a third-party vendor to acquire social media data, an organisation should ensure that the vendor meets all compatibility and accountability standards required for the research project as well as provide all needed software services. The regulatory and societal expectations of privacy with social media data are rapidly changing and should be considered in earnest to maintain the credibility and viability of the research effort.

More specifically, Appendix 11.1 provides an introduction to the data protection regulation applicable in the European Union (EU) and derives some globally applicable principles.

11.4 Outlook: Relevance, Improvements and Future Potential

As a field, we are at a crossroads in pharmacovigilance. The potential of social media is hard to deny, but the execution in relation to the collection of adverse reactions has born little fruit (Rees et al. 2018; Convertino et al. 2018; Caster et al. 2018). Yet, many researchers regularly derive new insights from monitoring social media content (Lardon et al. 2018; Kurzinger et al. 2018; Patel et al. 2018; Keller et al. 2018; Chen et al. 2018). One research article's title summarises this succinctly: "Descriptions of adverse drug reactions are less informative in forums than in the French pharmacovigilance database but provide more unexpected reactions." (Karapetiantz et al. 2018). This may very well be the key insight from the past decade of efforts to understand the role of social media for collecting adverse reaction data; given that any surveillance system is inherently designed to identify what is expected, as broadly defined among the scope of outcomes. The challenge for the future will be to narrow the scope of inquiry and to focus on social media mining applications that are most likely to generate new *knowledge*; our focus to date has been on *information* more generally. When considering an assessment of a new safety concern with a medicine, evidence from animal studies, laboratory findings, clinical trials, pharmacoepidemiological studies, and treatment experience all come into play. Machines do not appear to be on the cusp of replacing this complex human assessment in the immediate future; perhaps, harvesting new knowledge from the exuberant promise of social media will require the development of automated multifactorial safety reviewing.

A further objective of social media research for pharmacovigilance purposes is to capture information about patients and medicinal products through a patient-centric lens. This is achieved by turning to social media to amplify the patient voice to understand patients' knowledge, attitudes, and behaviours—to understand them as audiences of our communication—and to collect data which help evidence-based planning and evaluating of communication interventions that support informed therapeutic choice and safe use of medicines. Social media is a communication channel, which is an important research topic in itself. Such research may determine who uses social media and how, with a view to inform communication strategies for incorporating the social media not only for listening but also messaging. Beyond pharmacovigilance *per se*, social media data present the tantalising possibility of providing insight into how physicians communicate with each other (Albarqouni et al. 2019; Graff et al. 2018; Falzon et al. 2016), topics that patients want to know more about (Charlie et al. 2018), and how the public reacts to health news in real time (Adams and Schiffers 2017). These broader dimensions of medicines safety and communication have not yet been evaluated in social media adequately.

In conclusion, social media listening and crowdsourcing of information provide a timely and insightful complement to traditional methods for medicinal product risk communication research, and is applicable globally. Given people's increasing use of the internet and social media, and patients' views on the prospects of its utility for data gathering in support of patient-centred care (see Chap. 16), the emerging discipline of social media research is becoming an essential part of a multidisciplinary and multilayered approach to medicinal product risk communication research (see Chap. 1). As a source for data on real-time patient discussions, social media can be used to understand aspects of use of medicines in healthcare, information needs and adverse reactions as characterised by patients, as well as to monitor and improve risk communication efforts. Online discussions among patients about medicines often extend to wider aspects of use, such as off-label use, and issues with product quality, formulation and handling and disposal, and even reluctance to adhere to treatment regimens due to adverse reactions experienced by the patient. Social media can also be used to identify specific patient groups for soliciting perspectives on certain safety concerns and risk communication needs. Lastly, as social media listening and crowdsourcing information gains traction as a viable source for insights, it will become necessary to acknowledge its myriad challenges—in particular inherent noise, incomplete data when follow-up is impossible, privacy and patient protection, and lack of regulatory guidance. More coordinated research among academics, regulators, pharmaceutical industry, and subject matter experts is needed to develop best practice guidance. Practical solutions that adequately address these social media research challenges without impacting the usefulness of the data for pharmacovigilance, including improving communication about risks and safe use of medicines, will be of utmost importance.

Conclusions

- Social media research can provide a timely and insightful complement to traditional data sources for pharmacovigilance as well as medicinal product risk communication research, in particular for planning and evaluating of communication interventions.
- As a source for real-time patient discussions, social media listening can facilitate understanding aspects of use of medicines in healthcare, adverse reactions as characterised by patients, audiences and their information needs as well as help monitor and improve risk communication efforts. Online discussions among patients about medicines often extend to wider aspects of use, such as off-label use, as well as issues with product quality, formulation, handling and disposal, sensitive or stigmatised topics, and reluctance to adhere to treatment due to adverse reactions.
- Social media can also be used to identify specific patient groups for soliciting perspectives on certain safety concerns and risk communication needs, an approach called crowdsourcing for information.
- Social media is an evolving global communication channel. Understanding who uses these media and how is important for informing communication strategies, for both listening and tailoring messaging.
- Social media research needs to consider specific potential for bias as well as ethical and legal concerns. Therefore, more collaboration is needed among researchers, regulators, the pharmaceutical industry, and subject matter experts. This collaboration is critical to develop best practice guidance and practical solutions that adequately address these challenges without impacting the usefulness of the data for pharmacovigilance and communication about risks and safe use of medicines.

Appendix 11.1: Legal Aspects Relevant to Internet-Based and Social Media Research

Researchers making use of data from the internet and the social media need to consider legal aspects. The applicable law will vary depending on where relevant actors, e.g. internet and social media users and researchers, are located. The relevant rules are usually those of the country where researchers are based. The European Union (EU) data protection rules, found in General Data Protection Regulation (GDPR) (Regulation (EU) 2016/679), can have "extra-territorial effect"—that is they bind researchers outside the EU when they target those within the EU.

Types of Law to Consider

In addition to adhereing to legislation on personal data protection, confidentiality and privacy, other legal aspect may be of relevance to the research project. Other legal concerns include contracts (e.g. with data vendors), intellectual property (e.g. onwership of digital content, reproduction and transfer rights, ownership of algortihms developed), sector-specific regulation (e.g. medical product marketers), as well as civil and criminal law (e.g. stalking, bullying, etc.).

Personal Data Protection Law

Personal data protection law—discussed here in more detail as the most relevant law to consider for internet-based and social media research related to health matters—does in general not prohibit the processing of data, but it lays down conditions for when, on what basis and how the processing of personal data should take place, and it gives enforceable rights to persons who are data subjects. Reference is made here to the EU GDPR, which is recognised by many—consumer organisations notably too—as a global standard. There, personal data are defined as any information relating to an identified or identifiable natural person. Researchers will often work with data that have been pseudo-anonymised by the data provider. That means that the data subject is not identified but there can still be a risk of possibly identifying the person through combining data or using additional information. This is particularly a risk when a patient has a rare disease. Where however information is truly anonymous, i.e. where the information does not relate to an identified or identifiable natural person or to personal data rendered anonymous in such a manner that the data subject is not or no longer identifiable, data protection legislation is not necessary to be applied. Statistics on the number and the length of visits of people on a website, stratified by country, age and sex, are examples of data likely to be anonymous data.

Grounds for Processing of Personal Data Relevant to Health Research

The EU GDPR specifies the grounds on which personal data may be processed—consent, performance of a contract, performance of a legal obligation, protecting the vital interests of the data subject, necessary for the performance of a task in the public interest, and the legitimate interests of the processor (subject to fundamental interests of the data subject). The EU GDPR also specifies strict rules as to what consent means. The EU GDPR prohibits the processing for special categories of personal data, including ethnic data, genetic and biometric data for the purpose of uniquely identifying a natural person, as well as data concerning health, sex life and sexual orientation. Such data are however allowed to be processed on defined exempting grounds, which include:

- explicit consent by the data subject has been given; or
- the personal data have manifestly been made public by the data subject; or
- the data processing is necessary for the purposes of preventive or occupational medicine and provision of care, whether for an individual or populations; or
- processing is necessary for reasons of public health, including ensuring high quality and safety of healthcare, medicinal products or medical devices.

These exemptions can be given for medicinal product risk communication research making use of data from the internet and the social media for understanding, planning, evaluating or improving communication. For example, patients may have identified themselves in comments on websites or publically accessible social media posts, or patients of a closed social media group may have given consent for their data to be used for the purpose of such research, to, e.g. identify their risk perceptions or questions for the safe use of medicines. Where patients publish their information under a pseudonym, researchers should not make attempts to identify that person through combining data, but may attempt to contact them if needed for a specific research project.

Principles for the Processing of Personal Data

Where the processing of personal data is allowed, the EU GDPR requires the data processing (i.e. collection, recording, organisation, structuring, storage, adaptation or alteration, retrieval, consultation, use, disclosure by transmission, dissemination or otherwise making available, alignment or combination, restriction, erasure or destruction) to be:

- lawful, fair and transparent in relation to the data subject (principle of lawfulness, fairness and transparency);
- for the specified purpose only (principle of purpose limitation);
- adequate, relevant and limited to what is needed (principle of data minimisation);
- based on accurate data (principle of accuracy);

- performed in a way that permits identification of data subjects for no longer than is necessary (principle of storage limitation);
- secure, which includes that the data should be protected against unauthorised or unlawful processing and accidental loss, destruction or damage (principle of integrity and confidentiality).

Rights of Data Subjects

As mentioned before, data protection law gives enforceable rights to persons who are data subjects towards the data controller. When planning research, the protocol needs to guarantee the following rights of data subjects, either because locally applicable legislation requires this or because it can be considered ethical good research practice:

- right of access to the data subject's data and information on the conditions of data processing;
- right to rectification in order to correct or complete data;
- right to erasure of data, i.e. the right to be forgotten;
- right to restriction of processing;
- right to data portability, i.e. to obtain the data in a readable format and to transfer them to another data controller; and
- right to object to data processing at any time.

The rights of data subjects—here the users of social media—may be limited in respect of processing for archiving purposes in the public interest, scientific or historical research purposes or statistical purposes. This will be specified by each EU member state (which could mean that the position will be different across member states) and must be subject to safeguards—again these will be specified by each member state.

Concluding Remarks

Researchers making use of data from the internet and the social media need to consider various types of law applicable in the given jurisdictions of all actors involved. Researchers need to in particular adhere to personal data protection, confidentiality and privacy legislation and are accountable in this respect towards data subjects. In jurisdictions where such legislation does not exist, the principles presented here can be considered good research practice. Research protocols and data processing need to be designed accordingly (Woods 2017). Regularly updated guidance on the EU GPRD is provided by the European Data Protection Board (EDPB) (European Data Protection Board (EDPB) 2018).

Acknowledgements The authors thank Lorna M Woods at the School of Law, University of Essex, United Kingdom for the review of this appendix.

Appendix 11.1

European Data Protection Board (EDPB) (2018) [guidance documents published on website]. Brussels: EDPB; Accessible at: https://edpb.europa.eu/edpb_en.

Regulation (EU) 2016/679 of the European Parliament and of the Council of 27 April 2016 on the protection of natural persons with regard to the processing of personal data and on the free movement of such data, and repealing Directive 95/46/EC (General Data Protection Regulation). Official Journal of the European Union; 4 May 2016: L 119/1-88.

Woods LM (2017) Legal considerations relevant to social media and health [lecture]. Pharmacovigilance and social media [training course on 15 October 2017]. Liverpool: 17th Annual Meeting of the International Society of Pharmacovigilance; 15-18 October 2017.

References

Abdellaoui R, Schück S, Texier N, Burgun A (2017) Filtering entities to optimize identification of adverse drug reaction from social media: how can the number of words between entities in the messages help? JMIR Public Health Surveill 3(2):e36. Accessible at: https://publichealth.jmir.org/2017/2/e36/

Abou Taam M, Rossard C, Cantaloube L, Bouscaren N, Roche G, Pochard L, Montastruc F, Herxheimer A, Montastruc JL, Bagheri H (2014) Analysis of patients' narratives posted on social media websites on benfluorex's (Mediator®) withdrawal in France. J Clin Pharm Ther. 39:53–55. Accessible at: https://onlinelibrary.wiley.com/doi/abs/10.1111/jcpt.12103

Adams S, Schiffers P (2017) Co-constructed health narratives during a 'media event': the case of the first Dutch Twitter heart operation. Digit Health 3:2055207617712046. Accessible at: https://www.ncbi.nlm.nih.gov/pmc/articles/PMC6001202/.

Albarqouni L, Hoffmann T, McLean K, Price K, Glasziou P (2019). Role of professional networks on social media in addressing clinical questions at general practice: a cross-sectional study of general practitioners in Australia and New Zealand. BMC Fam Pract 20(1):43. Accessible at: https://bmcfampract.biomedcentral.com/articles/10.1186/s12875-019-0931-x

Alvaro N, Conway M, Doan S, Lofi C, Overington J, Collier N (2015) Crowdsourcing Twitter annotations to identify first-hand experiences of prescription drug use. J Biomed Inform 58:280–287. Accessible at: https://www.sciencedirect.com/science/article/pii/S1532046415002415?via%3Dihub

Anderson LS, Bell HG, Gilbert M, Davidson JE, Winter C, Barratt MJ, Win B, Painter JL, Menone C, Sayegh J, Dasgupta N (2017) Using social listening data to monitor misuse and nonmedical use of bupropion: a content analysis. JMIR Public Health Surveill 3:e6

Bahk C, Goshgarian M, Donahue K, Freifeld CC, Menone CM et al (2015) Increasing patient engagement in pharmacovigilance through online community outreach and mobile reporting applications: an analysis of adverse event reporting for the Essure device in the US. Pharm Med 29:331–341

Barry F (2014) Pfizer: how Facebook can 'unblind' a clinical trial. Outsourcing-pharma.com. June 9. Accessible at: https://www.outsourcing-pharma.com/Article/2014/06/09/Pfizer-How-Facebook-can-unblind-a-clinical-trial#

Bian J, Topaloglu U, Yu F (2012) Towards large-scale Twitter mining for drug-related adverse events. SHB12. Accessible at: https://www.ncbi.nlm.nih.gov/pmc/articles/PMC5619871/

Bousquet C, Audeh B, Bellet F, Lillo-LeLouet A (2018) Comment on "Assessment of the utility of social media for broad-ranging statistical signal detection in pharmacovigilance: results from the WEB-RADR Project". Drug Saf 41:1371–1373. Accessible at: https://link.springer.com/article/10.1007%2Fs40264-018-0747-y

Carbonell P, Mayer MA, Bravo A (2015) Exploring brand-name drug mentions on Twitter for pharmacovigilance. Stud Health Technol Inform, 210. Accessible at: https://www.ncbi.nlm.nih.gov/pubmed/?term=25991101

Caster O, Dietrich J, Kurzinger ML, Lerch M, Maskell S, Noren GN, Tcherny-Lessenot S, Vroman B, Wisniewski A, van Stekelenborg J (2018) Assessment of the utility of social media for broad-ranging statistical signal detection in pharmacovigilance: results from the WEB-RADR project. Drug Saf 41:1355–1369

Charlie AM, Gao Y, Heller SL (2018) What do patients want to know? Questions and concerns regarding mammography expressed through social media. J Am Coll Radiol 15(10):1478–1486. Accessible at: https://www.jacr.org/article/S1546-1440(17)31170-5/fulltext

Chary M, Genes N, McKenzie A, Manini AF (2013) Leveraging social networks for toxicovigilance. J Med Toxicol 9:184–191. Accessible at: https://www.ncbi.nlm.nih.gov/pmc/articles/PMC3657021/

Chen X, Faviez C, Schuck S, Lillo-Le-Louët A, Texier N et al (2018) Mining patients' narratives in social media for pharmacovigilance: adverse effects and misuse of methylphenidate. Front Pharmacol 9:541

Cocos A, Fiks AG, Masino AJ (2017) Deep learning for pharmacovigilance: recurrent neural network architectures for labeling adverse drug reactions in Twitter posts. J Am Med Inform Assoc 24:813–821. Accessible at: https://academic.oup.com/jamia/article-abstract/24/4/813/3041102?redirectedFrom=fulltext

Comfort S, Perena S, Hudson Z, Dorrell D, Meireis S, Nagarajan M, Ramakrishnan C, Fine J (2018) Sorting through the safety data haystack: using machine learning to identify individual case safety reports in social-digital media. Drug Saf 41:579–590. Accessible at: https://www.ncbi.nlm.nih.gov/pmc/articles/PMC5966485/

Convertino I, Ferraro S, Blandizzi C, Tuccori M (2018) The usefulness of listening social media for pharmacovigilance purposes: a systematic review. Expert Opin Drug Saf 17:1081–1093. Accessible at: https://www.ncbi.nlm.nih.gov/pubmed/?term=30285501

Demner-Fushman D, Elhadad N (2016) Aspiring to unintended consequences of natural language processing: a review of recent developments in clinical and consumer-generated text processing. Yearb Med Inform 10:224–233. Accessible at: https://www.ncbi.nlm.nih.gov/pubmed/?term=27830255

Dizon D, Graham D, Thompson M, Johnson L, Johnston C et al (2012) Practical guidance: the use of social media in oncology practice. Bus Oncol 8(5):e113–e124

Donahue M (2012) Patient recruitment via social media: lessons learned. Pharm Exec. February 13. Accessible at: http://www.pharmexec.com/patient-recruitment-social-media-lessons-learned

Edwards IR, Lindquist M (2011) Social media and networks in pharmacovigilance: boon or bane? Drug Saf 34:267–271. Accessible at: https://www.ncbi.nlm.nih.gov/pubmed/?term=21417499

Emadzadeh E, Sarker A, Nikfarjam A, Gonzalez G (2018) Hybrid semantic analysis for mapping adverse drug reaction mentions in tweets to medical terminology. AMIA Annu Symp Proc 16:679–688. Accessible at: https://www.ncbi.nlm.nih.gov/pmc/articles/PMC5977584/

Eshleman R, Singh R (2016) Leveraging graph topology and semantic context for pharmacovigilance through twitter-streams. BMC Bioinformatics 17(Suppl 13):335. Accessible at: https://bmcbioinformatics.biomedcentral.com/articles/10.1186/s12859-016-1220-5

Falzon D et al (2016) Digital health for the End TB Strategy: developing priority products and making them work. Eur Respir J 26(48):29–45

Freifeld CC, Brownstein JS, Menone CM, Bao W, Filice R, Kass-Hout T, Dasgupta N (2014) Digital drug safety surveillance: monitoring pharmaceutical products in twitter. Drug Saf 37:343–350. Accessible at: https://link.springer.com/article/10.1007%2Fs40264-014-0155-x

Ghosh R, Lewis D (2015) Aims and approaches of Web-RADR: a consortium ensuring reliable ADR reporting via mobile devices and new insights from social media. Exp Opin Drug Saf 14:1845–1853. Accessible at: https://www.tandfonline.com/doi/abs/10.1517/14740338.2015.1096342?journalCode=ieds20

Golder S, Norman G, Loke YK (2015) Systematic review on the prevalence, frequency and comparative value of adverse events data in social media. Br J Clin Pharmacol 80(4):878–888. Accessible at: https://bpspubs.onlinelibrary.wiley.com/doi/full/10.1111/bcp.12746

Graff SL, Close J, Cole S, Matt-Amaral L, Beg R, Markham MJ (2018) Impact of closed Facebook group participation on female hematology/oncology physicians. J Oncol Pract 4(12):e758–e769

Grajaless F III, Sheps S, Ho K, Novak-Lauscher H, Eysenbach G (2014) Social media: a review and tutorial of applications in medicine and health care. J Med Internet Res 16(2):e13

Gupta S, Pawar S, Ramrakhiyani N, Palshikar GK, Varma V (2018) Semi-supervised recurrent neural network for adverse drug reaction mention extraction. BMC Bioinformatics 19(Suppl 8):212. Accessible at: https://bmcbioinformatics.biomedcentral.com/articles/10.1186/s12859-018-2192-4

International Telecommunication Union (ICU). ICT Facts and Figures The World in 2015. Accessible at: http://www.itu.int/en/ITU-D/Statistics/Documents/facts/ICTFactsFigures2015.pdf

Jiang K, Chen T, Calix RA, Bernard GR (2018a) Identifying consumer health terms of side effects in Twitter posts. Stud Health Technol Inform 251:273–276. Accessible at: https://www.ncbi.nlm.nih.gov/pmc/articles/PMC6041256/

Jiang K, Feng S, Song Q, Calix RA, Gupta M, Bernard GR (2018b) Identifying tweets of personal health experience through word embedding and LSTM neural network. BMC Bioinformatics 19(Suppl 8):210. Accessible at: https://bmcbioinformatics.biomedcentral.com/articles/10.1186/s12859-018-2198-y

Kang GJ, Ewing-Nelson SR, Mackey L, Schlitt JT, Marathe A, et al (2017) Semantic network analysis of vaccine sentiment in online social media. Vaccine 35:3621–3638. Accessible at: https://www.ncbi.nlm.nih.gov/pmc/articles/PMC5548132/

Karapetiantz P, Bellet F, Audeh B, Lardon J, Leprovost D et al (2018) Descriptions of adverse drug reactions are less informative in forums than in the French pharmacovigilance database but provide more unexpected reactions. Front Pharmacol 9:439

Keller MS, Mosadeghi S, Cohen ER, Kwan J, Spiegel BMR (2018) Reproductive health and medication concerns for patients with inflammatory bowel disease: thematic and quantitative analysis using social listening. J Med Internet Res 20(6):e206. Accessible at: https://www.jmir.org/2018/6/e206/

Kheloufi F, Default A, Blin O, Micallef J (2017) Investigating patient narratives posted on Internet and their informativeness level for pharmacovigilance purpose: The example of comments about statins. Therapie 72:483–490. Accessible at: https://www.ncbi.nlm.nih.gov/pubmed/?term=28065444

Knezevic MZ, Bivolarevic IC, Peric TS, Jankovic SM (2011) Using Facebook to increase spontaneous reporting of adverse drug reactions. Drug Saf 34:351–352

Kuhn M, Campillos M, Letunic I, Jensen LJ, Bork P (2010) A side effect resource to capture phenotopic effects of drugs. Mol Syst Biol 6:343. Accessible at: https://www.embopress.org/doi/full/10.1038/msb.2009.98

Kuhn M, Letunic I, Jensen LJ, Bork P (2016) The SIDER database of drugs and side effects. Nucleic Acids Res 44(D1):D1075–D1079. Accessible at: https://academic.oup.com/nar/article/44/D1/D1075/2502602

Kurzinger ML, Schuck S, Texier N, Abdellaoui R, Faviez C, Pouget J, Zhang L, Tcherny-Lessenot S, Lin S, Juhaeri J (2018) Web-based signal detection using medical forums data in France: comparative analysis. J Med Internet Res 20:e10466. Accessible at: https://www.jmir.org/2018/11/e10466/

Lardon J, Abdellaoui R, Bellet F, Asfari H (2015) Adverse drug reaction identification and extraction in social media: a scoping review. J Med Internet Res 17:e171. Accessible at: https://www.ncbi.nlm.nih.gov/pubmed/?term=26163365

Lardon J, Bellet F, Aboukhamis R, Asfari H, Souvignet J, Jaulent MC, Beyens MN, Lillo-LeLouet A, Bousquet C (2018) Evaluating Twitter as a complementary data source for pharmacovigilance. Exp Opin Drug Saf 17:763–774. Accessible at: https://www.tandfonline.com/doi/abs/10.1080/14740338.2018.1499724?journalCode=ieds20

Larkin M (2014) Social media for pharma: an expert's view. Elsevier. December 2. Accessible at: http://www.elsevier.com/connect/social-media-for-pharma-an-expertsview

Lengsavath M, Dal Pra A, de Ferran AM, Brosch S, Härmark L, Newbould V, Goncalves S (2017) Social media monitoring and adverse drug reaction reporting in pharmacovigilance: an overview of the regulatory landscape. Ther Innov Regul Sci 51(1):125–131

Lipset C (2014) Engage with research participants about social media. Nat Med 20:231

Liu J, Wang G (2018) Pharmacovigilance from social media: an improved random subspace method for identifying adverse drug events. Int J Med Inform 117:33–43. Accessible at: https://www.sciencedirect.com/science/article/abs/pii/S1386505618304416?via%3Dihub

Liu J, Zhao S, Zhang X (2016) An ensemble method for extracting adverse drug events from social media. Artif Intell Med 70:62–76. Accessible at: https://linkinghub.elsevier.com/retrieve/pii/S0933-3657(15)30037-3

Liu J, Zhao S, Wang G (2018) SSEL-ADE: a semi-supervised ensemble learning framework for extracting adverse drug events from social media. Artif Intell Med 84:34–49. Accessible at: https://www.sciencedirect.com/science/article/pii/S0933365717301847?via%3Dihub

Medical Dictionary for Regulatory Activities (MedDRA). Accessible at: http://www.meddra.org

Naik P, Umrath T, van Stekelenborg J, Ruben R, Abdul-Karim N, et al (2015) Regulatory definitions and good pharmacovigilance practices in social media: challenges and recommendations. Ther Innov Regul Sci 49:840–851. Accessible at: https://journals.sagepub.com/doi/abs/10.1177/2168479015587362?rfr_dat=cr_pub%3Dpubmed&url_ver=Z39.88-2003&rfr_id=ori%3Arid%3Acrossref.org&journalCode=dijc

Nikfarjam A, Sarker A, O'Connor K, Ginn R, Gonzalez G (2015) Pharmacovigilance from social media: mining adverse drug reaction mentions using sequence labeling with word embedding cluster features. J Med Am Inform Assoc 22:671–681

O'Connor A, Jackson L, Goldsmith L, Skirton H (2014) Can I get a retweet please?: health research recruitment and the Twittersphere. J Adv Nurs 70:599–609

Park HA, Jung H, On J, Park SK, Kang H (2018) Digital epidemiology: use of digital data collected for non-epidemiological purposes in epidemiological studies. Healthc Inform Res 24:253–262. Accessible at: https://www.ncbi.nlm.nih.gov/pubmed/?term=30443413

Patel R, Belousov M, Jani M, Dasgupta N, Winokur C, Nenandic G, Dixon WG (2018) Frequent discussion of insomnia and weight gain with glucocorticoid therapy: an analysis of Twitter posts. NPJ Digit Med, 1. Accessible at: https://www.ncbi.nlm.nih.gov/pmc/articles/PMC6364798/

PatientsLikeMe. About us. patientslikeme.com. 2019. And: Okun S, Goodwin K (2017) Building a learning health community: By the people, for the people. Learn Health Sys 1:e10028. Both accessible at: https://www.patientslikeme.com/about

Peacock E (2014) Global forum special section: transforming recruitment for clinical trials via patient social networks. DIA. October 1. Accessible at: http://www.diaglobal.org/en/resources/news#article=65afd337-6fc3-4abf-8d43-797172fc1314

Peacock E (2015) Engaging patient social networks in clinical trials and burden of disease studies. Drug Information Association (DIA). October 1

Perrin A (2015) Social media usage: 2005–2015. Pew Research Center. Accessible at: http://www.pewinternet.org/2015/10/08/social-networking-usage-2005-2015/

Pierce CE, Bouri K, Pamer C, Proestel S, Rodriguez HW, Ven Le H, Freifeld CC, Brownstein JS, Walderhaug M, Edwards IR, Dasgupta N (2017) Evaluation of Facebook and Twitter monitoring to detect safety signals for medical products: an analysis of recent FDA safety alerts. Drug Saf 40:317–331. Accessible at: https://link.springer.com/article/10.1007%2Fs40264-016-0491-0

Powell GE, Seifert HA, Reblin T, Burstein PJ, Blowers J et al (2015) Social media listening for routine post-marketing safety surveillance. Drug Saf 39:443–454

Rees S, Mian S, Grabowski N (2018) Using social media in safety signal management: is it reliable? Ther Adv Drug Saf 9:591–599. Accessible at: https://www.ncbi.nlm.nih.gov/pubmed/?term=30283627

Rothman M, Gnanaskathy A, Wicks P, Papadopoulos E (2015) Can we use social media to support content validity of patient-reported outcome instruments in medial product development? Value Health 18:1–4

Sarker A, Ginn R, Nikfarjam A, O'Connor K, Smith K et al (2015) Utilizing social media data for pharmacovigilance: a review. J Biomed Inform 54:202–212

Sarker A, Nikfarjam A, Gonzalez G (2016) Social media mining shared task workshop. Pac Symp Biocomput 21:581–592. Accessible at: https://www.worldscientific.com/doi/abs/10.1142/9789814749411_0054

Segura-Bedmar I, Martinez P, Revert R, Moreno-Schneider J (2015) Exploring Spanish health social media for detecting drug effects. BMC Med Inform Decis Mak 15(Suppl 2):S6. Accessible at: https://bmcmedinformdecismak.biomedcentral.com/articles/10.1186/1472-6947-15-S2-S6

Sharpe T (2014) Global forum special section: patient perspective on social media. Drug Information Association (DIA). October 1. Accessible at: http://www.diaglobal.org/en/resources/news#article=7b3df92f-82b7-443a-a759-ad46b203f0b3

Sloane R, Osanlou O, Lewis D, Bollegala D, Maskell S, Pirmohamed M (2015) Social media and pharmacovigilance: a review of the opportunities and challenges. Br J Clin Pharmacol 80:910–920. Accessible at: https://www.ncbi.nlm.nih.gov/pubmed/?term=26147850

Smart Patients, Inc. (2015) Accessible at: https://www.smartpatients.com/about

Smith M, Benattia I (2016) The patient's voice in pharmacovigilance: pragmatic approaches to building a patient-centric drug safety organization. Drug Saf 39:779–785

Snipes K (2015) Using social media and digital media to increase patient recruitment and retention. Clinical Leader. June 15

Stergiopoulos S (2014) Global forum special section: social listening to enhance clinical research. Drug Information Association (DIA). October 1. Accessible at: http://www.diaglobal.org/en/resources/news#article=c0736ec3-2280-4261-b621-f756d3a4bf6e

Sullivan R, Sarker A, O'Connor K, Goodin A, Karlsrud M, Gonzalez G (2016) Finding potentially unsafe nutritional supplements from user reviews with topic modeling. Pac Symp Biocomput 21:528–539

Thompson M (2014) Social media in clinical trials. ASCO p E101. Accessible at: https://www.researchgate.net/publication/262608279_Social_Media_in_Clinical_Trials

Tricco AC, Zarin W, Lillie E, Jeblee S, Warren R, Khan PA, Robson R, Hirst G, Straus SE (2018) Utility of social media and crowd-intelligence data for pharmacovigilance: a scoping review. BMC Med Inform Decis Mak 18:38. Accessible at: https://www.ncbi.nlm.nih.gov/pubmed/?term=29898743

Tufts Center for the Study of Drug Development (2014) Industry usage of social and digital media communities in clinical research. White Paper, Boston. Accessible at: http://csdd.tufts.edu/files/uploads/TCSDD_Social_Media_Final.pdf

Wong A, Plasek JM, Montecalvo SP, Zhou L (2018) Natural language processing and its implications for the future of medication safety: a narrative review of recent advances and challenges. Pharmacotherapy 38:822–841. Accessible at: https://www.ncbi.nlm.nih.gov/pubmed/?term=29884988

Wu H, Fang H, Stanhope SJ (2013) Exploiting online discussions to discover unrecognized drug side effects. Methods Inf Med 52:152–159

Design Science with a Focus on User-Centred Evaluation of Written Information

12

Jörg Fuchs

Abstract

Written information about medicines is commonplace and has been used worldwide for decades to communicate risks and safe use advice for medicines. This chapter describes ways to optimise these important information materials using a design science approach—a structured process that starts with awareness of a problem, continues to development of a proposal/artefact up to its evaluation, and ends with a conclusion, including increased design science knowledge and/or awareness of unresolved or new issues relevant to communication. As illustrated here, creation and optimisation of information about medicines still has much room for improvement, to be enacted considering the totality of issues integral to the quality of information—in particular comprehensibility, usability, typography and layout. In this context, the systematic use of quality criteria is highly recommended. Evaluation is a key step of the design process; therefore, several evaluation methods are presented, with consideration of their advantages and limitations. Crucially, the evaluation should focus on improving the entire information material rather than simply attaining the success criteria of a couple of tested key messages. In addition, this chapter is meant to opens eyes and provide ideas for future perspectives and pathways for user-centred information materials.

J. Fuchs (✉)
Department of Drug Regulatory Affairs, Institute of Pharmacy, University of Bonn, Bonn, Germany
e-mail: joerg.fuchs@paint-consult.com

© Springer Nature Singapore Pte Ltd. 2020

P. Bahri (ed.), *Communicating about Risks and Safe Use of Medicines*,
https://doi.org/10.1007/978-981-15-3013-5_12

12.1 The Discipline of Design Science: Scope, Theories and Principles

Written communication of risks and safe use advice for medicines, whether disseminated in print or via the internet and digital electronic devices, bear a fundamental role in ensuring appropriate medicine use. For patients, they come in the format of package leaflets/inserts, drug/medication guides or consumer medication information (CMI); for healthcare professionals, as summary of product characteristics within the European Union (EU) and several African countries, prescribing information in the United States of America (USA), package inserts in Japan, or in the many forms of additional educational materials for either of these user groups. The fundamental role of the package leaflet for patients, for example, in the EU, is stated in the EU Directive 2001/83/EC, Articles 58 to 64 as an obligatory requirement for every medicine (The European Parliament and the Council of the European Union 2012). While the pharmaceutical industry and regulatory authorities put great effort into achieving precise and detailed instructions, it must be asked whether our legally required information about medicines, including information about risk minimisation measures, reaches the desired audience and aims.

This chapter focuses on written information, as in the context of reaching users, motivation to read and use the provided content is seen as the basis of ensuring clear communication of risk and safe medicine use. A key factor is the perception of the instructions—driven by the clarity of the layout, legibility and comprehensibility of information and the resultant awareness and motivation of the user to take correct actions when using medicines. The success of information material is determined by each step of its creation, production and distribution; ultimately, in how it meets user needs. Such requirements are constantly in flux and must be permanently adapted to current information needs and habits. In this context, involving end users in the creation and testing process is a beneficial approach—initiated in the last century with research into using information about medicines, such as readability testing of CMI in Australia in the 1990s, and since 2005, for example, compulsory readability testing of package leaflets in the EU (Sless and Wiseman 1997; The European Parliament and the Council of the European Union 2004). Listening to the public to fulfil their information interests is a new approach to translate communication research about risks and safe medicine use results into guidelines, such as for regulators (Bahri and Castillon Melero 2018; European Medicines Agency and Heads of Medicines Agencies 2019). The involvement of end users in the creation of written information about risks and safe use of medicines can be compared to the description by van Beusekom et al. for patient involvement in pictogram creation (Van Beusekom et al. 2018):

1. End users are involved as passive objects of observation for researchers only.
2. End users are invited to comment on predefined written and visual information.
3. End users actively take part in the compilation process and have decision power regarding the creation of written and visual information.

Those applying design sciences need to understand some cognitive processes, namely perception and motivation:

Perception with regard to using written information about medicines is comprised of uptake, selection, processing (e.g. comparison with prior knowledge) and interpretation of contents. Not all stimuli create perceptions, only those that are cognitively processed and serve to orientate a subject. Perception enables meaningful actions and the development of mental models and thus, anticipatory and planned thought. However, perception may also cause overstimulation, confusion and disorientation. The visual perception of written information works via our eyes and is composed of texts and illustrations or pictograms, whereby the latter can be used as interpretation or visual explanation of a text, stand-alone information source or for decorative purposes. They help to simplify complex instructions, increase user attraction and motivation to read provided information, convey alarming effects or, at a more basic level, better inform users with poor reading skills (for perception specifically of risks, see Chap. 7 on the cognitive and behavioural sciences).

Motivation is defined as the totality of reasons that lead to the willingness to act, including desire, emotions and needs (Ellliot and Covington 2001). It can be divided into intrinsic (internal or inherent) motivation and extrinsic (external) motivation. Intrinsic motivation is exemplified in the self-desire of a patient to seek more information about own diseases or used medicines. Such natural tendency better motivates patients to read information about medicines than external motivations, such as the advice of package leaflets to read the provided instructions. Stronger examples of external motivation to read this type of medical information include advices from healthcare professionals or friends, or treatment successes achieved by other people. Despite the presence of positive stimuli in information materials—such as a clear, coloured and interesting layout, including illustrations (Fuchs et al. 2017; Shiyanbola et al. 2017)—negative stimuli are known to demotivate users when attempting to read instructions. Factors such as an unattractive layout, bad legibility (e.g. small font size), poor comprehensibility, unstructured information presentation and use of long paragraphs, as well as large volumes of text, can prove daunting to users (Fuchs 2010a, b; Van Beusekom et al. 2016; Vander Stichele et al. 1991) (for motivation theories, see Chap. 7 on the cognitive and behavioural sciences).

Linguistics aspects are an important element of using texts, but the scientific study of language, which involves an analysis of language form, meaning and context (Halliday and Webster 2006; Martinet and Palmer 1967), is outside the scope of this chapter. Other important text factors are (Deutsches Institut für Normung (German Institute for Standardisation) 2013):

- *Recognisability:* the property of single characters that allows the characters to be recognised and distinguished.
- *Legibility:* the property of a sequence of recognisable characters, which makes it possible to capture these characters in the context within a text.
- *Readability:* the property of recognisable and legibly arranged characters that allow the information to be clearly understood. It depends on the:
  - complexity of text vocabulary and syntax (content)
  - text presentation (typography, formatting).

- *Comprehensibility:* the readers' ability to understand the text, to process text, understand its meaning and to integrate it with that what the reader already knows.
- *User-friendliness:* the fact or quality of being simple for people to use. In the case of texts, it is influenced by the four previous factors.

Design science focuses on research for the development and performance of designed artefacts (e.g. products, processes or information about risks and safe use of medicines) and is used in areas such as information technology (IT) solutions, in the engineering of technical products and in management and business processes. In a sequence of expert activities, it is targeted at improving the functional performance of these artefacts, finding solutions and developing knowledge, such that experts can apply the design solutions to problems within their field. Design science not only creates artefacts, but also evaluates their benefits to respective problem areas and intended users. Thereby, the re-evaluation and field testing of any problem improve the quality of the artefacts (Vaishnavi et al. 2019; Van Aken 2005).

Vaishnavi and Kuechler termed designing new artefacts as innovative, where the knowledge required to create the artefact exists as routine design. However, routine design can also lead to innovative form—the so-called design science research. Innovative research is cyclic and sometimes called "improvement research" (Vaishnavi et al. 2019) (see Fig. 12.1).

According to Vaishnavi and Kuechler, the issue of awareness of a problem looms at the beginning of each design science research and originates from different sources, such as new industry developments, findings in an allied discipline or new results in a researchers' field. Both term the output of this step a proposal for a new research effort. During the creative suggestion step, a tentative design and/or prototype—or at the very least the germ of an idea—for problem solution is created as part of the proposal.

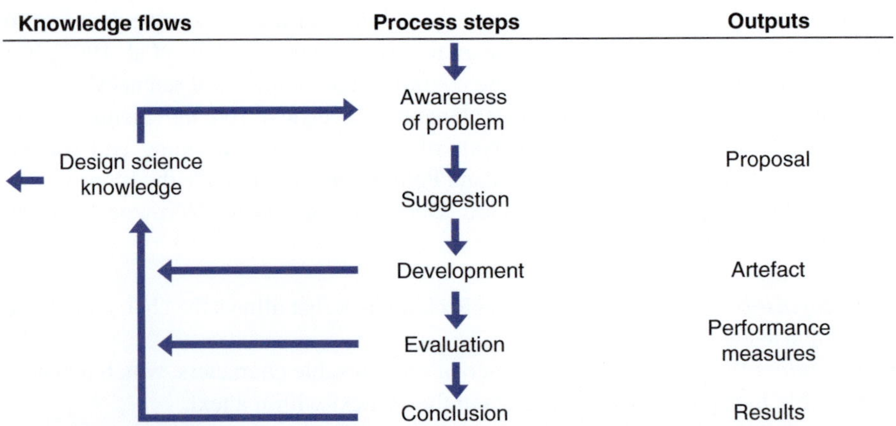

Fig. 12.1 Design science research cycle (general process model) according to Vaishnavi and Kuechler (Vaishnavi et al. 2019)

The tentative design is further developed and implemented in the development step, whereby its implementation does not necessarily involve novelty beyond the state-of practice, as the novelty is contained primarily within the design rather than in the construction of the artefact. Afterwards, the usefulness, quality and efficacy of an artefact must be demonstrated via well-executed evaluation methods. The final process of conclusion typically contains the results (e.g. a finished product), while the output of design science research is the newly acquired science knowledge (Vaishnavi et al. 2019). Other design science research models are available, although with similarities, such as the circulating design science processes according to Pfeffers et al. (2008), Hevner et al. (2004), Purao (2002), Gregg et al. (2001), March and Smith (1995).

12.2 Research Approaches and Methods

As previously stated, design science research can be applied to a plurality of areas; however, it is often described in a very theoretical manner (Vaishnavi et al. 2019; Van Aken 2005). The following endeavours to present design science research in a practical way with the example of approaches and methods for creating written information about medicines—mining the author's daily experience in this area as well as his own and others' research. Print materials—especially package leaflets/inserts, drug/medication guides or consumer medication information/CMI (all named in the following for simplification as package leaflets)—have been selected, as they are very common and have been used worldwide for decades in the ongoing effort to communicate risks and advice for safe medicine use (Bernardini et al. 2000; PizzolI et al. 2019; Fuchs et al. 2005; Hamrosi et al. 2014; Koo et al. 2005; Weitbrecht and Voßkämper 2002). Given that package leaflets are usually delivered to patients in direct conjunction with the medicine (The European Parliament and the Council of the European Union 2012; Hamrosi et al. 2014; Koo et al. 2005; Dawoodi and Bhosale 2016; East African Community Secretariat 2014; Fujita et al. 2014), it is not surprising that they are globally one of the most investigated forms of written information about medicines. Using package leaflets as a print material example also allows the transfer of provided methods, approaches and applications to other written forms of risk and safe medicine use communication, including those via internet, modern IT or mobile technology solutions.

12.2.1 Problem Awareness Step in the Design Science Cycle

Formative own and/or external research, and/or literature reviews are necessary at the beginning of the design science process to achieve awareness of problems that will be addressed through applying a design science approach.

The following problem is used in Sects. 12.2.1, 12.2.2, 12.2.3, 12.2.4 and 12.2.5 as one example to illustrate the different steps of the cyclic design science process, based on the author's own research:

Example: The Volume of Text Problem
Package leaflets are constantly criticised as being too long, difficult to read and hard to understand (PizzolI et al. 2019; Weitbrecht and Voßkämper 2002; Caldeira et al. 2008; Fuchs et al. 2007; Papay et al. 2010; Tong et al. 2018; Van Dijk et al. 2014a). Despite the repeated demands of patients and healthcare professionals for significantly shorter versions, their word count continues to increase; currently, the average package leaflet in the EU registers at 2600 words (Fuchs et al. 2007, 2017; Wolf et al. 2016).

In a cross-over readability test study from September 2002 to April 2003, each of the 1105 participants tested in two rounds with minimum 4 weeks break, one of five original package leaflets available on the German market and the corresponding versions of five model package leaflets. The models were developed by using a set of over 100 quality criteria, such as compressed text (originals: 563–2433 words, models: 514–643 words), optimised wording and a layout with a larger font size of 11pt They contained the same content required to sufficiently inform patients as their corresponding originals (Fuchs 2010a; Fuchs and Hippius 2007). Within the group of original package leaflets and also in the direct comparison between each package leaflet version of both groups, it was shown that increasing the number of words led to a significant decrease in participants':

- Motivation to read the provided information.
- Ability to locate the tested content, with participants requiring significantly more time to find the information.
- Trust to use the described medicine if needed.
- Feeling well informed by the package leaflet.
- Desire to have similar package leaflets in the future.

However, there was no general relationship between the comprehensibility and the volume of text, indicating that long texts can also be comprehensible (Fuchs 2010a). These results show an existing major problem that the current volume of text and its ongoing increase in package leaflets exert a significant negative effect on communicating risks and safe use of medicines via this patient information.

12.2.2 Suggestion Step in the Design Science Cycle

The next step of the design science process consists of creating research-evidence-based suggestions.

Example: Suggestions for Solving the Volume of Text Problem
The awareness of the volume of text problem led to the suggestion to reduce or limit the word count of package leaflets—and of medical information in general—with the principle being to provide short and concise information about medicines without deleting essential content.

So, how can we come from the problem awareness to the suggested text compression without deleting essential information? A key suggestion based on the readability test study presented in Sect. 12.2.1 (Fuchs 2010a; Fuchs and Hippius 2007) is to reduce the word count of templates used for package leaflets—these are text frames consisting of headings and standard texts and usually do not contain specific medical information. They are intended for large groups of different or all medicines of a region or country. For example, a core template in accordance with the Therapeutic Goods Regulation applies to the CMI in Australia (Aslani et al. 2010; Australian Government, Department of Health, Therapeutics Goods Administration 2019; Australian Government 1990). For package leaflets, the Quality Review of Documents (QRD) template applies in the EU (and some non-EU countries in Europe), the Swiss template in Switzerland and the template currently used in East African countries, which is similar to a previous version of the QRD template used in the EU (East African Community Secretariat 2014; Institutsrat des Schweizerischen Heilmittelinstituts 2019; European Medicines Agency 2019). Replacing the EU's current 840-word QRD template (version 10.1 published in June 2019 for EU-centralised procedures and version 4.1 published in February 2020 for mutual recognition and decentralised procedures—both are almost identical in texts for package leaflets) with the 200-word alternative developed in the suggestion step, yields a significant text compression of around 15% in all EU package leaflets, without deleting specific medical information. This alternative was first published in 2012 and is based on the QRD template, but optimised by avoiding repetitions and long sentences, akin to the template used to create the models for the study mentioned in Sect. 12.2.1 (Fuchs et al. 2012).

Furthermore, in communication science the following five general rules of communicating more with fewer words exist:

- Picture the receiver (audience) in your mind before you begin to write, as a written communication is a link between people.
- Choose simple words and use the shorter word if more than one is appropriate ("Automobile or car? > Car!").
- Be polite and clear, as this makes the message stronger with a clear impact.
- Make the message brief and direct by trimming redundant words or phrases.
- Choose strong, active verbs. "I suggest…" instead of "It would seem to me that we might…" (Bauer and Erdogan 2012).

Table 12.1 lists recommendations based on the author's daily practice, own and others' research. As found for package leaflets approved by authorities in EU countries, the application of all issues presented in Table 12.1 would reduce the number of words on average by a further 20% (Fuchs 2010a) (note: The text reduction achieved using the 200-word template is not contained in this 20%). This table also contains methods for the evaluation step, which are further discussed in Sects. 12.2.4 and 12.3. The technique to implement the text compression can be manual- or software-based; software solutions can be simpler and faster—even more so with ever-improving artificial intelligence.

Table 12.1 Recommendations to compress the volume of text of written information about medicines without deleting essential information

Recommendations	Explanations and evidence	Evaluation methods[a]
Use bullet points	Usually a couple of words can be deleted in comparison to full sentences. At the same time the clarity and comprehensibility may increase—particularly in enumerations.	Method used by the author of this chapter for the first six recommendations of Table 12.1: An original text is reworked by another writer applying the recommendation listed in the first column and the word counts are compared. Afterwards, a readability test is used to check the usability of the revised text.
Use maximum 20 words in sentences and bullet points	The first EU readability guideline (European Commission 1998) and the "Always read the leaflet" guideline of the United Kingdom (Medicines and Healthcare Products Regulatory Agency 2005) recommend the threshold of maximum 20 words per sentence or bullet point, although this is less specific in the current EU readability guideline as "Long sentences should not be used" (European Commission 2009). This threshold is also recommended by Australian communication researchers (Sless and Shrensky 2006). The 20-word recommendation has the advantage of being an unambiguous threshold. This is an agreement rather than evidence-based and the optimum may differ between languages. However, the average length of sentences was found in several studies for English and German to be 20 and 22 words, respectively (Amstad 1978). See also Table 12.3.	
Use short words	Use the shorter word if more than one is appropriate as already explained in the five general rules of communicating in Sect. 12.2.2 (Bauer and Erdogan 2012).	
Avoid text brackets	Although text brackets can be helpful in providing further information, too often they contain repetition rather than additional information. In the case of medical terms, for example, the mention of difficult medical terms offers no further information to patients when precise and comprehensible explanations are already provided (Fuchs 2005). The thresholds of an acceptable number and length of text brackets could differ between languages and type of information. Furthermore, Amstad wrote that text brackets interrupt the syntactic and semantic unit. The beginning of the text bracket must be remembered until the solution appears. This is of special importance if a significant part of the semantic information appears at the end of text brackets and thus at the end of the sentence (Amstad 1978).	
Avoid information irrelevant for intended users	In a patient information leaflet, for example, this applies to contents relevant for healthcare professionals only, such as the aseptic preparation of an infusion for hospital use.	
Avoid filler words	Filler words have usually low meaningfulness, do often not convey additional information and are not necessary for understanding the context. Examples are "in principle", "basically" or "aware of the fact". Instead of "be aware of the fact that dampness may affect the device and cause rust", the version "dampness may affect the device and cause rust" is recommended (US Department of Health and Human Services, Food and Drug Administration, Center for Devices and Radiological Health 2001).	

Avoid repetitions	A readability test study of English and German package leaflets with 241 participants, published in 2014, shows that repetitions do not generally increase the locating and understanding of information. This study tested three template texts on different enalapril package leaflet texts, whereby each participant tested one enalapril text using two different QRD template versions (the text frame of headings and standard texts used in the EU that contains several repetitions), and a 200-word model template without repetitions. No other differences existed between the leaflet texts tested per participant (Wolf et al. 2014). This finding has been confirmed by another readability test study with package leaflets of three different medicines—again each leaflet was tested using the QRD template and 200-word template (Fuchs et al. 2012). The findings of both studies reject the Food and Drug Administration (FDA) guidance applicable in the USA for medical device patient labelling "repeat important points and summarise important information, to increase the reader's recall and reading comprehension. The reader will remember the message when key points are reinforced"; particularly, as the FDA provides no evidence for this recommendation (US Department of Health and Human Services, Food and Drug Administration, Center for Devices and Radiological Health 2001). Furthermore, no evidence was found that a summary of key information/headline section at the beginning of package leaflets increases patients' ability to locate and understand provided information (Dickinson et al. 2016; Dickinson 2014; Dolk et al. 2011; Van Dijk et al. 2014b). Therefore, if the information is of special importance it should be highlighted (e.g. using bold print) rather than repeated.	Readability test of texts with identical content and layout—once with repetitions and once without (Fuchs et al. 2012; Wolf et al. 2014).
Use short text templates	Text templates consisting of headings and general advices without medical or therapy specific information should be as short as possible (Fuchs et al. 2012; Wolf et al. 2014). See Sects. 12.2.2–12.2.5 and the recommendation "avoid repetitions" for further details.	Creating different templates; afterwards readability test of the templates using identical layout and medical specific wording (Fuchs et al. 2012; Wolf et al. 2014).

[a]Please note: Despite extensive literature research, more evaluation methods may exist than listed here

12.2.3 Development Step in the Design Science Cycle

In the next step of the design science process, the proposal created in the suggestion step is further developed and implemented to construct the artefact, underpinned by hypotheses and research. Techniques for implementation will vary depending on the tentative design and/or artefact of the written information proposal. For example, a development algorithm may require the construction of a formal proof showing its correctness; a pilot study can establish proof of concept and software solutions used to implement novel assumptions about human cognition in an area of interest (Vaishnavi et al. 2019). During artefact construction, one should not only focus on the identified problem but consider other issues too.

Example: Considerations for Artefact Construction for Solving the Volume of Text Problem

The further development of the volume of text suggestion and subsequent evaluation of the usefulness and efficacy of short package leaflets demand the consideration of all conditions/processes, influencing factors, etc. applied during the creation of the information. Focussing solely on the identified problem without wider consideration is insufficient; the volume of text is an extremely important factor, but only one of many influencing the use of information about risks and safe medicine use. In aiming to create optimal information materials, each influencing factor should lie within its optimal range according to the current evidence. This is essential to best determining the volume of text's influence and avoids disturbances due to sub-optimal variables. The issues discussed below merit consideration for solving the volume of text problem.

Known issues to be considered for artefact construction for information about medicines include:

- *General considerations*: General recommendations for written and also visual information are listed in Table 12.2.
- *Comprehensibility issues*: Table 12.3 provides a selection of standard quality requirements for creating comprehensible information about medicines, including methods for their evaluation.
- *Typographic issues*: Typography is the art and technique of arranging type in a legible, readable and appealing manner. It comprises, for example, the typeface, type size, line length, line spacing (leading) and letter-spacing (tracking) (Bringhurst 2005). Table 12.4 lists a selection of typographic standard quality requirements.
- *Layout issues*: The use of a clear and attractive layout in information about medicines is essential to motivate reading. Table 12.5 illustrates standards for layout recommendations, including methods for evaluation, while Table 12.6 provides recommendations for creating pictograms, illustrations and images.
- *Content-specific quality requirements*: Information about risks and safe medicine use comprises an enormous diversity of content, such as side effects, contraindications, dosage instructions, warnings and precautions. Their requirements

Table 12.2 Important general recommendations for creating written and visual information about medicines

Recommendations for clarification	Explanations	Evaluation methods[a]
What information must be communicated?	E.g. information about risks and safe medicine use. The recommendation is that the required information is provided. Missing information cannot be used by the recipient (DiSantostefano et al. 2014).	Expert evaluation
Who are the recipients?	E.g. patients, healthcare professionals, authorities, employees of pharmaceutical companies, outdoor or hotline staff.	Expert evaluation
Which skills and characteristics of recipients must be considered?	E.g. reading skills, country-specific issues that reflect the user group.	Literature research
Which guidelines and other legal rules must be considered?	E.g. guidelines and legislation valid for the intended countries, including recommendations published by the relevant authorities.	Literature research
What is the most appropriate order of contents, if not legally determined?	Start with the most important content, followed by content in order of decreasing importance, which is in line with users' preferred order. However, the order must follow a logical system, such as contraindications before dosage instructions (Fuchs et al. 2005, 2007). Both young and old people favour a similar order (Fuchs et al. 2007; Morrow et al. 1996). In addition, users can better remember content if their preferred order is used (Morrow et al. 1991).	Consultations to ask users what is important for them and their preferred order (Fuchs et al. 2005, 2007; Pander Maat et al. 2015)
Which manuals, references or publications are available to ensure best quality of required information?	Literature research is a recommended method; however, it should not be confined to big databases like PubMed or Embase; research about medical information evaluation is often published in less high-ranking journals. Thus, the use of secondary literature sources or search engines are alternative options. Use of predefined inclusion and exclusion criteria is recommended.	Literature research

[a]Please note: Despite extensive literature research, more evaluation methods may exist than listed here

Table 12.3 Comprehensibility recommendations for written information about medicines

Recommendations	Explanations and evidence	Evaluation methods[a]
Avoid contradictory information	An example is when a contraindication is stated for using the medicine in patients with kidney or liver problems, while elsewhere is stated "the medicine can be used in patients with kidney or liver problems if absolutely necessary".	Readability test (Fuchs 2005)

(continued)

Table 12.3 (continued)

Recommendations	Explanations and evidence	Evaluation methods[a]
Avoid sentences or bullet points longer than 20 words	In addition to the impact on the volume of text and the available evidence explained in Table 12.1, the sentence and bullet point length influence the comprehensibility and locating of information. However, the influence of exceeding the threshold of maximum 20 words on the comprehensibility or locating of contents is unknown (e.g. a minor increase of the maximum word count in bullet points/sentences, or increased number of long bullet points/ sentences). Nevertheless, using shorter sentences in a sub-optimal package leaflet improved the comprehensibility in a test of 71 participants aged 60 years and older (Hohgräwe 1988).	Proposed methods: Readability test and measuring reading speed are options to determine an optimal threshold of sentence and bullet point length, using texts with identical wording and layout that only vary in the sentence and bullet point length.
Avoid difficult terms, abbreviations, acronyms	Terms, abbreviations and acronyms difficult for the information user must be avoided as these can cause medication errors (European Commission 2009; Brunetti et al. 2007; Institute for Safe Medication Practices 2015). According to Table 12.1, difficult terms and abbreviations should not additionally be provided, as mentioning these medical terms offers no further information to the user when short, precise and comprehensible explanations are available.	Comprehensibility tests described in Sect. 12.3.3
Avoid difficult scientific and unusual symbols	Symbols, such as $<$, $>$, $\leq$, $\geq$, are not familiar to everyone and can be confused; therefore, their replacement by more appropriate texts is recommended (European Commission 2009). This also applies to unusual symbols that are difficult to understand (Sless and Shrensky 2006).	Comprehensibility tests in Sect. 12.3.3
Use active speech	Active speech is recommended, starting with instructions followed by explanations. Using English as an example, this usually means starting with the verb (European Commission 2009; Sless and Shrensky 2006; Raynor 1992). However, the readability test of Dutch oxazepam and tetracycline package leaflets with 70 participants did not show an effect on comprehensibility due to change from passive to active voice (Franck et al. 2011).	Readability test (Franck et al. 2011), usability test

Table 12.3 (continued)

Recommendations	Explanations and evidence	Evaluation methods[a]
Avoid non-quantifiable phrases	Words such as "recently", "many" or "very rare" are non-quantifiable phrases which do not enable users to clearly understand the content of the information being communicated. E.g. the phrase "recently" can be interpreted as either a period lasting at least 14 days or a period of 1 month or more (Fuchs 2005; Fuchs et al. 2006). In a questioning of 200 people relating to meaning of side effect frequencies, "very rare", for example, was overestimated by a factor of four hundred—frequency of 4% instead of <0.01% (Berry et al. 2002). Use quantifiable numerical data instead of non-quantifiable phrases alone, or minimum both in conjunction; however, percentages should be avoided due to their poorer comprehensibility (Knapp et al. 2009). Various numerical explanations may differ in their comprehensibility. For example, the side effect frequency explanation for EU package leaflets used since July 2011 has a significantly lower comprehensibility than the previous version published in September 2007. In addition, people overestimate the current EU frequency explanation by up to a factor of 10 (European Medicines Agency 2007; Wolf et al. 2014).	Readability test (Fuchs and Hippius 2007; Fuchs et al. 2012; Wolf et al. 2014), comprehensibility test (Berry et al. 2002; Knapp et al. 2009)
Avoid different terms to describe the same issue	Always use the same term for one issue (Raynor 1992). Different terms for the same issue may cause readers to believe different aspects are described, e.g. reduced kidney function, renal impairment, renal insufficiency, kidney problems or renal problems. Using the most common, short and comprehensible term for intended users is recommended.	Proposed method: Readability test combined with comprehensibility tests described in Sect. 12.3.3
Use Arabic numerals	Use Arabic instead of Roman numerals. These can be more quickly read and better understood, as found in a comparison speed and accuracy reading test with 30 students (Perry 1952).	Reading speed, accuracy of reading (Perry 1952)

[a]Please note: Despite extensive literature research, evaluation methods other than the listed examples are applicable to assess the comprehensibility. Other methods are questioning, multiple choice test, usability test, memorability/memory factor, subjective perception (Tillmann 2014) or methods like the cloze test. In the cloze test every fifth word is blanked out and readers are asked to fill in the gaps (Taylor 1953)

Table 12.4 Typography recommendations for written information about medicines

Recommendations	Explanations and evidence	Evaluation methods[a]
Font characteristics		
Use fonts with humanist characteristics	The characters of the selected font type must be easily distinguishable. Critical characters are, for example, 0 (number) and O (capital letter o) as well as 1 (number), I (capital letter i), l (lower-case letter L) (Deutsches Institut für Normung (German Institute for Standardisation) 2013; European Commission 2009). Typefaces with humanist characteristics are recommended as their characters are more open and more quickly recognisable (Deutsches Institut für Normung (German Institute for Standardisation) 2013).	Reading speed (reading a text and measuring the required time) (Connolly 1998), reading errors (Burtt and Basch 1923), reading amount (the volume of text read within a given time).
Serif and sans serif fonts are appropriate	Serif and sans serif font types showed similarly good reading properties in a 200-word text, based on assessments of 12 young and 12 older people using a 7-point Likert scale and reading time (Connolly 1998). Using 10 content questions after 90 seconds reading of 450 words, 375 adults also had no general advantage in text comprehension when using serif or sans serif fonts (Poulton 1965). Although some researchers prefer serif fonts, and others sans serif fonts, many studies are available illustrating equal legibility between both fonts (Soleimani and Mohammadi 2012).	Reading speed (Connolly 1998), reading errors (Burtt and Basch 1923), reading amount.
Use 9 to 12pt font size	The optimum of 9 to 12pt for people without major limitations was found in different studies, based on measurements of reading speed (Paterson and Tinker 1929, 1940; Tinker and Paterson 1931a), reading amount (Aberson and Bouwhuis 1997), users' opinions (Bernardini et al. 2001), skimming items (Poulton 1967a, 1969) and through readability testing of identical text versions printed in font sizes between 7 and 16pt, and afterwards calculating the rank sum of results in locating information, comprehensibility and participants' opinions (Fuchs et al. 2010a). Font sizes over 12pt are usually not recommended as legibility properties decrease significantly when further increasing the font size. One explanation is that users can see less words in one view, and require more eye fixations and perceptual time when using font sizes over 12pt, in comparison to the optimum range (Paterson and Tinker 1942).	Reading speed (Paterson and Tinker 1929), reading amount (Aberson and Bouwhuis 1997), user opinion (Bernardini et al. 2001), readability testing (Fuchs et al. 2010a), eye movements (Paterson and Tinker 1942), skimming items (Poulton 1967a, 1969).
Carefully select font colour	The use of colour in package leaflets can improve information and be used to highlight key messages; however, it does not generally induce higher motivation to read the contents (Fuchs et al. 2018; Hemphill 1996). The reduced contrast and legibility of coloured texts other than black font (see next line), present problems for people with reduced colour sensitivity or colour blindness (Moudgil et al. 2016; Pickford 1963). Users' associations and emotions to colours, which can be negative (Bernardini et al. 2001; Hemphill 1996), must be considered before using this option to emphasise content. Therefore, no reason exists for a general favouritism for coloured medical information, such as in package leaflets, over their black/greyscale equivalent (Fuchs et al. 2018).	Reading speed (Tinker and Paterson 1931a), readability test (Fuchs et al. 2018), reading amount.

Use high contrast between font and paper colour	Black font on white paper has the highest contrast of all possible colour combinations (Fuchs and Kutscha 2015). Tinker and Paterson investigated the reading speed of 10 combinations of font and background colours, dividing 850 college students into 10 equal groups. Black font on white background was the most quickly legible; green and blue font on a white background and black font on a yellow background were almost as good. Combinations of orange on black or white background, red on green, and black on purple were difficult to read (Tinker and Paterson 1931a). Both authors also investigated eye movements of 20 students and found that black font on white background in comparison to red font on green has: • 24.8% less eye fixation. • 20.2% more words per eye fixation. • 14.5% fewer pauses between eye fixations. • 42.6% lower perceptual time (Tinker and Paterson 1944). Moreover, adults from 45 years onwards require more contrast between font and background than younger people, with those aged over 70 requiring three times more contrast than 20-year-olds (Ekstrom 1993).	Reading speed (Tinker and Paterson 1931a), eye movements (Tinker and Paterson 1944), contrast measurement (Fuchs and Kutscha 2015).
Use dark font on bright background instead of reversed versions	Paterson and Tinker found a 10.5% quicker reading speed in a study with 280 students when using black font on white background in comparison to white font on black background (Paterson and Tinker 1931), whereby words printed in black on white can be perceived at a greater distance than words printed in white on black (difference: 14.7%) (Holmes 1931).	Reading speed (Paterson and Tinker 1931), perception at different distances (Holmes 1931).
Avoid capitals, italics and underlined print	Capitals have slower legibility because their upper and lower contours form a straight line, thus contour differences of character heights, such as with the letter "g", are not recognisable (Poulton and Brown 1968; Tinker and Paterson 1928). A siginificant 9% slower reading speed was found with headings in capitals compared with bold emphasised texts in lower cases, under involvement of 264 adults ($p < 0.01$) (Poulton 1967b). This was also found for short headings, whereby headings in upper and lower cases can be better remembered than those in capitals (Breland and Breland 1944). This applies similarly to underlined text. Italic print has also been shown to be less legible than texts in upper and lower cases (Tinker and Paterson 1928). For example: **package leaflet**, PACKAGE LEAFLET, PACKAGE LEAFLET, *package leaflet*. Based on ten open questions in a comprehensibility test, texts in upper and lower cases were on average 13% faster to comprehend than those in capitals (Poulton and Brown 1968). Thus, when key words require emphasis, use of bold print, for example, is more appropriate. However, a single capital letter can be seen from a greater distance than a lower-case letter due to its larger character height (Burtt and Basch 1923; Roethlein 1912).	Reading speed/amount (Tinker and Paterson 1928; Poulton 1967b), readability/ comprehensibility test (Poulton and Brown 1968), memory test (Breland and Breland 1944).

(continued)

Recommendations	Explanations and evidence	Evaluation methods[a]
Avoid reduced space between words	Removal of spaces between words reduces reading speed with higher impairment on lower-sighted than on normal-sighted people (Sass et al. 2006).	Reading speed (Sass et al. 2006).
Line characteristics		
Line spacing (leading)	The German norm DIN 1450 recommends a line spacing of around 120% of the font size (Deutsches Institut für Normung (German Institute for Standardisation) 2013), which is in line with recommendations of Tinker and Paterson after measuring the reading speed (Tinker and Paterson 1949).	Reading speed (Tinker and Paterson 1949).
Line length (column width)	The German norm DIN 1450 recommends maximum 80 characters per line for texts like package leaflets (Deutsches Institut für Normung (German Institute for Standardisation) 2013). However, line length should not be too short, as this could reduce legibility. Smaller font sizes require shorter line lengths than larger fonts (Tinker and Paterson 1929, 1931b, 1949. Despite the amendment of the line length, 10pt font size with around 80 mm line length showed, in a study of 5 groups with 80 students each, the fastest reading speed compared to the combinations of 12pt font size/97 mm line length, 14pt/115 mm, 8pt/72 mm and 6pt/67 mm (Tinker and Paterson 1931b). When a 10pt font type was printed with 12pt line spacing, line lengths ranging from 60 to 130 mm were equally legible (Tinker 1963).	Reading speed (Tinker and Paterson 1929, 1931b).
Use text attributes to emphasise key words, such as bold print	Text attributes include, for example, bold print, italic, underlined, capitals, illustrations, diagrams, frames, alternative font colour, tables and lists. They help to pick out content more quickly and to highlight key messages. However, capitals, italics or underlined texts significantly reduce legibility in comparison to normal texts printed in upper- and lower-case letters, as explained above. Recommended text attributes are bold print, a different font colour with high contrast to the underground and good differentiation to the remaining text, larger font sizes, bullet points and tables (Fuchs et al. 2017, 2018). Where information must be highlighted using bold print, for example, emphasise key words only, as emphasising entire sentences or paragraphs diminishes the effect, including the locating of contents (Azodi et al. 2002).	Readability test (Fuchs et al. 2018), Skimming items.

Left-justified and justified text are appropriate	Although the EU readability guideline suggests excluding justified text (European Commission 2009), there is no existing research supporting this general exclusion if columns are sufficiently broad, such as on average 12 words per line according to an English reading speed study (Gregory and Poulten 1970). Where the average line length is 7 words, justified English texts result in an inferior position compared to left-justified texts (Gregory and Poulten 1970). In a Swedish study with 48 adults and texts with 10 cm average line length, no significant differences in reading speed, eye fixations and regressions were found as total result between justified and unjustified texts, which is in line with other studies quoted by Zacchrisson. Only the least proficient readers showed a longer reading time for right-justified texts (Zachrisson 1965). However, justified text has the advantage that paragraph endings can be recognised more readily than with uncorrected left-justified text. Large spaces between words can be remedied through appropriate typesetting measures. Therefore, the use of only left-justified print cannot be generally recommended.	Reading speed (Gregory and Poulten 1970; Zachrisson 1965). Eye fixations and regressions (Zachrisson 1965).
Use horizontal texts	Use horizontal texts only, including also in figures and tables. As found with English texts, these can be read faster than vertical versions (Yu et al. 2010).	Reading speed (Yu et al. 2010).

[a]Please note: Despite extensive literature research, evaluation methods other than those examples listed to assess the typography are applicable. Method categories apply to:

- Eye movement: tachistoscope, electrooculography, eye tracking, eye movement registration
- Reading performance: kymograph, reading speed, reading time, reading quantity, reading accuracy, reading ability, content analysis, meaning extraction, comprehensibilitys
- Threshold measurement: reading distance, recognisability, visibility meter (Tillmann 2014)

Table 12.5 Layout recommendations for written information about medicines

Recommendations	Explanations and evidence	Evaluation methods[a]
Use layout that motivates reading	As stated in 12.1, the motivation to read the information is the basic issue. Therefore, apart from compressing the volume of text and a verbal invitation, clear appearance and sub-categorisation of texts, frequent use of text attributes, including colouration and use of illustrations elicits such motivation. Black/white layouts can also motivate (Fuchs et al. 2018).	Opinion survey (Fuchs 2010a; Fuchs et al. 2018)
Portrait and landscape format are appropriate	The current EU readability guideline recommends landscape format for package leaflets (European Commission 2009); however, no evidence exists for this general favouritism toward landscape format, as portrait format is also appropriate (Fuchs et al. 2016; Hartley and Johnson 2000). Moreover, using portrait format with two columns is most effective in saving printable area and probably the main reason that it is most frequently used in package leaflets (Fuchs et al. 2016, 2017). The 2-column portrait format also offers more appropriate column widths and significantly reduces the number of column breaks required (Fuchs et al. 2016). The latter exerts a large negative influence on the locating of information, thereby supporting the use of the portrait format (Fuchs and Hippius 2007).	Readability test (Fuchs et al. 2016; Hartley and Johnson 2000)
Format size	Use a format size that fits comfortably in the hand and consider that double-sided printed leaflets show 50% of information on each page compared to the lower rate when using booklets—such as 10% on two pages of a booklet with 20 pages (Fuchs et al. 2016).	Readability test (Fuchs et al. 2016)
Avoid page/column breaks in sections	Page breaks in a paragraph reduce the locating of provided information; therefore, these should be avoided (Fuchs and Hippius 2007; Azodi et al. 2003).	Readability test (Fuchs and Hippius 2007; Azodi et al. 2003)
Use consistent layout	A uniform layout style eases navigation through the document and generates an impression of professionalism. For example, this applies to text attributes, headings and the point form (Sless and Shrensky 2006).	Proposed methods: Reading speed, reading amount, readability test
Use consistent style in headings	Headings and subheadings improve the locating of information, comprehensibility and people can better remember provided content, as shown with 175 pupils (Hartley et al. 1980). Again, a uniform heading/subheading style eases navigation through the entire document. Recommended styles for headings are, for example: • use larger font size compared to the body text. • emphasise heading, e.g. using bold print, frames or other design elements.	Retention test (Hartley et al. 1980), speed and correctness of located contents (Spencer et al. 1974), readability test

(continued)

Table 12.5 (continued)

Recommendations	Explanations and evidence	Evaluation methods[a]
Use consistent style in bullet points	Uniform style in all bullet points eases navigation through the entire document. For example, use bullets for first level of bullet points as these can be more readily noticed than less prominent signs, such as dashes (Sless and Shrensky 2006). Less prominent signs are recommended where further subdivision is required. Uniform style is also recommended at the end of bullet points, whereby Australian communication researchers and the "always read the leaflet" guideline of the United Kingdom prefer to avoid unnecessary punctuation, such as semicolon, comma, dot (Medicines and Healthcare Products Regulatory Agency 2005; Sless and Shrensky 2006).	Speed and correctness of located contents (Spencer et al. 1974)
Use opacity of minimum 80% to assess paper quality	Use opacity to assess paper quality instead of paper weight or thickness, as paper with low grammage can have a similarly high opacity (the measure of impenetrability of visible light) to heavier or thicker paper (Fuchs and Kutscha 2015; Feldmüller et al. 2011). Furthermore, an opacity of minimum 80% is recommended. Opacity has a significant influence on the legibility, which applies, for example, to the contrast between font and paper colour (Fuchs and Kutscha 2015). However, opacity does not consider spreading, evaporation and penetration of the print. Therefore, measurement of the printed opacity (percentage of the original whiteness of the paper after printing, also known as print through or striking through test (IGT Testing Systems 2006)) becomes more and more of interest, as major changes are observed in the print technologies that are used (e.g. offset, inkjet); most leaflets are printed on both sides and ink may pass into the paper. The used print technology and print colours also influence the legibility and the printed opacity seems to better reflect this influence, even though it is not yet a standard.	Diffuse reflectance according to ISO 2471 (Fuchs and Kutscha 2015; Beuth Verlag 2008), printed opacity (print through or striking through tests) (IGT Testing Systems 2006)

[a]Please note: Despite extensive literature research, evaluation methods other than those examples listed to assess the layout quality could be applicable. Methods include those as listed in the note below Table 12.4

Table 12.6 Pictogram/illustration/image recommendations for information about medicines

Recommendations	Explanations and evidence	Evaluation methods[a]
Use only tested pictograms	Pictograms, illustrations and images can enhance the communication of information (Dowse and Ehlers 2004); however, pictograms have the problem of possible misinterpretation that can result in incorrect use of medicines—increasing the risk of adverse events as well as reduced therapy success as explained in Sect. 12.3.4 (Dowse and Ehlers 2004; Wolff and Wogalter 1993). Therefore, testing of pictograms with the intended user group is highly recommended (Van Beusekom et al. 2018; Wolff and Wogalter 1993).	Comprehensibility test (Wolff and Wogalter 1993), see Sect. 12.3.4
Use a pictogram, illustration and image in conjunction with explanatory text	The use of pictograms, illustrations and images with explanatory text is essential to achieve sufficient comprehensibility and reduces the risk of misinterpretation (Friedmann et al. 1997; Pires et al. 2015a). This was the preferred version for prescription medicine instructions according to user assessments using an 8-point Likert scale, compared to pictorial-only instructions (Sojourner and Wogalter 1997).	Comprehensibility test (Friedmann et al. 1997), user opinion (Sojourner and Wogalter 1997), see Sect. 12.3.4
Focus on main details	Avoid details not required to convey the intended information (Ekstrom 1993). This avoids a cognitive overload. For example, in an investigation of four internal organ presentations those with medium or less details were preferred; particularly, participants with low-literacy level favoured less details (Van Beusekom et al. 2015).	Comprehensibility test using questionnaires (Van Beusekom et al. 2015)
Use sufficient large size of pictogram, illustration and images	Sufficiently large size is essential to allow users to notice the content provided (Mansoor and Dowse 2007).	Usability and comprehensibility tests described in Sects. 12.3.2 and 12.3.4
Use sufficient contrast	Similar to texts, sufficient contrast to the background is essential to capture the provided content.	Usability and comprehensibility tests described in Sects. 12.3.2 and 12.3.4

[a]Please note: Despite extensive literature research, more evaluation methods may exist than listed here

vary with the type of medical information and recipient. Table 12.7 provides important requirements of dosage instructions used in package leaflets as an example, as these instructions are regarded as very important information (Dawoodi and Bhosale 2016; Fuchs et al. 2007).

It must be highlighted that several issues listed in Tables 12.1, 12.2, 12.3, 12.4, 12.5, 12.6, and 12.7 influence more than one aspect, e.g. the recommended use of

Table 12.7 Dosage instruction recommendations for package leaflets

Recommendations	Explanations and evidence	Evaluation methods[a]
Specify every dose in the number of tablets, capsules, drops, the volume or any other form of the ready to use medicine	According to a readability test study with 1105 participants, dosages provided in the number of tablets, capsules, drops or volume of the medicine have significantly better comprehensibility than those provided using the amount of active substances. One main reason is that patients must not calculate the dose using the composition information if it is provided in the proposed form (Fuchs and Hippius 2007). This is confirmed by a questioning of 92 participants on the dosage instruction of three OTC products (Patel et al. 2002). The results of the PAINT3 study—involving 4835 participants and testing 295 package leaflets using the written readability test—showed that dosage instructions provided in the number of tablets only, have—with an average 80.9%—a significantly higher comprehensibility level than dosage instructions providing both the number of tablets and the amount of active substance (average of located and understood dosage instructions: 72.0%) (Fuchs 2010b).	Readability test (Fuchs and Hippius 2007)
Provide single and maximum daily doses	Dosages provided in daily doses only, that require calculations by patients to achieve single doses, are difficult to understand according to a study with 92 participants of dosage instructions of three OTC products (Patel et al. 2002) and a questioning with 67 participants of 10 dosage instructions (Mazzullo et al. 1974).]. Therefore, dosages in package leaflets must always be provided in a way that does not require any additional calculation.	Readability test (Patel et al. 2002)
Provide dosages that depend on age or body weight, but not on both	In a readability test with 205 participants of an antibiotic dosage table that provided doses per age and corresponding body weight, 62.0% determined the dose of an antibiotic for an 8-year-old child weighing 40 kg according to the body weight, while 17.8% chose the lower dose according to the age. 9.3% tried to calculate a compromise between both the doses by age and body weight, while a further 9.8% were unable to assess the correct dose themselves and referred to the doctor or pharmacist. Therefore, dosage instructions for patients need to be based on only one and the most appropriate system, such as according to age or body weight—but not on both (Fuchs et al. 2010b).	Readability test (Fuchs and Hippius 2007; Fuchs et al. 2010b)
Use a table or other clear separation of dosages	If different dosages must be provided for different user groups, indications, etc. a clear separation is recommended, using such as a table, different subsections with subheadings, bullet points (Fuchs and Hippius 2007).	Readability test (Fuchs and Hippius 2007)
Avoid margins in dosage instructions	Negative examples are "1 to 3 times 2 to 4 tablets" or "several times daily" as they are non-quantifiable phrases. They are not recommended, other than with an explanation as to when each scope has to be used (Fuchs and Hippius 2007).	Readability test (Fuchs and Hippius 2007)

[a]Please note: Despite extensive literature research, more evaluation methods may exist than the listed readability test

bullet points reduces the word count, but also increases the ability to locate and comprehend provided information. Furthermore, the recommendations listed in Tables 12.1, 12.2, 12.3, 12.4, 12.5, 12.6, and 12.7 can be used as quality criteria, e.g. in the form of an evaluation checklist, which is presented in greater detail in Sect. 12.3.4.

12.2.4 Evaluation Step in the Design Science Cycle

The evaluation step contains an analytic part in which hypotheses are made about the behaviour of the artefact. The evaluation either confirms or rejects a hypothesis. Often, evaluation findings and additional information gained during the preceding suggestion and development steps result in another cycle of suggestions, development and evaluation (see Fig. 12.1). This may suggest a new design, frequently preceded by new library research in the case of deviation from the original approach (Vaishnavi et al. 2019).

Example: Evaluation of the Suggestion for Solving the Volume of Text Problem

In our example, the hypothesis might be that a shorter volume of text improves the locating and use of information in package leaflets—the specific subject of the design process. A common method to measure the impact of a problem and a suggested solution is that all variables are fixed in different versions of the draft written information and only the design feature under evaluation varies. Therefore, package leaflets of three common medicines—repaglinide, enalapril, insulin—were optimised using a set of quality criteria reflecting Tables 12.1, 12.2, 12.3, 12.4, 12.5, 12.6, and 12.7, and printed in colour on light yellow paper and also in black on white paper using:

1. The QRD template version 1.2 (published in October 2006 for mutual recognition and decentralised procedures), resulting in word counts between 1093 and 1333,
2. The 200-word template described in Sect. 12.2.2 resulting in word counts between 682 and 849.

The package leaflets within each of the six pairs were identical in wording and design, except for the differences in the two templates. This means only the volume of text of non-medical specific information was variable (Fuchs et al. 2012). The six pairs were studied between September 2008 and May 2009 using the written readability test (Fuchs et al. 2012).

As the major finding of this study, the text compression of 400–500 words through use of the shorter 200-word template caused a significant reduction of 18.1% in time required to locate the 25 pieces of information tested and in a 15.7% increase in located and understood contents. Disadvantages due to the shorter template were not found (Fuchs et al. 2012). Moreover, these improvements could not be achieved by layout optimisations, such as colouring package leaflets. Another finding was that the motivation to read the package leaflets and the desire by participants to have similar package leaflets in the future was still positive for all longer versions using the QRD template, regardless of whether they were coloured or black/white versions (Fuchs et al. 2018).

Rarely in design science research, an initial hypothesis is completely borne out (Vaishnavi et al. 2019). In the case of the volume of text problem in package leaflets, a new hypothesis was that package leaflets up to 1500 words might still have a positive acceptance. Another hypothesis was that the benefit of a shorter template might also be seen in languages other than German and in longer versions than investigated.

12.2.5 Conclusion Step in the Design Science Cycle

The conclusion step is usually the end of a design science cycle and associated research effort, which is typically a stage of satisfaction even if there are still deviations from the artefact from the revised hypothetical predictions. The knowledge gained during the design science steps is frequently categorised as:

- Facts or behaviour that have been learned and can be applied repeatedly, or
- Anomalies that defy explanation and require further research (Vaishnavi et al. 2019).

The knowledge gained then feeds into new design science cycles for future information materials.

Example: Conclusion of the Design Science Cycle for the Volume of Text Problem

The results presented in Sect. 12.2.4 confirm the hypothesis and underpin the benefits as well as the necessity of short package leaflets. In a newer study on three templates—the QRD template version 8 (published July 2011 for centralised procedures), its precursor and the 200-word template, all tested in English and German, with the examples of a short and a long enalapril package leaflet text and using the written readability test method—the advantages for the short 200-word template were confirmed (Wolf et al. 2014).

The results of a study using the written readability test with 4835 participants and testing 295 package leaflets show increasing the word count has the most negative influence on the use of package leaflets. The threshold up to which patients are still motivated to read package leaflets is 1500 words—optimally 1000 words—meaning a rethink is essential with regard to the current significantly longer versions (Fuchs 2010b). It can be expected that a large volume of text has a similar negative influence on all written information about medicines covering risks and safe use advice—whether intended for patients or healthcare professionals.

12.3 Evaluation Methods of Written Information About Medicines and Their Utility

As simple as it may sound, the core requirement of all information materials about risks and safe use of medicines is that the information required for users is provided therein (see Table 12.2). Major information gaps for patients and healthcare professionals have been identified in current materials worldwide and should be avoided (DiSantostefano et al. 2014; Fuchs et al. 2010c; Ramadas et al. 2013; Sawalha et al. 2008; Shruti et al. 2016; Sillo et al. 2018; Tayyem and Takrouri 2009). It is important to note, complete information must not necessarily lead to an increase in the volume of text (Fuchs 2010a). After verification that the necessary content is provided, the quality of information materials needs evaluation. Sect. 12.3 provides important evaluation methods.

12.3.1 Readability Tests

An important and frequently used evaluation method is readability testing, also known as user testing, readability user test, readability proof, comprehension study, consultation with target patient groups or user consultation. Readability tests were first developed in the 1990s by Australian communication researchers in the form of verbal face-to-face interviews for diagnostic testing of medical information, such as CMI. The intention was to detect difficulties in locating, understanding and using provided information during their development process and fostering improvements; however, this is not a legal requirement in Australia (Sless and Wiseman 1997; Sless 2007). In contrast, readability testing has been a legal requirement for package leaflets in the EU since 2005 (The European Parliament and the Council of the European Union 2004) and in the Eurasian Economic Union since 2016 (Eurasian Economic Commission Council 2016). In the USA, comprehension studies/readability proofs have been demanded for medical device patient labelling since 2001 and for leaflets of non-prescription medicines in defined cases since 2009 (US Department of Health and Human Services, Food and Drug Administration, Center for Devices and Radiological Health 2001; US Department of Health and Human Services, Food and Drug Administration, Center for Drug Evaluation and Research (CDER) 2009). Besides the described original Australian intention, readability tests are often used, for example, in the EU, to demonstrate that the success criteria required to secure medicine approval from authorities have been achieved (The European Parliament and the Council of the European Union 2012; European Commission 2009; Eurasian Economic Commission Council 2016). Readability tests are also used in research to enhance patient information by comparing different versions (Fuchs and Hippius 2007; Franck et al. 2011; Dickinson et al. 2001; Jarernsiripornkul et al. 2019; Pander Maat and Lentz 2010), but also to compare patient information of different countries and continents (Tong et al. 2018; Raynor et al. 2007).

Different readability test methods with different success criteria can be used. This also applies to countries were readability tests are a legal requirement—meaning that no legally binding or specific best test method exists (Medicines and Healthcare Products Regulatory Agency 2005; European Commission 2009; US Department of Health and Human Services, Food and Drug Administration, Center for Devices and Radiological Health 2001; Eurasian Economic Commission Council 2016; US Department of Health and Human Services, Food and Drug Administration, Center for Drug Evaluation and Research (CDER) 2009). The two methods that are officially accepted in all EU countries through guidelines are compared in Table 12.8 (European Commission 2009; Co-ordination Group for Mutual Recognition and Decentralised Procedures—Human (CMD(h)) 2016). Other methods may be acceptable if they ensure suitable measurement of the legibility, locating, comprehensibility and usability of information provided (European Commission 2009). Examples of other methods—however, currently without general acceptance by authorities—are psychological analysis of patient information (P.A.P.I), communication science methods, multiple choice tests (Federal Institute for Drugs and Medical Devices 2013; Hieber 2008).

Laypersons are involved in both readability test methods of patient information described in Table 12.8, while past participants from the previous 6 months as well as healthcare professionals are excluded. The involvement of participants from the targeted patient population might be helpful but is not a requirement (Medicines and Healthcare Products Regulatory Agency 2005, 2008; European Commission 2009; Sless and Shrensky 2006; Eurasian Economic Commission Council 2016; Health Products Regulatory Authority 2018). Furthermore, results can be influenced by

Table 12.8 Comparison of readability test methods accepted in the EU (Co-ordination Group for Mutual Recognition and Decentralised Procedures—Human (CMD(h)) 2016)

Test steps	Verbal face-to-face interview (Australian method)	Written readability test (self-completion method)
Pre-test	**Pilot test** with three to six participants before main test to ensure the questions are appropriate.	**Systematic review** to evaluate and optimise the entire medical information before the main test, using: • a set of 200 quality criteria. • results of more than 1500 scientific and regulatory publications. • study results of over 2000 medical term comprehensibility classifications.
Main test	**Verbal** interview using a set of questions.	**Written** questioning via questionnaire.
	• Minimum **two test rounds** of 12–15 key messages with minimum ten participants each. • **Monitoring** through tester(s).	
Success criteria	Minimum 90% correctly located information and of that 90% understood information, resulting in minimum 80% correct answers per tested information item (**“90% of 90% rule”).**	Minimum **80% correct answers** per tested information item (located and understood).

participants' demographic characteristics, such as age, education level, literacy and health literacy. Therefore, a broad mix of participants is recommended, mirroring the intended user group (Fuchs and Hippius 2007; Paech et al. 2011; Wolf et al. 2012). The selected questions are intended to evaluate the key messages (European Commission 2009). Rather than simply depicting provided information, the questions should be created in such a way as to display readers' understanding of the content and assess whether they would take the correct actions in critical situations when using the medicine.

Advantages of Readability Tests

- With an acceptable effort the comprehensibility, user-friendliness and ease of locating information materials are tested.
- According to Beusekom et al., end users are invited to comment on predefined written and visual information (Van Beusekom et al. 2018), as mentioned in Sect. 12.1.

Limitations of Readability Tests

- Readability tests do not measure any change in knowledge, the therapy success, or what users do in practice. While the content can be located and understood in a readability test, there are possibilities for distraction in a real-world setting, causing patients to deviate from instructions.
- The number of minimum ten participants per test round is low for statistically significant results; however, this is sufficient to identify problems in tested information and initiate subsequent optimisation (Sless and Shrensky 2006).
- Results can be influenced by the kind of questions asked during the test, such as open/closed questions, explicit/implicit contents, positive/negative framing, neutral/judgemental questions, generally understandable/technical language. The influence and the participants' unconscious or preconscious associations and subsequent bias may remain undetected.
- Usually 12–15 key messages are tested, which the Australian communication researchers assess to be sufficient (European Commission 2009; Sless and Shrensky 2006). Sometimes, more key messages are tested (Fuchs et al. 2012; Wolf et al. 2014; National Agency for Medicines and Medical Devices of Romania 2010). However, significantly more information is normally provided in package leaflets and it is impossible to test all at once. To counter this, the initial step of the written readability test is a systematic review to evaluate and optimise the entire leaflet, before conducting the main test with laypersons (see Table 12.8). This strategy reduces the number of difficult words per package leaflet on average by 84% and even the word count by 20% (Fuchs 2010a).
- "External negative influences ... may occur in a face-to-face interview" as stated a position paper from the EU regulatory network (Co-ordination Group for Mutual Recognition and Decentralised Procedures—Human (CMD(h)) 2016). Examples include influences via the interviewer's facial expressions and gestures, participants' hearing problems and interview logging errors, caused by incorrect interpretation and/or documentation of the participants' verbal answers. The competence to read the tested information must be presupposed in both methods when investigating written information.

- Sless, one of the Australian researchers responsible for developing the verbal face-to-face interview readability test stated that "...the application of the 90% of 90% rule in the EU is totally inappropriate, and probably unattainable without some fudging of results", as a lower success rate seems to be a more reasonable level (Sless 2007). Data collected to validate the written readability test further demonstrate this point (Fuchs and Hippius 2007; Fuchs et al. 2012).
- A few verbal face-to-face interviewers additionally measure participant's time taken to answer every individual question (Foster 2013; Tong et al. 2014). For example, according to Forster: "'Information found with difficulty' is defined as requiring more than 2 min or more than 2 permitted prompts from the interviewer in order to find the relevant information" (Foster 2013). However, given the small number of participants per test round and the absence of evidence, using this variable and threshold must be rejected, as the time taken to locate a specific information:
  - Is significantly influenced by the length of the package leaflet (Fuchs 2010a; Fuchs et al. 2012; Wolf et al. 2014)
  - Differs extremely between participants (Fuchs and Hippius 2007; Fuchs et al. 2012) and older people require significantly more time (Fuchs and Hippius 2007; Foster 2013)
  - Is influenced by the positioning of the questions in the questionnaire; questions asked at the end of the readability test retain an advantage, as participants may recall location and content through searches for previous answers.

Regardless of the criticisms made here regarding the current use of readability tests within the EU, the EU is the pioneer of implementing this important package leaflet evaluation method. Readability tests represent the current gold standard and everyone on the globe can benefit from the achievements in the EU.

12.3.2 Usability Tests

Usability testing is a very helpful method for evaluating the appropriate use and design of an extremely wide range of products, such as medicines, medical devices or software, as well as their instructions for use in the form of text and illustrations. The goal is to determine the extent to which the instructions support the safe and effective use of the product, identify design-related problems and user expectations and take improvement actions. As such, it is part of risk management. This differs from usability inspections (e.g. heuristic evaluation, cognitive or pluralistic walk-through) where specialists evaluate the user interface without involving users (Nielsen 1994). Usability testing can be applied to package leaflets, but also to many other issues, such as splitting tablets or opening packaging materials (e.g. according to the norm CEN/TS 15945); for example, in the case of new tablet forms or childproof closures and packaging materials (Deutsches Institut für Normung (German Institute for Standardisation) 2011; Fuchs and Finke 2008; Kopyto et al. 2018).

Usability testing includes creating a realistic scenario or realistic situation, wherein participants (potential or real users) have to carry out tasks using the

Table 12.9 Selected usability test methods for safe use instructions

Method	Description
Think aloud protocol	Users provide all of their thoughts aloud about the device during use of the product (Medicines and Healthcare Products Regulatory Agency 2017; Lewis and Rieman 1994). Think aloud facilitates the evaluators in that the users' train of thought can be followed and erroneous assumptions of instructions during use can be noted.
Co-discovery learning	This is an adaptation of the think aloud protocol. Users are grouped in pairs and talk aloud naturally to each other while completing a task.
Hallway testing	Randomly-selected users are asked to use the product under observation of the tester(s) to identify problems, such as where users incorrectly or cannot perform tasks due to problems in locating and understanding instructions.
Contextual inquiry	Representatives of the intended users are observed when interacting with a marketed device as they would in a normal environment (Medicines and Healthcare Products Regulatory Agency 2017; US Department of Health and Human Services, Food and Drug Administration, Center for Devices and Radiological Health, Office of Device Evaluation 2016). In addition to observing, this can include asking users questions while or after they use the product or its instructions.
Remote usability testing	The tester(s) do not directly observe users while they use the product, but the users' activities are recorded for subsequent evaluation (Andreasen et al. 2007). For example, this method could be used where usability evaluators, developers and users are located in different countries and time zones, or that users are more relaxed and behave more naturally with the product.
Eye tracking	While using the product or information, either the point of gaze (where one is looking) or the motion of an eye relative to the head is measured, such as using video images (Rayner 1998). Eye tracking is often coupled with other methods.
Focus group	A moderator guides a discussion with a group of participants when using the product (Medicines and Healthcare Products Regulatory Agency 2017). This can also be used to check for necessary instructions (essential or missing information).
Interview	Single or groups of users are interviewed to establish their experience and expectations in using the product and/or its instructions (Medicines and Healthcare Products Regulatory Agency 2017; US Department of Health and Human Services, Food and Drug Administration, Center for Devices and Radiological Health, Office of Device Evaluation 2016).

product under controlled conditions while the tester(s) systematically supervise and take notes. Other usability test instruments can be used, such as scripted instructions and validated questionnaires.

Several authorities have published guidelines, such as the FDA in the USA ("Applying Human Factors and Usability Engineering to Optimize Medical Device Design") and the Medicines and Healthcare products Regulatory Agency (MHRA) in the United Kingdom (UK) ("Human Factors and Usability Engineering Guideline") (Medicines and Healthcare Products Regulatory Agency 2017; US Department of Health and Human Services, Food and Drug Administration, Center for Devices and Radiological Health, Office of Device Evaluation 2016). The intended usability test method must suit the product, task and potential problem. Table 12.9 provides examples of methods.

Advantages of Usability Tests

- Usability tests enable assessment of whether users can correctly and easily use the products and instructions within the product-specific requirements. This allows the identification of problems, users' expectations and options for improvements.
- Even if readability tests show that users can locate and understand the content of instructions, usability tests can identify handling problems, according to the author's experience, such as due to:
  - human carelessness, psychological and physiological limitations
  - unusual product handling steps in comparison to similar products
  - product-specific difficulties.

Limitations of Usability Tests

- Some usability test methods require a large effort in performance.
- Several usability test methods miss the natural user environment, such as think aloud protocols or tests with a focus group.
- Similar to readability tests, the number of participants is usually low with regard to achieving sufficient statistical evidence; however, this is assessed as sufficient to identify problems in tested information and initiate subsequent optimisation.

12.3.3 Comprehensibility Tests of Medical/Pharmaceutical Terms, Abbreviations, Non-Quantifiable Phrases and Symbols, Including Explanations

Several guidelines stipulate that difficult terms, abbreviations and symbols should be avoided in medical information for laypersons (Medicines and Healthcare Products Regulatory Agency 2005; European Commission 2009; Sless and Shrensky 2006; Brunetti et al. 2007), as this improves the comprehensibility (Fuchs and Hippius 2007; Franck et al. 2011).

Hohgraewe defined difficult medical terms by the fact that they have been included in a medical dictionary or encyclopaedia (Hohgräwe 1988). To explain medical terms and abbreviations, encyclopaedias and medical dictionaries are available in most languages. In addition, free glossaries with proposed lay terms are published online for many languages (Medicines and Healthcare Products Regulatory Agency 2005; Institute for Safe Medication Practices 2015; Austrian Federal Office for Safety in Health Care 2013; Feinstein Institute for Medical Research 2013; Lebanese American University 2011; Medicines Evaluation Board 2019). However, explanations in glossaries, encyclopaedias and medical dictionaries are usually generated by way of expert consensus rather than comprehensibility tests. It has not been established whether medical terms contained in the quoted catalogues are familiar to laypersons and could therefore be used in patient information—or not, nor have their proposed lay terms been tested.

To bridge this gap, the author of this chapter has created and presents here a method to categorise medical terms (including abbreviations and symbols), into those familiar to laypersons or not. A questionnaire of this comprehensibility test contains up to 60 different terms for which the participants are requested to provide an explanation, without any aid or time restriction. The additional questions for each term are "Do you know this term?" (answer options: yes/no) and "How sure are you with your explanation?" (answer options: sure/other/unsure). As determined by the unilateral binominal test with alpha = 0.05, the minimum number of participants required per tested term is 15 (Bock 1998). However, minimum 20 participants are recruited per term in this comprehensibility test, akin to the recommended number for readability tests in the EU (European Commission 2009; Co-ordination Group for Mutual Recognition and Decentralised Procedures—Human (CMD(h)) 2016). Identical to readability tests, the group of selected participants must reflect the population of tested language, while healthcare professionals excluded. Similar to EU readability test success criteria, a term is defined familiar to laypersons in this comprehensibility test if 80% of the 20 participants provide a correct explanation. If the comprehensibility rate is 50 to <80%, an additional test is carried out with 20 new participants, such that results from a total of 40 participants per term can be used for the categorisation. Since 2008, the author and his team have investigated over 2000 English and over 500 German medical terms, abbreviations and symbols in the United Kingdom and Germany (Fuchs et al. n.d.). The results show that common terms such as allergy (German: Allergie) and depression (German: Depression) are familiar to laypersons and can thus be used in patient information without explanation. However, terms with a comprehensibility rate below 80% must be explained (e.g. vasculitis with comprehensibility rate of 60.0% in English using "inflammation of blood vessels", or 2.4% for its German translation "Vaskulitis" using "Entzündungen der Blutgefäße") (Fuchs et al. n.d.; Scheunpflug 2008). The results also show language-specific differences in comprehensibility rates, whereby comprehensibility rates found in the UK are in many cases higher than for the German equivalent.

The development of a system used by healthcare professionals to create patient-friendly lay terms of pharmaceutical and medical terms, including a method for their evaluation, was additionally performed by the author of this chapter. For evaluation, a multiple choice questionnaire with five medical terms as answer options per explanation is used, with a recheck in another part of the questionnaire with the medical term against five explanation options—whereby per questionnaire up to 30 medical term/explanation pairs can be tested. The participant and test requirements are similar to those outlined above for the comprehensibility test of medical terms. The results illustrate a significant advantage for short explanations of not more than 50 characters (spaces excluded), over longer versions. To be acceptable, explanations to replace difficult terms must be precise and without other difficult terms. For example, the German explanation of vasculitis "Entzündungen der Blutgefäße" (inflammation of blood vessels) registered a comprehensibility rate of 95.5% (Fuchs et al. n.d.; Scheunpflug 2008).

Further, recommendations to create user-friendly lay terms (other than those presented in this paragraph based on the author's research) are available; however, usually not validated, such as that published in annex 8 of the Guidance "Always Read the Leaflet" (Medicines and Healthcare Products Regulatory Agency 2005).

A similar test method to assess the comprehensibility of abbreviations and symbols used in package leaflets was applied in a Portuguese study. The questionnaire used listed the abbreviation or symbol in the first column (e.g. MAO) and in the second its corresponding full wording (e.g. monoamine oxidase inhibitor). The participants had to indicate in the third column whether they knew the meaning of the abbreviation/symbol (answer options: yes/no) and if yes, they were asked to provide a brief description of the meaning of the abbreviation/symbol. Null answers and wrong explanations were classified as incorrect and all the others as correct by two specialists, working independently. There was no time limit for completing the questionnaire, but all participants completed the questionnaire in less than 1 h. Furthermore, control questions (one per page) were included to check participants' attention. Control items were selected from abbreviations/symbols commonly appearing in package leaflets. The tested (186 or 187) and control (11 or 12) abbreviations/symbols were in alphabetical order and administered in two undergraduate non-biomedical classes, which were significantly better educated than the average Portuguese population, and led to results from 18 participants (Pires et al. 2015b, 2017a).

Another method, published in 2000, involved a study in the USA with 249 patients to determine the understanding of common medical terms used by healthcare providers. The patients were asked whether six pairs of terms had the same or different meanings and scored on the number of correct answers. For example, the percentage of patients who recognised the use of analogous terms for bleeding versus haemorrhage was 21% (Lerner et al. 2000).

In a Sri Lankan study involving 600 patients, the knowledge of the anatomical location of ten organs in the human body was investigated by marking in a diagram which showed the contour of a person (Ramanayake et al. 2014). This method also helps to understand which wording for organs is familiar to patients.

Advantages of Comprehensibility Tests of Difficult Terms, Abbreviations, Non-Quantifiable Phrases and Symbols, Including Explanations

- More accurate classification into terms familiar to laypersons and those that need explanations in patient information can be achieved compared to expert assessments only.
- Systematic creation of lay terms by healthcare professionals, with subsequent evaluation via comprehensibility testing, may better improve patient information in comparison to developments without testing.

Limitations of Comprehensibility Tests of Difficult Terms, Abbreviations, Non-Quantifiable Phrases and Symbols, Including Explanations

- Greater investment in time and cost is needed compared to expert assessments without testing.
- Comprehensibility tests must be performed per language as differences are possible.
- The number of participants per tested medical term, abbreviation, non-quantifiable phrase, symbol or created explanation is relatively low; therefore, representativeness must be achieved: the group should reflect the average population of laypersons in the tested language and region intended for the use of information.

- The test conditions do not totally reflect the real-life situation of understanding a term in medical information. Understanding and explaining an individually presented medical term is more difficult than when it appears within a meaningful text. However, it can be assumed that a medical term that is recognised and understood outside any context will be understandable within a text.

12.3.4 Tests for Illustrations, Images, Pictograms and Other Graphics

In some jurisdictions, pictograms, symbols, images or other graphics are allowed in package leaflets and on outer packaging to aid comprehension of information, for example, in the EU (The European Parliament and the Council of the European Union 2012). According to the EU readability guideline: "They should only be used to aid navigation, clarify or highlight certain aspects of the text and should not replace the actual text. Evidence may be required to ensure that their meaning is generally understood and not misleading or confusing" (European Commission 2009). This is supported by Sojourner and Wogalter who examined five instruction leaflets—(a) text-only, (b) pictograms-only, (c) text with all pictograms, (d) partial pictograms and (e) without instructions—with 35 participants aged 18–59 years, with each version rated by each participant using an 8-point Likert scale. Version "(c) with text and pictograms" was most preferred and rated more effective as well as easier to understand and remember. Furthermore, version (a) with text-only was rated as more suitable compared to version (b) pictogram-only (Sojourner and Wogalter 1997).

Although pictograms, illustrations and images can enhance the communication of information even for people with poor reading skills/literacy or non-native speakers (Dowse and Ehlers 2004), as well as increase the reader's curiosity and motivation to engage with the provided content, they have disadvantages, such as:

- Risk of misinterpretation that can result in incorrect use of medicines—increasing the risk of adverse events as well as reduced therapy success; therefore, additional text and testing are necessary (Wolff and Wogalter 1993; Pires et al. 2015a).
- Sensitivity to cultural differences, age and personal experiences of the users, including health conditions such as eyesight (Van Beusekom et al. 2018; Dowse and Ehlers 2004); pictograms that are comprehensible in one culture may be misinterpreted in another, as shown in a comprehensibility test with 304 low-literacy interviewees in South Africa of 23 USA versus 23 locally developed pictograms (Dowse and Ehlers 2004).
- Limitation of content a pictogram/image can convey; therefore, these design elements should be limited to particularly important content.

Usability tests (see Sect. 12.3.2) and comprehensibility tests (see Sect. 12.3.3) can also be used to evaluate the appropriateness of pictograms and images. Specific study designs measure behavioural outcomes to determine whether an image is helpful. One example is the uniformity of the masses measure in accordance with the European Pharmacopoeia, where different people split tablets and the appropriateness of pictograms or images illustrating how the tablet should be split is assessed (Fuchs and Finke 2008). For images and pictograms advising on closure or packaging systems, usability testing according to the norm CEN/TS 15945 (a norm containing criteria and test methods for evaluating consumer packaging) can also help to assess images and pictograms based on the success rate (Deutsches Institut für Normung (German Institute for Standardisation) 2011; Kopyto et al. 2018). Thereby, the role of end users in testing can be, as described by van Beusekom (see Sect. 12.1): passive up to active participation in creating design solutions with decision power regarding design solutions (Van Beusekom et al. 2018).

Van Beusekom et al. carried out a systematic review of 73 studies from different countries, such as the USA, South Africa, India and Canada. They found that the involvement of end users in creation and/or evaluation of pictograms has a positive influence on the comprehensibility and opinions of pictograms, including information memory. Repeated involvement of end users in the iterative design improvement cycle could be most effective. Yet the comprehensibility of pictograms differs greatly between countries, cultures, the age of the users and the degree of literacy, suggesting that—at least in the final pictogram evaluation—preferably the desired target group should be included (Van Beusekom et al. 2018).

Friedman et al. studied three cholestyramine labels/package leaflets with 2225 participants in 40 different regions of the USA, via questionnaire. The comprehensibility of the version with symbols/graphics only was significantly lower for participants without a university degree than for a text-only and a graphic/text version. No significant differences were found between the graphic/text and the text-only versions (Friedmann et al. 1997).

In 1993, 28 USA pictograms were studied, at first with 143 participants aged 9–60 years, who were asked to write down their interpretation of each pictogram, which were subsequently assessed by three people. Five pictograms did not reach the success rate of 85% correct explanations. A second study with 112 participants aged 18–48 years assessed 16 pictograms, including improved versions of the five pictograms that had failed in the first study. Again, two pictograms did not reach the 85% rate. The pictograms of the second study were re-assessed in a further study with stricter criteria, whereby pictograms which had originally been tested positive no longer reached the success rate (Wolff and Wogalter 1993).

The presented studies show how difficult it is to evaluate and improve pictograms. Even if they have been optimised, not all problems can be solved and new difficulties may occur. Therefore, pictograms should always be combined with short explanatory text.

Advantages of Testing Illustrations, Images, Pictograms and Other Graphics

- This may improve illustrations, images, pictograms and other graphics and avoid misinterpretations.

Limitations of Testing Illustrations, Images, Pictograms and Other Graphics

- The testing is limited in generalisability and transferability of results to other intended users, as illustrations, images, pictograms and other graphics are generally vulnerable to misinterpretation problems, especially when used in cultures other than tested.

12.3.5 Quality Criteria-Based Evaluations

Using quality criteria for evaluation and improvement of layout, legibility and comprehensibility of information about medicines, as well as for a systematic creation, ensures a high quality of patient information, as shown on a set of over 100 quality criteria in a cross-over-readability-test study with 1105 participants (Fuchs 2010a; Fuchs and Hippius 2007). Therefore, this is recommended by authorities and an established standard in the first step of the written readability test method (Medicines and Healthcare Products Regulatory Agency 2005; European Commission 2009; Co-ordination Group for Mutual Recognition and Decentralised Procedures—Human (CMD(h)) 2016; Medicines and Healthcare Products Regulatory Agency 2012). Quality criteria can be used to evaluate that required contents are contained (Fuchs et al. 2010c; Ramadas et al. 2013; Sillo et al. 2018; Tayyem and Takrouri 2009; Pires et al. 2015c) and to assess the way the specific information is provided (see Table 12.7, for an example, on dosage instructions), including comprehensibility, layout and typography parameters (see Tables 12.1, 12.2, 12.3, 12.4, 12.5, and 12.6) (Fuchs et al. 2017; Fuchs 2005; Pires et al. 2015a; Medicines and Healthcare Products Regulatory Agency 2012).

It is also conceivable to use quality criteria for evaluation instead of readability or usability tests and hence without involving participants from the intended users. However, this firstly requires justification by means of evidence that the results would be comparable and is therefore currently not universally accepted by authorities (Federal Institute for Drugs and Medical Devices 2013).

Quality criteria can be used manually or automatically, whereby software solutions may have advantages over manual handling in such as providing more comfort, being faster and, with future enhancement through artificial intelligence, also more efficient in detecting problems with contents, missing information, legibility and comprehensibility.

The creation of quality criteria demands careful consideration that each criterion is (Fuchs 2005):

- Comprehensible, precise and without non-quantifiable specifications; for example, the criterion "Use minimum 9 pt font size" should be preferred in comparison to "Clear and legible font",
- Evidence-based; for example, the recommendation to use only landscape format is not acceptable, as no evidence exists that this format is always more appropriate than portrait format; quality criteria derived from current evidence are presented in Tables 12.1, 12.2, 12.3, 12.4, 12.5, 12.6, and 12.7,
- Focussed to one issue per criterion only, which eases assessment of whether the criterion is fulfilled or not; a yes/no-assessment per quality criterion (fulfilled/not fulfilled) of criteria created according to the three bullet points above is recommended (Fuchs et al. 2006, 2010c).

Sometimes, scores have been used to evaluate fulfilment of each quality criterion, such as "Font choice, size and style: score 0 for difficult to read; 1 for clear and legible" (note: Both score definitions use non-quantifiable phrases and more than one issue is contained in the criterion "Font choice, size and style"). In other cases up to 5 penalty points were given for a large volume of text, a large number of long sentences, repetitions and also for many difficult terms, or penalty points for font sizes (below 8pt: 1 point for 7.5pt, for 7pt 2 points, 6.5pt 3 points, 6pt 4 points and under 6pt 5 points) (Medicines and Healthcare Products Regulatory Agency 2012, Beime and Menges 2012; Beime 2010; Haug et al. 2011). The goal has been a final score for each evaluated material to enable comparison. However, no evidence exists that, for example, a difference of 0.5pt always has the exact value of 1 penalty point, or that 1 penalty point for inadequate font size truly equals in negative influence on usability as 1 penalty point applied for extensive volume of text or a certain number of difficult terms. Furthermore, the number of long sentences, repetitions and difficult terms significantly increases with increasing the volume of text (Fuchs et al. 2006), hence such scoring for each of these four issues punishes associated problems multiple times. Moreover, the usability of information about medicines differs between materials, languages, user groups, etc. (Tong et al. 2018; Wolf et al. 2014; Raynor et al. 2007). All these considerations do not support the use of the described score systems.

Advantages of Quality Criteria-Based Evaluations

- The use of quality criteria has an added value for achieving high quality of information materials.

Limitations of Quality Criteria-Based Evaluation

- The use of scoring systems, as described above, is not recommended.
- Quality criteria-based evaluation can currently not replace readability and usability tests.

12.3.6 Opinion and Perception Surveys

Surveys of opinions or perceptions collect assessments from a chosen population group (in case of information about medicines: patients, healthcare professionals or both), including their needs and wishes. Surveys can be conducted either in a person-to-person contact (Calamusa et al. 2012; Wolka et al. 2015)], via phone (Hamrosi et al. 2014; Aikin et al. 2004; Vinker et al. 2007), in writing (Hamrosi et al. 2014; Vander Stichele et al. 1996) or through an online questionnaire (Bell and Sullivan 1981; McAvoy et al. 2007) as a one-time survey (cross-sectional study) or, more rarely in the area of information about medicines, as repeated surveys (longitudinal study).

The number of participants required for statistical power should be calculated as part of the study protocol. Inclusion and exclusion criteria of participants need to be carefully defined as well as the selected questions and mode of participants' response). Modes of response include:

- Free opinions, e.g. expressed via free-text fields.
- Agreement/rejection of predefined statements with single or multiple answer options, e.g. used in the PIL-S-study to assess the participants' preference and weighting of different topics related to content and layout of package leaflets (Van Dijk et al. 2014a).
- Response using an evaluation scale for predefined statements, e.g. a Likert scale as a multi-level response scale as can be used in readability tests in addition to the key message questions, or to assess legibility properties of font types or frequency information of side effects (Fuchs 2010a; Connolly 1998; Knapp et al. 2004).

More details on survey methods and studies are provided in Chap. 8 on the social sciences.

Advantages of Opinion and Perception Surveys

- They can provide further information for deeper understanding of intended users; in particular, in conjunction with methods like readability and usability tests.
- They are important to understand users' opinions, needs and preferences.

Limitations of Opinion and Perception Surveys

- Results of such surveys depend on the quality and objectivity of methods used. Without knowledge of the research design (research question, study situation, choice of participants, interviewer behaviour, etc.) the quality of the results is difficult to assess.
- Results do not always conform with results from other evaluation methods, such as readability, usability and comprehensibility tests, or they may differ from the real-life experience. For example, in a readability test study with 1105 participants, no correlation was found between the comprehensibility of tested package leaflets (percentage of correct answers to key message questions) and participant opinions about comprehensibility (Fuchs 2010a).
- User groups of different demographic characteristics can provide different opinions and perceptions. In a Portuguese questioning with 503 participants using a Likert scale to evaluate 12 package leaflets, significant differences were attributed to the education, income, reading habits and frequency of medicine use, that are all interlinked via socioeconomic status. Participants with lower education, lower income, reduced reading habits and taking more medicines provided a significantly better global opinion about the package leaflets (Pires et al. 2017b). As a result, inappropriate participant selection may falsify the results.
- Results can be influenced by response bias, such as socially desirable answer behaviour or when participants do not understand the questions, but may not ask for clarification to avoid embarrassment, or misinterpret questions. In the case of socially undesirable issues, participants may tend not to admit in surveys or to give advanced answers. Furthermore, the "say-yes tendency" plays a distorting role. Further sources of response bias may be the framing and order of the questions and predefined answers, as well as the interviewer's behaviour. Furthermore, it is possible to provoke certain answers through suggestive questions.

- As participants only respond to the questions asked, other relevant opinions or perceptions may remain undetected. This includes associations and unconscious or preconscious opinions or perceptions.
- Results may have a broad range of interpretability, for example, when gathering opinions and perceptions using free-text fields.
- Selection bias may jeopardise representativeness. For example, those who are negative about such surveys usually do not participate or pass the survey on to others; therefore, falling out of the sample (self-selection or non-response bias), a bias particularly relevant in telephone and online surveys. The bias described in the example does not become smaller with larger sample sizes.

12.3.7 Readability Formula-Based Evaluations

A variety of formulas are used to assess the readability of written materials, whereby no consensus exists as to which formula is best suited to assess patient information about risks and safe use of medicines. Therefore, it is favourable to use a variety of formulas (Fullmann et al. 2017; University of Hohenheim 2010). Furthermore, different languages require specific or adapted readability formulas. As such the Flesch-Reading-Ease formula, the Flesch–Kincaid Grade Level readability formula, the Gunning Fog Index, the SMOG Index, for example, are often used for English texts (Flesch 1948; Gunning 1952; Kincaid et al. 1975; McLaughlin 1969). For German texts, the Amstad formula, the "Wiener Sachtextformel" (Viennese factual formula), the German Flesch-Reading-Ease and SMOG Index are used, and for Persian the Flesch–Dayani formula (Amstad 1978; University of Hohenheim 2010; Dayani 2000).

Readability formulas or indexes use average sentence and word length and the number of syllables with different weighting factors to calculate a reading ease or a reading grade level (Amstad 1978; Flesch 1948; Gunning 1952; Kincaid et al. 1975; McLaughlin 1969; Dayani 2000). The average reading grade of the population in the USA and United Kingdom is the eighth grade (13- to 14-year-olds) and patient information should be at grades 5 to 6 (10- to 11-year-olds), as considered in studies investigating information about medicines using readability formulas (Fullmann et al. 2017; National Center for Education Statistics, and US Department of Education, Office of Educational Research and Improvement 2002; Pinero-Lopez et al. 2019).

Advantages of Readability Formulas

- These formulas are easy to use without great effort and are usually software-based.

Limitations of Readability Formulas

- Readability formulas do not consider the cohesion of a sentence. For example, two sentences with the same words in different order have the same results using readability formula, but may have different comprehensibility.
- The volume of text, style of writing, typography and layout also greatly influence the readability according to Tables 12.1, 12.2, 12.3, 12.4, 12.5, 12.6, and 12.7; however, these factors are not considered by a readability formula. Therefore, assessment only via readability formula is questionable and they are usually used:

  - with previous deletion of all headings, tables, graphics, images, figures, the commercial name of the medicine, all bullet points (hyphens, numbers, asterisks, etc.), and
  - with all abbreviations, acronyms, units, magnitudes and numbers replaced by their meaning in words.

  See, for example, the study of 35 biosimilar package leaflets published in 2019 (Pinero-Lopez et al. 2019).
- According to the FDA of the USA "...readability indexes can predict, but do not measure the reader's actual ability to comprehend labelling. Because of the complexity of the process by which individuals interact with hazard alerts, you should not rely on readability indexes to predict warning and precaution comprehension." (US Department of Health and Human Services, Food and Drug Administration, Center for Devices and Radiological Health 2001).
- The predicators and criteria by which readability formulas are developed are not anchored in any text processing theory. Moreover, correlative relationships are taken into account instead of cognitive text processing. These formulas only measure syntactic characteristics, but do not take the content of the texts into account (Felsch 2004).

12.4 Outlook: Relevance, Improvements and Future Potential

Three different types of human communication exist: (a) verbal, (b) written and (c) non-verbal via perceiving a person's body language and behaviour and inferring meaning. Written communications are printed messages on paper or appearing on a screen in digital media. They are most suited to conveying facts, complex and/or extensive contents, or if a permanent document and no immediate reply is needed. The recipient of a written message can read it at any time; however, as a general rule, concise writing equals most effective communication (Fuchs 2010a; Bauer and Erdogan 2012; Mansoor and Dowse 2007).

In the case of written information about risks and safe use of medicines, design science offers an appropriate option for their structured user-centred development and improvement. Starting from the awareness of a problem in such written information material, a proposal and artefact are created through a design science cycle and evaluated. The evaluation step is essential to improve the quality of the information material and to assess in the conclusion step the usefulness of the developed artefact, or refuse or redesign it if results show insufficient benefit (Vaishnavi et al. 2019; Van Aken 2005). It is the overall aim of the design science process that messages about risks and safe use of medicines reach the intended recipients (patients, healthcare professionals, or both), are understood and result in the intended outcomes.

Written information can also be the proposal and artefact in a design science process to reduce risks or resolve problems that have become apparent in using medicines or medical devices. The idea is to prevent user errors by design. The usefulness, quality and efficacy of created information about medicines must be demonstrated via well-executed evaluation methods, such as through measurement of risk awareness, knowledge levels, comprehensibility of messages, impact on behaviour or the number and type of occurred risk issues (e.g. blood levels, metabolic parameters, reporting of side effects or incorrect use) (European Network of Centres for Pharmacoepidemiology and Pharmacovigilance 2020). This evaluation leads to the final design science cycle step of conclusion, which contains the results of final written information material and new knowledge adding to the evidence base for design science (Vaishnavi et al. 2019).

Methods of generating this evidence through testing for readability, usability, comprehensibility, perceptions and quality of information are presented in this chapter. Methods from other sciences are needed to further study cognitive and behavioural outcomes, like following instructions and safe use advice. The multilayered research framework presented in Chap. 1 brings different methods together for comprehensive research into medicinal product risk communication.

Future Challenges

There are a number of future challenges, and applying design science thinking is supposed to support tackling them. The constantly increasing number of information materials per medicinal product poses a major challenge. Beyond the statutory product information, e.g. in the EU the package leaflet, summary of product characteristics and labelling of the inner and outer packaging—as the minimum material for each product, risk management programmes may become part of the product license and demand the dissemination of further materials about risks and safe use and, sometimes, also informed consent forms. Multiple materials mean high text volume with the risks of repetition, inconstancy, confusion and overtaxing of users. Newly developed materials may compete with existing ones. Further, one must consider that these multiple materials add to the omnipresence (see Chap. 1) and the abundance of information that exists within society. On the other hand, patients and healthcare professionals want shorter information about medicines than currently exists, and every increase in the volume of text reduces the motivation of users to read it (Fuchs 2010a; Weitbrecht and Voßkämper 2002; Caldeira et al. 2008; Fuchs et al. 2007; Papay et al. 2010; Van Dijk et al. 2014a; Wolf et al. 2016). According to the motto "less is more", a new design science cycle has to be initiated to achieve a more effective approach, e.g. we need to optimise existing information tools and resolve identified weaknesses instead of developing umpteen new materials! For example, an optimal, compressed package leaflet that contains all product information relevant for patients and avoids unnecessary information could then be disseminated via different channels (in the package, online, mobile, audio, etc.).

Design Science-Based Suggestions for the Future

Materials required by the regulatory authorities, like package leaflets for patients or summaries of product characteristics for healthcare professionals, are bound to guidelines. These regulatory guidelines should take into account existing scientific evidence-based knowledge and contain only evidence-based recommendations. One negative example is recommending landscape format in package leaflets (see Table 12.5).

Also, the requirements and recommendations in guidelines should be tested, whereby authorities and other competent institutions should be obliged to remedy any shortcoming immediately it becomes evident. For example, the QRD template had never been tested before implementation and research shows that a notably shorter version of 200 words would bestow significant benefits and shorten each package leaflet used in the EU without loss of medicine specific information (see Sect. 12.2) (Fuchs et al. 2012; Wolf et al. 2014)—also a very important factor in the enhancement of electronic product information (ePI) (European Medicines Agency et al. 2019a, b). Other countries, such as the USA in the case of medication guides, use only a short template and the first QRD template from 1996 contained just 94 words (US Food and Drug Administration 2018; Wolf 2015).

In the case of patient package leaflets used in the EU and Eurasian Economic Union, for example, a new leaflet must be readability tested (The European Parliament and the Council of the European Union 2004; Eurasian Economic Commission Council 2016). Readability tests represent the gold standard and everyone on the globe can benefit from the achievements in the EU. However, these tests are now used more to demonstrate that the success criteria of 12–15 tested key messages have been achieved, rather than to improve the entire information—the original intention of Australian readability tests (Sless 2007). The improvement of the quality of the entire package leaflet must be the focus in the future, applying evidence-based design features as quality standard. The quality criteria of Tables 12.1, 12.2, 12.3, 12.4, 12.5, 12.6, and 12.7 may serve as a basis for quality checklists used before testing with laypersons. Therefore, this is a solid component in the first step of written readability tests and results in significant improvements (see Sect. 12.3.1) (Fuchs and Hippius 2007; Wolf et al. 2014).

Another suggestion is the combination of evaluation methods like readability and usability testing (e.g. if instructions for use of a device are contained) and additionally applying comprehensibility tests as described in Sect. 12.3.3 if medical terms with an unclear level of comprehensibility are used. The latter enables clear decisions on which terms can be used or need an explanation.

Frequently, participants' opinions and perceptions about the tested package leaflet are additionally collected in readability tests, which can lead to helpful information. However, this is assessed to be more of an add-on evaluation rather than a replacement of readability or usability testing, due to the fact that opinions can differ to the reality (Knapp et al. 2004; Pires et al. 2017b). This same add-on evaluation value is also seen in readability test formulas, as these do not measure the cohesion of texts, as explained in Sect. 12.3.7. Readability formulas must be rejected if all calculation steps applied to the formula being used are not published and they are not acceptable as stand-alone evaluations.

Currently, after successful readability testing, package leaflets are frequently changed by pharmaceutical companies and authorities in EU approval procedures. Often, these changes are not content-related, such as insertions of blank lines after headings or reinserting difficult terms and long sentences. In future, if a package leaflet has been successfully tested without showing weakness in the final version, the wording and layout used should be retained, unless there are content-related needs. Furthermore, it is recommended to prepare a best possible package leaflet using quality criteria before submission to the authorities and to test it in the latter stages of the approval procedure; therein minimising the risk of major changes after the readability test.

The idea of iterative testing was born in 2017 (European Commission 2017; European Medicines Agency 2017); however, it could reverse the positive intention of readability testing. Moreover, such regular retesting is assessed to be not productive, as:

- A readability test usually covers not more than 12–15 pieces of key information.
- Testing makes less sense if texts may not be amended, or general problems, such as the overly extensive volume of text, cannot be solved.
- Evidence is missing that such repeated testing substantially benefits patients.

For future method development, exploring and using outcome evaluation (effectiveness of communication) should be discussed, despite achieving best possible legibility, comprehensibility and evaluation of information about medicines, such as:

- Administration parameters: e.g. correct time, quantity (such as the number of tablets, capsules, drops used), frequency of use, which evaluate the dosage instructions using measuring systems to remove the medicine from the packaging (Claxton et al. 2001).
- Increase of knowledge: e.g. about disease, treatment, including medicines and adverse events. The increase of knowledge can be measured through comparison of knowledge before and after using information materials, or comparison of groups using different materials, including placebo-controlled groups (Mansoor and Dowse 2007; Jarernsiripornkul et al. 2019; Humphris and Field 2003).
- Treatment success parameters: e.g. measurement of laboratory levels (blood pressure, glucose levels, number of epileptic seizures, pain [strength and frequency of attacks]), active substance levels in the body.
- Treatment safety parameters: e.g. occurrence of adverse events, including laboratory levels (e.g. liver enzymes, kidney function), cases of emergency.

These additional assessment parameters are the author's personal suggestions, which are currently more time and cost expensive than other evaluation methods provided above and could require ethical approval. They are also influenced by other issues, such as the effectiveness of the individual product or therapy procedure. However, in 2011 Garner et al. also published the idea of outcome evaluation as success measurement of package leaflets "... in terms of patients' reactions, expectations and decisions in the light of writers' intention..." (Garner et al. 2011). Achieving a certain readability level is only the starting point of evaluation. After complete reading and constructing a meaning, the ultimate evaluation of information about medicines is the reader's cognitive, affective or behavioural response (Garner et al. 2011).

Conclusions

- Written information about risks and safe use of medicines can be seen as a product that can benefit from being created and optimised by a design science-based approach. However, such information material can also be the proposal/artefact to solve a problem occurring in use of medicines and medical devices.
- A design science-based approach includes a user-centred design process, generation and application of evidence-based design features as quality criteria standard and testing with the participation of representatives of intended users.
- Applicable evaluation methods include tests for readability, comprehensibility and usability as well as quality-criteria evaluations and user surveys.
- The creation and optimisation of written information about the risks and safe use of medicines still has much room for improvement, in particular regarding the volume of text, comprehensibility, typography and layout.
- Improvements should be targeted at the upgrading of the entire information material as a product in all aspects, rather than testing a couple of key messages.
- Only evidence-based, user-centred recommendations should be implemented in guidelines on such information materials, and shortcomings should be remedied in evidence-based and timely manner.

References

Aberson DHA, Bouwhuis DG (1997) Silent reading as determined by age and visual acuity. J Res Read 20:184–204

Aikin KJ, Swasy JL, Braman AC (2004) Patient and physician attitudes and behaviors associated with OTC promotion of prescription drugs, summary of FDA survey results. http://www.fda.gov/downloads/aboutfda/centersoffices/officeofmedicalproductsandtobacco/cder/ucm600276.pdf. Accessed 28 Sept 2019

Amstad T (1978) Wie verständlich sind unsere Zeitungen? (How comprehensible are our newspapers?). Universität Zürich, Zurich

Andreasen MS, Nielsen HV, Schrøder SO, Stage J (2007) What happened to remote usability testing?: an empirical study of three methods. Proceedings of the SIGCHI conference on Human factors in computing systems ACM DL. https://doi.org/10.1145/1240624.1240838

Aslani P, Hamrosi K, Feletto E, Raynor DKT, Knapp P, Huges J, et al. (2010) Investigating Consumer Medicine Information (I-CMI) Project: Australian Government, Department of Health and Ageing; The Pharmacy Guild of Australia. http://6cpa.com.au/resources/fourth-agreement/investigating-consumer-medicine-information-i-cmi-project/. Accessed 27 Sept 2019

Australian Government (1990) Therapeutic goods regulations. https://www.legislation.gov.au/Details/F2018C00897. Accessed 27 Sept 2019

Australian Government, Department of Health, Therapeutics Goods Administration (2019) Consumer information (CMI). https://www.tga.gov.au/consumer-medicines-information-cmi. Accessed 28 Sept 2019

Austrian Federal Office for Safety in Health Care (2013) Wie sollen medizinische Fachbegriffe für die Gebrauchsinformation übersetzt werden?—Empfohlene Übersetzungen. https://www.basg.gv.at/index.php?eID=tx_nawsecuredl&u=0&g=0&t=0&hash=7e5eb47e4c76a9e6064a5e

9c87f2625100edec1f&file=fileadmin/redakteure/A/Arzneimittel/FAQ_Arzneimittel/130327_Layterms.pdf. Accessed 27 Sept 2019

Azodi K, Himstedt S, Hinrichs A, Krüger M, Schrader S, Schulz M (2002) Testing of the readability of package leaflets as an initial step under the pharmaceutical care initiative towards increasing the safety of medicinal products. Pharm Ind 64:1119–1125

Azodi K, Himstedt S, Hinrichs A, Krüger M, Schrader S, Schulz M (2003) Test auf Lesbarkeit läuft in Apotheken. Pharm Ztg 148:3296–3298

Bahri P, Castillon Melero M (2018) Listen to the public and fulfil their information interests: translating vaccine communication research findings into guidance for regulators. Br J Clin Pharmacol 84:1696–1705

Bauer T, Erdogan B (2012) Communication—different types of communication and channels. In: Bauer T, Erdogan B (eds) An introduction to organizational behavior (v.1.0). Creative commons, pp 347–366. https://www.academia.edu/28038582/An_Introduction_to_Organizational_Behavior_v._1.0. Accessed 27 Sept 2019

Beime B (2010) BfArM im Dialog—Aktionsplan AMTS—Arzneimitteltherapiesicherheit durch bessere Lesbarkeit von Packungsbeilagen? http://www.bfarm.de/SharedDocs/Downloads/DE/Service/Termine-und-Veranstaltungen/dialogveranstaltungen/dialog_2010/100414/12_Beime.pdf?__blob=publicationFile&v=2. Accessed 27 Sept 2019

Beime B, Menges K (2012) Does the requirement of readability testing improve package leaflets? Evaluation of the 100 most frequently prescribed drugs in Germany marketed before 2005 and first time in 2007 or after. Pharmaceut Reg Affairs 1:1–6

Bell RC, Sullivan JL (1981) Student preferences in typography. J Programmed Learning Educ Technology 18:57–61

Bernardini C, Ambrogi V, Perioli L, Tiralti MC, Fardella G (2000) Comprehensibility of the package leaflets of all medicinal products for human use: a questionnaire survey about the use of symbols and pictograms. Pharmacol Res 41:679–688

Bernardini C, Ambrogi V, Fardella G, Perioli L, Grandolini G (2001) How to improve the readability of the patient package leaflet: a survey on the use of colour, print size and layout. Pharmacol Res 5:437–443

Berry DC, Knapp P, Raynor DK (2002) Provision of information about drug side-effects to patients. Lancet 359:853–854

Beuth Verlag (2008) ISO2471:2008–12 paper and board—determination of opacity (paper backing)—diffuse reflectance method. https://www.beuth.de/en/standard/iso-2471/115477155. Accessed 27 Sept 2019

Bock J (1998) Bestimmung des Stichprobenumfangs. R. Oldenbourg Verlag, München, Wien

Breland K, Breland MK (1944) Legibility of newspaper headlines printed in capitals and in lower case. J Appl Psychol 28:117–120

Bringhurst R (2005) The elements of typographic style, 4.0 ed. Hartley & Marks, Vancouver

Brunetti L, Santell JP, Hicks RW (2007) The impact of abbreviations on patient safety. Jt Comm J Qual Patient Saf 33:576–583

Burtt HE, Basch C (1923) Legibility of bodoni, baskerville roman and Cheltenham type faces. J Appl Psychol 7:237–245

Calamusa A, Di Marzio A, Cristofani R, Arrighetti P, Santaniello V, Alfani S et al (2012) Factors that influence Italian consumers' understanding of over-the-counter medicines and risk perception. Patient Educ Counsel. 87:395–401

Caldeira TR, Neves ERZ, Perini E (2008) Historical evolution of package inserts in Brazil. Cad Saúde Pública 24:737–743

Claxton AJ, Cramer J, Pierce C (2001) A systematic review of the associations between dose regimens and medication compliance. Clin Ther 23:1296–1310

Connolly GK (1998) Legibility and readability of small print: effects of font, observer age and spatial vision. Thesis, Department of Psychology, University of Calgary, Calgary

Co-ordination Group for Mutual Recognition and Decentralised Procedures—Human (CMD(h)) (2016). Position paper on user testing of package leaflet—consultation with target patient groups (Compliance with article 59(3) of Council Directive 2001/83/EC); Doc. Ref: CMDh/234/2011, Rev. 01. http://www.hma.eu/fileadmin/dateien/Human_Medicines/CMD_h_/procedural_guidance/Consulation_PatientsGroups/CMDh_234_2011_Rev01_2016_12_clean.pdf. Accessed 27 Sept 2019

Dawoodi I, Bhosale UA (2016) Evaluation of knowledge and awareness of patients about prescribed drugs and their package inserts: a cross-sectional study. Asian J Pharm 10:S96–S99

Dayani MH (2000) A criteria for assessing the Persian texts' readability. J Soc Sci Hum 10:35–48

Deutsches Institut für Normung (German Institute for Standardisation) (2011) Packaging—ease of opening—criteria and test methods for evaluating consumer packaging; German version DIN CEN/TS 15945:2011. https://www.beuth.de/en/technical-rule/din-cen-ts-15945/133884093. Accessed 27 Sept 2019

Deutsches Institut für Normung (German Institute for Standardisation) (2013) DIN 1450: lettering—legibility. https://www.beuth.de/de/norm/din-1450/170093157. Accessed 27 Sept 2019

Dickinson RJ (2014) The inclusion of a headline section and information about the benefits of medicines in written medicines information. The University of Leeds, School of Healthcare, Leeds

Dickinson D, Raynor DK, Duman M (2001) Patient information leaflets for medicines: using consumer testing to determine the most effective design. Patient Educ Counsel 43:147–159

Dickinson RJ, Raynor DK, Knapp P, MacDonald J (2016) Do patients use a headline section in a leaflet to find key information about their medicines? Findings from a user-test study. Ther Innov Regul Sci 50:581–591

DiSantostefano RL, Beck M, Yeakey AM, Raphiou I, Stempel DA (2014) Patient comprehension of medication guides for asthma and chronic obstructive pulmonary disease medications. Ther Innov Regul Sci 48:574–582

Dolk S, Knapp P, Maat HP, Lentz L, Raynor T (2011) Headline section in patient information leaflets: does it improve reading performance and perception? Information Design Journal 19:46–57

Dowse R, Ehlers M (2004) Pictograms for conveying medicine instructions: comprehension in various south African language groups. S Afr J Sci 100:687–693

East African Community Secretariat (2014) The Compendium of medicine evaluation and registration for medicine regulation harmonization in the East African Community—Document no: EAC/TF-MED/MER/FD/COM/N1R0. https://apps.who.int/medicinedocs/documents/s22312en/s22312en.pdf. Accessed 29 Sept 2019

Ekstrom I (1993) Printed materials for an aging population: design considerations. J Biocommun 20:25–30

Ellliot AJ, Covington MV (2001) Approach and avoidance motivation. Educ Psychol Rev 13:73–92

Eurasian Economic Commission Council (2016) On the rules of marketing authorization and assessment of medicinal products for medical use, Resolution No. 78. http://www.eurasiancommission.org/en/act/texnreg/deptexreg/LS1/Documents/EEC%20Decision%2078_Rules%20of%20authorization%20and%20assessment%20of%20medicinal%20products%20for%20human%20use_eng.pdf. Accessed 27 Sept 2019

European Commission (1998) A guideline on the readability of the label and package leaflet of medicinal products for human use, Brussels. http://www.pharma-eu.com/pdfs/Guideline%20on%20Readbaility%20EMEA.pdf. Accessed 27 Sept 2019

European Commission (2009) Guideline on the readability of the labelling and package leaflet of medicinal products for human use. Brussels, Rev. 1. http://ec.europa.eu/health/files/eudralex/vol-2/c/2009_01_12_readability_guideline_final_en.pdf. Accessed 27 Sept 2019

European Commission (2017) Report from the Commission to the European Parliament and the Council in accordance with Article 59(4) of Directive 2001/83/EC of the European Parliament and of the Council of 6 November 2001 on the Community code relating to medicinal products for human use. http://ec.europa.eu/health/sites/health/files/files/documents/2017_03_report_smpc-pl_en.pdf. Accessed 28 Sept 2019

European Medicines Agency (2007) Minutes of the fourth meeting of the EMEA human scientific committees' working party with patients' and consumers' organisations (PCWP). https://www.paint-consult.com/fileadmin/editorial/downloads/z_textverlinkungen/guideline-einfluss/haeufigkeitsangaben_nebenwirkungen/EMEA_new_wording_for_section_4.pdf. Accessed 27 Sept 2019

European Medicines Agency (2017) EMA action plan related to the European Commission's recommendations on product information. https://www.ema.europa.eu/documents/other/european-medicines-agency-action-plan-related-european-commissions-recommendations-product_en.pdf. Accessed 12 Oct 2019

European Medicines Agency (2019) Product information templates: centralised procedures—version 10.1; MR/DC/Referral procedures—version 4.1, 2020. http://www.ema.europa.eu/ema/index.jsp?curl=pages/regulation/document_listing/document_listing_000134.jsp&mid=WC0b01ac0580022c59. Accessed 6 Mar 2020

European Medicines Agency, Heads of Medicines Agencies (2019) Guideline on good pharmacovigilance practices (EU-GVP). EMA, Amsterdam

European Medicines Agency, Heads of Medicines Agencies, European Commission (2019a) Electronic product information for human medicines in the EU—draft key principles; A joint EMA-HMA-EC collaboration; EMA/849614/2018. https://www.ema.europa.eu/documents/regulatory-procedural-guideline/electronic-product-information-human-medicines-european-union-draft-key-principles_en.pdf. Accessed 28 Sept 2019

European Medicines Agency, Heads of Medicines Agencies, European Commission. (2019b) Electronic product information for medicines in the EU—report from an EMA-HMA-EC workshop held on 28 November 2018. https://www.ema.europa.eu/documents/report/report-european-medicines-agency-ema/heads-medicines-agencies-hma/european-commission-ec-workshop-electronic-product-information-epi_en.pdf. Accessed 28 Sept 2019

European Network of Centres for Pharmacoepidemiology and Pharmacovigilance (2020) The European Union electronic Register of Post-Authorisation Studies (EU PAS register). http://www.encepp.eu/encepp/studiesDatabase.jsp. Accessed 28 Sept 2019

Federal Institute for Drugs and Medical Devices (2013) FAQ Packungsbeilagenprüfung—Welche Methoden sind vom BfArM für die Durchführung einer solchen Untersuchung akzeptiert? https://www.bfarm.de/DE/Service/FAQ/_functions/Arzneimittelzulassung/pal/_node.html. Accessed 27 Sept 2019

Feinstein Institute for Medical Research (2013) Human research protection program guidance document—glossary of lay terminology. http://www.feinsteininstitute.org/wp-content/uploads/2013/02/Glossary-of-Lay-Terminology_12-15-14.pdf. Accessed 29 Dec 2018

Feldmüller T, Wesch M, Kutscha M, Die EU (2011) Readability guideline: Auswirkungen auf die Packungsbeilage. Pharm Ind 73:441–446

Felsch C (2004) Frequentielle Lesbarkeitsanalyse—Studienarbeit (frequential readability analysis—student research project). Grin Verlag für akademische Texte, Jena

Flesch R (1948) A new readability yardstick. J Appl Psychol 32:221–233

Foster CS (2013) An analysis of volunteer age and level of education on performance in 'Readability' testing for patient information leaflet. J Health Med Inform 4:2–4

Franck MCJ, Foulon V, Van Vaerenbergh L (2011) ABOP, the automatic patient information leaflet optimizer: evaluation of a tool in development. Patient Educ Counsel 83:411–416

Friedmann CP, Romeo D, Hinton SS (1997) Healthcare decisions and product labeling: results of a consumer comprehension study of prototype labeling for proposed over-the-counter cholestyramine. Am J Med 102:50–56

Fuchs J (2005) Die Packungsbeilagen als ein Mittel zur gezielten information und Handlungsanleitung für Patienten—Entwicklung und Testung eines Instrumentes zur Beurteilung und Optimierung der Packungsbeilagen von Arzneimitteln [package inserts as medium to convey targeted information and directions for use to patients: developing and testing a tool to rate and optimise pharmaceutical product package inserts. Dissertation, Humboldt University, Berlin

Fuchs J (2010a) The way forward in package insert user tests from a CROs perspective. Drug Inf J 44:119–129

Fuchs J (2010b) Patient information via package inserts within the European Union—results of the PAINT3 study. http://www.paint-consult.com/fileadmin/editorial/downloads/vortraege/PAINT-Consult_Presentation_chin_Deligation_Bonn_2010_engl.pdf. Accessed 27 Sept 2019

Fuchs J, Finke A (2008) Hippius M. Wie genau lassen sich Tabletten teilen? (How exact can tablets be divided?). Arzneimittel-Therapie-Kritik & Medizin und Umwelt 48:147–159

Fuchs J, Hippius M (2007) Inappropriate dosage instructions in package leaflets. Patient Educ Counsel. 67:157–168

Fuchs J, Kutscha M (2015) How best to assess paper quality for package leaflets – weight or opacity? Pharm Ind 77:1380–1383

Fuchs J, Hippius M, Schaefer M (2005) A survey of package inserts use by patients. Hosp Pharm Eur 21:29–31

Fuchs J, Hippius M, Schaefer M (2006) Analysis of German package inserts. Int J Clin Pharmacol Ther 44:8–13

Fuchs J, Banow S, Görbert N, Hippius M (2007) The importance of package insert information in the European Union. Pharm Ind 69:165–172

Fuchs J, Heyer T, Langenhan D, Hippius M (2010a) New font size requirements in package inserts of medicines. Pharm Ind 72:2032–2036

Fuchs J, Finke A, Hippius M (2010b) Ambivalent dosage instructions for children. Pharm Ind 72:606–610

Fuchs J, Werner S, Scheunpflug C, Götze EA, Elsterman K, Scheffel K et al (2010c) Excessive medical information increase in package inserts. Int J Clin Pharmacol Ther 48:781–790

Fuchs J, Scheunpflug C, Götze EA (2012) The influence of the European Union's template on the use of package inserts compared with a shorter model template. PharmInd 74:126–136

Fuchs J, Götze EA, Voigt C (2016) Landscape versus portrait format in package leaflets—which format is more suitable according to readability test results from the PAINT3 study? Pharm Ind 78:1174–1184

Fuchs J, Kraft S, Vettermann A, Reiche M (2017) Typographic changes in package leaflets of the European Union based on the example of German versions between 2005 and 2015. Ther Innov Regul Sci 51:431–438

Fuchs J, Götze EA, Voigt C (2018) Should package leaflets be coloured in the future? Pharm Ind 80:1428–1435

Fuchs J, Scheunpflug C, Götze EA PAINT-consult medical term, abbreviation and symbol test results. Unpublished information

Fujita PL, Machado CJS, de Olivera Teixeira M (2014) The medicine package leaflet and the regulation of its configurations in terms of form and content in Brazil. Saúde e Sociedade 23:166–180

Fullmann K, Blackburn DF, Fenton ME, Mansell H (2017) Readability and suitability of COPD consumer information. Can Respir J. https://doi.org/10.1155/2017/2945282

Garner M, Zhenye N, Francis J (2011) A framework for the evaluation of patient information leaflets. Health Expect 15:283–294

Gregg DG, Kulkarni UR, Vinze AS (2001) Understanding the philosphical underpinnings of software engineering research in information systems. Inform Syst Front 3:169–183

Gregory M, Poulten EC (1970) Even versus uneven right-hand margins and the rate of comprehension in reading. Ergonomics 13:427–434

Gunning R (1952) The technique of clear writing. McGraw-Hill, New York

Halliday MAK, Webster J (2006) On language and linguistics, 3rd edn. Continuum International Publishing Group, London

Hamrosi KK, Raynor DK, Aslani P (2014) Enhancing provision of written medicine information in Australia: pharmacist, general practitioner and consumer perceptions of the barriers and facilitators. BMC Health Serv Res 14:1–10

Hartley J, Johnson M (2000) Portrait or landscape? Typographical layouts for patient information leaflets. Visible Lang 34:296–309

Hartley J, Kenely J, Owen G, Truemann M (1980) The effect of headings on children's recall from prose text. Br J Educ Psychol 50:304–307

Haug O, Box G, Kohn M, Streiftau N, Haseloff A (2011) Prüfung der Verständlichkeit und Lesbarkeit von Arzneimittelinformationen anhand aktuell am Markt befindlicher Packungsbeilagen. http://www.langcor.de/PDF/Packungsbeilagen-Studie-OTC-2010.pdf. Accessed 27 Sept 2019

Health Products Regulatory Authority (2018) Guide to labels and leaflets of human medicines. http://www.hpra.ie/docs/default-source/publications-forms/guidance-documents/aut-

g0034-guide-to-labels-and-leaflets-of-human-medicines-v18.pdf?Status=Master&sfvrsn=39. Accessed 27 Sept 2019
Hemphill MA (1996) Note an adults' color-emotion associations. J Genet Psychol 157:275–280
Hevner AR, March ST, Park J, Ram S (2004) Design science in information systems research. Manag Inf Syst Q 28:75–105
Hieber C (2008) Lesbarkeitstest—Methoden, Bridging, Ausnahmen. https://www.paint-consult.com/fileadmin/editorial/downloads/z_textverlinkungen/lesbarkeitstest/AGES-Empfehlung_Lesbarkeitstest_Methoden.pdf. Accessed 27 Sept 2019
Hohgräwe U (1988) Verständlichkeit von Instruktionstexten und das Informationsverhalten von Arzneimittel-Verbrauchern. Wuppertal: Fachbereich 1—Gesellschaftswissenschaften der Bergischen Universität—Gesamthochschule Wuppertal
Holmes G (1931) The relative legibility of black print and white print. J Appl Psychol 15: 248–251
Humphris GM, Field EA (2003) The immediate effect on knowledge, attitudes and intentions in primary care attenders of a patient information leaflet: a randomized control trial replication and extension. Br Dent J 194:683–688
IGT Testing Systems (2006) IGT Information leaflet W43, printing through (85 Shore A), IGT AIC2-5T2000, Global Standard Tester 2/3/3H. https://www.igt.nl/wp-content/uploads/W43.pdf. Accessed 27 Sept 2019
Institute for Safe Medication Practices (2015) ISMP's list of error-prone abbreviations, symbols and dose designations. https://www.ismp.org/sites/default/files/attachments/2017-11/Error%20Prone%20Abbreviations%202015.pdf. Accessed 27 Sept 2019
Institutsrat des Schweizerischen Heilmittelinstituts (2019). Verordnung des Schweizerischen Heilmittelinstituts über die Anforderungen an die Zulassung von Arzneimitteln (Arzneimittel-Zulassungsverordnung, AMZV), 9 Nov 2001 (last update 1 Jan 2019). http://www.admin.ch/ch/d/sr/8/812.212.22.de.pdf. Accessed 27 Sept 2019
Jarernsiripornkul N, Phueanpinit P, Pongwecharak J, Krska J (2019) Development and evaluation of user-tested Thai patient information leaflets for nonsteroidal anti-inflammatory drugs: effect on patients' knowledge. PLoS One 14:1–15
Kincaid JP, Fishburn RP, Rogers RL, Chissom BS (1975) Derivation of new readability formulas (automated readability index, fog count, and flesch reading ease formula) for navy enlisted personnel. University of Central Florida, Institute for Simulation and Training. https://stars.library.ucf.edu/cgi/viewcontent.cgi?article=1055&context=istlibrary. Assessed 18 Oct 2019
Knapp P, Raynor DK, Berry DC (2004) Comparison of two methods of presenting risk information to patients about the side effects of medicines. BMJ 13:176–180
Knapp P, Raynor DK, Woolf L, Gardner P, McMillan B (2009) Evaluating the effects on side-effect risk estimates by people when given single- versus double-ended frequency expressions. Int J Pharm Pract 17(2):B32–B33
Koo M, Krass I, Aslani P (2005) Consumer use of consumer medicine information. J Pharm Pract Res 35:94–98
Kopyto N, Braun-Münker M, Ecker F (2018) Importance of opening advices with novel packaging concepts. Pharm Ind 80:1123–1127
Lebanese American University (2011) Medical to lay terminology. http://gsr.lau.edu.lb/irb/forms/medical_lay_terms.pdf. Accessed 27 Sept 2019
Lerner EB, Jehle DVK, Janicke DM, Moscati RM (2000) Medical communication: do our patients understand? Am J Emerg Med 18:764–766
Lewis C, Rieman, J (1994) Task-centered user interface design: a practical introduction. http://hcibib.org/tcuid/tcuid.pdf. Accessed 18 Oct 2019
Mansoor L, Dowse R (2007) Written medicines information for south African HIV/AIDS patients: does it enhance understanding of co-trimoxazole therapy? Health Educ Res 22:37–48
March ST, Smith GF (1995) Design and natural science research on information technology. Decis Support Syst 15:251–266
Martinet A, Palmer E (1967) Elements of general linguistics, 3nd edn. University of Chicago Press, Chicago

Mazzullo JM, Lasagna L, Girner PF (1974) Variations in interpretation of prescription instructions—the need for improved prescribing habits. JAMA 227:929–931

McAvoy DR, Pitts PJ, Holdsworth SM, Elsner MW, Dowsett SA, Rotelli MD et al (2007) A new model for communicating risk information in direct-to-consumer print advertisements. Drug Inf J 41:111–127

McLaughlin HG (1969) SMOG grading: a new readability formula. J Read 12:639–646

Medicines and Healthcare Products Regulatory Agency (2005) Always read the leaflet—getting the best information with every medicine. https://www.gov.uk/government/uploads/system/uploads/attachment_data/file/391090/Always_Read_the_Leaflet___getting_the_best_information_with_every_medicine.pdf. Accessed 27 Sept 2019

Medicines and Healthcare Products Regulatory Agency (2008) Questions and answers on PLPI PIL user testing. http://webarchive.nationalarchives.gov.uk/20141205150130/http://www.mhra.gov.uk/home/idcplg?IdcService=GET_FILE&dDocName=CON014586&RevisionSelectionMethod=Latest. Accessed 27 Sept 2019

Medicines and Healthcare Products Regulatory Agency (2012) Best practised guidance on patient information leaflets. https://www.gov.uk/government/uploads/system/uploads/attachment_data/file/328405/Best_practice_guidance_on_patient_information_leaflets.pdf. Accessed 27 Sept 2019

Medicines and Healthcare Products Regulatory Agency (2017) Human factors and usability engineering—Guidance for medical devices including drug-device combination products, version 1.0. https://assets.publishing.service.gov.uk/government/uploads/system/uploads/attachment_data/file/645862/HumanFactors_Medical-Devices_v1.0.pdf. Accessed 27 Sept 2019

Medicines Evaluation Board (2019) Patiëntvriendelijke termen. https://www.cbg-meb.nl/binaries/college-ter-beoordeling-van-geneesmiddelen/documenten/beleidsdocumenten/2019/01/01/patientvriendelijke-termen/190628+Lijst+met+pati%C3%ABntvriendelijke+termen+voor+bijsluiter.pdf. Accessed 27 Sept 2019

Morrow D, von Leirer O, Altieri P, Tanke E (1991) Elder's schema for taking medication: implications for instruction design. J Gerontol 46:378–385

Morrow DG, von Leirer O, Andrassy JM, Decker Tanke E, Stine-Morrow EAL (1996) Medical instruction design: younger and older adult schemas for taking medication. Hum Factors 38:556–573

Moudgil T, Arora R, Kaur K (2016) Prevalance of color blindness in children. Int J Med Dental Sci 5:1252–1258

National Agency for Medicines and Medical Devices of Romania (2010) HOTÃRÂREA Nr. 6/23.03.2010 referitoare la aprobarea Ghidului privind modalitatea de efectuare a consultãrii cu grupurile þintã de pacienþi în vederea elaborãrii prospectului. http://www.anm.ro/_/HCS/HCS_6_2010.rar. Accessed 16 Oct 2019

National Center for Education Statistics, US Department of Education, Office of Educational Research and Improvement (2002) Adult literacy in America, a first look at the findings of the National Adult Literacy Survey (NALS). https://nces.ed.gov/pubs93/93275.pdf. Accessed 18 Oct 2019

Nielsen J (1994) Usability inspection methods. Wiley, New York

Paech T, Ihnken B, Menges K, Dobmeyer T (2011) Readability of package leaflets according to age and level of education. Pharm Ind 73:1387–1398

Pander Maat H, Lentz L (2010) Improving the usability of patient information leaflets. Patient Educ Counsel. 80:113–119

Pander Maat H, Lentz L, Raynor D (2015) How to test mandatory text templates: the European patient information leaflet. PLoS One. https://doi.org/10.1371/journal.pone.01392501-17

Papay J, Fritz D, Contu T, Ellis M, Debussey S (2010) Assessment of a simplified format of written patient prescription drug information. Drug Inf J 44:375–391

Patel VL, Branch T, Arocha JF (2002) Errors in interpreting quantities as procedures: the case of pharmaceutical labels. Int J Med Inform 65:193–211

Paterson DG, Tinker MA (1929) Studies of typographical factors influencing speed of reading; II. Size of type. J Appl Psychol 13:120–130

Paterson DG, Tinker MA (1931) Studies of typographical factors influencing speed of reading, VI. Black type versus white type. J Appl Psychol 13:241–247
Paterson DG, Tinker MA (1940) How to make type readable. Harper, Oxford
Paterson DG, Tinker MA (1942) Influence of size of type on eye movements. J Appl Psychol 26:227–230
Perry DK (1952) Speed of accuracy of reading Arabic and Roman numerals. J Appl Psychol 36:346–347
Pfeffers K, Tuunanen T, Rothenberger M, Chatterjee S (2008) A design science research methodology for information systems research. J Manag Inf Syst 24:45–77
Pickford RW (1963) Natural selection and colour blindness. Eugen Rev 55:97–101
Pinero-Lopez MA, Figueiredo-Escriba C, Modamio P, Lastra CF, Marino EL (2019) Readability assessment of package leaflets of biosimilars. BMJopen 9:e024837. https://doi.org/10.1136/bmjopen-2018-024837
Pires C, Vigário M, Cavaco A (2015a) Graphical content of medicinal package inserts: an exploratory study to evaluate potential legibility issues. Health Inf Libr J 33:121–129
Pires C, Vigário M, Martins F, Cavaco A (2015b) Abbreviations and symbols in a large sample of medicinal package leaflets: automatic detection and comprehension assessment. Procedia Computer Sci 64:683–690
Pires C, Vigário M, Cavaco A (2015c) Package leaflets of the most consumed medicines in Portugal: safety and regulatory compliance issues. A descriptive study. Sao Paulo Med J 133:91–100
Pires C, Martins F, Cavaco A, Vigário M (2017a) Automatic quantification of abbreviations in medicine package leaflets and their comprehension assessment. Int J E-Health Medical Commun 8:47–64
Pires C, Cavaco A, Vigário M (2017b) How sociodemographic features impact subjects' opinion on packages leaflets of medicines? Australasian Medical J 10:774–784
Pizzoll TSD, Moraes CG, Arrais PSD, Bertoldi AD, Ramos LR, Farias MR et al (2019) Medicine package inserts from the users' perspective: are they read and understood? Rev Bras Epidemiol 22:1–12
Poulton EC (1965) Letter differentiation and rate of comprehension in reading. J Appl Psychol 49:358–362
Poulton EC (1967a) Skimming (scanning) news items printed in 8-point and 9-point letters. Ergonomics 10:713–716
Poulton EC (1967b) Searching for newspaper headlines printed in capitals or lower-case letters. J Appl Psychol 51:417–425
Poulton EC (1969) Skimming lists of food ingredients printed in different sizes. J Appl Psychol 53:55–58
Poulton EC, Brown CH (1968) Rate of comprehension of an existing teleprinter output and of possible alternatives. J Appl Psychol 52:16–21
Purao S (2002) Design research in the technology of information systems: truth or dare. Working paper. GSU Department of CIS, Georgia State University, Atlanta. http://www3.cis.gsu.edu/vvaishnavi/9220Sp07/Documents/truth-dare-Purao%202002.pdf. Accessed 28 Sept 2019
Ramadas D, Chakrabordy A, Swaroop HS, Syed F, Praveen KV (2013) Spinivas BN. A study of package inserts in southern India. J Clin Diagn Res 7:2475–2477
Ramanayake BS, Liyanagoda NE, Dahanayake PK, Hemachandra MAD (2014) Do patients understand medical communication? Patients' knowledge on anatomical location of organs in human body. Sci Res J 2:12–15
Rayner K (1998) Eye movements in reading and information processing: 20 years of research. Psychol Bull 124:372–422
Raynor DK (1992) Writing patient information—a pharmacist's guide. Pharm J 254:180–182
Raynor DKT, Svarstad B, Knapp P, Aslani P, Rogers MB, Koo M et al (2007) Consumer medication information in the United States, Europe and Australia: a comparative evaluation. J Am Pharm Assoc 47:717–724
Roethlein BE (1912) The relative legibility of different faces of printing types. Am J Psychol 23:1–36

Sass SM, Legge GE, Lee H-W (2006) Low-vision reading speed: influences of linguistic inference and aging. Optom Vis Sci 83:166–177
Sawalha AF, Sweileh WM, Zyoud SH, Jabi SW (2008) Comparative analysis of patient package inserts of local and imported anti-infective agents in Palestine. Libyan J Med 34(4):181–185
Scheunpflug C (2008) Entwicklung eines Testsystems, um pharmazeutische und medizinische Fachbegriffe patientenverständlich zu erklären (development of a test system for explaining pharmaceutical and medical terms to patients). Thesis, Friedrich Schiller University, Jena
Shiyanbola OO, Smith PD, Huang YM, Mansukhani SG (2017) Pharmacists and patients feedback on empirically designed prescription warning labels: a qualitative study. Int J Clin Pharm 39:187–195
Shruti DA, Sarala NS, Bhuvana K (2016) Analysis of package inserts of drugs utilized in a tertiary care hospital. J Young Pharm 8:275
Sillo HB, Masota NE, Kisoma S, Rago L, Mgoyela V, Kaale EA (2018) Conformity of package inserts information to regulatory requirements among selected branded and generic medicinal products circulating on the east African market. PLoS One 13:1–13
Sless D (2007) PIL testing: misapplied and out of context. Regulatory Rapporteur J 11:14–15
Sless D, Shrensky R (2006) Writing about medicines for people. Communication Research Institute, Canberra
Sless D, Wiseman R (1997) Writing about medicines for people: usability guidelines for consumer medicine information, 2nd edn. Department of Health and Family Services, Canberra
Sojourner RJ, Wogalter MS (1997) The influence of pictorials on evaluations of prescription medication instructions. Drug Inf J 31:963–972
Soleimani H, Mohammadi E (2012) The effect of text typographical features on legibility, comprehension, and retrieval of EFL learners. Engl Lang Teach 5:207–216
Spencer H, Reynolds L, Coe B (1974) Typographic coding in lists and bibliographies. Appl Ergonomics 5:136–141
Taylor WL (1953) Cloze procedure: a new tool for measuring readability. Journalism Mass Commun Q 30:415–433
Tayyem MM, Takrouri MSM (2009) Patient's safety information available on drug package inserts used in neuroanesthesia. Internet J Anesthesiol 19:1–7
The European Parliament and the Council of the European Union (2004) Directive 2004/27/EC of the European Parliament and of the Council of 31 March 2004 amending Directive 2001/83/EC on the Community code relating to medicinal products for human use. OJ; L136:34–57
The European Parliament and the Council of the European Union (2012) Directive 2001/83/EC of the European Parliament and of the Council of 6 November 2001 on the Community code relating to medicinal products for human use (Consolidated version: 16 Nov 2012). https://ec.europa.eu/health/sites/health/files/files/eudralex/vol-1/dir_2001_83_consol_2012/dir_2001_83_cons_2012_en.pdf. Accessed 27 Sep 2019
Tillmann D (2014) Metaanalyse von Lesestudien (meta-analysis of reading studies). Thesis, Faculty of Media, HTWK/Leipzig University of Applied Sciences, Leipzig
Tinker MA (1963) Legibility of print. The Iowa State University Press, Iowa
Tinker MA, Paterson DG (1928) Influence of type form on speed of reading. J Appl Psychol 12:359–368
Tinker MA, Paterson DG (1929) Studies of typographical factors influencing speed of reading, III. Length of line. J Appl Psychol 13:205–219
Tinker MA, Paterson DG (1931a) Studies of typographical factors influencing speed of reading, VII. Variations in colour of print and background. J Appl Psychol 15:471–479
Tinker MA, Paterson DG (1931b) Studies of typographical factors influencing speed of reading, V. Simultaneous variation of type size and line length. J Appl Psychol 15:72–78
Tinker MA, Paterson DG (1944) Eye movements in reading black print on white background and red print on dark green background. Am J Psychol 1:93–94
Tinker MA, Paterson DG (1949) Speed of reading nine point type in relation to line width and leading. J Appl Psychol 33:81–82
Tong V, Raynor DK, Aslani P (2014) Design and comprehensibility of over-the-counter product labels and leaflets: a narrative review. Int J Clin Pharm 36:865–872

Tong V, Raynor DK, Aslani P (2018) Comparative user testing of Australian and UK over-the-counter labels and leaflets for Diclofenac. Ther Innov Regul Sci 52:38–48

University of Hohenheim (2010) Der Hohenheimer Verständlichkeitsindex (The Hohenheimer Comprehensibility index). https://www.uni-hohenheim.de/politmonitor/methode.php. Accessed 23 Dec 2018

US Department of Health and Human Services, Food and Drug Administration, Center for Devices and Radiological Health (2001) Guidance on medical device patient labeling; final guidance for industry and FDA reviewers. https://www.fda.gov/media/71030/download. Accessed 27 Sept 2019

US Department of Health and Human Services, Food and Drug Administration, Center for Devices and Radiological Health, Office of Device Evaluation (2016) Applying human factors and usability engineering to medical device—guidance for industry and food and drug administration staff. https://www.fda.gov/media/80481/download. Accessed 27 Sept 2019

US Department of Health and Human Services, Food and Drug Administration, Center for Drug Evaluation and Research (CDER) (2009) Guidance for industry—label comprehension studies for non-prescription drug products—draft guidance. https://www.fda.gov/media/75626/download. Accessed 27 Sept 2019

US Food and Drug Administration (2018) 21CFR280.20 content and format of a medication guide. https://www.accessdata.fda.gov/scripts/cdrh/cfdocs/cfcfr/CFRSearch.cfm?fr=208.20. Accessed 28 Sept 2019

Vaishnavi V, Kuechler W, Petter S, De Leoz G (2019) Design science research in information systems. http://desrist.org/design-research-in-information-systems. Accessed 28 Sept 2019

Van Aken JE (2005) Management research as a design science: articulating the research products of mode 2 knowledge production in management. Br J Manage 16:19–36

Van Beusekom M, Bos M, Wolterbeek R, Guchelaar H-J, van den Broek J (2015) Patients' preferences for visuals: differences in the preferred level of detail, type of background and type of frame of icons depicting organs between literate and low-literate people. Patient Educ Counsel. 98:226–233

Van Beusekom MM, Grootens-Wiegers P, Bos MJW, Guchelaar HJ, van den Broek JM (2016) Low literacy and written drug information: information-seeking, leaflet evaluation and preferences, and roles for images. Int J Clin Pharm 38:1372–1379

Van Beusekom MM, Kerkhoven AH, Bos MJW, Guchelaar HJ, van den Broek JM (2018) The extent and effects of patient involvement in pictogram design for written drug information: a short systematic review. Drug Discov Today 23:1312–1318

Van Dijk L, Monteiro SP, Vervloet M, de Bie J, Raynor DKT (2014a) Study on the package leaflets and the summary of product characteristics of medicinal products for human use—PIL-S study. http://ec.europa.eu/health/files/committee/75meeting/pil_s.pdf. Accessed 27 Sept 2019

Van Dijk L, Vervloet M, Monteiro SP, van der Burgt S, Raynor DKT (2014b) Feasibility and value of a possible "key information section" in patient information leaflets and summaries of product characteristics of medicinal products for human use—the PILS-BOX study. http://ec.europa.eu/health/files/committee/75meeting/pilbx.pdf. Accessed 27 Sept 2019

Vander Stichele RH, Van Haecht CH, Braem MD, Bogaert MG (1991) Attitude of the public toward technical package inserts for medication information in Belgium. Ann Pharmacother 25:1002–1006

Vander Stichele RH, De Potter B, Vyncke P, Bogaert MG (1996) Attitude of physicians toward patient package inserts for medication information in Belgium. Patient Educ Counsel. 28: 5–13

Vinker S, Eliyahu V, Yaphe J (2007) The effect of drug information leaflets on patient behaviour. Isr Med Assoc J 9:383–386

Weitbrecht WU, Voßkämper C (2002) Influence of the drug package information paper on compliance of neurological and psychiatric outpatients. Fortschr Neurol Psychiatr 70:178–184

Wolf A (2015) An analysis and evaluation of the development of the QRD human product information template used in package leaflets—theses. University of Bonn, Bonn

Wolf MS, King J, Wilson EAH, Curtis LM, Bailey SC, Duhig J et al (2012) Usability of FDA-approved medication guides. J Gen Intern Med 27:1714–1720

Wolf A, Fuchs J, Schweim HG (2014) Readability of the European QRD template—the European QRD template version 8 in comparison to its predecessor and a shorter model template. Pharm Ind 76:1312–1322
Wolf A, Fuchs J, Schweim HG (2016) Implementation of the European QRD template in package leaflets of centralized approved medicines. Ther Innov Regul Sci 50:106–114
Wolff JS, Wogalter MS (1993) Test and development of pharmaceutical pictorials. In: Monica S (ed) Human factors and ergonomics society, interface 93—humanizing technology proceedings, pp 187–192
Wolka A, Simpson K, Lockwood K, Neuhauser L (2015) Focus on health literacy: recommendations to improve European Union risk management plan public summaries. Ther Innov Regul Sci 49:369–376
Yu D, Park H, Gerold D, Legge GE (2010) Comparing reading speed for horizontal and vertical English text. J Vis 10:1–17
Zachrisson B (1965) Studies in the legibility of printed text. Almqvist & Wiksell, Stockholm, Göteborg, Uppsala

13 Dissemination and Implementation Science

Elaine H. Morrato and Meredith Y. Smith

Abstract

The dissemination and implementation of health interventions is the active and targeted distribution of information and intervention materials to a specific public health, healthcare professional or patient audience with the goal of transferring knowledge and/or promoting changes in health attitudes and behaviours. In this chapter, we present key tenets of effective health dissemination and implementation in the context of medicinal product risk minimisation and communication. We review best practices and recommendations from dissemination and implementation (D&I) science and discuss their application to risk minimisation programme design, implementation and evaluation stages. To illustrate these concepts, we examine the evolution of the valproate risk minimisation programme in Europe.

E. H. Morrato (✉)
Parkinson School of Health Sciences and Public Health, Loyola University Chicago, Chicago, IL, USA

Colorado School of Public Health, University of Colorado Anschutz Medical Campus, Aurora, CO, USA
e-mail: EMorrato@luc.edu

M. Y. Smith
Alexion Pharmaceuticals, Inc., Boston, MA, USA

School of Pharmacy, University of Southern California, Los Angeles, CA, USA

© Springer Nature Singapore Pte Ltd. 2020

P. Bahri (ed.), *Communicating about Risks and Safe Use of Medicines*,
https://doi.org/10.1007/978-981-15-3013-5_13

13.1 The Discipline of Dissemination and Implementation Science: Scope, Theories and Principles

13.1.1 Rationale for Applying Dissemination and Implementation (D&I) Science to Medicinal Product Risk Communication Research

This chapter focusses on the application of dissemination and implementation science (D&I) to medicinal product risk communication and risk minimisation. D&I science is an inter-disciplinary field in health intervention research that seeks to support effective adoption and integration of evidence-based health interventions within particular healthcare, public health or community settings (Brownson et al. 2017). Towards that end, it emphasises the development and application of methods and strategies to facilitate adoption of interventions by healthcare professionals, patients and other affected stakeholders. Two concepts fundamental to D&I science are:

(1) *Dissemination*, the active approach of spreading an intervention to the targeted recipients using one or more planned strategies and communication channels; and
(2) *Sustainability*, the extent to which an evidence-based intervention delivers its intended benefits and is maintained over the long-term (Rabin and Brownson 2017; Shelton et al. 2018).

Dissemination and sustainability are equally central to the field of medicinal product risk communication and risk minimisation (Smith and Morrato 2014). Medicinal product risk communication and minimisation represent a form of health intervention disseminated broadly and scaled to the population level. Its public health goal is to support the safe and appropriate use of medicinal products and to optimise the benefit-risk balance of the products. In Europe, companies are required to submit a risk management plan (RMP) at the time of application for marketing authorisation approval which includes information on how product-related risks will be prevented or minimised in patients. In the United States (US) under certain conditions, risk minimisation may take the form of a formal risk evaluation and mitigation strategy programme (REMS) and include a set of required elements to ensure safe use of the medicinal product (see Chap. 1).

Well-conducted dissemination planning and execution are vital to the success of risk communication efforts as the latter is heavily dependent on whether and to what extent the key messages reach the target audience, are understood and are appropriately acted upon. Sustainability planning is a key consideration as well, because risk communication messaging for a product must continue throughout the post-authorisation period. Sustainability is a direct function of how effectively the programme has been integrated into the healthcare delivery process. Specifically, programmes which have been designed to fit within existing processes are more likely to be continued over time than those which have not been. As such, sustainability strategies can also help minimise the "burden" of the risk communication programme on the healthcare system itself, another goal of regulatory risk minimisation efforts (Center for Drug Evaluation and Research and Center for Biologics Evaluation and Research 2019a; European Medicines Agency and Heads of Medicines Agencies 2017a).

To date, regulators have provided extensive guidance regarding the content and format of risk communication tools as well as how to assess their effectiveness (Center for Drug Evaluation and Research and Center for Biologics Evaluation and Research 2011, 2019a, b; European Medicines Agency and Heads of Medicines Agencies 2015a, 2017a, b). Comparatively little attention, however, has been paid to issues of designing for dissemination, implementation and sustainability, either in existing guidance or in the actual practice and evaluation of therapeutic risk communication and minimisation programmes. By comparison, within the broader context of the healthcare system, there is a growing recognition that a well-designed dissemination plan is essential for successful programme delivery (Glasgow and Chambers 2012; Glasgow et al. 2012).

The purpose of this chapter is to describe and apply D&I science to medicinal product risk minimisation and communication research. Specifically, it seeks to: first, explain how the concepts of dissemination and sustainability can inform the design, implementation and evaluation of risk communication and related risk minimisation activities; and second, critically appraise the valproate risk minimisation efforts in Europe through the lens of D&I science. To advance the science of therapeutic risk minimisation, pragmatic considerations from D&I science are provided for improving adoption and sustainability of interventions to support safe use behaviours and minimise specific product risks.

13.1.2 D&I Science in Health: Scope and Definition

A key dissemination challenge is that scientific knowledge about best care can take decades to become integrated into clinical practice, and even then adoption can be highly uneven (Institute of Medicine Committee on Quality of Health Care in America 2001).

The challenge of expediting adoption can be attributed to both the time it takes to generate and synthesise the evidence, and the decisional processes required to integrate such evidence into practice within complex health systems. Green and colleagues conceptualised knowledge translation from scientific research to health practice, and ultimately to health policy, as a diffusion process through a "leaky pipe" (Green et al. 2009). Key decisional steps, i.e. potential leaks slowing diffusion, include: making decisions on research priorities and funding; forming consensus around the best available scientific evidence; planning dissemination programmes; engaging the community and practitioners in the implementation process; and adapting dissemination strategies over time in response to implementation barriers. Green et al. further characterised stages of clinical decision-making affecting the integration of evidence-based medicine into health services. Stages include healthcare professionals' awareness, acceptance and agreement, perceived applicability, ability, behavioural intention to comply and actual adherence (Glasziou and Haynes 2005).

The application of D&I science has emphasised the requirement for having scientific evidence as the starting point for dissemination (Proctor et al. 2012). An emerging view posits that stakeholders, such as healthcare professionals and patients, should be involved early in the diffusion planning process so that dissemination strategies can address the health needs, capabilities and circumstances of the specific target audiences. The "Designing for Dissemination" movement seeks to accelerate knowledge translation and the integration of evidence into practice by collaborating with stakeholders early on in the design process (Brownson et al. 2013; Chambers 2019; Ho and Peter Wall Workshop 2014; Ramsey et al. 2019). In this context, health dissemination can be re-framed as a social marketing and distribution challenge using a customer-centred approach to inform intervention design and selection of dissemination strategies (Chambers 2019; Kreuter and Wang 2015). Planning with stakeholder partnership early in the development and dissemination process has been shown to enhance reach, receptivity and effectiveness (Westfall et al. 2016).

13.1.3 D&I Science in Health: Key Tenets of Theory

Effective health intervention implementation and dissemination, regardless of the intervention, has several common features (see Fig. 13.1).

First, dissemination is a *goal-directed* process. The US National Research Council emphasises the need to link risk communication with goals and outcomes: "A risk communication is successful to the extent that it contributes to the outcomes its sponsor desires" (Committee on Risk Perception and Communication 1989). As described by Brewer, there are three potential goals of risk communication: to share information, to change beliefs and to change behaviour" (Brewer 2011).

In the context of medicinal product risk minimisation, the goal of sharing information includes objectives to raise awareness and knowledge in healthcare professionals and patients regarding a medicine's risk and what can be done to minimise, mitigate or prevent the risk. The goal of changing beliefs can be operationalised to include affecting beliefs about the importance of performing certain clinical actions, such as patient monitoring. Behaviour change goals include, for example, patient counselling, documenting informed decision-making, promoting safe medicines use, making appropriate patient selection, discontinuation of prescribing a medicine for particular patients when its benefits no longer outweigh its risks.

- Goal-directed
- Context-grounded
- Theory-driven
- Responsive and adaptive

Fig. 13.1 Key elements of effective dissemination of health evidence

A second feature of effective health dissemination is that it is *context-grounded* and attuned to the clinical situation and circumstances in which the risk minimisation is occurring. At the individual level, context includes current knowledge, attitudes, norms and behaviours of healthcare professionals and patients given the medicine's indicated use. At the healthcare setting or clinic level, context includes culture, implementation climate, available resources and readiness for implementation (Damschroder et al. 2009; Keith et al. 2017). At the health system level of programme planning, context can include predisposing, reinforcing and enabling factors and incentives affecting delivery of healthcare (Green and Kreuter 2005). Clinical practice guidelines, payer and reimbursement requirements, and health policies and laws are all examples of ecological factors that can affect the effectiveness of health dissemination.

Effective health dissemination is also *theory-guided* and utilises knowledge and methods acquired from behavioural and social sciences that are discussed in Chaps. 7 and 8. Theories, models and frameworks encourage systematic application of knowledge to guide dissemination planning, implementation and evaluation (Morrato 2018). They provide a social science mechanism of action to guide the causal pathway for risk minimisation in much the same way that a biological mechanism of action guides the clinical development of new medicines. Even risk minimisation programmes that address only a subset of constructs within a theoretical model should be framed conceptually, so that regulators and society perceive the larger context (and body of literature) guiding the programme. Ultimately, the use of theories and frameworks helps enable cross programme comparisons and fosters generalisable knowledge to advance the science of health dissemination.

A variety of models, frameworks and theories have been developed and used for D&I in healthcare (Nilsen 2015; Nilsen and Bernhardsson 2019; Tabak et al. 2012). Collectively, these models can be categorised into five groups: (1) process models, which specify the processes of transferring empirical research findings into actual real world practice; (2) determinant frameworks, which identify barriers and facilitators that can explain or otherwise influence programme implementation and its outcomes; (3) classic theories drawn from such disciplines as psychology and organisational behaviour which can be used to explain implementation efforts; (4) implementation theories, which have been developed by implementation science researchers; and (5) evaluation frameworks, which identify which implementation measures to evaluate in order to gauge implementation effectiveness (Nilsen 2015). Elements from multiple different theories, frameworks and/or models can be combined to guide intervention design (Damschroder et al. 2009; Birken et al. 2017). A review of social science theories applicable for risk minimisation programmes has been described by Morrato (2018).

Lastly, effective health dissemination is *responsive and adaptive* to changing context and audience needs. Diffusion of innovation theory states that adoption is a time-based process with early adopters having different informational needs than later adopters (Dearing and Cox 2018). Thus, health dissemination messaging is expected to evolve over time and be adaptable. This is consistent with how risk management has been conceptualised across a medicine's product lifecycle (benefit-risk assessment, communication and evaluation (BRACE) cycle) (Radawski et al. 2015).

- Multi-level audiences and multiple communication channels
- Need for balancing both benefit and risk messaging
- Need for identifying core risk messaging (global consistency) while allowing adaptation (local customisation)
- Highly regulated environment

Fig. 13.2 Factors that increase dissemination and implementation complexity in medicinal product risk communication

13.1.4 Dissemination Considerations in Medicinal Product Risk Communication

Several factors make the dissemination of medicinal product risk communication and minimisation particularly complex and challenging (see Fig. 13.2).

First, risk minimisation programmes are *multi-level* and seek to reach a variety of *target audiences* across a variety of *communication channels*. For example, these programmes are multi-level because they operate at policy level and affect health system-, healthcare professional- and patient-level safe use behaviours. They can encompass a wide array of activities and tools, and typically target a range of audiences (e.g. healthcare professionals, patients, informal care providers, the general public) and interventions settings (e.g. in-patient and out-patient healthcare settings, home). Ongoing engagement of patients and healthcare professionals is for successful dissemination of risk communication and other risk minimisation activities (Brown and Bahri 2019).

While the label and packaging represent the primary source of information about a medicinal product's risks for patients and healthcare professionals, numerous other risk communication tools can also be used as well. Common examples of such tools include safety alerts from regulatory authorities, direct healthcare professional communications (DHPCs), also referred to as Dear Healthcare Provider/Professional-letters, medication guides, educational brochures, patient reminder and/or alert cards and checklists. Complexity increases when one also considers secondary sources of information, such as the news media, medical societies, patient organisations and personal social networks and various social media platforms.

In addition, risk communication speaks to only one aspect of a product's overall benefit-risk profile; therefore, there is need for *balancing benefit and risk messaging* to healthcare professionals and patients. Major regulatory agencies have adopted the use of benefit-risk templates to document and assess a medicine's profile and guide more transparent regulatory decision-making (Leong Wai Yeen et al. 2014; Muhlbacher et al. 2016).

Because medicines are typically marketed across multiple countries under different regulatory authorities, global pharmaceutical companies face the added challenge of identifying *core risk messaging* and risk minimisation measures while also allowing *flexible adaptation* of message delivery and implementation at the local level (Smith and Morrato 2014). Adaptation is also a natural part of innovation adoption over time. Types of adaptation can include: language and cultural differences, mode of delivery, target audience(s) and service setting variation (Chambers and Norton 2016). Recognising this fact, the United States Food and Drug

Administration (US FDA) issued guidance to industry on processes and procedures for REMS modifications and revisions (Field et al. 2002). Stirman and colleagues have developed a research framework for cataloguing adaptations and modifications to health interventions in D&I research, including specifying the type of modification and identifying reasons for the change at the socio-political, setting, provider and recipient levels (Wiltsey Stirman et al. 2019).

Lastly, it must be underscored that medicinal risk communication occurs within a *regulated environment*. Not only does this affect the messaging, but the regulated context also affects the type of strategies available for risk minimisation across countries and regions. For example, US statute defines when REMS can include Elements to Ensure Safe Use (ETASU) and when routine risk communication (i.e. the label and packaging) alone is insufficient to mitigate a risk (Center for Drug Evaluation and Research and Center for Biologics Evaluation and Research 2019a). The statute also defines the types of ETASU that can be implemented: prescriber and pharmacist training or certification; controlled dispensing the medicine (e.g. only in certain healthcare settings or with evidence of safe use conditions such as laboratory results) and requirements that patients using the medicine will be monitored or enrolled in a registry. The importance to have full awareness of the legal framework applicable to a communication intervention for its planning or evaluation is discussed in Chap. 15.

13.2 Research Approaches and Methods

This section presents best practices from D&I science as a framework for strengthening risk minimisation programmes at the design, implementation and evaluation stages. Figure 13.3 summarises key steps for each stage.

Reporting standards for the evaluation of risk minimisation programmes have been proposed and collectively referred to as the RIsk Minimization Evaluation Study (RIMES) Statement (Smith et al. 2018). These standards were developed to

Designing for dissemination and implementation
1. Identify risk minimisation goals and objectives
2. Analyse the situational context
3. Identify anticipated risk minimisation care gaps
4. Select appropriate risk minimisation strategies
5. Develop communication and risk minimisation materials and tools

Programme implementation
1. Identify responsible organisations and implementation agents
2. Establish quality assurance and control policies and procedures
3. Document adaptations and modifications

Evaluation
1. Identify *a priori* hypotheses and primary success metrics
2. Identify secondary (explanatory) measures
3. Select study design(s) and population(s), balancing considerations of internal and external validity

Fig. 13.3 Key steps for strengthening risk minimisation programmes at the design, implementation and evaluation stages using best practices from D&I science

facilitate comprehensive, consistent and transparent reporting of risk minimisation evaluation studies, including those assessing the effectiveness of risk communication interventions. In this section we will also describe how the three stages relate to the various RIMES criteria.

13.2.1 Designing for Dissemination and Implementation

Designing for dissemination embodies design-thinking and the principle of beginning with the end in mind. Designing for dissemination can be conceptualised as the process of ensuring that the dissemination products (messages, materials) are developed in ways that closely correspond to the needs, resources, workflows and contextual characteristics of the target audience and setting. Designing for the spread, or diffusion, of a programme means that the implementer actively employs specific strategies early in the process of creating and refining a health programme to increase its chances of being noticed, positively perceived, accessed and tried and subsequently adopted, implemented and sustained in practice (Dearing et al. 2013). Ultimately, dissemination planning involves specifying the set of processes and activities (strategies) to be implemented in order to increase the dissemination potential of a health intervention or programme (Rabin and Brownson 2017).

Design planning for risk communication and risk minimisation programmes is a multi-step process including specifying the programme goals and objectives, understanding the clinical context and target audiences, identifying anticipated care gaps, selecting appropriate dissemination and risk minimisation strategies and developing communication materials and tools (see Fig. 13.3). These considerations correspond with specific RIMES criteria of pertaining to programme design, specification of target population, selection and development of risk minimisation tools, and identification of success metrics.

Chap. 12 explains the generic design process and its application to medicinal product risk communication in greater detail. The following elaborates on the process from a D&I science perspective.

13.2.1.1 Identify Goals and Objectives

Goals establish the overall direction and focus of a risk minimisation programme and serve as the foundation for developing programme objectives. For example, consider a product ("Drug X") with known teratogenic risk. A knowledge dissemination goal might include: "*All patients are to be aware that Drug X causes serious birth defects*". An attitudinal dissemination goal affecting benefit-risk decision-making might be: "*All prescribers agree to prescribe Drug X to women between the ages of 18 and 50 years only if they have no other treatment alternatives*". A safe use behaviour goal to mitigate teratogenic risk might be: "*To prevent foetal exposure to Drug X, all prescribers must perform a pregnancy test before initiating Drug X in all women between the ages of 18 and 50 years*".

Objectives operationalise the goals and serve as ways to assess progress toward meeting the goal. A common mnemonic device for writing good objectives is

SMART (Centers for Disease Control and Prevention 2018). The objective should be: Specific—Who is the target population? What is to be accomplished?; Measurable—Is it quantifiable? How much change is expected?; Achievable—Can the objective be accomplished in the proposed time frame given available current status?; Realistic—Will the objective have an impact on the goal?; Time-bound—Does the objective propose a timeline when the objective will be met?

To illustrate the application of SMART objectives, consider a "Drug Y" whose goal is *"To prevent a fatal drug–drug interaction by preventing concomitant use with Drug Z"*. An objective assessing progress toward this goal with physicians could be: *"To educate at least 80% of US-based prescribers and dispensing pharmacists about the risk of a fatal drug–drug interaction that is associated with use of Drug Y by December 1, 2020; and 100% by March 1, 2021"*. An objective assessing progress toward the goal with patients could be: *"To educate 100% of patients receiving Drug Y that they should not take Drug Y with Drug Z"*.

13.2.1.2 Analyse the Situational Context

The next step in dissemination planning is to analyse the situational context in which the risk minimisation efforts will occur, including system-, provider- and patient-level factors that might affect D&I success:

- *System-level factors* include current standards of care, existing policies and procedures, and resources available in the healthcare delivery system for managing the risk. System-level structures can vary widely between countries, states/provinces, and settings of care in terms of supporting implementation capability and capacity for adopting and integrating risk minimisation procedures into practice.
- *Provider-factors* include baseline knowledge and attitudes about the risk among physicians, pharmacists and other healthcare professionals and current risk minimisation behaviours and capabilities.
- *Patient-level factors* include patient (and where appropriate caregiver) knowledge and attitudes about the risk and their ability to perform certain risk minimisation behaviours. Knowledge, attitudes and skills may vary across patients, especially among vulnerable and special populations, and thus necessitate audience segmentation in order to maximise the effectiveness of risk messaging and the distribution of risk materials.

A variety of resources can be used to pragmatically assess the situational context for a given risk minimisation programme:

- The scientific literature may provide relevant insights and assessments from related clinical quality improvement initiatives, health services research and/or dissemination and implementation programmes and evaluation.
- Market data and administrative claims data on medicines and healthcare utilisation is another resource that can be used to quantify current behaviours, applying pharmacoepidemiological methods as discussed in Chap. 14.

- For manufacturers, the collective wisdom from the clinical development, commercialisation and medical affairs teams can provide a working mental model, i.e. thought process, about how clinical care delivery works in the real world. Advisory boards, comprised of key opinion leaders or patient stakeholders, can also provide valuable insight into real world norms.
- Lastly, formative research involving qualitative interviewing, observation and/or surveys might be needed to provide the granularity necessary for dissemination design.

A flow diagram can be useful for synthesising and visualising the clinical care process and for identifying the contextual factors and stakeholders that may affect prescribing, dispensing and monitoring. A flow diagram can also be helpful for identifying gaps, or possibly existing controls in place, in regard to safe use behaviours and risk minimisation goals. These types of visualisations have been used in clinical quality improvement. They go by many names, including value stream mapping (Gellad and Day 2016), activity diagrams and process mapping (Harel et al. 2016), patient care pathways (Rosstad et al. 2015), action effect diagrams (Reed et al. 2014) and driver diagrams (Issen et al. 2018).

13.2.1.3 Identify Anticipated Risk Minimisation Care Gaps

Based on risk minimisation goals and the situation analysis, the next step is to identify the anticipated healthcare delivery system gaps to target. For example, there might be gaps in knowledge and the skills necessary to perform key risk minimisation behaviours. Critical resources might only be available in certain healthcare settings. Consensus on appropriate patient selection and tools supporting shared decision-making may be lacking. Limited skills, ability and resources might be available in routine clinical practice to mitigate the risks and there is a need to establish new norms for monitoring and follow-up.

13.2.1.4 Select Appropriate Risk Minimisation Strategies

Table 13.1 shows how general risk minimisation strategies can be mapped to specific risk minimisation goals for a medicine given anticipated care gaps. Designing specific communication and risk minimisation interventions is most effective when guided by social science theory. As previously discussed, behavioural and social science theory, models and frameworks help elucidate the mechanisms involved for achieving safe use behaviours and provide the evidence-based scientific justification supporting intervention selection. The case study at the end of this chapter will demonstrate how this can be done.

Another emerging consideration at the design phase is the desire to select strategies that minimise the potential burden of the programme on the healthcare delivery system and patient access to the medicine (Center for Drug Evaluation and Research and Center for Biologics Evaluation and Research 2019a). For example, the US FDA cites strategies that have the potential to result in treatment interruption or delays, particularly problematic in situations where patients have serious or life-threatening conditions.

Table 13.1 Mapping risk minimisation goals, care gaps and strategies

Communication goal	Care gap	Potential risk minimisation strategies	
		Healthcare professionals	Patients
Affect Knowledge	Awareness of the risk	• Product labelling, SmPC • Communication campaign	• Patient Package Insert, MedGuide • Packaging • Outreach campaign
	Safe use behaviours necessary to minimise the risk	• Education • Clinical guidelines • Advocacy partnership with professional societies	• Outreach campaign • Advocacy partnership with patient organisations and associations
Affect Attitudes	Who is an appropriate patient for receiving the medicine (ensuring the benefits outweigh the risks)	• Patient counselling and shared decision-making tools and materials • Prior authorisation policies and procedures before dispensing	• Patient counselling and shared decision-making tools and materials
Affect Safe use behaviours	Appropriate patient selection	• Electronic Health Record alerts • Documentation of safe use conditions before dispensing	• Patient attestation (informed consent)
	Specialised dosing and administration	• Training, certification • Restricted healthcare settings of use	• Training
	Monitoring	• Point-of-Care Electronic Health Record alerts • Audit-and-Feedback reporting • Patient registry	• Patient reminders materials and systems
	Coordination of care (prescriber + other professionals involved in risk minimisation)	• Shared Electronic Health Record systems	• Patient support materials and systems

13.2.1.5 Develop Risk Communication and Minimisation Materials and Tools

Best practices in message development include iterative stakeholder engagement with the target audience to test and refine messaging, with special attention to issues of health literacy for patient-directed communication. There are several sources on best practices in message development for healthcare professionals and patients, including resources provided by the US FDA (Fischoff et al. 2011), the Agency for Healthcare Research and Quality (Agency for Healthcare Research and Quality

2016), and the US Centers for Disease Control (US CDC) and Prevention (Office of the Associate Director for Communications 2016). The US CDC also developed a widget, "The Clear Communication Index", which is a research-based tool to assess specific text for health literacy (see: www.cdc.gov/ccindex).

Trevena and colleagues provide a risk communication primer for patient decision aid developers emphasising the importance of focusing on the task required of the user; defining the relevant reference class (i.e. competing alternatives) for each decision; providing a consistent format and addressing the numeracy and graph literacy of the audience (Trevena et al. 2013). An assessment of US FDA REMS programmes found that although most of the patient education materials met criteria for being understandable, less than half met criteria for actionability (Chan et al. 2018). Moreover, graphics are not necessarily more intuitive than text and should be carefully considered for each situation (Ancker et al. 2006).

13.2.2 Programme Implementation

Implementation is the process of engaging stakeholders and executing the necessary steps required to achieve the risk minimisation goals. The US FDA defines programme implementation and operations as the extent to which the intended stakeholders are participating in the risk minimisation programme as designed, including the receipt and use of risk minimisation materials and tools (Center for Drug Evaluation and Research and Center for Biologics Evaluation and Research 2019a). Care should also be given to avoid unintended consequences as a result of implementation that could affect patient access or create a potential burden to the healthcare system related to programme operations.

Implementation considerations correspond with the RIMES reporting items for "Setting" and "Fidelity" and centre around clearly identifying responsibilities, establish quality policies and procedures, and planning for documenting adaptations and modifications that occur during the implementation process (see Fig. 13.3).

13.2.2.1 Identify Responsible Organisations and Implementation Agents

In any given risk minimisation programme, roles and responsibilities should be clearly delineated among implementing bodies (e.g. regulatory agencies, pharmaceutical companies and healthcare systems). For example, a regulatory agency might be responsible for disseminating a medicines safety alert; whereas, the manufacturer might be responsible for distributing patient counselling materials to physicians, while the healthcare system might be responsible for ensuring pharmacists also appropriately counsel patients when the medicine is dispensed.

At the micro-level, organisational implementation roles and responsibility should also need to be defined within organisations, for example, defining roles and responsibilities internally across organisational units and professionals within pharmacovigilance, medical affairs and sales departments. Documenting how implementers of risk minimisation interventions were selected, including required qualifications, helps ensure implementation reproducibility and continuity over time as turnover in personnel occurs. Identifying and addressing training needs of the implementers is also a critical step.

13.2.2.2 Establish Quality Assurance and Quality Control Policies and Procedures

Quality management principles can be readily applied to risk minimisation implementation and operations. Quality assurance activities focus on preventing mistakes and avoiding problems and quality control activities focus on ensuring standards are met when the product or service is delivered (ASQ 2015). For example, clinical quality indicators, established by governmental and non-governmental organisations, are quality control measures intended to measure and track clinical performance and outcomes and improve healthcare delivery.

International Organization for Standardization (ISO) standards are embraced in many areas of medicines development, e.g. for management of clinical trials and for the chemical processes involved in the manufacture of medicines. ISO quality assurance and control standards have also been fundamental to guidance on quality management of pharmacovigilance in the European Union (EU) (European Medicines Agency and Heads of Medicines Agencies 2017c). An example of using quality assurance standards for risk minimisation activities is the use of a formal protocol to ensure fidelity across settings. An example of quality control is the use of metrics to track for the delivery of specific risk communication materials or metrics for safe use clinical behaviours.

13.2.2.3 Document Adaptations and Modifications

Variation in implementation over time and whether intentional modifications were made to risk minimisation intervention should be documented. These implementation considerations are particularly relevant when implementing across countries and regions and in assessing intervention effectiveness over time. In dynamic learning healthcare systems focused on continuous quality improvement and innovation, adaptations will naturally occur. It is critical to understand heterogeneity in implementation and the degree to which it might be enhancing, or deterring, intervention effectiveness.

Stirman and colleagues have developed a useful framework and coding system for capturing modifications in and adaptation of interventions during programme implementation (Wiltsey Stirman et al. 2019). Sources of risk minimisation adaptation can include adjusting risk messaging due to cultural differences or health literacy needs; changing modes of message delivery due to varying communication preferences and infrastructure capabilities; and changing who implements and delivers the risk minimisation intervention due to varying medical practice norms (Chambers and Norton 2016).

13.2.3 Evaluation of Risk Communication Programmes

An implementation science approach seeks to determine not only *how* effective a programme is, but *why* a given programme is effective (or ineffective), under what circumstances, in which target population (or subpopulations) and for which types of outcomes (Glasgow et al. 2019). Such information can help clarify whether programme failure was due to inadequacies in its implementation or to the aspects of the intervention itself. It can also provide valuable insight into what specific programme content or components may need to be re-designed, enhanced or eliminated, and the degree to which evaluation results are generalisable (Glasgow et al. 2019).

Similarly, risk minimisation evaluation planning also includes identifying success metrics, selecting the appropriate study designs and study populations and specifying primary and secondary measures, ideally within the context of the relevant social science theory informing the programme (see Fig. 13.3). These evaluation considerations correspond to the RIMES reporting items for hypotheses, participants, measures and statistical analyses. Several of the RIMES criteria also address measures of sustainability and healthcare integration.

13.2.3.1 Identify *A Priori* Hypotheses and Primary Success Metrics

In order to determine whether a risk minimisation programme is meeting its goals or not, it is imperative that there is an a priori specification of which measure(s) are the primary endpoint(s) of interest versus which are explanatory measures used to assess the dissemination process. Best practice in D&I research is to prespecify metrics of effectiveness at the programme planning, or design, stage. Primary success metrics should relate directly back to the risk communication and minimisation goals, objectives and design assumptions specified during the designing for dissemination stage. Hypotheses concerning possible unintended consequences, e.g. reducing patient access, should also be pre-specified.

The US FDA defines metrics as the "measures (such as quantity, quality, duration, size or frequency) of an aspect of the [risk management] program that provide a systematic basis for assessing how well a program has performed" (Center for Drug Evaluation and Research and Center for Biologics Evaluation and Research 2019a). Evaluation hypotheses should be informed by the dissemination strategies deployed. For example, a hypothesis might be stated as: "*We hypothesised that, as a result of distributing an educational brochure, the percentage of physicians who prescribed <drug> and who correctly identify the 3 key steps involved in screening patients for <risk factor> prior to initiating <drug> therapy would increase from 20% to 80%.*"

The US FDA has begun requiring pharmaceutical companies to provide a scientific justification for specific performance thresholds for programme success metrics. One challenge in the field of medicinal risk minimisation is that there are not absolute success metrics or numeric standards that can be readily applied across programmes. Rather, performance metrics must be tailored to the situational context for each programme in order to assess unique healthcare delivery processes and safe use behaviours (Center for Drug Evaluation and Research and Center for Biologics Evaluation and Research 2019a; Willy et al. 2014).

13.2.3.2 Identify Secondary (Explanatory) Measures

If one conceptualises risk minimisation implementation as a time-dependent process, then a range of secondary measures can be identified to assess implementation temporally and to understand its effect on proximal and distal measures of safe use behaviours, processes and outcomes (Prieto et al. 2012). Measure specification can be greatly facilitated by visualising the causal relationships between measures in the form of a logic model or causal pathway diagram. This can be informed by the social science mechanism of action or theory being used to guide risk minimisation planning and design.

Examples of implementation measures include metrics to assess programme fidelity; programme participation and adoption among healthcare professionals (agents of risk minimisation adoption) and reach of the programme to patients (recipients of risk minimisation intervention). Implementation process measures assess the degree to which the risk communication intervention reached the intended target audience, the extent to which the intervention was adopted within the relevant healthcare delivery settings, the quality of the implementation process itself (e.g. the extent to which the programme was consistently delivered as designed across settings and geographic locales, in terms of content, "dose" and duration).

Process indicators are proximal measures that provide evidence that the implementing steps of risk minimisation measures occurred; and in turn, provide insight into whether the predicted impacts of these processes on safe use behaviour and health outcomes actually occurred or not (European Medicines Agency and Heads of Medicines Agencies 2015b).

Examples of distal measures, or long-term effectiveness, include measures of sustained implementation fidelity, knowledge retention and institutionalisation of safe use behaviours. Whether safety outcomes are a proximal or distal measure will largely depend upon whether the risk manifests quickly or through sustained use. Outcomes may include both intended outcomes (e.g. reduction in inappropriate prescribing) or unintended outcomes (e.g. barriers to patient access).

Best practices in D&I science also include evaluating the cost of implementation, at the healthcare system, healthcare professional and patient level in terms of time and absolute resources required including start-up investment and sustaining costs of risk minimisation activities (Ritzwoller et al. 2009). This is one means by which healthcare burden can be assessed and the relative cost effectiveness of risk minimisation interventions can be compared.

13.2.3.3 Select Study Design and Study Population

The selection of study design flows naturally from the additional risk measures that need to be assessed and the feasibility of assessing those measures. Common methods for evaluating risk communication and the adoption of minimisation measures include:

- *Healthcare audits* to track compliance with dispensing and counselling processes (Smith et al. 2017);
- *Surveys* to assess knowledge, attitudes and self-reported safe use behaviours among patients, physicians and other healthcare professionals (Brewer et al. 2019; Knox et al. 2015; Morrato et al. 2016). The US FDA has recently issued guidance to industry on best practices for survey methodology in the context of risk minimisation programmes (Center for Drug Evaluation and Research and Center for Biologics Evaluation and Research 2019b);
- *Pharmacoepidemiological studies like retrospective cohort studies, medical chart and health records reviews* and *drug utilisation studies* to assess observed safe use behaviours, including appropriate prescribing and monitoring (Alrwisan et al. 2019; Bian et al. 2017; Morrato et al. 2008); and
- *Patient registries* and *adverse event reporting systems* to prospectively evaluate observed safe use behaviours and their relationship with health outcomes (McGettigan et al. 2019; Tkachenko et al. 2019).

Mixed methods research has received increasing attention over the past decade in dissemination and implementation research given its ability to provide a more complete understanding (both in terms of breadth and depth) of the translation of health evidence into clinical practice and policy (Green et al. 2015. Mixed methods are defined as the integration of qualitative, e.g. key informant interviews and focus groups, and quantitative approaches into a single programme of evaluation research.

Methodologically rigorous qualitative assessment can be integrated with quantitative data in several ways: by merging data during the analytic phase; by connecting disparate quantitative and qualitative findings to inform one another and by embedding qualitative assessment as a sub-study within a quantitative study (Albright et al. 2013). Mixed methods are well suited for evaluating the health impact of medicinal risk minimisation interventions given their complexity as they enable researchers to triangulate findings from multiple data sources, and to evaluate heterogeneity of effects across settings and geographies.

The issue of external validity, i.e. the extent to which the results of an evaluation can be generalised to other situations and settings, is also of importance for risk communication and risk minimisation programmes (Huebschmann et al. 2019). Pragmatic and quasi-experimental designs using real world data are increasingly being employed to achieve a balance between internal and external validity when determining the effects of health policies (Handley et al. 2018).

13.3 Utility of Applied Methods for Researching Medicinal Product Risk Communication

To illustrate the application of D&I research methods, this section discusses a real world case study of a risk minimisation programme that was mandated in the EU for valproate.

13.3.1 Case Study on Applying a D&I Research Approach to Risk Minimisation and Communication for Valproate in the European Union

Valproate-containing medicinal products have been authorised in the EU since 1967 and are indicated for the treatment of epilepsy, and in some countries, for bipolar disorder and migraine headaches as well. Valproate is also a known teratogen, and the product label carries a warning to this effect. For some patients, however, valproate is the most effective treatment option. As a result, prior to taking valproate, women of child-bearing potential should be fully informed of the benefit-risk trade-offs involved in using the product. In 2014, in response to the publication of new data on the risks to children of valproate exposure in utero, the Pharmacovigilance Risk Assessment Committee (PRAC) of the European Medicines Agency (EMA) required that additional risk minimisation measures be implemented for valproate products in addition to an updated warning in the product information regarding use during pregnancy (European Medicines Agency 2014). In 2017, the PRAC started a new assessment procedure and convened a public hearing on risk communication and risk minimisation of valproate products (European Medicines Agency and Heads of Medicines Agencies 2017d). The public hearing yielded key insights regarding the dissemination and sustainability of the 2014 valproate risk minimisation programme across EU member states based on evaluations using various research designs. In 2018, the PRAC recommended further expanding risk minimisation measures to avoid valproate exposure in pregnancy. This decision was taken after examining the available epidemiologic evidence, consulting with healthcare professionals and patients, including women and their children who have been affected by valproate use during pregnancy, through extensive stakeholder engagement mechanisms, most prominently via the public hearing (European Medicines Agency and Heads of Medicines Agencies 2018a).

In the following case study, scientific considerations and reflection are presented for valproate risk minimisation and communication in light of evolving regulatory requirements in the EU. The discussion is organised in three parts relating to D&I research methods for designing for dissemination, implementation and evaluation. At each step, we highlight opportunities where the application of D&I methods could add further value to the risk minimisation programme.

13.3.1.1 Designing for Dissemination Considerations

1. Goals and objectives:

The overarching safety goal for valproate has been consistent between the 2014 and 2018 programmes—to avoid foetal exposure because of the increased risk of ensuing malformations and developmental problems post-birth. For female patients of child-bearing potential, the risk minimisation recommendation was not to use valproate unless pregnancy prevention requirements were met. This recommendation was the same whether the medicine was being used for the treatment of migraines, bipolar disorder, or epilepsy. However, for patients who had nonetheless become pregnant while on valproate, the specific risk minimisation recommendations in 2018, and the associated behavioural objectives, varied somewhat by indication. For migraines or bipolar disorder, it was required that valproate would not be used during pregnancy at all; whereas for epilepsy it was recognised that some women for whom valproate was the only effective treatment might need to continue valproate (with appropriate specialist care) during pregnancy.

D&I opportunity: Variations in recommendations across different indications and clinical care scenarios make risk communication more complex, and D&I approaches have specifically been developed to address complexity.

2. Situational context:

Several of the most critical contextual challenges faced in disseminating the valproate risk minimisation programme, at both times, are highlighted below (Smith and Raynor in press).

Implementation across diverse EU member states: The valproate risk minimisation programme was required to be implemented across 28 member states in the EU. Each country differed in terms of key factors affecting programme uptake: the healthcare delivery system, physician prescribing patterns, language, culture and local legal requirements affecting the practice of medicine. Effective implementation should thus entail an understanding of the barriers and facilitators to programme adoption unique to each country, and the development of strategies to address each accordingly.

Implementation across different socioecological levels: Within each country, implementation of the valproate risk minimisation programme involved multiple different socioecological levels—ranging from the pharmaceutical companies' affiliate offices down to local healthcare delivery settings (hospital, out-patient, etc.), prescribers and other healthcare professionals, and finally, to the patients themselves.

Multiple target audiences: Given the range of indicated usages for the medicine, risk communication information needed to be delivered to a range of audiences, including different types of healthcare professionals (e.g. general practitioners, specialists, nurses, midwives, pharmacists) as well as patients and their parents, in the case of paediatric patients. Moreover, the valproate patient population itself was heterogeneous in terms of medical condition being treated, sex, age and relationship status.

D&I opportunity: As a result of the heterogenicity of the target audiences, different messages and delivery modalities should be considered in order to more effectively reach different subgroups through risk communication.

3. Clinical care gaps:

The potential points for clinical care gaps were numerous given the fact that valproate treatment occurs over an extended period or even lifetime and requires

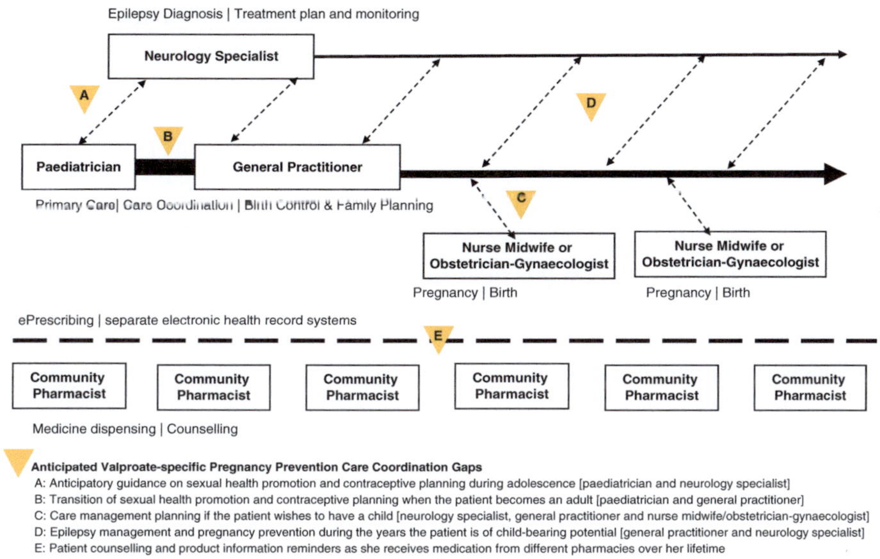

Fig. 13.4 Patient life course diagram for a female diagnosed with epilepsy in childhood and anticipated valproate risk minimisation care gaps

risk minimisation coordination at multiple time points between general practitioners, specialists, nurses, midwives and pharmacists.

D&I opportunity: A map of the clinical care journey of valproate patients can support the risk minimisation programme designing. Figure 13.4 shows one such patient pathway diagram for the treatment course of a female patient with epilepsy initiating valproate therapy as an adolescent. The visualisation of this patient pathway underscores the importance of both sustaining continuity in risk messaging over time and of integrating risk minimisation behaviours into routine care across multiple settings and with multiple healthcare professionals.

4. Minimisation strategies:

The risk minimisation strategies evolved between 2014 and 2018 as communication shifted from focusing on risk knowledge and attitude communication goals to encompassing specific behaviour goals.

2014 risk minimisation strategies:

Communication materials addressing risk knowledge goals included a patient booklet on the risks of valproate, especially when taken when a woman was pregnant, and a prescriber guide emphasising the teratogenic risk of valproate and the need to counsel women of child-bearing potential. In addition, a direct healthcare professional communication (DHPC) letter was designed to inform healthcare professionals of the risk of teratogenicity associated with valproate use and changes to the product information and conditions of use. With regard to influencing attitudes about appropriate use of valproate, an acknowledgement of risk form for prescribers to share with female patients following counselling was proposed.

2018 expanded risk minimisation strategies:

The revised risk minimisation strategies for valproate introduced in 2018 placed greater emphasis on behaviour-focussed communication goals. The pregnancy prevention programme aimed to ensure several behavioural steps had taken place to address potential care gaps, including:

- Assessing patients for the potential of becoming pregnant and involving the patient in evaluating her individual circumstances and supporting informed decision-making;
- Conducting pregnancy tests before starting and during treatment as needed;
- Counselling patients about the risks of valproate treatment;
- Explaining the need for effective contraception throughout treatment;
- Carrying out reviews of treatment by a specialist at least annually;
- Completing a risk acknowledgement form that patients and prescribers will go through at each such review to confirm that appropriate advice has been given and understood;
- Updating product information (package leaflet for patients and SmPC for healthcare professionals) to reflect the new guidance and including a visual warning in the form of boxed text which may be accompanied by other elements such as a symbol;
- Providing educational materials in the form of guides for patients and physicians to provide age-appropriate advice; and
- Including a patient alert card attached to the packaging so that pharmacists can counsel patients when the medicine is dispensed.

D&I opportunity: The implementation of these communication goals could be strengthened further through the application of relevant social science models or frameworks. In the case of the valproate risk minimisation programme, a determinant model such as the Dissemination of Evidence-Based Policy (DEBP) framework might be especially applicable. DEBP specifies domains and strategies for identifying and addressing programme barriers at multiple socioecological levels (e.g. at the level of the patient, the healthcare professional, the healthcare delivery setting, the local health authority and at the regional health authority level). Social marketing techniques can also be used to assess ways to strengthen and expand the programme's dissemination (Harris et al. 2012). Similarly, to improve uptake and impact of the risk communication messages, segmentation methods could be applied to identify key subgroups within the target audiences for whom messages and distribution modalities required specific tailoring.

5. Communication materials:

As the ultimate approval of the additional risk communication materials rested with the national health authority within each EU country, there was latitude for tailoring these materials (including translation in the local language(s)) for local needs. As an example, following the 2014 EU regulatory decision, the Medicines and

Healthcare Products Regulatory Agency (MHRA) in the United Kingdom (UK), developed a valproate toolkit based on input from patients and healthcare professionals and formal user testing. Aside from the toolkit developed by the MHRA, which received a lot of appreciation by stakeholders at the hearing, public testimony revealed that there had been a lack of involvement of healthcare professionals and valproate patients in the development of other risk communication materials. Similarly, tailoring of the risk communication messages to address unique concerns or considerations of specific segments of the valproate patient population (e.g. pre-pubescent girls, adolescent females, married women who were seeking to become pregnant) appears to have been lacking as well. To address the need for sustained risk messaging, communication materials were strengthened by the 2018 regulatory decision to include recommendations that the outer packaging of all valproate-containing products carry a visual warning about the risks in pregnancy. In addition to boxed text, this might include a symbol/pictogram, with the details to be adapted within each country. In addition, a patient reminder card should be attached to the outer package for pharmacists to discuss with the patient each time the medicine is dispensed.

D&I opportunity: Diffusion theory suggests that interventions which offer relative advantage to the end user, are easy to use, and have "trialability" are more likely to be adopted than those which do not (Dearing and Cox 2018). One way to ensure that interventions possess these characteristics is to involve end-users (including an array of different healthcare professionals and patients) in the development and testing of the risk communication messages, tools and overall programme design. Another tactic to support the adoption of safe use behaviors is to actively engage with local opinion leaders who, in the capacity of change agents, can advocate for and socially role model these behaviors within their professional networks.

13.3.1.2 Implementation Considerations

1. Responsibility and accountability:

In the EU, responsibility for medicinal product communication activities is fragmented. Depending on the type of marketing authorisation and safety review procedure, the EMA mandates risk communication content centrally, but national regulatory authorities approve the actual risk communication tools developed by the pharmaceutical companies accordingly in the local language. Within each country, the pharmaceutical companies are also charged with the actual distribution of the risk communication materials as "non-promotional" (i.e. not advertising) materials. Companies must rely on healthcare professionals to distribute the materials to patients and counsel them. This multi-level communication process adds considerable complexity to programme implementation (Smith and Raynor in press). For example, at the companies' country affiliate office level, staff were responsible for translating the risk communication materials, submitting them to the national regulatory authority for approval, training sales and medical liaison representatives to deliver the materials and overseeing the production, stocking and updating of the materials. At the country-level, multiple professional societies also needed to be engaged to develop and disseminate joint consensus statements and coordinated risk messaging. At the practice level, prescribers and other healthcare professionals needed to receive the materials, read them, inform patients regarding the key risk messages and counsel them regarding the benefit-risk trade-offs associated with taking valproate.

2. Quality assurance and quality control processes and procedures:

During the 2017 valproate public hearing, the UK Epilepsy Society testified that little to no provisions appeared to have been established for ongoing monitoring of programme implementation after the 2014 recommendations and for sharing feedback regarding programme impact in "real time" (European Medicines Agency and Heads of Medicines Agencies 2018b).

D&I opportunity: Based on best practices in D&I science, guidance and technical assistance for programme implementation monitoring and evaluation should be incorporated into risk minimisation planning, particularly at the level of the healthcare professional and healthcare setting. Examples of such guidance and support can be seen in the successful use of public health detailing teams which visit different community healthcare centres to introduce and reinforce evidence-based preventive care measures (Brownson et al. 2018). In addition, those responsible for programme implementation typically have multiple (sometimes competing) professional duties and responsibilities over and above the implementation of a risk minimisation programme. Relatedly, many lack expertise in programme implementation, and have few, if any, dedicated resources to assist them in this regard. For change to occur, knowledge, skills and expertise in programme implementation practices are crucial. Establishing "communities of practice" forums are one way to provide a structured venue for engaging implementers, exchanging best practices and discussing successful (or non-successful) implementation strategies and tactics.

3. Adaptations and modifications:

Notably, few provisions were established to document and evaluate adaptations and modifications of the programme across countries.

D&I opportunity: Best practices in dissemination science would recommend adaptations be systematically reviewed and compared against health outcome measures within each country in order to advance knowledge on which risk minimisation strategies are most effective (Chambers and Norton 2016).

13.3.1.3 Evaluation Considerations

Patient and healthcare professional testimony provided during the 2017 valproate public hearing yielded rich information regarding the dissemination of the valproate risk communication and minimisation measures across the EU, and the impact of such measure on the targeted outcomes. Using the lens of D&I science, one can view the testimony as providing insight into the causal pathway affecting dissemination of valproate risk information and knowledge transfer, the adoption of risk minimisation behaviours and ultimately the incidence of exposed pregnancies and birth defects. Key themes that emerged included the following:

- *Limited dissemination of risk information to healthcare professionals:*
  As highlighted in several testimonials at the public hearing, many healthcare professionals had low awareness of their role in counselling patients about the teratogenic risks of valproate and in distributing the risk communication materials. Examples cited included physicians working in hospital settings in Paris and general practitioners prescribing valproate in the UK (European Medicines Agency and Heads of Medicines Agencies 2018b). This low awareness may have been due to limited distribution of the risk communication materials themselves to healthcare professionals. To that point, a representative of the Pharmaceutical Group of the European Union (PGEU) representing community pharmacists also testified that many UK pharmacies had never received the valproate patient cards.
- *Limited distribution of valproate risk information materials and messages to the target patient populations:*
  Evidence from survey research and patient testimonials indicated that many patients had not received the valproate risk communication materials. In the UK, a 2017 survey of 2000 females diagnosed with epilepsy under the age of 50 showed that of the 475 respondents who were currently taking the medicine, 68% stated that they had not received the new valproate toolkit. While a majority (86%) of females using valproate reported having seen their prescriber within the past year, 27% stated that they had received no information about risks of foetal exposure (European Medicines Agency and Heads of Medicines Agencies 2018b). Other patients, both within the UK and elsewhere in the EU, gave similar testimonials.
- *Birth defect rates:*
  In a study presented by French health authorities, valproate use was estimated to be responsible for severe malformations in up to 4100 children in France since the medicine was first marketed in the country 50 years ago (BBC News 2017). However, a registry-based multi-centre study involving 15 countries reported that the prevalence of valproate congenital anomalies in Europe has actually decreased over the past decade from 0.22 per 10,000 births in 2005/6 to 0.03 per 10,000 births in 2013/14 (Morris et al. 2018). This decline may be due to effects of risk minimisation efforts and/or other temporal trends.
- *Future evaluation:*
  In its most recent review of 2018, the PRAC recommended that the companies marketing these medicines carry out additional studies to further characterise the nature and extent of the risks posed by valproate and to monitor ongoing valproate use and the long-term effects on affected pregnancies.

D&I opportunity: D&I science recommends that evaluators also evaluate the causal pathway from message delivery to health outcomes in order to diagnose and improve the risk communication and minimisation process. Questions to investigate might include: Did clinicians adopt counselling and testing recommendations? What proportion of female patients of child-bearing potential actually received the counselling? How consistently were recommended packaging and pharmacy dispensing interventions implemented across different EU member states? How effective were the risk communication and materials in changing knowledge, attitudes and behaviours among patients and healthcare professionals? What evidence is there that medical practice guidelines were changed by each of the affecting medical professions for each country such that risk minimisation recommendations might be maintained?

13.4 Outlook: Relevance, Improvements and Future Potential

D&I science offers an important contribution to multidisciplinary research in medicinal product communication (see Chap. 1) and risk minimisation, and to the pragmatic application of these interventions in the real world context. Specifically, it provides strategies, tools and tactics to facilitate the effective implementation and uptake of risk communication messages and risk minimisation activities, and to support their continued delivery over time.

As illustrated in the valproate case study, risk minimisation programmes are complex interventions that feature multiple components, target multiple audiences and must be implemented in diverse geographies and healthcare settings. As a result, their success is contingent on robust implementation and dissemination efforts. Ultimately, incorporating approaches from D&I science can enhance the quality of intervention implementation and dissemination, and highlight contextual factors that may produce variation in programme outcomes, thereby advancing knowledge in the field and improving the effectiveness of future such programmes to support safe and appropriate use of medicinal products.

Conclusions

- Health dissemination and implementation (D&I) is the active and targeted distribution of information and intervention materials to a specific public health, healthcare professional or patient audience with the goal of transferring knowledge and/or promoting changes in health-related attitudes and behaviours. D&I science can be applied to tackle the challenges of medicinal product risk minimisation and communication and inform intervention design, implementation and evaluation planning.
- Steps for designing for dissemination include identification of risk minimisation goals and objects, analysis of the situational context, identification of anticipated care gaps, selection of appropriate risk minimisation strategies and the development of communication materials and tools.
- Steps for implementation planning include identification of organisations and individuals who will be the dissemination and implementation agents, establishment of quality assurance and quality control policies and procedures and determining plans for documenting adaptations and modifications to the programme over time and across geographies.

- Steps for evaluation planning include specification of success metrics and hypotheses, identification of primary and secondary measures to assess implementation processes, risk knowledge and comprehension, safe use behaviour and health outcomes, and selection of study design and populations.
- The case example of valproate risk minimisation in the European Union illustrates implementation and dissemination complexities for medicinal products. Research approaches from D&I science can be applied to support interventions that improve the adoption and maintenance of safe and appropriate use of medicinal products.

References

Agency for Healthcare Research and Quality. Health Literacy Measurement Tools (Revised) [updated February 2016]. Available from: https://www.ahrq.gov/health-literacy/quality-resources/tools/literacy/index.html

Albright K, Gechter K, Kempe A (2013) Importance of mixed methods in pragmatic trials and dissemination and implementation research. Acad Pediatr 13(5):400–407

Alrwisan AA, Wei YJ, Brumback BA, Antonelli PJ, Winterstein AG (2019) Concomitant use of quinolones and stimulants and the risk of adverse cardiovascular symptoms: a retrospective cohort study. Pharmacotherapy

Ancker JS, Senathirajah Y, Kukafka R, Starren JB (2006) Design features of graphs in health risk communication: a systematic review. J Am Med Inform Assoc 13(6):608–618

ASQ (2015) ASQ/ANSI/ISO 9000:2015: quality management systems - fundamentals and vocabulary. American Society for Quality, Milwaukee

BBC News (2017) New evidence in France of harm from epilepsy drug valproate. April 20, 2017

Bian J, Chen B, Hershman DL, Marks N, Norris L, Schulz R et al (2017) Effects of the US food and drug administration boxed warning of erythropoietin-stimulating agents on utilization and adverse outcome. J Clin Oncol 35(17):1945–1951

Birken SA, Powell BJ, Presseau J, Kirk MA, Lorencatto F, Gould NJ et al (2017) Combined use of the Consolidated Framework for Implementation Research (CFIR) and the Theoretical Domains Framework (TDF): a systematic review. Implement Sci 12(1):2

Brewer NT (2011) Goals. In: Fischoff B, Brewer NT, Downs JS (eds) Communicating risks and benefits: an evidence-based user's guide. Food and Drug Administration, U.S. Department of Health and Human Services, Silver Spring, pp 3–10

Brewer SE, Campagna EJ, Morrato EH (2019) Advancing regulatory science and assessment of FDA REMS programs: a mixed-methods evaluation examining physician survey response. J Clin Transl Sci 3(4):199–209

Brown P, Bahri P (2019) 'Engagement' of patients and healthcare professionals in regulatory pharmacovigilance: establishing a conceptual and methodological framework. Eur J Clin Pharmacol 75(9):1181–1192

Brownson RC, Jacobs JA, Tabak RG, Hoehner CM, Stamatakis KA (2013) Designing for dissemination among public health researchers: findings from a national survey in the United States. Am J Public Health 103(9):1693–1699

Brownson RC, Colditz GA, Proctor EK (eds) (2017) Dissemination and implementation research in health: translating science to practice, 2nd edn. Oxford University Press, New York

Brownson RC, Fielding JE, Green LW (2018) Building capacity for evidence-based public health: reconciling the pulls of practice and the push of research. Annu Rev Public Health 39:27–53

Center for Drug Evaluation and Research, Center for Biologics Evaluation and Research (2011) In: US Department of Health and Human Services (ed) Guidance medication guides DOUBLEHYPHEN distribution requirements and inclusion in Risk Evaluation and Mitigation Strategies (REMS)

Center for Drug Evaluation and Research, Center for Biologics Evaluation and Research (2019a) In: US Department of Health and Human Services (ed) REMS assessment: planning and reporting. Guidance for industry (draft guidance). Food and Drug Administration, Silver Spring

Center for Drug Evaluation and Research, Center for Biologics Evaluation and Research (2019b) In: US Department of Health and Human Services (ed) Survey methodologies to assess REMS goals that relate to knowledge. Guidance to industry (draft guidance)

Centers for Disease Control and Prevention (2018) Writing smart objectives. Available from: https://www.cdc.gov/healthyyouth/evaluation/pdf/brief3b.pdf

Chambers DA (2019) Sharpening our focus on designing for dissemination: lessons from the SPRINT program and potential next steps for the field. Transl Behav Med

Chambers DA, Norton WE (2016) The adaptome: advancing the science of intervention adaptation. Am J Prev Med 51(4 Suppl 2):S124–S131

Chan HW, Russell AM, Smith MY (2018) What is the quality of drug safety information for patients: an analysis of REMS educational materials. Pharmacoepidemiol Drug Saf 27(9): 969–978

Committee on Risk Perception and Communication (1989) Improving risk communication. The National Academies Press, Washington, D.C.

Damschroder LJ, Aron DC, Keith RE, Kirsh SR, Alexander JA, Lowery JC (2009) Fostering implementation of health services research findings into practice: a consolidated framework for advancing implementation science. Implement Sci 4:50

Dearing JW, Cox JG (2018) Diffusion of innovations theory, principles, and practice. Health Aff (Millwood) 37(2):183–190

Dearing JW, Smith DK, Larson RS, Estabrooks CA (2013) Designing for diffusion of a biomedical intervention. Am J Prev Med 44(1 Suppl 2):S70–S76

European Medicines Agency. PRAC recommends strengthening the restrictions on the use of valproate in women and girls [press release]. October 10, 2014

European Medicines Agency and Heads of Medicines Agencies (2015a) Guideline on Good Pharmacovigilance Practices (GVP) Module XVI Addendum I - educational materials

European Medicines Agency and Heads of Medicines Agencies (2015b) Guideline on Good Pharmacovigilance Practices (GVP) Module XVI - risk minimisation measures: selection of tools and effectiveness indicators (Rev 2)

European Medicines Agency and Heads of Medicines Agencies (2017a) Guideline on Good Pharmacovigilance Practices (GVP) Module V - risk management systems (Rev 2)

European Medicines Agency and Heads of Medicines Agencies (2017b) Guideline on Good Pharmacovigilance Practices (GVP) Module XV - safety communication (Rev 1)

European Medicines Agency and Heads of Medicines Agencies (2017c) Guideline on Good Pharmacovigilance Practices (GVP) Annex I - definitions (Rev 4)

European Medicines Agency and Heads of Medicines Agencies (2017d) Summary of the EMA public hearing on valproate in pregnancy

European Medicines Agency and Heads of Medicines Agencies (2018a) New measures to avoid valproate exposure in pregnancy endorsed. Member State representatives agree new restrictions and pregnancy prevention programme

European Medicines Agency and Heads of Medicines Agencies (2018b) Public hearing on valproate: written interventions

Field TS, Cadoret CA, Brown ML, Ford M, Greene SM, Hill D et al (2002) Surveying physicians: do components of the "Total Design Approach" to optimizing survey response rates apply to physicians? Med Care 40(7):596–605

Fischoff B, Brewer NT, Downs JS (eds) (2011) Communicating risks and benefits: an evidence-based user's guide. Food and Drug Administration, U.S. Department of Health and Human Services, Silver Spring

Gellad ZF, Day TE (2016) What is value stream mapping, and how can it help my practice? Am J Gastroenterol 111(4):447–448
Glasgow RE, Chambers D (2012) Developing robust, sustainable, implementation systems using rigorous, rapid and relevant science. Clin Transl Sci 5(1):48–55
Glasgow RE, Vinson C, Chambers D, Khoury MJ, Kaplan RM, Hunter C (2012) National Institutes of Health approaches to dissemination and implementation science: current and future directions. Am J Public Health 102(7):1274–1281
Glasgow RE, Harden SM, Gaglio B, Rabin B, Smith ML, Porter GC et al (2019) RE-AIM planning and evaluation framework: adapting to new science and practice with a 20-year review. Front Public Health 7:64
Glasziou P, Haynes B (2005) The paths from research to improved health outcomes. ACP J Club 142(2):A8–A10
Green L, Kreuter M (2005) Health program planning: an educational and ecological approach, 4th edn. McGraw Hill, New York
Green LW, Ottoson JM, Garcia C, Hiatt RA (2009) Diffusion theory and knowledge dissemination, utilization, and integration in public health. Annu Rev Public Health 30:151–174
Green CA, Duan N, Gibbons RD, Hoagwood KE, Palinkas LA, Wisdom JP (2015) Approaches to mixed methods dissemination and implementation research: methods, strengths, caveats, and opportunities. Adm Policy Ment Health 42(5):508–523
Handley MA, Lyles CR, McCulloch C, Cattamanchi A (2018) Selecting and improving quasi-experimental designs in effectiveness and implementation research. Annu Rev Public Health 39:5–25
Harel Z, Silver SA, McQuillan RF, Weizman AV, Thomas A, Chertow GM et al (2016) How to diagnose solutions to a quality of care problem. Clin J Am Soc Nephrol 11(5):901–907
Harris JR, Cheadle A, Hannon PA, Forehand M, Lichiello P, Mahoney E et al (2012) A framework for disseminating evidence-based health promotion practices. Prev Chronic Dis 9:E22
Ho K, Peter Wall Workshop P (2014) Harnessing the social web for health and wellness: issues for research and knowledge translation. J Med Internet Res 16(2):e34
Huebschmann AG, Leavitt IM, Glasgow RE (2019) Making health research matter: a call to increase attention to external validity. Annu Rev Public Health 40:45–63
Institute of Medicine Committee on Quality of Health Care in America (2001) Crossing the quality chasm: a new health system for the 21st century. National Academies Press (US), Washington (DC)
Issen L, Woodcock T, McNicholas C, Lennox L, Reed JE (2018) Criteria for evaluating programme theory diagrams in quality improvement initiatives: a structured method for appraisal. Int J Qual Health Care 30(7):508–513
Keith RE, Crosson JC, O'Malley AS, Cromp D, Taylor EF (2017) Using the Consolidated Framework for Implementation Research (CFIR) to produce actionable findings: a rapid-cycle evaluation approach to improving implementation. Implement Sci 12(1):15
Knox C, Hampp C, Willy M, Winterstein AG, Dal Pan G (2015) Patient understanding of drug risks: an evaluation of medication guide assessments. Pharmacoepidemiol Drug Saf 24(5): 518–525
Kreuter MW, Wang ML (2015) From evidence to impact: recommendations for a dissemination support system. New Dir Child Adolesc Dev 2015(149):11–23
Leong Wai Yeen J, Salek S, Walker S (2014) Strategy for communicating benefit-risk decisions: a comparison of regulatory agencies' publicly available documents. Front Pharmacol 5:269
McGettigan P, Alonso Olmo C, Plueschke K, Castillon M, Nogueras Zondag D, Bahri P et al (2019) Patient registries: an underused resource for medicines evaluation: operational proposals for increasing the use of patient registries in regulatory assessments. Drug Saf
Morrato EH (2018) Social science theory as a framework for designing and evaluating pharmaceutical risk mitigation dissemination and implementation strategies. In: Sietsema WK, Sprafka JM (eds) Risk management principles for devices and pharmaceuticals: global perspectives on the benefit: risk assessment of medicinal products, 2nd edn. Regulatory Affairs Professional Society, Rockville

Morrato EH, Libby AM, Orton HD, Degruy FV 3rd, Brent DA, Allen R et al (2008) Frequency of provider contact after FDA advisory on risk of pediatric suicidality with SSRIs. Am J Psychiatry 165(1):42–50

Morrato EH, Brewer SE, Campagna EJ, Dickinson LM, Thomas DS, Druss BG et al (2016) Glucose testing for adults receiving Medicaid and antipsychotics: a population-based prescriber survey on behaviors, attitudes, and barriers. Psychiatr Serv 67(7):798–802

Morris JK, Garne E, Loane M, Addor MC, Barisic I, Bianchi F et al (2018) Prevalence of valproate syndrome in Europe from 2005 to 2014: a registry based multi-centre study. Eur J Med Genet 61(9):479–482

Muhlbacher AC, Juhnke C, Beyer AR, Garner S (2016) Patient-focused benefit-risk analysis to inform regulatory decisions: the European Union perspective. Value Health 19(6):734–740

Nilsen P (2015) Making sense of implementation theories, models and frameworks. Implement Sci 10(1)

Nilsen P, Bernhardsson S (2019) Context matters in implementation science: a scoping review of determinant frameworks that describe contextual determinants for implementation outcomes. BMC Health Serv Res 19(1):189

Office of the Associate Director for Communications (2016) In: U.S. Department of Health and Human Services (ed) Everyday words for public health communication

Prieto L, Spooner A, Hidalgo-Simon A, Rubino A, Kurz X, Arlett P (2012) Evaluation of the effectiveness of risk minimization measures. Pharmacoepidemiol Drug Saf 21(8):896–899

Proctor EK, Powell BJ, Baumann AA, Hamilton AM, Santens RL (2012) Writing implementation research grant proposals: ten key ingredients. Implement Sci 7(1):96

Rabin BA, Brownson RC (2017) Terminology for dissemination and implementation research. In: Brownson RC, Colditz GA, Proctor EK (eds) Dissemination and implementation research in health: translating science to practice, 2nd edn. Oxford University Press, New York, pp 19–45

Radawski C, Morrato E, Hornbuckle K, Bahri P, Smith M, Juhaeri J et al (2015) Benefit-Risk Assessment, Communication, and Evaluation (BRACE) throughout the life cycle of therapeutic products: overall perspective and role of the pharmacoepidemiologist. Pharmacoepidemiol Drug Saf 24(12):1233–1240

Ramsey AT, Proctor EK, Chambers DA, Garbutt JM, Malone S, Powderly WG et al (2019) Designing for Accelerated Translation (DART) of emerging innovations in health. J Clin Transl Sci 3(2–3):53–58

Reed JE, McNicholas C, Woodcock T, Issen L, Bell D (2014) Designing quality improvement initiatives: the action effect method, a structured approach to identifying and articulating programme theory. BMJ Qual Saf 23(12):1040–1048

Ritzwoller DP, Sukhanova A, Gaglio B, Glasgow RE (2009) Costing behavioral interventions: a practical guide to enhance translation. Ann Behav Med 37(2):218–227

Rosstad T, Garasen H, Steinsbekk A, Haland E, Kristoffersen L, Grimsmo A (2015) Implementing a care pathway for elderly patients, a comparative qualitative process evaluation in primary care. BMC Health Serv Res 15:86

Shelton RC, Cooper BR, Stirman SW (2018) The sustainability of evidence-based interventions and practices in public health and health care. Annu Rev Public Health 39:55–76

Smith MY, Raynor DKT. Improving the effectiveness of drug safety measures in the EU: the public hearing on valproate. BMC Health Serv Res (in press)

Smith MY, Morrato EH (2014) Advancing the field of pharmaceutical risk minimization through application of implementation science best practices. Drug Saf 37(8):569–580

Smith ZR, Makowski CT, MacDonald NC (2017) Inpatient pharmacy experience with an audit for a risk evaluation and mitigation strategy for riociguat. Am J Health Syst Pharm 74(21):1762–1763

Smith MY, Russell A, Bahri P, Mol PGM, Frise S, Freeman E et al (2018) The RIMES Statement: a checklist to assess the quality of studies evaluating risk minimization programs for medicinal products. Drug Saf 41(4):389–401

Tabak RG, Khoong EC, Chambers DA, Brownson RC (2012) Bridging research and practice: models for dissemination and implementation research. Am J Prev Med 43(3):337–350

Tkachenko E, Singer S, Sharma P, Barbieri J, Mostaghimi A (2019) US food and drug administration reports of pregnancy and pregnancy-related adverse events associated with isotretinoin. JAMA Dermatol

Trevena LJ, Zikmund-Fisher BJ, Edwards A, Gaissmaier W, Galesic M, Han PKJ et al (2013) Presenting quantitative information about decision outcomes: a risk communication primer for patient decision aid developers. BMC Med Inform Decis Mak 13(S2)

Westfall JM, Zittleman L, Felzien M, Norman N, Tamez M, Backlund-Jarquin P et al (2016) Reinventing the wheel of medical evidence: how the boot camp translation process is making gains. Health Aff (Millwood) 35(4):613–618

Willy ME, Graham DJ, Racoosin JA, Gill R, Kropp GF, Young J et al (2014) Candidate metrics for evaluating the impact of prescriber education on the safe use of extended-release/long-acting (ER/LA) opioid analgesics. Pain Med 15(9):1558–1568

Wiltsey Stirman S, Baumann AA, Miller CJ (2019) The FRAME: an expanded framework for reporting adaptations and modifications to evidence-based interventions. Implement Sci 14(1):58

Pharmacoepidemiology 14

Hubert G. Leufkens

Abstract

Pharmacoepidemiology is the study of the use of medicines in populations and their use as determinants of health. As such pharmacoepidemiological research is also subject to medicinal product risk communication and also provides methods for investigating the impact of communication—whether from official bodies, in the media or in healthcare—on the use of medicines and its health outcomes. The results of such evaluations constitute major evidence for planning and improving product information, communication components of risk minimisation measures and other actions of regulatory bodies and healthcare systems alike. As such pharmacoepidemiology has been called the fundamental science of medicines safety in patient care and is also seen as a corner stone of regulatory science and decision-making. This chapter reviews appropriateness and potential of pharmacoepidemiological research methods for the purpose of medicinal product risk communication research.

H. G. Leufkens (✉)
Utrecht Institute for Pharmaceutical Sciences, Utrecht, Netherlands
e-mail: h.g.m.leufkens@uu.nl

© Springer Nature Singapore Pte Ltd. 2020

P. Bahri (ed.), *Communicating about Risks and Safe Use of Medicines*,
https://doi.org/10.1007/978-981-15-3013-5_14

14.1 The Discipline of Pharmacoepidemiology: Scope, Theories and Principles

14.1.1 Considering Why Pharmacoepidemiology Is Important

Pharmacoepidemiology is the study of the use and effects of medicines in large numbers of people, not always necessarily patients. The discipline has its roots in pharmacology, clinical pharmacology and epidemiology (Evans 2012; Lapeyre-Mestre et al. 2013). But today we see also a need for more alignment with the humanities, ethics and behavioural science in order to elucidate, understand and intervene in medicine exposure-outcome associations and related communication. Pharmacoepidemiology is population-based and quantitative in nature (Evans 2012; Wettermark 2013). Medicine exposure-outcome associations are characterised by quantitative measurements of both exposure and the outcome of interest with the aim to give an estimate of the likelihood of a causal association, if present. The field of pharmacoepidemiology emerged partly as a response to the notion that randomised clinical trials—very much accepted and appreciated as the gold standard to determine causal effects of medicines—have their limitations regarding picking up rare safety concerns and reflecting the real world of medicines usage. As in the early days pharmacoepidemiology mainly addressed adverse effects of medicines, the data access and methodological advances in later years also opened windows for studying intended beneficial effects at both patient and public health levels; not without fierce controversy and debate though on the risk of various types of bias and confounding, possibly affecting the conduct and interpretation of non-randomised comparisons (Lapeyre-Mestre et al. 2013; Kurz and Perez-Gutthann 2018). More on this later in this chapter.

Over the years, however, sophistication of methods to prevent or adjust for bias and confounding have paved the way for better robust evidence generation on medicines-induced effects, both adverse and beneficial. But the essentials have been almost the same over the years. Given exposure to a medicine, or a combination of medicines, and the occurrence of an outcome, clinical or otherwise, the question is whether this medicine exposure-outcome occurrence is the result of chance or whether a causal association drives what we see. A classic example: in users of one or more products (e.g. naproxen, ibuprofen, diclofenac) from the class of the non-steroidal anti-inflammatory drugs (NSAIDs) we see an increased incidence of gastropathy, i.e. ulcers and bleeding. There is overwhelming evidence that this observation is due to a causal association between the exposure and the outcome. There has been not only statistical justification for this association, but also clinical, pharmacological and mechanistic (Bakhriansyah et al. 2017; Carson et al. 1987).

14.1.2 Going Back into the History of Pharmacoepidemiology

The history of pharmacoepidemiology—the field started to evolve about 50 years ago—has been always marinated with controversy and debate, e.g. about the limitations of the data, the methods used, the interpretation of the findings and more importantly, about what to do with the results in a clinical or regulatory context (Kurz and Perez-Gutthann 2018; Klungel et al. 2016). To mention one of the early antecedents in the field, in the early 1970s the Boston Collaborative Drug Surveillance (BCDS) programme reported on identifying associations between oral contraceptives and various diseases, an intriguingly broad scope for one of the early pharmacoepidemiological studies (Boston Collaborative Drug Surveillance Programme 1973). "Associations", "commonly used" and "various" reflect the strong open surveillance nature of the BCDS in those days. The data were collected by stationed nurses and "stored on magnetic tape". Given the limited technical possibilities and resources of the BCDS, the landmark contributions to a better understanding of what medicines do in large populations have been impressive. The study confirmed earlier data of the risk of oral contraceptive-induced venous thromboembolism (VTE). Among patients with VTE, about three out of four used oral contraceptives, in the controls this was one out of five. The age-standardised relative risk was 11 (95% CI 5.2–25). Oral contraceptive-induced VTE, particularly the differential risk between the "third" and "second" generation oral contraceptives, the role of different progestins and other risk factors became later one of the most heavily debated controversies in pharmacoepidemiology and a major challenge for risk communication (Herings et al. 1999; Vandenbroucke et al. 2001) (see Chaps. 1 and 2). But this early BCDS study already highlighted virtually all of the pertinent critical issues in almost every pharmacoepidemiological study, e.g. hazard of risk over time, proper ascertainment of exposure and outcome as well as impact of dose, duration of use, (previous) use of other medicines, underlying disease and how to deal with various biases, such as referral and information bias. And not to forget, how to disseminate the results in a balanced fashion, i.e. acknowledging and weighing the possible limitations of the data and the methods, but also acknowledging the valid and relevant implications of the findings for the clinical and the regulatory space.

Convincing focus on epidemiological and statistical methods has always been important in pharmacoepidemiology (Lapeyre-Mestre et al. 2013; Wettermark 2013). But without understanding the molecular basis of effects of medicines, both beneficial and adverse, statistical medicine exposure-outcome associations become rather disconnected from the real problems and challenges of learning about effects of medicines. This has been particularly become visible in the 1990s when the use of automated databases emerged. The power of such automated databases for pharmacoepidemiology has been immense. Without these databases, the science of pharmacoepidemiology would probably still be in its infancy. Getting timely and reliable answers is essential for prescribers, regulators, industry and patients, particularly when it comes to safety concerns. Where rare events in the past could only be studied in a case–control fashion, and virtually always in a time and resource consuming way, automated databases allow for building large cohorts and for following such pre-defined exposure groups over time, searching for the occurrence of the outcomes of interest (Van Staa et al. 2000). But these databases also brought challenges of data access, quality, governance and privacy, with inherent questions on the robustness of results and their communication to healthcare professionals, patients, industry and regulators.

14.1.3 Reflecting on the Role of Pharmacoepidemiology Today

Although pharmacoepidemiology has many academic antecedents, particularly when it comes to methodology development and validation, the field has always been connected to delivering evidence for regulatory and clinical decision-making. In addressing complex questions about differential risk of NSAIDs-induced gastropathy or oral contraceptives-induced VTE, pharmacoepidemiology has really contributed many times over the last decades to informed decision-making (Bakhriansyah et al. 2017; Vandenbroucke et al. 2001). Not always without controversy, but always with data, methods and directions on how to proceed and act. From that perspective, pharmacoepidemiology should not be seen as distinct, nor from upstream development of medicines, nor from downstream post-approval activities including pharmacovigilance and risk management plans. Over the last decades, the regulatory environment of post-approval commitments for the industry and its impact for academia has changed dramatically. In Europe, but also elsewhere in the world, getting a licence to market a medicine goes along with extensive legal obligations for the industry of monitoring, pro-active surveillance and post-approval safety (or efficacy) studies when needed (Kurz and Perez-Gutthann 2018).

These developments have changed the landscape of pharmacoepidemiology radically. Studies are required by regulatory authorities from industry or studies are done by academia, and sometimes also by regulatory or public health bodies themselves. Both industry and the regulatory authorities have to respond to the results, wherever the data come from. Studies are conducted by the various stakeholders on the same safety concern, and they may not come to the same conclusions. Many of such scenarios have been observed and they have all in common that transparency and regulatory context put high demands on communication and dialogue with specific stakeholders and the general public (Pitts et al. 2016).

Communicating about risks and safe use of medicines in the context of increasing data from pharmacoepidemiology requires balanced rules of engagement, public trust and an open mind towards dealing with the inherence uncertainties, i.e. both known and unknown unknowns. To improve dialogue at the interface between pharmacoepidemiology research and various interested audiences, we see increasingly guidance and directions from regulatory and professional associations on the why and how of communicating study results. For instance, the European Network of Centres for Pharmacoepidemiology and Pharmacovigilance (ENCePP), initiated by the European Medicines Agency (EMA), gives various types of guidance and policy advice on transparency on funding and conflicts of interest when communicating pharmacoepidemiology study results (Kurz and Perez-Gutthann 2018).

There are particular challenges for pharmacoepidemiology, and the communication of possibly found health hazards, when well-established medicines classes we know for decades and are used in large populations, e.g. medicines used against high blood pressure, such as diuretics, are at stake. This was the case when a subclass of diuretics, hydrochlorothiazides, were linked to an increased risk of skin cancer by pharmacoepidemiologists from Denmark (Pedersen et al. 2018). In the fall of 2018, the Pharmacovigilance Risk Assessment Committee (PRAC) of the EMA concluded—also taking into account other data sources—on a biologically plausible mechanism of an increased risk of non-melanoma skin cancer, particularly in those with high-dose exposures to hydrochlorothiazides (EMA 2018). Again, pharmacoepidemiology of well-established medicines revealed increased risks raising many questions on what to do with the findings. The fact that these medicines show convincing clinical benefits and are used by large populations make such findings not easy to handle in terms of regulatory and clinical decision-making. A similar case occurred not long ago when gliclazide, a sulphonylurea of first choice in many clinical guidelines across the globe for the treatment of type II diabetes, was linked to a higher risk of hypoglycaemia compared with metformin, but also with other sulphonylureas (van Dalem et al. 2016). Again, such products are widely used and implementing and communicating the results of the study would raise many questions on the overall benefit-risk balance of oral antidiabetics and some individual products in particular. But also changing a regulatory or prescribing policy (e.g. therapeutic guidelines) would be full of risks. For sure, we may expect more of this kind of studies in the future, given the increased access to automated databases, and the communication complexities are compelling (Radawski et al. 2015). All the ingredients for a heavy scientific, regulatory and clinical debate are there, i.e. low relative risks in susceptible populations of high base-line risk (e.g. patients who are older have multiple diseases and/or heavy disease burden), massive prescribing of low cost medicines with established benefits and possible differential risks between products (Giezen et al. 2008; Segec et al. 2015).

14.1.4 The Prospect of Real World Learning About Medicines

The evolution of pharmacoepidemiology over the last decades has been a summed result of advances in epidemiology, data science, clinical and molecular pharmacology, but also (legal) transitions in the regulatory space. These transitions have fuelled joined approaches like we see Europe, e.g. European Network of Centres for Pharmacoepidemiology and Pharmacovigilance (ENCePP), Pharmacoepidemiological Research on Outcomes of Therapeutics by a European ConsorTium (PROTECT), but also elsewhere in the world (e.g. United States (US), Canada, Asia, sub-Saharan Africa, just to mention a few); data platforms have been built successfully and a broad spectrum of studies on medicines safety are being conducted (Kurz and Perez-Gutthann 2018; Klungel et al. 2016). As a result, there is increasing interest in sophistication of methods, data science and statistical analysis.

Along with this, two other major developments with an impact on the future of pharmacoepidemiology should be mentioned. First, there is keen interest in "learning" about medicines effects during a product lifecycle. Decisions on medicines need both "learning" and "confirming", and both are relevant and complementary (Sheiner 1997). No "confirming" without "learning", and vice versa. Pharmacoepidemiology, very often non-experimental in terms of study design, is the science of "learning" about medicines, where randomised trials usually have the purpose to "confirm", although we see increasingly sophistic observational data that are strong robust enough to "confirm". Regulatory instruments like risk management plans (RMPs) and risk evaluation and mitigation strategies (REMS) are driving the field successfully on this notion (Potts et al. 2019). A second key development driving the direction of pharmacoepidemiology, and particularly relevant for this book on risk communication, has been the interaction and dialogue with the end-users of medicines, i.e. patients and consumers. All the examples of pharmacoepidemiological studies discussed earlier in this chapter have shown the critical role of the end-users, their uncertainties, expectations, risk perception and trust in data.

Both developments depicted here have aligned pharmacoepidemiology intensely with society dynamics and values, probably more than any other discipline of the pharmaceutical sciences or life sciences. Studying medicines effects is not purely "academic" anymore. It is about interactions with patients—Why should they believe the results of a case—control study? regulators—Can they ignore an academic study with different results than their own analysis? or industry—Are they willing to bring a medicine to the market with obvious safety concerns, claiming that a risk management system will solve this? All these questions require data and methods for real world learning, not only to complement the evidence that comes out of trials, but also to enable translation of study results and interpretation of the data study back into drug development, regulation and practice. It may be too early to evaluate the full potential of real world learning to decision-making during the lifecycle of a medicine (Skovlund et al. 2018). But more advanced methods and sophisticated data platforms will come and will add to the array of possible resources for informed decisions on the safety or benefit-risk of medicines. A key perspective will be the trade-off between internal and external validity (Evans 2012; Klungel et al. 2016). Whereas randomised comparisons are inherently strong on internal validity, they are often weak on external validity. Observational comparisons, due to their size and ability to reflect the real medical practice, are usually strong on external validity, but maybe weak on internal validity. There is no single best approach for addressing these trade-offs. It depends very much on research question, availability of data and other resources. In the field of oncology, for instance, we see increased use of blended data platforms, i.e. randomised trials, pragmatic trials and observational, non-randomised comparisons (Skovlund et al. 2018).

14.2 Research Approaches and Methods

14.2.1 Medicine Exposure-Outcome Associations

When it comes to research methods, better insight into how medicine exposure-outcome associations are shaped over time requires knowledge about the taxonomy of treatment allocation. Medicines are prescribed with a certain dose, are, for instance, dispensed as 30 tablets with directions to take these every day in the morning before breakfast and may be actually used according to these directions only during the first week and in an erratic and deliberate way the weeks after (Bergman 2006). The taxonomy of these different and highly variable scenarios of treatment allocation and actual exposure is critical to every pharmacoepidemiological study. What pharmacoepidemiologists coin as "medicine exposure" or "medicine utilisation" or "use" is the accumulated result of a non-random, often also irrational and non-scientific mixture of decisions, actions, communication and interventions to bring an individual medicinal product to a patient. The actual use of a medicine can vary in many ways, such as the medical condition and other circumstances of its use, dosing, length of use and how it is administered by or to the patient. Advances of pharmacoepidemiology have always been linked to safety issues and debates where medicine exposure and use have been critical to the elucidation and understanding of the issue at stake.

Defining a relevant medicine exposure-outcome association to be studied constitutes the basis of any pharmacoepidemiological research question, whatever study design for evaluating an exposure-outcome association is chosen (Evans 2012). Generic principles of epidemiological research have already been established for decades, and they still apply today in virtually every phase of studies in which an association, thought to be causal or not, is investigated. Pivotal principles provide, among other elements to consider, criteria for judging the strength of evidence, time relationships, plausibility with actual biological knowledge and the consistency with other research (Bradford Hill criteria).

In a *cohort study*, the definition of exposure drives the inclusion of cohort (and control) subjects. We see increasing interest in new users design or inception cohorts, meaning that only subjects that qualify for a certain exposure definition are included, e.g. new users of product "A" and no use of any other products from the class product "A" belongs to in the 6 months before.

In a *case–control study*, exposure ascertainment is driven by the hypothesised causal association of interest, the choice of an exposure window wherein the exposure is assessed and the definition of what exposure defines, e.g. within the exposure window at least one prescription or cumulative use of >15 defined daily doses (DDDs) of the product at interest.

We see also increasing interest in studying exposure variation over time and addressing the question whether that variation has been the result of any regulatory intervention, a communication strategy or a reimbursement change (Goedecke et al. 2018; Piening et al. 2012; Santa-Ana-Tellez et al. 2013). The research community has adopted increasingly interrupted time series analysis as a powerful statistical technique to study such questions. More on this later in this chapter.

In order to conduct and interpret pharmacoepidemiological research and communicate findings properly, one needs knowledge on major study designs, potential methodological pitfalls and careful consideration of whether identified associations are of temporal or causal nature. As principles of randomised controlled trials for experimental research on communication, "natural experiments" as a quasi-experimental research approach and cross-sectional surveys are covered in Chap. 8 on the social sciences, this chapter focuses on studying use of medicines, cohort study designs and time series analyses.

14.2.2 Medicines Use Studies and Fundamental Taxonomies

Proper taxonomy of the medicine exposure is key to evaluate any exposure change that is sensitive enough to enable picking up any effect of a communication or

Research question > Study design > Data collection and analysis > Interpretation and conclusion

Research question > **Taxonomy** > Study design > Data collection and analysis > Interpretation and conclusion > **Communication and implementation**

Fig. 14.1 The role of taxonomy of medicine exposure in pharmacoepidemiological research, its communication and implementation of research results

regulatory intervention. The field of drug utilisation or medicines use studies has built over the years sound methodology to do an important part of this job (Bergman 2006). While such studies usually are not directed typically at quantifying inferences and to determine causal effects, they provide the metrics for multiple taxonomies needed to study not only medicines use, but also medicine exposure-outcome associations (Vermeer et al. 2016).

Key have been medicines classification methods, e.g. the widely used Anatomical-Therapeutic-Chemical (ATC) coding system, volume of use metrics, e.g. number of prescriptions or packages, or defined daily dose (DDD), i.e. the assumed average maintenance dose calculated per day for its main indication in adults, and exposure windows, i.e. to log timing of start and end of therapy. The ATC system has various applications including lumping individual medicines together in logical, e.g. pharmacological, mechanistic or therapeutic groups (Bergman 2006). The DDD metrics is a population measure and is particularly used when only cumulative sales or dispensing data are available for a given local or global population. With the surge of pharmacoepidemiological studies using automated databases including individual medicines use data, the need for a population measure as the DDD has become less obvious.

The value of taxonomy for the problem at stake has been often undervalued, as it is not always considered as hard science. Even while accepting that a debate on what is science and what is not, robust taxonomy is a perquisite for sound hypothesis formulation, study design and conduct. The same shift we have seen over the years regarding the need for creating a follow-up of the conclusions of a pharmacoepidemiological study. This follow-up has two critical elements: communication (in multiple directions) and implementation (what to do with the results, both up- and downstream the development of medicines) (see Fig. 14.1).

14.2.3 Cohort Studies

Cohort studies are widely used in pharmacoepidemiology (Klungel et al. 2016; Van Staa et al. 2000). They are typically used to compare exposed patients, or other study subjects, with non-exposed subjects looking for differences in their outcome.

Earlier in this chapter, we already referred to NSAIDs-induced increased incidence of gastropathy. One of the early cohort studies in pharmacoepidemiology evaluated the risk of upper gastrointestinal bleeding from NSAIDs in a retrospective cohort study using data from 47,136 exposed patients and 44, 634 unexposed patients (Carson et al. 1987). Patients exposed to NSAIDs had about 50% more chance (relative risk of 1.5) to have the outcome of interest, i.e. upper gastrointestinal bleeding, in the 30 days after exposure compared to the unexposed controls. The study showed also an exposure dose-response and a duration response relationship. This cohort study was performed retrospectively, i.e. data were collected from existing 1980 billing data from Medicaid in the US states Michigan and Minnesota. A cohort study can also be conducted prospectively, i.e. cohorts are assembled simultaneously with the events under study (Evans 2012; Wettermark 2013). Prospective cohort studies are conceptually alike clinical trials with the major exception that treatment allocation is not random, i.e. exposure occurs "naturally" as a result of medical practice with all its clinical, cultural and socioeconomic correlates.

Cohort studies have many methodological advantages (e.g. less susceptible for bias or confounding) compared to case–control studies, which are rarely used to evaluate public health impact of communication or regulatory interventions. Moreover, over the years various methodical advances have been introduced (e.g. propensity-score matching) making unbiased comparisons between cohorts more feasible (Rassen et al. 2013). An international group of researchers used a cohort design to evaluate the impact on stroke incidence after two safety warnings targeting elderly patients using antipsychotics in the United Kingdom (UK) and Italy (Sultana et al. 2019). After each safety warning, elderly antipsychotic new initiators were propensity-score matched 1:1:1 on antipsychotic initiators before any safety warning. Stroke incidence within 6 months of antipsychotic initiation was the main outcome. The study showed a clear impact in terms of stroke incidence reduction in the UK, but not in Italy. In terms of usefulness of the cohort design, Goedecke et al. in a systematic review of 153 studies measuring the impact of medicines regulatory interventions found that the cohort design was not very often (in <5% of all studies) applied (Goedecke et al. 2018)]. More on this later in this chapter.

14.2.4 Interrupted Time Series Analyses

Another approach in studying the impact of communication or a regulatory intervention are interrupted time series analyses (ITS). In ITS essentially two time trends are compared (Bernal et al. 2017; Jandoc et al. 2015). First the underlying, or expected, trend of a particular outcome (e.g. prescribing of a certain medicine, knowledge about a particular safety concern) in the absence of the intervention of interest (e.g. safety warning, regulatory communication). The second time trend reflects the outcomes in a post-intervention period in the presence of an intervention. When this trend is "interrupted" in comparison with the expected time trend after the intervention this may provide a graphical impact model (e.g. slope change, level change or both). Regression techniques are used to evaluate whether post-intervention changes, if there, have any statistical meaning. The design of ITS has the big advantage compared to the generic before-after measurement that the expected time trend (often hidden) is taken into account, but is only possible when certain conditions are met. The most important ones are, firstly, that the intervention should be short and distinct in time allowing before and after measurements of the outcome. This means also that the outcome should have distinct moments in time, i.e. counts or the like. And third, sufficient data points should be available before and after the intervention allowing robust construct of the expected and “interrupted” time trends. In an ITS study looking at the impact of over-the-counter restrictions on antibiotic consumption in Brazil and Mexico, it was found that in Brazil the over-the-counter antibiotic consumption was still on a rise, but at a lower level after the intervention (Santa-Ana-Tellez et al. 2013). In Mexico the decrease continued as before the restriction, but also at lower level. Komen and colleagues used ITS to evaluate the impact of various policy interventions, i.e. reimbursement and various clinical guidelines, on the prescribing of oral anticoagulants for atrial fibrillation in the region of Stockholm in Sweden (Komen et al. 2017). This study was able to differentiate between the impacts of different policy interventions and the prescribing of oral anticoagulants. Overall, the application of ITS for evaluating the impact of regulatory and communication interventions reflects still ample heterogeneity in terms of methodological approach, data used and interpretation, as also shown by the previously mentioned systematic review of Goedecke et al. (Goedecke et al. 2018).

14.3 Utility of Applied Methods for Researching Medicinal Product Risk Communication

14.3.1 The Connection Between Pharmacoepidemiology and Communication

Communication around medicinal product risks may have various connections to pharmacoepidemiology (Radawski et al. 2015; Weatherburn et al. 2019). Communication can be the publication of a pharmacoepidemiological study in a scientific journal, media attention related to the publication or regulatory intervention (and implementation), such as for risk minimisation, based on the evidence provided by a study. This sequence is also depicted in Fig. 14.1, i.e. communication follows conduct of a study and relates to the dissemination of its results. How this connection turns of for a specific study is very much determined by the quality of the study, the confidence in its accuracy and robustness, the uncertainties about the results and its clinical relevance and health impact—i.e. does the study really matter? We have seen over the last decades many examples, e.g. the VTE risk of oral contraceptives, cardiovascular risks of oral antidiabetics and the suicide risk of antidepressants (Vandenbroucke et al. 2001; Blind et al. 2011; Hernandez et al. 2012). In all these cases, communication—the way this was done—was the dependent variable.

Communication can also be the independent variable, i.e. the intervention in the medicines use system, with research questions about the impact of communication on prescribing behaviour, patient adherence to therapy, reporting of suspected adverse reactions, trust in medicines and underlying research, regulation and healthcare, or on how media coverage is shaped. The critical methodological issue of studying the impact of product risk communication has always been that this impact may have many other determinants as well, making any (causal) inferences complex and not always feasible. In fact, a communication intervention virtually never happens as an isolated event. Many other factors contribute to any change in prescribing, adherence, adverse reaction reporting, trust and media coverage. Researching communication outcomes in terms of exposure and use of medicines is therefore a vital component of a multilayered research approach to medicinal product risk communication (see Chap. 1).

14.3.2 The Utility of Pharmacoepidemiology for Evaluating the Impact of Communication

It is noteworthy that various communication and risk perception aspects influence the nature of medicine use in various, sometime unpredictable ways (Radawski et al. 2015; Segec et al. 2015; Hernandez et al. 2012). This may happen through the authorised product information, the scientific literature or by what is being discussed about certain medicines in public spaces—(social) media in particular—or most fundamentally by the communication encounters between patients and healthcare professionals. These communication encounters lead to diagnoses and therapeutic decision-making, often involving medicines. In fact, in principle the aim of communication about medicines is to support safe and effective use.

A recent worldwide review identified the methods currently applied to evaluate the impact of regulatory action, which are most often safety advisory statements on the website of the regulatory body, boxed warnings in the product information and direct healthcare professional communications (DHPCs), hence most often communication-related (Goedecke et al. 2018). Studies eligible for review came mainly from Europe and North America, but also other places, such as Australia and Japan. In 55% of the reviewed studies ($N = 153$) measured changes in medicines use patterns over time, 27% health outcomes and 18% other outcomes, such as knowledge. Study designs and analytical approaches applied were before-after time series (66% of reviewed studies), cross-sectional studies with before-after comparisons (16%), cross-sectional studies at a single time-point (14%), some cohort studies and one randomised clinical trial.

Situations where the effects of communication, media coverage or regulatory interventions are studied, have been in a number of cases "natural experiments", i.e. one part of the population is exposed and the remaining part is considered as control. Examples of these include the reports of adverse events related to the use of the hypnotic triazolam (Halcion®) and the geographic distribution of media coverage of the possible health hazards related to triazolam (Van der Kroef 1991). Or more recently, the trends in the use of specific antidepressants, i.e. selective serotonin reuptake inhibitors (SSRIs), in the context of safety warnings in the UK and the Netherlands (Hernandez et al. 2012). All these examples show variable, and sometimes unintended, effects of communication activities. This was also seen by Piening et al., who reviewed 50 studies on the impact of safety-related regulatory actions over a 15 years period (1996–2010) and concluded that such actions could have some impact on clinical practice, but firm conclusions were difficult to draw (Piening et al. 2012). This review also revealed many methodological weaknesses (e.g. inadequate before/after designs, heterogeneity in analyses and outcome measures, limited use of adequate interrupted time series designs) of the studies. Furthermore, the review stressed the importance of measuring both intended and unintended effects of safety warnings. Unintended effects may include switching to alternative products outside the scope of the safety warning, but with a less favourable benefit-risk or at higher economic costs.

A more positive view was recently presented from the UK. Weatherburn et al. re-analysed outcome data relevant to UK regulatory risk communication using interrupted time series regression 12 months after each communication, i.e. DHPCs and communication via drug bulletins (Weatherburn et al. 2019). According to this study these communications seemed to be associated with significant changes in targeted prescribing and potential changes in clinical outcomes. But the previously already mentioned study by Sultana et al. comparing how safety warnings relating to antipsychotic-associated stroke among older persons were differentially followed by prescribers in the UK and Italy is another example of how variable safety warnings are picked up in real clinical practice (Sultana et al. 2019).

Evaluating the impact of communication remains a challenge, both in terms of applying the most suitable pharmacoepidemiological or other methods and translating the findings of the evaluations in concrete utility, e.g. change in practice, input to policy measures or other interventions. Available evidence so far indicates mixed findings when it comes to quantifying impact and utility. Further methodological improvements in study design, conduct and interpretation of the results are needed (Pitts et al. 2016; Radawski et al. 2015). But there is another strong message. No robust evaluation is possible without proper and a-prior taxonomy of the regulatory risk communication action.

14.3.3 The Need for Awareness of Confounding by Indication

There are many sources of bias and confounding in pharmacoepidemiological research. But by all means, confounding by indication, also coined as channelling bias, is one of the most pivotal ones. An iconic case illustrating confounding by indication has been the controversy about inhaled beta-agonists, prescribed against asthma, and asthma mortality. One of the first pivotal studies on this association was a case–control study in New Zealand comprising 117 patients who died of asthma between 1981 and 1983 (Crane et al. 1989). In patients prescribed fenoterol by metered dose inhaler, one of the inhaled beta-agonists, the relative risk (RR) of asthma death was 1.55 (95% confidence interval (CI) 1.04–2.33), and this risk was increased in patients with most severe asthma. This association was not seen in patients using other inhaled beta-agonists, i.e. salbutamol and terbutaline. Later, pharmacoepidemiologists from Canada published a nested case–control study on the risk of inhaled beta-agonists-induced fatal or near-fatal asthma based on data from the province of Saskatchewan, from 1980 to 1987 (Spitzer et al. 1992). They found also an increased risk of (near) asthma death, but with different point estimates for fenoterol and salbutamol. Further analyses of this dataset revealed important information on the question whether the comparison was confounded by indication, because of channelling of fenoterol to more severely ill patients. These findings fuelled an intense debate on how channelling of certain medicines to patients with prognostic differences can result in attributing incorrectly increased risk to the use of these medicines, an issue that is also today very topical (Segec et al. 2015).

Confounding by indication is not only important to consider when studying associations between medicines and health outcomes, but is likewise relevant when monitoring or investigating medicines use and harm in relation to communication events, such as safe use advice or a media debate. For example, the rate of a certain adverse reaction (i.e. number of cases over the number of exposed patients) might go up after a safe use advice. However, rather than immediately concluding that the safe use advice was ineffective—either for its content or dissemination—it needs to be considered whether the safe use advice was actually effective in raising risk awareness and led physicians to only prescribe the medicine in severely ill patients. Exactly these patients could also be more susceptible to this particular adverse reaction. So, it could be that the communication was effective, but led to unintended channelling of the medicine and relative increase of adverse reactions (i.e. in relation to the number of exposed patients). As the communication might have effectively reduced the number of exposed patients, the number of adverse reactions in absolute terms could still have gone down too. Advanced studies into medicines use and exposure would maybe confirm this and further benefit-risk assessment by the regulatory body would then look in this patient population specifically, and further risk minimisation measures would be introduced as appropriate (Pitts et al. 2016; Potts et al. 2019).

14.4 Outlook: Relevance, Improvements and Future Potential

14.4.1 Medicine Exposure as a Social Construct

Much of what has been said before exemplifies that medicine exposure can be seen as a kind of a social construct, requiring smart blending of pharmacology, epidemiology and social sciences in order to understand the dynamics over time, the communication and regulatory context, and the consequences of all these for the correct use of taxonomies (see Sect. 14.2.2). This has inherent effects on the way study designs, measurements and analyses in pharmacoepidemiological studies are planned and conducted (Evans 2012; Lapeyre-Mestre et al. 2013). The hazard function of the medicine exposure-outcome association at interest over time as well as the methods for exposure and outcomes ascertainment, comparing new with old medicines and landscaping of the market place where the studies are conducted, together with the taxonomies of all these elements require an informed understanding for appropriate conduct and interpretation of research.

An interesting example in this respect relates to the hepatotoxicity of nimesulide, a selective cyclo-oxygenase-2 inhibitor (a type of NSAIDs) used for inflammatory and pain conditions. The usage of this medicine varies widely across Europe. In about half of the countries of the EU nimesulide has not been authorised at all, while in some other countries, e.g. Italy, France and Poland, the product is among the most popular NSAIDs prescribed. Worldwide exposure of nimesulide between 2005 and 2007 accounted for 16% of all DDDs for NSAIDs, thereby being the second most frequently used product in this class. In 2012 the SALT study, this was a European non-interventional retrospective study at seven centres (2005–2007) to provide estimates of the rates of acute liver failure (ALF) leading to liver transplantation, showed no difference in event rates for abnormal liver function between major NSAIDs, including nimesulide (Gulmez et al. 2013). The overall conclusion of the EMA was that the benefit-risk balance of short-term usage of nimesulide remained positive (EMA 2012).

This has been also the case when the question was on the table whether pandemic vaccines are associated with narcolepsy. Not long after the European pandemic influenza vaccination in the spring of 2010 had started—this happened not in all European countries in the same way—case reports of narcolepsy, a permanent condition with frequent sudden sleep onset, were received by the Swedish and Finish authorities. In the aftermath more reports across Europe were received, but quantitatively most of the reports came from the countries where the signal initially occurred. In 2014 a research group from Sweden reported from a pharmacoepidemiological study showing an increased and age-related risk of narcolepsy in individuals vaccinated with one of the pandemic vaccines, i.e. Pandemrix®. This association was not univocally confirmed in other, i.e. non-signalling countries (Feltelius et al. 2015). Gadroen et al. contrasted over the period from 2010 to 2014 reporting to EudraVigilance, the EU database of adverse reactions, of narcolepsy after pandemic flu vaccination between signalling countries (i.e. Sweden, Finland) and non-signalling countries (12 EU/European Economic Area (EEA) countries and 4 non-EU/non-EEA countries) and showed how such safety concerns may vary across geographic regions (Gadroen et al. 2016).

Both examples show clearly the interplay between science, the regulatory context and intriguing role of how non-medical factors affect how medicine exposure may vary between countries and how risks, concerns and communication needs are different between and within societies. Medicine exposure, and related safety concerns, in both cases has been the summed results of a broad array of scientific, clinical, regulatory, economic and societal factors.

14.4.2 Future Potential of Pharmacoepidemiology for Medicinal Product Risk Communication Research

All these experiences with complex weighing of the benefits and risks of medicines, with the search for the best evidence to support (regulatory) decision-making, and with the communication of the decision show the importance of deepening insight into the taxonomies of medicines use, both quantitatively and qualitatively. This insight is needed for the design and proper conduct and interpretation of pharmacoepidemiology studies, but also for the impact evaluation of any intervention that follows, e.g. changes to the product information, DHPCs, communication campaigns, or other interventions impacting on the use of medicines (Kurz and Perez-Gutthann 2018; Goedecke et al. 2018). This is also needed for studying the impact on medicines use of other communication events, like coverage of a safety concern in the mass news or social media. Better alignment between pharmacoepidemiology and medicinal product risk communication—operations and research—will benefit both. In pharmacoepidemiology, evaluating and understanding the impact of various determinants of medicine exposure, including communication, is a multidisciplinary research field. Further integration of pharmacoepidemiology, communication science, health service research and the humanities is needed (see Chap. 1). A communication or regulatory intervention virtually never occurs in isolation. Such interventions are often part of a chain of events, analyses, policy interventions or political manoeuvring. For improving medicinal product risk communication, pharmacoepidemiological methods, including cohort studies and interrupted time series analysis, may be instrumental to evaluate and to improve, eventually, communication and patient outcomes. This will never be a binary or simple exercise. The multidimensional nature requires an open mind towards an array of methodological approaches, data and learning (Sheiner 1997). The future will bring more of these, for good reasons.

Conclusions

- Pharmacoepidemiology is about quantifying and understanding medicine exposure-outcome associations.
- Medicine exposure, i.e. treatment allocation, is not binary. It is a multivariate construct with various pharmacological, regulatory, economic and social dimensions.
- Pharmacoepidemiological methods (e.g. cohort studies, interrupted time series) can be used for evaluating the impact of product risk communication or other (regulatory) interventions.
- However, such interventions virtually never happen as isolated events, many other factors may modify its effects. Hence making causal inferences on intervention and impact remain complex and challenging.

References

Bakhriansyah M, Souverein PC, de Boer A, Klungel OH (2017) Gastrointestinal toxicity among patients taking selective COX-2 inhibitors or conventional NSAIDs, alone or combined with proton pump inhibitors: a case-control study. Pharmacoepidemiol Drug Saf 26(10):1141–1148

Bergman U (2006) The history of the drug utilization research group in Europe. Pharmacoepidemiol Drug Saf 15(2):95–98

Bernal JL, Cummins S, Gasparrini A (2017) Interrupted time series regression for the evaluation of public health interventions: a tutorial. Int J Epidemiol. 46(1):348–355

Blind E, Dunder K, de Graeff PA, Abadie E (2011) Rosiglitazone: a European regulatory perspective. Diabetologia 54(2):213–218

Boston Collaborative Drug Surveillance Programme (1973) Oral contraceptives and venous thromboembolic disease, surgically confirmed gallbladder disease, and breast tumours. Lancet 1(7817):1399–1404

Carson JL, Strom BL, Soper KA, West SL, Morse ML (1987) The association of nonsteroidal anti-inflammatory drugs with upper gastrointestinal tract bleeding. Arch Intern Med 147(1):85–88

Crane J, Pearce N, Flatt A, Burgess C, Jackson R, Kwong T, Ball M, Beasley R (1989) Prescribed fenoterol and death from asthma in New Zealand, 1981–83: case-control study. Lancet 1(8644):917–922

EMA Assessment report for nimesulide containing medicinal products for systemic use (2012) https://www.ema.europa.eu/en/documents/referral/nimesulide-article-31-referral-assessment-report_en.pdf

EMA PRAC recommendations on signals (2018) https://www.ema.europa.eu/en/documents/prac-recommendation/prac-recommendations-signals-adopted-3-6-september-2018-prac-meeting_en-0.pdf

Evans SJ (2012) Pharmacoepidemiology. Br J Clin Pharmacol 73(6):973–978

Feltelius N, Persson I, Ahlqvist-Rastad J, Andersson M, Arnheim-Dahlström L, Bergman P, Granath F, Adori C, Hökfelt T, Kühlmann-Berenzon S, Liljeström P, Maeurer M, Olsson T, Örtqvist Å, Partinen M, Salmonson T, Zethelius B (2015) A coordinated cross-disciplinary research initiative to address an increased incidence of narcolepsy following the 2009–2010 Pandemrix vaccination programme in Sweden. J Intern Med 278(4):335–353

Gadroen K, Straus SMJM, Pacurariu A, Weibel D, Kurz X, Sturkenboom MCJM (2016) Patterns of spontaneous reports on narcolepsy following administration of pandemic influenza vaccine; a case series of individual case safety reports in Eudravigilance. Vaccine 34(41):4892–4897

Giezen TJ, Mantel-Teeuwisse AK, Straus SM, Schellekens H, Leufkens HG, Egberts AC (2008) Safety-related regulatory actions for biologicals approved in the United States and the European Union. JAMA 300(16):1887–1896

Goedecke T, Morales D, Pacurariu A, Kurz X (2018) Measuring the impact of medicines regulatory interventions: systematic review and methodological considerations. Br J Clin Pharmacol 84:419–433

Gulmez SE, Larrey D, Pageaux GP, Lignot S, Lassalle R, Jové J, Gatta A, McCormick PA, Metselaar HJ, Monteiro E, Thorburn D, Bernal W, Zouboulis-Vafiadis I, de Vries C, Perez-Gutthann S, Sturkenboom M, Bénichou J, Montastruc JL, Horsmans Y, Salvo F, Hamoud F, Micon S, Droz-Perroteau C, Blin P, Moore N (2013) Transplantation for acute liver failure in patients exposed to NSAIDs or paracetamol (acetaminophen): the multinational case-population SALT study. Drug Saf 36(2):135–144

Herings RM, Urquhart J, Leufkens HG (1999) Venous thromboembolism among new users of different oral contraceptives. Lancet 354(9173):127–128

Hernandez JF, Mantel-Teeuwisse AK, van Thiel GJ, Belitser SV, Warmerdam J, de Valk V, Raaijmakers JA, Pieters T (2012) A 10-year analysis of the effects of media coverage of regulatory warnings on antidepressant use in the Netherlands and UK. PLoS One 7(9):e45515. https://doi.org/10.1371/journal.pone.0045515

Jandoc R, Burden AM, Mamdani M, Lévesque LE, Cadarette SM (2015) Interrupted time series analysis in drug utilization research is increasing: systematic review and recommendations. J Clin Epidemiol 68(8):950–956

Klungel OH, Kurz X, de Groot MC, Schlienger RG, Tcherny-Lessenot S, Grimaldi L, Ibáñez L, Groenwold RH, Reynolds RF (2016) Multi-centre, multi-database studies with common protocols: lessons learnt from the IMI PROTECT project. Pharmacoepidemiol Drug Saf 25(Suppl 1):156–165

Komen J, Forslund T, Hjemdahl P, Andersen M, Wettermark B (2017) Effects of policy interventions on the introduction of novel oral anticoagulants in Stockholm: an interrupted time series analysis. Br J Clin Pharmacol 83(3):642–652

Kurz X, Perez-Gutthann S (2018) ENCePP steering group strengthening standards, transparency, and collaboration to support medicine evaluation: ten years of the European Network of Centres for Pharmacoepidemiology and Pharmacovigilance (ENCePP). Pharmacoepidemiol Drug Saf 27(3):245–252

Lapeyre-Mestre M, Sapède C, Moore N et al (2013) Pharmacoepidemiology studies: what levels of evidence and how can they be reached? Therapie 68(4):241–252

Pedersen SA, Gaist D, Schmidt SAJ, Hölmich LR, Friis S, Pottegård A (2018) Hydrochlorothiazide use and risk of nonmelanoma skin cancer: a nationwide case-control study from Denmark. J Am Acad Dermatol 78(4):673–681

Piening S, Haaijer-Ruskamp FM, de Vries JTN, van der Elst ME, de Graeff PA, Straus SMJM, Mol PGM (2012) Impact of safety-related regulatory action on clinical practice: a systematic review. Drug Saf 35:373–385

Pitts PJ, Louet HL, Moride Y, Conti RM (2016) 21st century pharmacovigilance: efforts, roles, and responsibilities. Lancet Oncol 17(11):e486–e492

Potts J, Genov G, Segec A, Raine J, Straus S, Arlett P (2019) Improving the safety of medicines in the EU: from signals to action. Clin Pharmacol Ther. https://doi.org/10.1002/cpt.1678. [Epub ahead of print]

Radawski C, Morrato E, Hornbuckle K, Bahri P, Smith M, Juhaeri J, Mol P, Levitan B, Huang HY, Coplan P, Li H, BRACE Special Interest Group (2015) Benefit-risk assessment, communication, and evaluation (BRACE) throughout the life cycle of therapeutic products: overall perspective and role of the pharmacoepidemiologist. Pharmacoepidemiol Drug Saf 24(12):1233–1240

Rassen JA, Shelat AA, Franklin JM, Glynn RJ, Solomon DH, Schneeweiss S (2013) Matching by propensity score in cohort studies with three treatment groups. Epidemiology 24(3):401–409

Santa-Ana-Tellez Y, Mantel-Teeuwisse AK, Dreser A, Leufkens HG, Wirtz VJ (2013) Impact of over-the-counter restrictions on antibiotic consumption in Brazil and Mexico. PLoS One 8(10):e75550. https://doi.org/10.1371/journal.pone.0075550

Segec A, Keller-Stanislawski B, Vermeer NS, Macchiarulo C, Straus SM, Hidalgo-Simon A, De Bruin ML (2015) Strategy in regulatory decision-making for management of progressive multifocal Leukoencephalopathy. Clin Pharmacol Ther 98(5):502–505

Sheiner LB (1997) Learning versus confirming in clinical drug development. Clin Pharmacol Ther 61(3):275–291

Skovlund E, Leufkens HGM, Smyth JF (2018) The use of real-world data in cancer drug development. Eur J Cancer 101:69–76

Spitzer WO, Suissa S, Ernst P, Horwitz RI, Habbick B, Cockcroft D, Boivin JF, McNutt M, Buist AS, Rebuck AS (1992) The use of beta-agonists and the risk of death and near death from asthma. N Engl J Med 326(8):501–506

Sultana J, Fontana A, Giorgianni F, Tillati S, Cricelli C, Pasqua A, Patorno E, Ballard C, Sturkenboom M, Trifirò G (2019) Measuring the effectiveness of safety warnings on the risk of stroke in older antipsychotic users: a Nationwide cohort study in two large electronic medical records databases in the United Kingdom and Italy. Drug Saf. https://doi.org/10.1007/s40264-019-00860-z. [Epub ahead of print]

van Dalem J, Brouwers MC, Stehouwer CD, Krings A, Leufkens HG, Driessen JH, de Vries F, Burden AM (2016) Risk of hypoglycaemia in users of sulphonylureas compared with metformin in relation to renal function and sulphonylurea metabolite group: population based cohort study. BMJ 354:i3625

Van der Kroef C (1991) Triazolam. Lancet 338(8758):56

Van Staa TP, Leufkens HG, Abenhaim L, Zhang B, Cooper C (2000) Use of oral corticosteroids and risk of fractures. J Bone Miner Res 15:993–1000

Vandenbroucke JP, Rosing J, Bloemenkamp KW, Middeldorp S, Helmerhorst FM, Bouma BN, Rosendaal FR (2001) Oral contraceptives and the risk of venous thrombosis. N Engl J Med 344(20):1527–1535

Vermeer NS, Ebbers HC, Straus SM, Leufkens HG, Egberts TC, De Bruin ML (2016) The effect of exposure misclassification in spontaneous ADR reports on the time to detection of product-specific risks for biologicals: a simulation study. Pharmacoepidemiol Drug Saf 25(3):297–306

Weatherburn CJ, Guthrie B, Dreischulte T, Morales DR (2019) Impact of medicines regulatory risk communications in the United Kingdom on prescribing and clinical outcomes: systematic review, time series analysis and meta-analysis. Br J Clin Pharmacol. https://doi.org/10.1111/bcp.14104. [Epub ahead of print]

Wettermark B (2013) The intriguing future of pharmacoepidemiology. Eur J Clin Pharmacol 69(Suppl 1):43–51

15 Legal Frameworks

Burkhard Sträter

Abstract

Understanding the legal obligations of pharmaceutical companies and regulatory authorities in relation to medicines information in any given jurisdiction is vital for appropriate preparation of medicinal product-related communication. Likewise, any evaluation of a communication intervention a posteriori needs to check if content and timing have been compliant with these obligations in place for consumer and patient protection. In particular, the right of patients to receive compensation in the case harm occurs due to the pharmaceutical company being non-compliant or negligent, i.e. the marketing authorisation holder's liability, impacts on communication requirements. This chapter presents legal principles of global value, including the precautionary principle, with the historical but still fundamental case of the thalidomide disaster, and looks to challenging legal questions of the future.

B. Sträter (✉)
Rheinische Friedrich-Wilhelms-Universität Bonn, Master Study Course Regulatory Affairs – MDRA, Bonn, Germany
e-mail: mdra@uni-bonn.de

© Springer Nature Singapore Pte Ltd. 2020

P. Bahri (ed.), *Communicating about Risks and Safe Use of Medicines*,
https://doi.org/10.1007/978-981-15-3013-5_15

15.1 The Discipline of the Legal Sciences: Scope, Theories and Principles

Communication on the efficacy and safety of medicinal products must not only be based on the scientific evidence for the product but also on legal requirements laid down by the legislators in the countries concerned.

In the European Union (EU) as a relevant example, this applies primarily to the mandatory information contained in the legally required package leaflet, summary of product characteristics and labelling of the packaging (i.e. the so-called statutory information) and to additional risk management materials for patients and healthcare professionals, such as direct healthcare professional communications (DHPC), which the pharmaceutical company that holds the marketing authorisation sends either voluntarily or at the instigation of authorities. Although the regulatory requirements for these information carriers describe the type of information that must be included, they do not describe the procedure to be followed for inconclusive or controversial evidence on risks and adverse reactions. Information intended to ensure the correct use of medicinal products is of particular importance. As a rule, it is specifically geared to risk reduction, such as the information on indication, contraindication, warnings and precautions for use and dosing. However, the section on adverse reactions in package leaflets and summaries of product characteristics describes the risk—albeit extremely rare—taken by a patient. Rather, it takes the "informed consent concept" into account. Patient and physician should know what risks they are taking. For liability, however, the information on the correct use of the medicinal product, for example, by indication, contraindication, warnings and precautions and dosage, is of far greater significance, because mistakes in the information bear the probability to cause damage to patients.

15.1.1 Lessons Learnt from the Thalidomide Disaster

Thalidomide, authorised in 1956 in Germany under the brand name of Contergan® and many other European countries as a sleeping pill, was the unfortunate cause for death and severe birth defects in children of women who had used this medicine during pregnancy (Science Museum 2017). This has gone down in medical history as the so-called thalidomide disaster of the 1960s and has lastingly altered the assessment of risks and benefits of medicinal products as well as the requirements for warnings and precautions for use in their product information (see Chap. 1). It is therefore worth reflecting on this case, which has been so fundamental for the establishment of pharmacovigilance and risk communication.

At the time, the scientific assessment of teratogenic risks was objectively flawed. Accordingly, communicating the risks to the patients and women concerned was a disaster in itself because Contergan was promoted as a sleeping pill for pregnant women! The responsible scientists of the marketing authorisation holder claimed to have examined and evaluated the product according to the level of scientific findings available at the time. In Germany, the public prosecutor's office brought however charges against the scientists of the responsible company, accusing them of the worst conceivable form of bodily injury and homicide. The Regional Court of Aachen was required to decide whether the employees' conduct was culpable of not applying all available evidence—if not intentional, then negligent.

The criminal proceedings were dropped, because the responsible company, in cooperation with the authorities, found a solution for the children concerned by setting up a foundation, which still provides support today. With this settlement, however, the Regional Court made a groundbreaking decision that has had a lasting effect on legislation, especially in Germany (Kloesel/Cyran Arzneimittelrecht Kommentar E1 2019; Regional Court of Aachen 2014). The Court made it clear that the responsible company must not wait until there is certain knowledge of the causality between the use of a medicinal product and the occurrence of damage. If there is a reasonable suspicion of a possible causality, scientists may not wait in the hope that this suspicion is unfounded. Such conduct was found to have been negligent. The precautionary principle had already been established here by case law and made a lasting impression on legislation in Germany and in the EU. As a result, legislation was created in the EU in the 1960s and 1970s with Directives 65/65/EC, 75/318/EC and 75/319/EC, which were transposed by the EU member states through corresponding national laws. The same principle applies in the United States (US). Their Food and Drug Administration (US FDA) has clarified this in its labelling guidance (FDA 2006). These regulations and guidances established strict standards for safety testing and clinical trials before a medicinal product can be authorised for use in healthcare as well as pharmacovigilance processes for the continued safety surveillance for the products in the post-authorisation phase. This is now the international standard (e.g. at global level (Council for International Organizations of Medical Sciences (CIOMS) 1998), in the EU (EMA 2004) and in the US (FDA 2006).

15.1.2 The Precautionary Principle

The precautionary principle is applied in environmental and health policy. A uniform definition does not exist. The United Nations Conference on Environment and Development (UNCED) in Rio de Janeiro in 1992 clarified the precautionary principle in Chapter 35 (3) of Agenda 21, thereby creating an international understanding as follows:

> *"In the face of threats of irreversible environmental damage, lack of full scientific understanding should not be an excuse for postponing actions which are justified in their own right. The precautionary approach could provide a basis for policies relating to complex systems that are not yet fully understood and whose consequences of disturbances cannot yet be predicted."*

This means that damage to the environment and health is to be avoided, even if the knowledge base is still incomplete. The precautionary principle therefore aims at taking preventive action to avoid damage despite a lack of certainty about the nature and extent of the probability of occurrence of possible damage events. The precautionary principle contrasts with the scientific principle, according to which only those risks are to be considered that can be scientifically proven (Wikipedia 2020).

A comparable situation arises for regulatory authorities and pharmaceutical companies when they are required to assess unexpected and hitherto unknown risks of medicinal products. If a pharmaceutical company becomes aware of information about a new suspected serious unexpected adverse reaction, the following decision is to be made: is there a reasonable suspicion of causality, which consequences can be drawn from this and which measures must be taken? To wait until clarity exists according to the rules of science is negligent. Rather, measures must be taken to eliminate the potential risk, e.g. by refraining from authorisation and recalling medicinal products from the market or by taking measures to protect patients from new identified or potential risks. And this creates a legal obligation to communicate the measures taken.

In the example of thalidomide, the risk-benefit analysis was clear very quickly. The teratogenic risks to the embryo from the treatment of sleep disorders in pregnant women required a recall from the distribution chain with immediate effect. However, a risk-benefit analysis can also result in other consequences. This is shown likewise by thalidomide, as it was granted a marketing authorisation once again in the 2000s, namely in the EU and in other countries for the treatment of severe cancer conditions, multiple myeloma for patients aged 65 and over, and in younger patients if they cannot be treated with high-dose chemotherapy. This re-authorisation was possible because concrete risk minimisation measures have been ordered in the form of a pregnancy prevention programme. This needs to be followed by all healthcare professionals and female patients of child-bearing potential as well as, given the dissemination of thalidomide into the semen, by male patients and their female partners of child-bearing potential (EMA 2019) (see Chap. 1). The implementation of a pregnancy prevention programme requires a major communicative effort, and this shows the importance of risk communication between companies, doctors and patients in order to make the worst conceivable risk of teratogenicity an acceptable risk through the measures taken. Precisely the example of thalidomide therefore shows that the requirements under liability law have a direct impact on the type and content of communication about the risks of medicinal products.

15.1.3 Natural Sciences Versus Legal Sciences: Contrary or Complementary?

Liability and legal provisions in relation to risk assessment and communication for medicinal products are essential considerations when planning communication interventions or assessing whether such intervention is legally and hence overall appropriate.

The influence of the legal requirements for communication results from different areas of law. Legal experts distinguish between public law, civil law and criminal law. This distinction has been established throughout the world with some differentiations. Not explicitly mentioned is financial and social law, which is to be classified under public law. For the analysis of pharmaceutical law, however, the above-mentioned distinction is of decisive importance. Public law, also known as administrative law, regulates the relationship between the state and citizens. By contrast, civil law regulates claims between entities, which may be real private persons or private institutions. It is here that civil liability issues are primarily clarified, e.g. the claims of patients against pharmaceutical companies. Criminal law aims to sanction behaviour that is particularly harmful to individuals or society and, in addition to civil liability, to outlaw the act in a special way by imposing a penalty.

Pharmaceutical law regulates the marketing authorisation, distribution and statutory information of medicinal products and belongs to all three of these areas of law. Pharmaceutical law is a special field of the law of danger prevention. It logically follows the principle of prohibition subject to authorisation, i.e. clinical testing, manufacturing and distribution of medicinal products are prohibited unless authorised by the regulatory authorities. If medicines cause unacceptable damage to the patients concerned, the patient, as a private entity, is entitled to compensation from the marketing authorisation holder. If patients are culpably harmed by a medicinal product, criminal law provides for effective and severe penalties against the distribution of any such product. The decisive question is therefore whether legal considerations can provide guidance to the addressees of the law—frequently natural scientists—with regard to what should be communicated to the public and when. The introductory example of this chapter has already shown the essential principle that is firmly anchored in all three relevant areas of law and therefore has a lasting influence on risk-benefit assessment and communication: Those who have understood and followed the message of the thalidomide decision of the Regional Court of Aachen can plan communication interventions that are in accordance with the law. This will be further explained below.

15.1.3.1 Legal Perspective

Regulations governing package leaflets vary greatly throughout the world. It is practically impossible to present these in detail in a manner that compares the legal systems. The example of the EU will therefore be used in the following to illustrate the public law framework, as an important jurisdiction that also serves as a model for other countries.

EU law contains extensive and detailed regulations on the marketing authorisation, manufacture and clinical testing of medicinal products (Directive 2001/20/EC; Directive 2001/83/EC; Regulation (EC) No. 726/2004; Regulation (EU) No. 536/2014). We are in the area of administrative law here, something which is often not recognised by scientists, because the legislation also deals intensively with the criteria for scientific evaluation. The marketing authorisation application contains the pharmaceutical requirements in the areas of quality, safety and efficacy. These parts of the marketing authorisation application are undoubtedly characterised by the high scientific requirements of toxicology, pharmacology, pharmaceutical technology and medicine. However, they relate to a product whose marketing is subject to authorisation. The authorisation procedure itself is an administrative procedure, however, it follows the legal rules of administrative law. The same applies to the revocation of the marketing authorisation. Article 126 in conjunction with Article 116 of Directive 2001/83/EC specify the conditions under which a marketing authorisation may be revoked or restricted, together with the corresponding requirements for communication through the package leaflet, the summary of product characteristics and the educational materials. The decision on the continued existence of a marketing authorisation therefore also follows administrative law requirements.

15.1.3.2 The Relevance of Liability

Beyond this, the civil and criminal liability of a pharmaceutical company and its employees is governed in the EU by the rules of product liability, as shown in the following overview (see Fig. 15.1, slide from a presentation by Sträter Lawyers).

Civil liability primarily concerns the company that holds the marketing authorisation. The same applies to the consequences of the Penalty Regulation for medicinal products that hold a so-called central marketing authorisation in the EU. However, the consequences of criminal law usually concern the individual employees of a company. The case of the thalidomide disaster makes this very clear. The company was sued under civil law. However, individuals are always the targets for criminal law charges. For this reason, the employees of the company responsible were also involved in substantial and lengthy criminal proceedings. In Germany, product recalls regularly lead to numerous criminal investigations for personal injury and homicide. The recall of rofecoxib (Vioxx®) (see Chap. 3) and cerivastatin (Lipobay®) (Angelmar 2006) also led to numerous criminal proceedings in Germany and elsewhere.

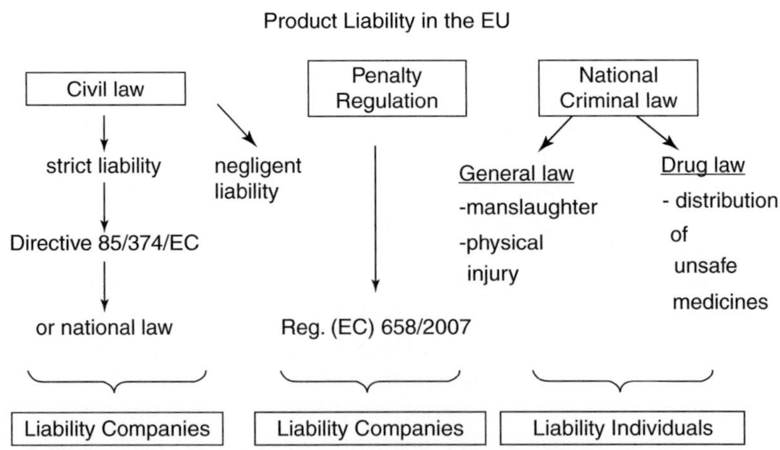

Fig. 15.1 Product liability in the European Union (EU). *Reg*, Regulation

Significance of the Marketing Authorisation for Liability
Regulatory affairs (RA) managers and scientists tend to defend themselves with the objection that the medicinal products had been approved and would have remained approved up to the recall. However, civil and criminal courts refer to the provisions EU legislation, namely in Article 25 of Directive 2001/83/EC and Article 15 of Regulation (EU) 726/2004. The provisions are almost identical:

> Article 15 Regulation (EC) 726/2004:
> "The granting of authorisation shall not affect the civil or criminal liability of the manufacturer or of the holder of the marketing authorisation pursuant to the applicable national law in Member States."
>
> Article 25 Directive 2001/83/EC:
> "Authorization shall not affect the civil and criminal liability of the manufacturer and, where applicable, of the marketing authorization holder."

This clearly shows that, in addition to the marketing authorisation, the legal framework conditions of liability also have a significant influence on the distribution and, above all, communication on medicinal products regarding risk issues, as the following will show.

15.1.3.3 The Relationship Between Scientific Assessment and Legal Judgement

What is the relationship between the acquisition and dissemination of knowledge by the natural scientists on the one hand and the law and legal sciences on the other? Roman law already distinguished between "scientia" and "prudentia", i.e. natural science and the humanities based on Aristotle's theory of science (Rühl 2005)—important to note that in 2016 we celebrated Aristoteles' 2400th birthday (Froese 2018), Uhlmann G (2016). This tense relationship is therefore age-old. It even goes back further than this. Hammurabi created the first codex in Babylon in the eighteenth century BC (!) and he wrote it in cuneiform (Encyclopaedia Britannica 2020), one of the earliest writing systems invented by the Sumerians. The first codified requirements for public order were therefore made in ancient Babylon. Since that time, medicine and law have co-existed, because both illness and conflict are part of human life, and particularly the teachings on how to heal diseases have repeatedly sparked dispute. Over these millennia, both sciences have highly developed to a point where they should treat each other with mutual respect and not with ignorance.

Marketing authorisation and pharmacovigilance assessors see themselves as scientists—and rightly so. The concept of science is also derived from this understanding of "scientia" in the sense of Roman law. However, legal science is also referred to as jurisprudence, i.e. a human science committed not only to formal rules but also to wisdom. Both sciences are therefore complementary to each other. Medicinal product marketing authorisation and accompanying information is a good example of the balancing act between natural science on the one hand and jurisprudence on the other.

This becomes all the more obvious when new adverse reactions occur. If natural scientists can neither deny nor rule out causality with the use of a product, then it is not rarely the case that plausible theories exist side by side within the meaning of epistemology. If, therefore, natural science cannot give a clear answer, then according to case law on the thalidomide disaster and the precautionary principle, the question whether there is an obligation to act, including communication, is not a scientific one but a legal one. In the thalidomide case, the Regional Court of Aachen was required to examine whether the behaviour of the employees of the responsible company was negligent, and developed the principle that in any such constellation of the coexistence of plausible scientific theories, the duty to act must be developed from the criteria of criminal law for the assessment of negligence and thus blame. This means that in communication planning, not only the scientific evaluation but also the legal framework conditions and requirements must always be taken into account.

This cannot mean that lawyers can now decide which of the scientific views or theories is the right one according to legal criteria. This is exclusively reserved for the natural sciences! However, this question must be distinguished from the consequences arising for risk minimisation measures and communication with physicians and patients if such a question, which has not yet been clarified from a scientific point of view, is now under discussion. The message of the thalidomide disaster and the thalidomide decision of the Regional Court of Aachen is as follows: from a criminal law point of view, it may be negligent and therefore culpable to wait until certainty is guaranteed. Action must be taken beforehand, and in particular information communicated! These principles are also followed by the precautionary principle described above in contrast to the scientific principle.

In authorities and companies, RA managers are therefore often required to accelerate the process of scientific evaluation and procedures. They must therefore develop an understanding of the scientific requirements according to the current level of knowledge and compare this with the regulatory and legal requirements that create duties to act with respect to the medicinal product and communication. Lawyers specialised in pharmaceutical law and experienced in administrative, civil and criminal law are therefore very helpful in the planning of communication.

15.2 Provisions and Applications

15.2.1 Regulation of Information About Medicines

15.2.1.1 Legal Requirements for Pharmaceutical Companies

The statutory, official so-to-say, product information in the EU consists of the package leaflet, the summary of product characteristics and also the labelling of the packaging and is specified in the marketing authorisation. Structure and content of the summary of product characteristics are specified by public law administrative provisions, e.g. in Article 11 of Directive 2001/83/EC, which is described below as a relevant example. In addition to the characterisation of the product according to active substances, excipients, strength, pharmaceutical forms and the name of the medicinal product, there are instructions on correct use and the section on adverse reactions. This division is remarkable for both the package leaflet and the summary of product characteristics. The first part deals with the question of how the medicinal product should be used, under which safety provisions and in which dosages for the right indication and for how long. Warnings and precautions, which are part of the instructions for correct use, are intended to create special attention to risks. This part of the information is of particular importance for the safety of patients and thus for the responsibility of marketing authorisation holders and regulatory authorities. Errors in this information can very easily cause damage to the patient and thus substantiate liability. The adverse reactions section, however, is intended to ensure an "informed consent" of the patient. The content reflects the outcome of the scientific evaluation and covers adverse reactions that may occur in both correct and other use of the medicine. Unlike the warnings and precautions for use section, which can also provide information on minimising theoretical risks in the sense of the precautionary principle, only those risks are listed in the adverse reactions section for which there are well-founded suspicions of causality. Here too, legal requirements and scientific evaluations interact. Title VIII on the advertising of medicinal products in Directive 2001/83/EC clarifies that the basic information of the assessment must be included and advertising must be limited to the conditions of use specified in the marketing authorisation, and may not contain statements contrary to the regulatory assessment or going beyond the contents of the product information or otherwise be misleading.

Technical public law requirements therefore set the framework for official information and that from companies, but at the same time also for the responsibility of the companies towards patients specifically, as will be shown in the following.

15.2.1.2 Global Responsibilities of Pharmaceutical Companies

Compliance with the regulatory requirements is comparatively simple if a medicinal product is authorised and distributed in only one jurisdiction. However, this tends to be the exception. Preparations of high therapeutic value are regularly used worldwide. This results in a range of variants of package inserts and summaries of product characteristics. This can be the result of problematic strategies of pharmaceutical companies. However, regulatory authorities also often try to develop their own profile independently of the assessments in other countries. The range of variants is thus large and often corresponds to different interpretations of the available evidence and its limitations, and sometimes companies or resource-poor authorities in low- and middle-income countries do not act according to the level of scientific knowledge. Sometimes, there are also genetic reasons or differences in locally established medical procedures and concomitant medications, or other prevalent diseases (e.g. infections) that justify different regulatory actions, or there is no approved or affordable alternative in a country.

This can have difficult liability consequences, especially for the affected companies and their employees. For example, if restrictions such as contraindications are established in one country but are not mentioned in the product information in another, a contra-indicated and injured patient will spontaneously ask why the information differs in other countries. The patient will say: "If I had lived in this country, I ought not to have received the medicine. And already the burden of proof turns to the detriment of the marketing authorisation holder who has to justify the discrepancies. The company is then exposed to a significantly increased liability risk.

Is there any chance of escaping these liability risks and of ensuring adequate information on the efficacy and safety of medicinal products in accordance with the latest scientific findings?

For the EU, the Guidelines on Good Pharmacovigilance Practices (EU-GVP) (European Medicines Agency 2012), in whose Annex I the definitions for the terms relevant in pharmacovigilance are found, offer orientation here as follows:

> Company core data sheet (CCDS)
>
> "For medicinal products, a document prepared by the marketing authorisation holder containing, in addition to safety information, material related to indications, dosing, pharmacology and other information concerning the product (see GVP Annex IV, ICH-E2C(R2) Guideline)."

According to this definition, which in its essence originally goes back to the CIOMS III Report of 1994 (Guidelines for Preparing Core Clinical-Safety Information on Drugs 1998), the company core data sheet comprises the information in the summary of product characteristics, which in the opinion of the pharmaceutical company is to be used everywhere in the world. One part of the company core data sheet is set out below and is particularly important to liability:

> Company core safety information (CCSI)
>
> "For medicinal products, all relevant safety information contained in the company core data sheet prepared by the marketing authorisation holder and which the marketing authorisation holder requires to be listed in all countries where the company markets the product, except when the local regulatory authority specifically requires a modification.
>
> It is the reference information by which listed and unlisted are determined for the purposes of periodic reporting for marketed products, but not by which expected and unexpected are determined for expedited reporting (see GVP Annex IV, ICH-E2C(R2) Guideline)." (emphasis added)

From a legal point of view, this definition accurately describes the requirement for pharmaceutical companies to harmonise information on medicinal products globally if they wish to avoid liability risks for the distribution of their medicinal products due to incorrect information. Within the company consensus must be ensured on how the package leaflets and summaries of product characteristics should be designed according to the latest scientific knowledge. A dialogue with the authorities on this subject should be documented. Based on this, the company must create a uniform company core data sheet "as a reference for the company". Employees in the respective affiliated companies must be forced to at least attempt to obtain approval for this version. Only if the authority expressly rejects it, can it be justified to remain on the market with this discrepancy. In the individual case of liability, the courts will have to decide whether the company has acted diligently and persistently enough. Therefore, if pharmaceutical companies neglect this forced harmonisation of the content of package leaflets and summaries of product characteristics, this will dramatically increase liability risks because the safety of patients is jeopardised.

Identity of the Medicinal Product: Responsibilities of the Pharmaceutical Company

For the reporting of adverse reactions (as an individual case safety report (ICSR)), the risk assessment and the company core safety information, it is also of decisive importance how the identity of the medicinal product is defined. Big products are often sold in more than 100 countries, in various strengths and dosage forms. The names of the medicinal products may vary, as do the legally responsible persons in the company. Given these variants in distribution, how can the identity of a company and a medicinal product be defined?

For the EU it has been clarified for this purpose that all companies belonging to the same group worldwide or interlinked by licencing agreements must be understood as one company. The European Commission has already clarified this in the Communication on Community Marketing Authorisation Procedures for Medicinal Products (98/C 229/03) and in the Notice to Applicants, Volume 2A (Council of European Communities 1998; European Commission 2016). The EU-GVP Module VI on "Collection, management and submission of reports of suspected adverse reactions to medicinal products" also refers to this Communication. This explains as follows in its section "VI.C.2.2 Responsibilities of the marketing authorisation holder":

> "The marketing authorisation holder shall ensure that any information and adverse reactions, suspected to be related to at least one of the active substances of its medicinal products authorised in die the EU, is brought to the attention by any company outside the EU belonging to the same mother company (or group of company). The same applies to the marketing authorisation holder, when having concluded a commercial agreement for the company outside the EU for one of its medicinal products authorised in the EU. [...] The clock for the submission [...] starts when a valid ICSR is first received by one of these companies outside the EU." (emphasis added)

The periodic safety update reports—PSURs—must also follow these requirements and the obligation to implement the company core safety information in accordance with the EU-GVP Module VII. It therefore ensures harmonised and consistent communication on medicinal product risks in global distribution of a medicinal product that must be understood as identical in this sense.

The situation is different for medicinal products with the same active substance in the relationship between originator and generic companies. These companies are *not* interlinked but are usually engaged in lively competition. Here, each of the companies is obliged to record and report the adverse reactions for its own product and, where necessary, to implement risk minimisation measures. The situation is different for subsidiaries, parent companies and licensees, however. Here, interlinked relationships and the legal basis for exerting influence are given, so that consistent information across products must also be guaranteed.

15.2.1.3 Duties of Regulatory Authorities for Harmonising Product Information

In their turn, the regulatory authorities must take official measures for products in terms of their active substance to ensure that the information for generic and original medicinal products is consistent.

In the EU, the harmonisation of summaries of product characteristics (SmPCs) within and across member states is forced by means of an annual list of substances whose SmPCs are to be harmonised, in accordance with Article 30 (2) of Directive 2001/83/EC. This list is based on proposals from the member states for follow-up by the European Commission and the European Medicines Agency (EMA). This process helps avoiding problems in the marketing authorisation of generic medicinal products. Generic product applicants make reference to originator products in so-called decentralised marketing authorisation procedures in the EU. If the originator's information is not consistent within the concerned member states of the EU, there will be problems in harmonising the product information for generic products across member states. If new SmPC texts are agreed far away from the inconsistency of the originator, there will be horizontal harmonisation of the product information across the generic medicinal products, but vertical disharmony in relation to the originator product. This is unacceptable, as it leads to the disorientation of the patients where pharmacists are obliged to make "aut idem" substitution (i.e. dispensing a different product than prescribed with the identical active substance in same strength and route of administration), often according to the specifications of the health insurance funds and other price regulations. Such inconsistencies in the product information received by patients can also occur during stays abroad, e.g. of tourists. Even in bi-national communities, different product use instructions between countries, e.g. for children, can lead to irritation and give rise to mistrust.

This phenomenon of inconsistency of product information for identical medicinal products is a widespread phenomenon and is due to a relationship characterised by competition and not by cooperation between companies. Global collaboration of both companies and regulatory authorities will be necessary to ensure harmonisation in the interest of fostering understanding and adherence of patients to the safe use instructions. An example is the EU referral concept whereby product information of mainly nationally authorised products is harmonised through a procedure at EU level with an outcome that is legally binding in all member states pursuant to Article 32 of Directive 2001/83/EC.

15.2.2 Information About Newly Identified Risks with Medicines: Considerations for Pharmaceutical Companies

According to the EU rules, the marketing authorisation holder must ensure that all information on its medicinal product is consistent throughout the world. It is obliged to report adverse reaction case reports as well as regulatory action taken anywhere in the world to the EU regulatory authorities. The companies concerned fulfil this obligation comprehensively through more than 100,000 notifications per year. However, notification is only one part of the relevant obligations. If the minimum criteria for reporting cases of suspected adverse reactions according to the EU-GVP Module VI are fulfilled, the reporting obligations are comparatively simple to define. However, the consequences to be drawn for the information and communication to patients and healthcare professionals is one of the most difficult questions in pharmacovigilance. The reasonable suspicion of a causal relationship between an adverse event and a medicinal product creates a legal obligation for marketing authorisation holders and the authorities to inform healthcare professionals and patients of the risks involved and to take appropriate measures.

The European Commission is at effort to achieve a high level of transparency here. With an access policy for EudraVigilance, i.e. the EU database of all reported cases of adverse reactions, patients, healthcare professionals, experts and other stakeholders are provided with access to the database content. Caveat statements on the webpage giving access to database content to the public explain that the information relates to suspected adverse reactions, but there is not necessarily a causal relationship, and that the information should not be interpreted as meaning that the medicine is unsafe to use. This welcome step guarantees transparency, but cannot answer the question of which concrete advice is required to patients and healthcare professionals in the case of an uncertain situation.

It should also be considered here that the requirements for reporting adverse reactions to authorities are lower than the requirements for specific safety measures. Companies report numerous adverse reactions and the assessments by the companies and the regulatory authorities come to the conclusion that no measures need to be taken. What are the decisive steps here? The assessment must be made in two stages, as the following figure illustrates (see Fig. 15.2, slide from a presentation by Sträter Lawyers): firstly, the causality assessment, and secondly, the assessment of the impact on the risk-benefit balance.

15.2.2.1 Assessment of Causality

Firstly, it must be clarified whether a new unknown risk must be taken into consideration in the assessment of the risk-benefit balance. The assessment of causality and the degree of suspicion is of decisive importance here (see Fig. 15.2). The decision of the Regional Court of Aachen in the thalidomide case described above provides pertinent guidance. As already explained, a decision had to be made within the

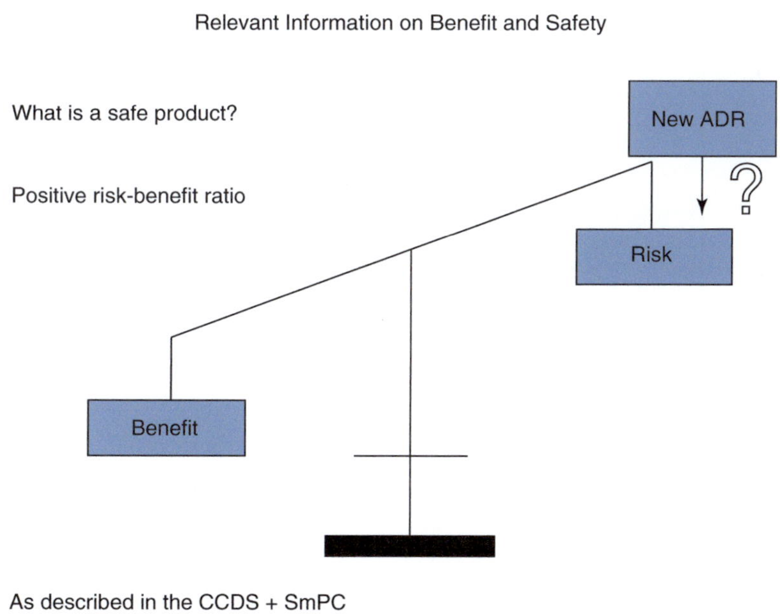

Fig. 15.2 Assessment of risk information. *ADR* adverse drug reaction, *CCDS* company core data sheet, *SmPC* summary of product characteristics

framework of criminal proceedings as to whether it was acceptable for the employees of the responsible company to wait to inform the public or whether this waiting was already to be considered as culpable. This question always arises for employees in companies when new unknown and especially serious adverse reactions arise. The Court's ruling within the framework of criminal responsibility is clear: it is not permissible to wait until there is certainty. Rather, indication of a reasonable suspicion of causal relationship is a relevant criterion.

The following figure illustrates this principle (see Fig. 15.3, slide from a presentation by Sträter Lawyers):

In the coordinated system of knowledge acquisition, a distinction can be made between the type of knowledge (see the x-axis) obtained in relation to its evidential value (see the y-axis). The classical process of epistemology according to Karl Popper (Popper 1934) starts with the formation of hypotheses. Clinical trials or other research, for example, are then initiated in order to verify or falsify the hypothesis made. We therefore call them "confirmatory studies". If the proof of the theory succeeds, the "sun of knowledge" is attained.

The assessment of causality must therefore be defined: Has the status of hypothesis and theory formation been achieved, but proof not yet been obtained? In such a case, two co-existent theories stand side by side, one favours causality whilst the other denies it. If the "sun of knowledge" has not yet been reached, no final conclusion can be drawn according to scientific criteria. It is important to recognise that *legal requirements* now determine the *duty to act*. The Regional Court of Aachen makes it clear that if there are reasonable grounds for suspicion, i.e. serious

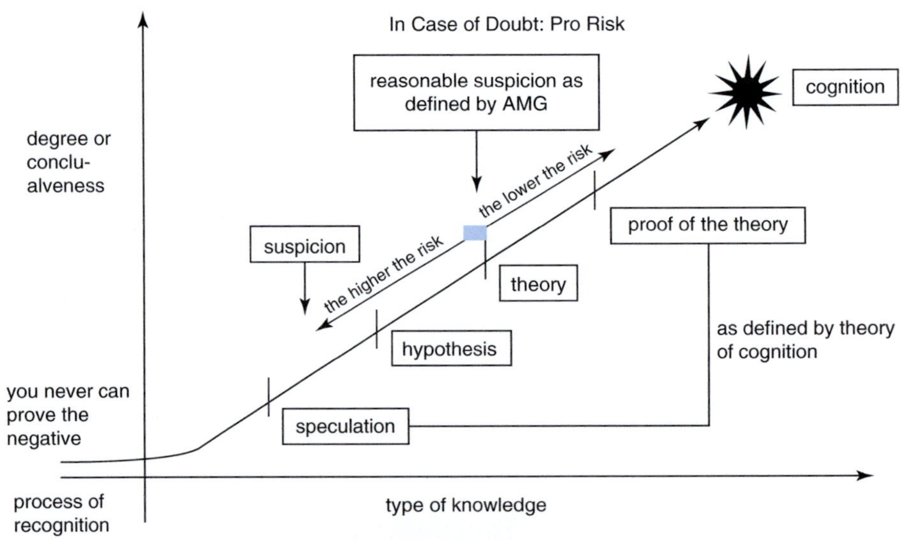

Fig. 15.3 Dealing with uncertainty in risk assessments—"In case of doubt: pro risk". *AMG* Arzneimittelgesetz, i.e. the German medicines law, which also implements EU Directives

indications, waiting is negligent. If a company does not wish to expose itself to the charge of culpable conduct, it must act despite the uncertain scientific situation. The precautionary principle described above also follows these principles.

On the other hand, it is important to recognise that not every suspicion arising from reports on suspected adverse reactions qualifies for triggering duties to act in relation to communication to the public. Below the threshold of *justified suspicion, pure speculation* cannot trigger duties to act. A typical and misleading question is: "Can you rule out the existence of a causal link?" It should be noted here that even according to the rules of epistemology and logic, the non-existence of a fact can never be proven—you can never prove the negative (Popper 1934)! Risks can never be ruled out. However, this cannot be the decisive criteria for duties to act. A suspicious case with minimum criteria triggers reporting duties. A reasonable suspicion of causality obliges the case to be incorporated in the risk-benefit assessment and may possibly require inclusion in the product information and other communication to patients and healthcare professionals.

For example, the regulatory authorities in Europe based their approval of the rofecoxib-containing medicinal product Vioxx® (see Chap. 3) on these criteria in relation to cardiovascular risks. At the time of the marketing authorisation, there was no evidence that rofecoxib has cardiotoxic effects. However, there was reason for suspicion. Corresponding warnings were included in the product information. This was based on the VIGOR study, which showed clear superiority compared to other non-steroidal anti-inflammatory drugs (NSAIDs) in terms of the gastro-intestinal adverse reactions. However, the study substantiated the suspicion that cardiotoxic effects are significantly increased. The pharmaceutical company interpreted this as a cardioprotective effect of the comparator substance naproxen (FDA Arthritis Advisory Committee 2001). This theory seemed plausible. However, the regulatory authorities in Europe and also the US FDA did not agree, as could be seen in their assessments and the description of these adverse reactions in the summary of product characteristics and package leaflet (ODDB 2002). When at a later date further studies on the treatment of colon carcinoma showed evidence of the causality of cardiological risks, there was no fundamental change in the assessment, but just a further step from reasonable suspicion to knowledge. Therefore, it can be argued that the responsible company "over-reacted" with the recall of the medicinal product from the market (whilst others criticised that the product should have been withdrawn earlier (see Chap. 1)). The risk-benefit balance was positive, also taking into account the cardiotoxic effects already described in the product information. In view of the coexistence of both theories—cardioprotective versus cardiotoxic effect—regulatory authorities had consistently assumed the worst case, namely a cardiotoxic effect, and nonetheless reached a positive risk-benefit assessment, above all because within the class of NSAIDs, the COX-2 inhibitors, such as rofecoxib, have a significantly lower gastro-intestinal risk. This also explains why other COX-2 inhibitors with similar risk-benefit profiles have remained on the market and have also been re-authorised, such as celecoxib and etoricoxib.

15.2.2.2 Assessment of Impact on the Risk-Benefit Balance and Information Requirements

This makes it clear that the second step following the causality assessment requires special attention. In this step, it must be examined what effects new risk information has on the risk-benefit balance. Questions arise as to whether the positive assessment of the benefit to risk "starts to falter", whether the benefit does still prevail, and which measures, restrictions—communicated by warnings and other information to patients and healthcare professionals—can justify a positive assessment of the risk-benefit balance? The following overview illustrates this (see Fig. 15.4, slide from a presentation by Sträter Lawyers):

If, as in the case of thalidomide, the indication of sleep disorders in pregnant women constitutes the benefit, the result of the decision on the suspicion of causality of the teratogenic risks is clear: immediate and rapid product recall and corresponding information to specialised doctors, other healthcare professionals and affected patients. However, if the indication is multiple myeloma (see Chap. 1) and a pregnancy prevention programme is already part of the terms of marketing authorisation, the risk-benefit assessment can be positive, in favour of the treatment of multiple myeloma.

The same situation arises with the use of the active substance isotretinoin (see Chap. 4) to treat acne, which often occurs in women of child-bearing age. However, this substance is teratogenic in the same way as thalidomide. Here, too, it is remarkable that the regulatory authorities see a positive risk-benefit balance despite teratogenic risks if pregnancy can be prevented with all conceivable risk minimisation measures and communication.

In such cases, package leaflets and summaries of product characteristics must be re-designed. A direct healthcare professional communication (DHPC), other communication materials or labelling of the packaging may be required. Details are provided in the EU-GVP Modules XV and XVI and EU-GVP Annex II.

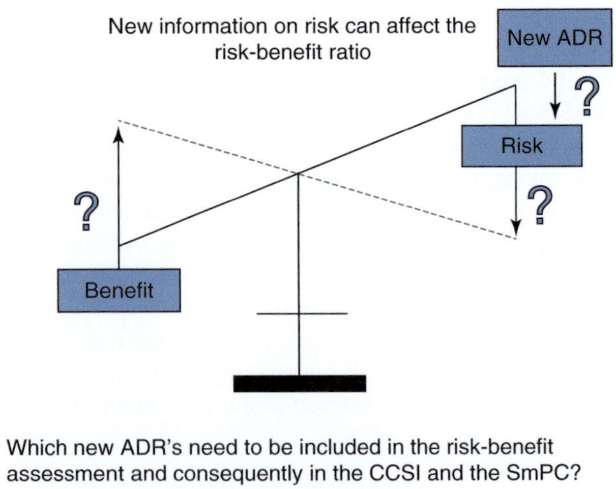

Fig. 15.4 Impact of new risk information on the assessment of the risk-benefit balance. *ADR* adverse drug reaction, *CCSI* company core safety information, *SmPC* summary of product characteristics

Interactions with Other Medicinal Products

New types of risk frequently result from the interaction between co-administrated medicinal products, particularly when new products are used in combination with established treatment schedules for a particular disease or in the treatment of multiple diseases. Although substances are thoroughly tested for interactions before marketing authorisation, new adverse reactions can suddenly occur due to not yet known interactions. However, the risks arising from interactions with other medicinal products can be addressed by appropriate measures such as mutual contraindications or warnings in the interaction sections of the package leaflet and the summary of product characteristics. If, in the case of newly identified risks, the physicians concerned are also informed by a direct healthcare professional communication (DHPC), the risk can be reduced to an acceptable level. A withdrawal of only one medicine due to interaction with another medicinal product may then be not the appropriate measure, but the provision of broad information about the interactions might be preferable.

15.2.2.3 Priorities in Implementing New Information and Risk Minimisation Measures

When a newly identified risk requires patients and healthcare professionals to be informed, the question arises as to how quickly they must be communicated. The following criteria should be considered:

- *Implementation in production of medicinal products*

Routine updates of package leaflets and summaries of product characteristics occur every once or twice a year, but are not sufficient including for urgent information. Even the next production of a new batch is often inappropriate because there are still larger quantities of packages on the market and the supply chain of wholesalers and pharmacies, so that new package leaflets only reach patients with a delay of 2–3 years. Moreover, patients and physicians may not implement the changes in safe use advice, because they do not constantly "scan" for changes in package leaflets they receive for their medicines, in particular for chronic diseases, or, respectively, summaries of product characteristics they can access as healthcare professionals. The recall of medicinal products from the market to replace old package leaflets is time consuming, may jeopardise the continuous supply of medicines and patient care, and still does not provide the relevant information to the target audience in good time if it is not made known wildly at the time of the recall.

It is particularly risky for companies to collect several new pieces of information on the correct use of medicines in order to implement them in a joint change much later. In such case the version of the package leaflet distributed in the current supply chain and read by patients clearly deviates from the current state of knowledge. If this is multiplied in the worldwide supply chain, the inconsistency with the current state of knowledge increases and becomes widespread. In order to avoid this, the company core safety information must be adapted to the current state of knowledge *and* be implemented at short notice in global sales. The priorities here should be risk-proportionate, and companies should follow appropriate standard operation procedures (SOPs) of a quality-assured pharmacovigilance system to ensure that in any case the attempt has been made to implement the stipulated information in the respective legal system of the country concerned. If national law does not allow this, it cannot, by its very nature, be forced. If, however, the attempt has not even been made, and warnings from European or US package leaflets have not been not implemented, harmed patients will have a good case to hold the company liable. Cooperation between regulatory and pharmacovigilance departments is therefore required to speed up the process, so that the necessary risk minimisation measures and communication can be implemented quickly.

Perhaps in the future it will also be possible to send "push mails" using mobile health apps for chronic diseases in order to provide the new information to physicians and patients. We are still a long way from this but I am convinced that it will come faster than anyone expects.

- *Impact on supply*

As hinted to already, when amending package leaflets and summaries of product characteristics, it must be considered that the recall of medicinal products from the market could endanger the care of patients, especially in the case of serious illnesses. Recalls can lead to supply bottlenecks! In such cases, the product must remain available on the market. Here, however, it is helpful to provide information to the healthcare professionals and patients directly in the form of a direct healthcare professional communication (DHPC).

- *Priorities for implementation according to the type of information*

The official texts in package leaflets and summary of product characteristics can be differentiated as follows: The first part deals with how to use the medicinal product correctly and in accordance with the requirements of the marketing authorisation. This covers the sections on indication, contraindication, warnings and precautions, and dosing. The second part includes adverse reactions. For including them, as said before, there must be a reasonable suspicion of the causal relationship between the adverse event and the medicine. As far as adverse reactions can be prevented, suitable risk minimisation measures are described in the first part, and preventability is a driving criterion to amend product information quickly. Preventability may also drive including a precautionary warning where there is uncertainty about the causal relationship.

A clear prioritisation can be derived from the point of view of liability in favour of the first part of the of the product information, as it contains crucial information for the safe use of the medicinal product. For example, if a patient receives information on a relevant contraindication too late, i.e. after having taken the medicinal product and suffering irreversible damage, the question that will spontaneously arise is: since when has the pharmaceutical company known about this and why was I not notified in good time? The patient has a good chance of proving that the incorrect and out-of-date information in the package leaflet has caused the damage, e.g. if a contraindication is missing. With a view to protecting the patient and reducing liability risks for the company and its employees, such kind of information therefore deserves absolute priority in its communication to healthcare professionals and patients.

By contrast and perhaps surprisingly, timely information on possible adverse reactions in the second part of the product information is of less importance. Not every missing piece of information on adverse reactions influences the therapeutic decision or leads to liability. Rather, the patient must make a convincing argument that he or she would not have taken a medicinal product, if having knowledge about this adverse reaction. Often, however, an indicated product is without alternative, especially in the case of serious diseases.

15.2.3 Information About Newly Identified Risks with Medicines: Considerations for Regulatory Authorities

The discussion so far has focussed on the responsibility and liability of companies and employees for appropriate communication with healthcare professionals and patients. The question arises as to whether regulatory authorities and their employees are subject to the same obligations.

The employees of the authorities are indeed obliged to implement their regulatory decisions and supervise companies to be compliant with the resulting requirements. It is quite possible that the regulatory procedures in accordance with legislation take a long time. If the company recognises earlier that certain measures are necessary, there may already be an obligation to implement them, even before the authority decides on measures. It would however certainly not be good practice of the company to "overtake the authorities on the inside" by unilateral measures. According to the legal requirements in the EU, a company must rather inform the authorities *before* taking any action. There is also a practical reason behind. How should an authority react adequately to the withdrawal of a product if it has not been adequately and sufficiently informed by the companies in advance?

It may well be a requirement of liability law to take early action on issues on which there is consensus between the authority and the company. If, for example, there is a proposal of ten measures to be taken and there is already consensus on five dealing with the safe use of the product, it cannot be justified to allow a long time to implement these because of the ongoing discussion on the other five points. In this respect, it may be necessary to inform healthcare professionals and patients on the agreed five measures and the ongoing discussions, e.g. by means of a direct healthcare professional communication (DHPC).

Conversely, employees in regulatory authorities must be aware that the rules on official liability can lead to claims for damages being brought against the state for employee negligence if no action is taken. Procedures of this kind are not frequent, but they are possible and can have very lasting effects for the employees concerned.

15.3 Outlook: Relevance, Improvements and Future Potential

15.3.1 Current Challenges and Developments

When planning risk communication, it is important—ideally within the framework of a multidisciplinary approach (see Chap. 1)—to also satisfy the legal obligations on patient protection. Similarly, in a review such as a court case, communication interventions made (or not made) are also evaluated to determine whether they satisfied legal obligations.

The approved package leaflet and summary of product characteristics describe the findings on benefit and risk of a medicinal product. They determine further communication and advertising. Since this information must correspond to the level of scientific knowledge, the obligation to guarantee consistent information on the medicinal product of the same company throughout the world results from this, ideally also independently of the manufacture in future. Consistent information satisfies the responsibility towards the patient and is suitable to reduce liability risks of a civil and criminal law nature. The definition of company core safety information as a global document accurately describes the matter.

Harmonising information on generic and original medicinal products is a particular challenge because they are not under the responsibility of the same company. The authorities are therefore called upon here to push for harmonisation between these products of identical type. Regional cooperation, as is increasingly established in the various regions of the world, may in future strengthen the authorities in this respect.

New, in particular serious, adverse reactions deserve special attention in pharmacovigilance, and the assessment must inevitably follow as to whether this new knowledge has consequences for the information provided to the patients and healthcare professionals and the distribution of the medicinal product, and whether the precautionary principle must be applied if the data situation is still uncertain. Neglecting this principle will rather result in very serious criminal law consequences for employees and civil liability risks for the company, because waiting until evidence is available may be considered negligent under criminal law, especially if major damage to potentially affected patients must be reduced. This is not only a requirement of decency in terms of the responsibility toward the patients. The huge challenge—and this will remain so in the future—is which evidence can legitimately trigger the precautionary principle.

The digitalisation of information and the widespread use of mobile health apps used in adherence programmes are promising. They open up the option of using push mails to inform chronically ill patients in particular and their attending physicians about new information and illnesses. The speed with which information is communicated is far ahead of the conversion of package leaflets and summary of product characteristics and their perception by patients.

15.3.2 Alert Information Overload Due to Liability Phobia?

The design of package leaflets, particularly in Europe, is a matter for concern. The information is extensive and often designed to make it difficult for patients to understand it. There is a danger that patients may not follow the doctor's prescriptions due to the wealth and type of information, and may interrupt necessary medication. The information can therefore cause risks to the patients due to incompliance. The EU guideline on readability (European Commission 2009) has made a first contribution here, and this is most welcome. For example, it can be observed that package leaflets and summaries of product characteristics for centrally authorised medicinal products are less comprehensive than those for products with purely national authorisations from EU member states. The European Commission has just launched an initiative for further improvement (Mezher 2017).

A final question: Do liability strategies have an inappropriate influence on the design of the package leaflets?

It is difficult to answer this because the process has many factors shaped by the marketing authorisation practice of over 100 regulatory authorities throughout the world and driven by different legal interpretations. Within the EU, a welcome harmonisation is to be observed on the basis of quite different cultures. The question that arises frequently in the context of the discussion on harmonising the package leaflets of originators and generic companies is the following: "Should we not continue to mention the wealth of adverse reactions for liability reasons?" The principles developed in this chapter can claim validity here according to which only the information on risks is of importance for which there is a reasonable suspicion of causality. Below this threshold, information is not legally required. If, therefore, package leaflets are to be updated, or "cleaned up", and superfluous information removed, this principle is suitable for the process. Transparency geared to patient protection must be ensured according to these criteria whilst avoiding a superfluous and often incomprehensible flood of information.

Conclusions

- Understanding the legal obligations of pharmaceutical companies and regulatory authorities in relation to medicines information and advertisement in any given jurisdiction is vital for appropriately preparing of medicinal product-related communication, and likewise for its evaluation.
- New, unexpected and in particular serious adverse reactions deserve special attention in the pharmacovigilance of the responsible companies, not only for risk assessment but also for communication purposes.
- As the case of the thalidomide has taught, the precautionary principle calls for rapid information if major potential harm needs to be mitigated where

there is a reasonable suspicion of a causal relationship with the medicine. This is not only a requirement of decency of responsibility towards the patients; waiting for evidence is to be judged as negligent under criminal law and triggers serious liability risks for companies and employees in the company.

- Current challenges lie in particular in the global consistency of the product information for a given medicinal product, but also the active substance, which should be addressed through the concept of the company core safety information (CSSI) and regional regulatory collaboration.
- The digitalisation of information and wide dissemination of push mails through mobile health apps, for example, are already used in adherence programmes and promise progress for medicinal product safety through the speed with which information is conveyed.
- The future should bring transparency and at the same time avoiding unnecessary and confusing information overload with a view to supporting patient safety.

Declarations After graduating, the author was a judge in Berlin for 5 years and then head of the legal department of the German Federal Health Agency for 5 years. He then established the Sträter law firm and is partner of this law firm which advises pharmaceutical companies and medical device manufacturers, as well as physicians, pharmacies, hospitals and universities. He co-founded the Master's Programme in Drug Regulatory Affairs (MDRA) at the University of Bonn 20 years ago and has headed its examination board for 10 years. Within the study programme, he leads one of the twelve modules, namely the "Pharma law" module, which addresses the balancing act between scientific evaluation and legal framework conditions for risk minimisation and other measures, i.e. also the legal framework described here for information to physicians, pharmacists and patients.

References

Angelmar R (2006) The rise and fall of Baycol/Lipobay. J Med Market 7(1):77–88

Council for International Organizations of Medical Sciences (CIOMS) (1998) Guidelines for preparing core clinical-safety information on drugs (Report of CIOMS Working Group III & V), 2nd edn. CIOMS, Geneva

Council of European Communities (1998) Commission communication on the Community marketing authorisation procedures for medicinal products, Ref. 98/C 229/03, 22.07.1998

Directive 2001/20/EC of the European Parliament and of the Council of 4 April 2001 on the approximation of the laws, regulations and administrative provisions of the member states relating the implementation of good clinical practice in the conduct of clinical trials on medicinal products for human use

Directive 2001/83/EC of the European Parliament and of the Council of 6 November 2001 on the Community code relating to medicinal products for human use

EMA (2004) Note for guidance on definitions and standards for expedited reporting (ICH topic E2D). EMA, London, https://www.ema.europa.eu/en/documents/scientific-guideline/international-conference-harmonisation-technical-requirements-registration-pharmaceuticals-human-use_en-12.pdf

EMA (2019) EU product information for Thalidomide Celgene, http://www.ema.europa.eu/ema/index.jsp?curl=pages/medicines/human/medicines/000823/human_med_001090.jsp&mid=WC0b01ac058001d124

Encyclopaedia Britannica (2020) Hammurabi: King of Babylonia. https://www.britannica.com/biography/Hammurabi

European Commission Guideline on the Readability of the Labelling and Package Leaflet of Medicinal Products for Human Use, Revision 1, 12 January 2009, https://ec.europa.eu/health/sites/health/files/files/eudralex/vol-2/c/2009_01_12_readability_guideline_final_en.pdf

European Commission Notice to Applicants Volume 2A Procedures for marketing authorisations, Chapter 1, December 2016, 2.8 Concept of "applicant" and "marketing authorisation holder"

European Medicines Agency and Heads of Medicines Agencies (2012) Guideline on Good Pharmacovigilance Practices (GVP). London/Amsterdam: European Medicines Agency, since 2012

FDA Arthritis Advisory Committee (February 8, 2001) "VIOXX Gastrointestinal Outcomes Research Trial (VIGOR)", Bonnie Goldmann, slide 39, "Conclusions" slide 49

FDA (2006) Guidance document: adverse reactions section of labelling for human prescription drug and biological products — content and format. FDA, Rockville, MD, United States, https://www.fda.gov/media/72139/download

Froese N (2018) Aristoteles: Logik und Methodik in der Antike, http://www.antike-griechische.de/Aristoteles.pdf

Kloesel/Cyran Arzneimittelrecht Kommentar E1 (2019) (Contergan-Entscheidung und A 1.0 Anmerkungen 12, 25, 26, 27, 29 zu § 5 AMG – Definition der Bedenklichkeit eines Arzneimittels)

Mezher M (2017) European Commission recommends changes to SmPCs, package leaflets. Regulatory Focus, https://www.raps.org/regulatory-focus™/news-articles/2017/3/european-commission-recommends-changes-to-smpc,-package-leaflets

ODDB (2002) Summary of product characteristics for Vioxx, section on "Clinical Efficacy", 5th paragraph, http://ch.oddb.org/de/gcc/fachinfo/reg/55050

Popper K (1934) Epistemology and philosophy of science in "The Logic of Scientific Discovery", https://en.wikipedia.org/wiki/Karl_Popper

Regional Court of Aachen in the Thalidomide decision, see remark 1, and very instructively the Administrative Court of Cologne on risk measures of the Federal Institute for Drugs and Medical Devices (BfArM) in PharmR 9/2014, page 410 ff

Regulation (EC) No. 726/2004 of the European Parliament and of the Council of 31 March 2004 laying down Community procedures for the authorisation and supervision of medicinal products for human and veterinary use and establishing a European Medicines Agency

Regulation (EU) No. 536/2014 of the European Parliament and of the Council of 16 April 2014 on clinical trials on medicinal products for human use, and repealing Directive 2001/20/EC

Rühl U (2005) Ist Rechtswissenschaft überhaupt eine Wissenschaft?, with further notes on the antique understanding of science and on the tense relationship between natural science and humanities, with further notes on the significance of categorising sciences according to Aristotle, https://www.jura.uni-bremen.de/uploads/Ulli_Ruehl/Ruhl-ReWi_Vortrag.pdf

Science Museum (2017) Brought to life – exploring the history of medicine: Thalidomide. London: Science Museum [webpage]. Accessed: 2 July 2017

Uhlmann G (2016) Ringvorlesung: 2400 Jahre Aristoteles und Aristotelismen. Freie Universität Berlin, https://www.geisteswissenschaften.fu-berlin.de/we02/griechisch/graezistik/aristotelismuszentrum/RVL2400.html

Wikipedia (2020) Vorsorgeprinzip, https://de.m.wikipedia.org/wiki/Vorsorgeprinzip

From Passive to Active: Patients as Contributors to Medicinal Product Risk Communication Research

16

François Houÿez

Abstract

Since the 1980s, as a result of the AIDS epidemic, we have witnessed the rise of patient movements that have successfully advocated for the development of new medicines, changes in pharmaceutical legislation and policies and increasing participation in governmental decision-making. Based on the concept of patient-centred healthcare, this chapter discusses that patients can and should be proactive in highlighting their information needs and interests, and come together in patient organisations that may initiate, contribute to or even conduct medicinal product risk communication research. This chapter shares the real life experiences of patient representatives and makes proposals for the future with a global outlook.

F. Houÿez (✉)
European Organisation for Rare Diseases (EURORDIS), Paris, France
e-mail: francois.houyez@eurordis.org

© Springer Nature Singapore Pte Ltd. 2020

P. Bahri (ed.), *Communicating about Risks and Safe Use of Medicines*,
https://doi.org/10.1007/978-981-15-3013-5_16

16.1 Patients at the Centre of Communication About Medicines

Making information available and in a timely manner so that patients and their families can make informed decisions is a principle of patient-centred healthcare. Patient-centred care has been defined as care where the individual's health needs and desired outcomes are the driving force behind all healthcare decisions and quality measurements. Patients are therefore seen as partners with their healthcare professionals, and treated not only from a clinical perspective, but also from emotional, mental, spiritual, social and financial perspectives (New England Journal of Medicine Catalyst 2017).

Patients—unlike scientific assessors of medicines, who separate the assessments of benefits and risks and weigh these in what is called a risk-benefit balance for deciding if the risks are acceptable—always weigh benefits and risks of treatment options together, based on the information they obtain. They perceive risks as higher or lower in light of the expected benefit. In addition, the more severe the disease, the more quickly—without too much reflection—patients accept higher risks as long as benefits are likely. On the other hand, once the disease is effectively controlled by the medication, the constraints and burdens arising from long-term medication prescriptions—such as organising one's daily life around fixed times of intake—and side effects the medicine may or may not have become more prominent in the patient's risk perception. A side effect, or adverse reaction in technical terminology, which was initially acceptable and tolerable, becomes unbearable when health of the patient returns to normal.

How patients perceive and accept risks in the context of the expected benefits has fundamental implications for their information and communications needs and expectations.

16.1.1 Adverse Reactions to HAART: A Key Experience

The typical ways of patients' risk perception became apparent through the discussion around adverse effects and long-term adherence to treatments against human immunodeficiency virus (HIV) and its manifestation, acquired immune deficiency syndrome (AIDS) (Boyle 2000). In retrospect, this constitutes a key experience for patients as well as specialists in safety surveillance and risk management of medicines or pharmacovigilance.

Effective medication against HIV/AIDS became available in 1996, as highly active antiretroviral treatment or in short HAART, consisting of a personalised combination of several active substances against the virus. This was one of the most important breakthroughs in pharmaceutical history, which changed within only a little more than a decade a deadly disease into a—as we know it now—manageable condition with the possibility of a normal life expectancy. However, not long after the regulatory marketing authorisation of these medicines for use in healthcare, many patients using HAART long-term experienced changes in body shape due to accumulation and/or loss of fat tissue. This metabolic disorder, later called lipodystrophy, had not been detected during the clinical trials that tested these substances before marketing authorisation. This was because the onset of the disorder occurs only after treatment longer than the usual duration of a clinical trial. The mean time to onset for lipodystrophy varies from 14 (Carr et al. 1998) to 38 (Price et al. 2015) months, whereas the clinical trials typically lasted for 24 weeks, during which the decrease, in the human body, of genetic material of the virus, i.e. the HIV's ribonucleic acid (RNA) was used as a surrogate marker for proving that the medicine was efficacious. At this early time of marketing, the lipodystrophy side effect had not yet been described, not even been named, and any long-term adverse consequences of HAART and their seriousness were generally unknown.

Patients experiencing or hearing about these new adverse effects that they suspected were being caused by HAART interrupted on a large scale their life-saving treatment. Even if understandable, this was a dangerous behaviour. These patients did not only risk an increase in the viral load in their bodies, but also risked that viruses that were genetically different and had not yet been successfully destroyed by the treatment multiplied in their bodies, rendering a later re-start of the medicine possibly ineffective—a phenomenon called resistance development of the virus.

Once patients had reported the lipodystrophy side effect to authorities—which was facilitated by global networking and exchange through the then increasing use of the internet—studies were initiated under the Oversight Committee on Metabolic Disorders of HAART, newly established by the regulatory bodies in the European Union (EU) and the manufacturers of the products (Carr et al. 2003) to investigate the causality. The Oversight Committee also involved researchers and data sources from the United States (US). The research resulted in updates to the product information with the risk of lipodystrophy, coordinated by regulators on both sides of the Atlantic.

Another risk of HAART identified after marketing authorisation and investigated under the Oversight Committee was the increase of the cardiovascular mortality for an individual after 5 years on HAART (Bozzette et al. 2003; Data Collection on Adverse Events of Anti-HIV Drugs (DAD) Study Group 2003), which the study estimated as a twofold risk increase. Yet, regulatory bodies considered the risk-benefit balance as remaining positive in favour of treating HIV patients. One must remember that studies from Australia, Europe and the United States of individuals diagnosed with AIDS before 1986 showed a median survival time past the initial diagnosis of 10–13 months (Bacchetti et al. 1988; Batalla et al. 1989; Stehr-Green et al. 1989; Whyte et al. 1989). A twofold increased risk of serious cardiovascular adverse effects also emerged a short time later for a different product, the anti-inflammatory medicine rofecoxib (Vioxx®), which resulted in a negative risk-benefit assessment and withdrawal of this product from the market (see Chap. 3). That means that a patient on HAART and rofecoxib would have been told that both products double the risk for a cardiovascular incident, but one, the HAART, should be continued, and the other one, rofecoxib, should be stopped. For a message of this kind to be understood correctly and adhered to by the patient, it is necessary to communicate and explain the criteria for considering a risk-benefit balance positive or negative and what are the consequences of stopping a treatment.

16.1.2 Research Questions of Relevance to Patient-Centred Communication

The experience with HAART shows that the generation, assessment and communication of evidence about the benefits and risks of medicines, including the scientific uncertainty due to missing data from long-term use or in specific concurrent medical conditions, are interlinked and make medicinal product risk communication for patients and the general public highly complex and challenging. To understand the underling factors and possible solutions to the challenges, the following research questions are of particular relevance:

- From where do patients get information about risks?
- What can they do when they consider the information as not sufficient?
- What risks really matter—the risk of getting an adverse reaction in the first place or the consequences of it—and how can one know how bad, i.e. serious and irreversible, the consequences can be?
- How should the information on the risks be appropriately balanced against the information on the benefits, particularly when the risks are not clearly identified and quantified?
- How can complex pharmacoepidemiological concepts and measurements be translated into concise information that patients can easily use?
- How can the information be tailored to different patient audiences?

This chapter discusses that patients can and should be a part of researching the answers to these questions; and that they are a part of the solution for improving medicinal product risk communication. This highlights which aspects are important to consider when designing research about how patients receive, perceive and use information. It further stresses that patients are not passive but active audiences and suggests that they should not only be subject to research observations but, in the fundamental sense of the term, possibly be researchers themselves, proactively providing their information needs and interests. This is in line with the concept of participatory action research (see Chap. 1) and could essentially support planning communication and evaluating its effectiveness. As individuals, patients should not only be observant, give feedback and participate in research projects, but may also come together in patient organisations and initiate, contribute to or even conduct relevant research, and provide input to research priorities and policies.

For this purpose, this chapter shares the real life experience of the author in his leading roles in patient groups for advocacy, pharmacovigilance and communication. Examples given stem from mainly from Europe, but it is acknowledged that many countries in the world have successful patient organisations.

16.1.3 Communication for Advocacy: How Patients Started to Fight for New Medicines

The active role of organised patients in the development of medicines and communication of their benefits and risks started in the US in 1980/81 with the AIDS epidemic. Patients and their peers immediately started to question researchers if any progress was on its way in identifying the cause of the syndrome and treating its consequences. Being called or stigmatised as an "AIDS victim" was clearly rejected by those affected; instead, many patients decided to have an active role.

16.1.3.1 The Denver Principles

In 1983, a group of fifteen people[1] living with HIV or AIDS gathered in the US city Denver for the Second National AIDS Forum at the National Lesbian and Gay Health Conference to agree on guiding principles for future action. They defined the philosophy of their engagement as: "We condemn attempts to label us as victims, a term which implies defeat, and we are only occasionally patients, a term which implies passivity, helplessness and dependence upon the care of others". Eleven principles followed this preamble, the so-called Denver Principles of HIV Advocacy (People with AIDS Advisory Committee 1983). While most of these were specific to the fight against HIV/AIDS, two can be generalised and are applicable to patients with any medical condition:

- To be involved at every level of decision-making for all decisions that affect patients' lives;
- To be included in all forums with equal credibility as other participants for sharing own experiences and knowledge.

These two principles can be considered as fundamental to patient-centred healthcare as well as the role of patients in advocacy and participation in governmental decision-making. Therefore, the term "patient" is adopted in this chapter for persons living with a medical condition, however, not with a passive connotation, but in the sense of patients actively engaging in their health, as far the condition and situation allows them of course. In this book it is overall acknowledged that anybody is or can become a patient (see Chap. 1). The Denver activists could probably not have known that their engagement would establish advocacy for new medicines driven by patients, which is now common in many disease areas.

[1] From San Francisco: Bobbi Campbell (1952–1984), Bobby Reynolds (–1987), Dan Turner (1948–1990), Michael Helquist representing his partner Mark Feldman, who had planned to attend but died shortly before the conference; from New York City: Michael Callen (1955–1993), Bob Cecchi (1942–1991), Phil Lanzaratta (–1986), Richard Berkowitz, Bill Burke, Artie Felson, Tom Nasrallah, Matthew Sarner; from Los Angeles: Gar Traynor; Elbert from Kansas City by way of Houston; and one individual from Denver whose name has been forgotten.

16.1.3.2 Health Advocacy

Advocacy in health is an activity for overcoming major barriers to public and occupational health improvements that are due to the current situation and societal conditions, which cannot be addressed at individual level. The modern use of the term "advocacy" for this purpose gained momentum from the Ottawa Charter on Health Promotion of 1986, which defines health promotion as aiming to make conditions favourable for health through advocacy, whereby these factors may be political, economic, social, cultural, environmental, behavioural or biological. As such advocacy shapes the societal and political climate (World Health Organization (WHO) Advocacy 2019). Advocacy is a strategic series of action designed to influence those who hold governmental, political, economic or private power, in order to effect change in favour of those of less power or else more vulnerable (Ayer and Bunn 2004). Strategies and communication for advocacy use emerging opportunities or create own events, and often apply imaginative, dramatic and newsworthy tactics (World Health Organization (WHO) Advocacy 2019). As this chapter shows, advocacy makes increasingly use of systematically collected data, e.g. from scientific publications, own surveys or social media forums.

16.1.3.3 The Impact of HIV Patient Advocacy on Regulation of Medicines

The Denver Principles inspired actions of many AIDS groups throughout the US, while in Europe the first groups were more oriented towards direct support to patients through the organisation of home care services as well as information and prevention campaigns.

The identification of the virus by Prof. Françoise Barré-Sinoussi and her team in France in 1985 attracted much public attention and hopes emerged that maybe the first effective treatment would be discovered too in the country where the virus was identified first. In July 1985, Rock Hudson, a famous US actor who had announced by way of a press statement in the previous month to be in France for treatment against AIDS (History.com 2009), said in public that he would "fly Concorde" to have access to a compound from a French pharmaceutical company, called HPA-23, as in his words "Only the country where HIV was discovered could find the magic cure". Within hours, transcontinental flights to France were fully booked by more than 100 US citizens wanting to enrol in clinical trials for HPA-23. This compound, antimonium tungstate by its chemical name, later proved to not be effective against AIDS (Van 1985; Wikipedia 2019).

In March 1987, concerned individuals in the US united to form the AIDS Coalition to Unleash Power (ACT UP) in New York, San Francisco and other large US cities. ACT UP and other HIV activist organisations accused the US Food and Drug Administration (US FDA) of unnecessarily delaying the approval of medications to fight HIV and subsequent opportunistic infections. Their campaigns communicated through posters (e.g. New York Public Library, Manuscripts and Archives Division, New York Public Library Digital Collections 1969–1997)—one example is shown in Figure 16.1—and ACT UP's first demonstration

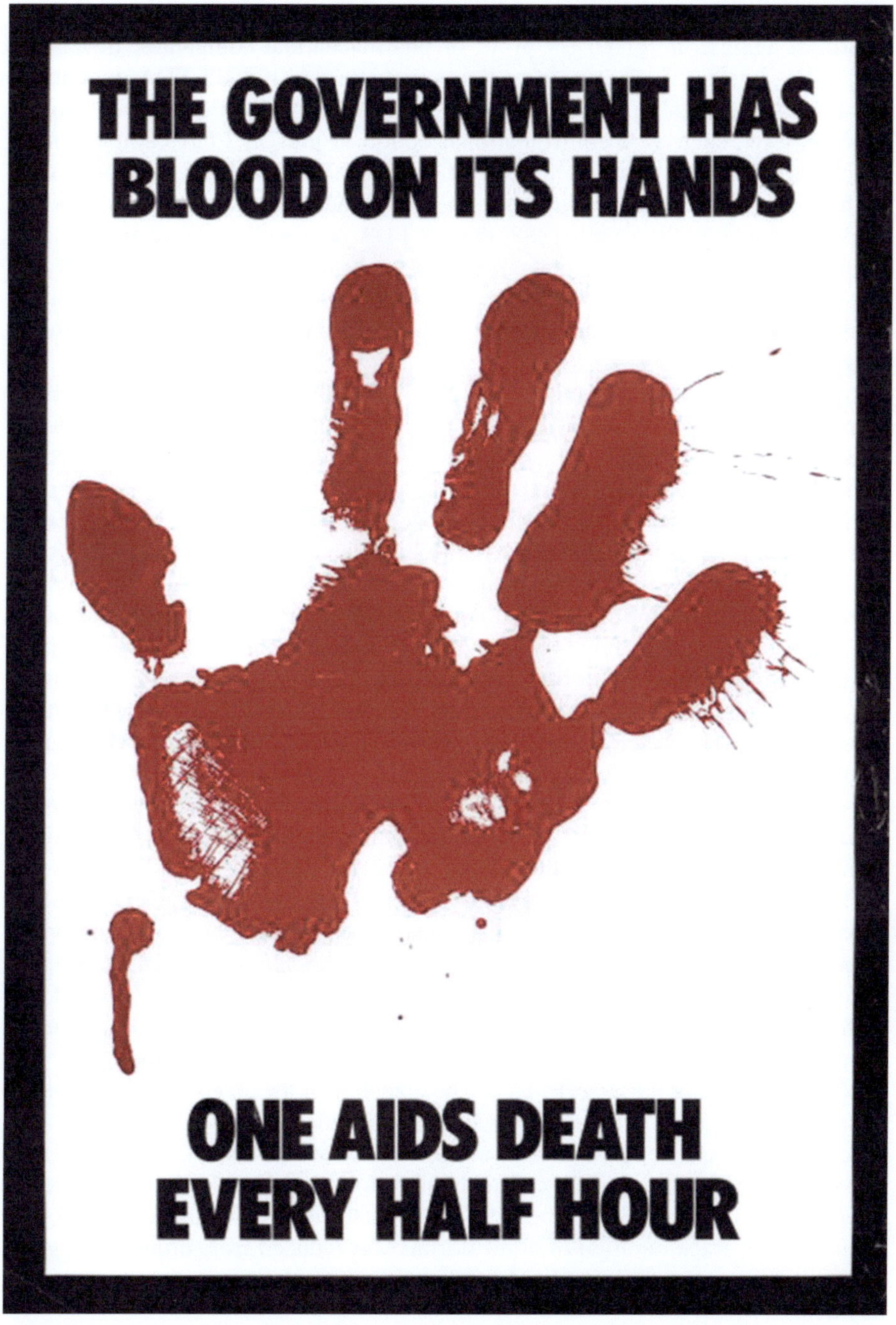

Fig. 16.1 Example of poster for patient advocacy communication (New York Public Library, Manuscripts and Archives Division, New York Public Library Digital Collections 1969–1997)

took place on New York's Wall Street 3 weeks after its foundation on 24 March, to protest against the greed for profit of pharmaceutical companies. Seventeen people were arrested. Shortly after the demonstration, the US FDA announced that it would shorten its approval process by 2 years. ACT UP continued staging large protests, such as a confrontational action at the US FDA campus on 11 October 1988, which resulted in nearly 180 arrests. The US FDA responded with further improvements of the situation for life-threatening diseases, such as AIDS and cancer, and on 20 March 1987, the US FDA approved zidovudine (AZT) as the first antiretroviral treatment against HIV via its new accelerated approval system (US Food and Drug Administration (US FDA) 2018). Marketing authorisations in Europe were issued shortly after, for example, in Germany in April (Würdemann 1987).

In July 1989, a sister organisation to US ACT UP, ACT UP Paris, was born in France. Although other groups had existed in France since the beginning of the epidemic, some individuals decided to unite for conducting new actions based on civil disobedience, because the AIDS mortality continued to ravage the at-risk populations. Parallel groups in the United Kingdom, i.e. the Terrence Higgins Trust, and in Germany, i.e. the Deutsche AIDS-Hilfe, shared the same analysis: despite the mobilisation of forces and large investments, effective treatments were not yet there. Zidovudine, unfortunately, did not work well, not in all patients and not for long, and if it did work, only for some months. In line with the Denver Principles, patient advocates therefore created community advisory boards to discuss with decision-makers in pharmaceutical industry and public sponsors important research aspects, such as the development plan for a new active substance, clinical trial protocols in terms of design and inclusion criteria, compassionate use of new active substances and fair pricing. In France, TRT5, a coalition of leading AIDS organisations, signed an agreement in 1992 with the Agence Nationale de Recherches sur le Sida (ANRS; now France Recherche Nord & Sud Sida-HIV hépatites), the national AIDS research institute, to review all clinical trials funded by the ANRS. At European level, the European Aids Treatment Group (EATG) set up the European Community Advisory Board (E-CAB) in 1997. An important achievement of European advocacy took place in April 1996, when a first patient delegation met with the Committee for Proprietary Medicinal Products (CPMP), the scientific committee of the European Medicines Evaluation Agency (EMEA; now the European Medicines Agency (EMA)). The objective of the meeting was to propose a change in the guidelines for the evaluation of anti-HIV products. Patients proposed to use surrogate markers such as HIV-RNA and CD4 T cells instead of progression to AIDS or mortality. The EMEA followed the advice, organised a scientific workshop in September 1997 and changed its guidelines. As a consequence, the average duration of clinical trials was reduced from around 3, 4 years with using clinical endpoints to 24 weeks with using the newly agreed surrogate markers.

16.1.4 Communication for Participation: How Patient Organisations Impact on Governmental Decision-Making Today

Today many patient organisations exist around the globe; they vary by status, but usually are not-for-profit. They are more numerous in countries with a long tradition of associations, meaning individuals coming together with the same mission, collecting resources to conduct actions to achieve their goals and with the understanding that members of the board of directors or other governing bodies are not paid. Some patient organisations are local, some are national, usually set up by patients with the same disease or a group of diseases. Patients, but sometimes also parents, carers or people at risk of developing a disease, can become member. Federations of all organisations advocating for a same disease may span across countries, e.g. in Europe, or internationally: their members are patient organisations rather than individuals. Funding varies a lot between organisations, depending on the level of public awareness, the ability of fundraisers to initiate effective methods to collect donations, the existence of funding instruments from public authorities, and on pharmaceutical companies investing in a particular disease. When receiving funds from sources other than their members, organisations adopt policies to preserve their independence vis-à-vis their funders. Some organisations in the EU have developed a code of practices between patient organisations and the healthcare industry, which enables these organisations to collaborate with the EMA without undue influences of industry on the EMA (European Organisation for Rare Diseases (EURORDIS) 2019). This responds to views that patients' organisations could be ground troops acting for the pharmaceutical industry (Herxheimer 2003).

In analysing objectives and methods of health advocacy in Europe, political science researchers like Janine Barbot (1998) stated that advocates' competence was not related to quasi-academic acquisition of biomedical knowledge (as opposed to Steven Epstein 1995), but rather by empirical discussion over clinical trial protocols. But questions on the relation between advocates and those they should represent remain. Is there a patient elite? The first generation of advocates acquired experience as well as medical and other relevant knowledge, but knowledge transfer to new generations may be problematic. Also, the more scientific the topics become, the more specialised patient representatives need to be. Is there a gap between "expert patients" and the "ordinary" patient group members and further the majority of patients, who are not organised in such groups? Do "expert patients" still understand and represent the "ordinary" patient?' Do patient group members obtain more frequently access to clinical trials or compassionate use programmes than non-organised patients? In reality though, apart from a few exceptions, the idea of patients becoming experts to the same extent as scientific experts, as described by Steven Epstein, is exaggerated. Even the objective to engage into an "equal-to-equal" dialogue with scientists might be questionable or even rejected.

16.2 Expectations and Needs for Communication About Risks with Medicines from the Perspective of Patients and the Public

In order to conduct research on medicinal product risk communication from the perspective of patients, understanding their needs and expectations is fundamental, no matter from which scientific discipline one comes and which research methods ones applies (see Chaps. 1–15).

In the EU, representatives of patient and citizen organisations involved at the level of the EMA have issued the following recommendations to improve the communication on the assessments of the risk-benefit balance of medicines:

- Benefits and risks should always be communicated together and the benefits of the medicine should be made more prominent and well explained in the package leaflet in order to provide a good balance between information on risks versus benefits.
- The description of benefits and risks should be provided both in qualitative and quantitative terms.
- Important aspects of adverse reactions to inform patients about are the time to onset (i.e. how long it may take for the reaction to occur after using the medicine for the first time and after which time of use an occurrence of an adverse reaction is unlikely), duration (i.e. how long the reaction may last) and reversibility (i.e. whether it will resolve completely) as well as impact of an adverse reaction on the patient.
- The information should be provided clearly to help choose the most appropriate treatment.
- Factors which may influence a benefit or a risk in an individual should be clearly described (EMEA/CPMP Working Group with Patients' Organisations 2004; European Medicines Agency (EMA) 2009).

These recommendations have become part of the strategy for the EU regulatory network across EU member states, emphasising explicitly: "Information on medicinal products can be further improved to encourage better use of medicines by taking better into account the expectations and needs of both patients and healthcare professionals" (European Medicines Agency (EMA) 2015). Although the recommendations represent a consensus of patient and citizen organisations for the EU, international organisations, namely the International Alliance of Patient Organisations (IAPO) and Health Action International (HAI) are part of the organisations involved by the EMA, and the principles may therefore be considered universal and specifiable to other world regions.

These recommendations of patients towards communication about medicines risks have to be taken into account when defining criteria for planning and evaluating communication interventions. In addition, some major aspects impacting on patients' needs and expectations for medicinal risk communication have to be considered, as discussed next, namely health literacy, numeracy and benefit perception.

16.2.1 Diverse Health Literacy

Health literacy has been defined as the cognitive and social skills which determine the motivation and ability of individuals to gain access to, understand and use information in ways which promote and maintain good health (Nutbeam 1998) or, more focussed on decision-making, the degree to which individuals have the capacity to obtain, process and understand basic health information and services needed to make appropriate health decisions (Selden et al. 2000). As such health literacy has been described as being critical for managing personal health and at the core of everything done in healthcare and public health (Nutbeam 2008; Rubinelli et al. 2009), with the central question of "what does it take to have the capacity to process and understand health information in order to make appropriate health decisions?" (National Academies of Sciences Engineering, and Medicine 2015).

Health literacy varies across different generations of citizens, their different education and socio-economic levels. In a survey in eight European countries (random sample of approximately 1000 citizens of 15 years and older in each country), about 12% of these populations had overall insufficient health literacy and 35% had problematic health literacy, i.e. allowing them to follow instructions but not to come to judgements of their own (HLS-EU Consortium 2012). Thus, it can be estimated that nearly every second citizen in the EU faces life- and health-related decisions with limited health literacy. The situation is even more severe in low- and middle-income countries, but with effort and help of communication and anthropological experts one can strive for informing even illiterate people for understanding and consent.

Any research for planning or evaluating communication interventions about medicines that intends to truly care for patients needs audience segmentation or stratification by health literacy and support communication that helps people making appropriate medication choices regardless of their general health literacy level.

16.2.2 Numeracy and Risk Perception

Among a number of skills, health literacy includes numeracy, i.e. the ability of an individual to reason with numbers and other mathematical concepts and to apply these in a range of contexts and to solve a variety of problems (National Numeracy (NN) 2014–2017). An even more specific skill of numeracy needed to understand risks is statistical literacy, often lacking not only in the general population but also in healthcare professionals. While proposals for clear presentations of data on frequencies and probabilities in healthcare have been made (Gigerenzer et al. 2008), patient advocates use different instruments when discussing a risk-benefit balance with their peers. Some examples are given here.

16.2.2.1 Hazard Cards

To present the quantitative dimension of risks, a card game has been developed at the School of Education, Aarhus University in Denmark called "Hazard Cards" (Hazard Cards 2019), which can help differentiating types of risks with a range of consequences—risks more or less caused by a variety of human activities and more or less avoidable. The cards link risk data with risk perception. To achieve this, the cards depict events that all had high publicity, but different features influencing the perception of the risk, i.e. different so-called cognitive factors. Cognitive factors include, among others, causal relationship with human interference, dreadfulness of outcome, avoidability of the risk and relatedness with reproduction (Bennett 1999). For example, cards provide data for a comparison of the Titanic sinking, the Chernobyl catastrophe, the thalidomide disaster (see Chap. 1) and the risks of the hip surgery cement Boneloc®.

16.2.2.2 Risk Scales

Another useful tool to help understanding the magnitude of a risk is a visual risk scale in the context of other life risks. Patients often express difficulties with verbal and numerical risk quantification, such as the frequencies of adverse reactions of medicines as provided in EU package leaflets. There, adverse reaction frequencies are provided in terms of categories, distinguishing between “very common (may affect more than 1 in 10 people)”, “common (may affect up to 1 in 10 people)”, “uncommon (may affect up to 1 in 100 people)”, “rare (may affect up to 1 in 1,000 people)” or very rare (may affect less than 1 in 10,000 people) (European Commission (EC) 2009). Some patients find this grouping based on a multiplying factor of 10 (i.e. “ten times the risk”) confusing and inappropriate in terms of the ranges covered, i.e. they may find it inappropriate that, e.g. for the category “common” a 1% risk and a 9% risk are grouped together. The covered ranges become apparent when presenting the frequency groups in natural numbers with a constant denominator of 10,000 (see Table 16.1). A risk scale as a visual tool (e.g. (e.g. National Safety Council (NSC) 2017)) supports understanding of these ranges more easily, as shown by Figure 16.2.

16.2.3 Contextualising Risk with Benefit Information

The expectation of patients that risk information should be communicated in relation to information about the expected benefit poses a number of issues of appropriate contextualisation. From a patient’s perspective, the most important question is about the personal likelihood, extent and relevance of the expected benefit, rather than the likelihood and characteristics of the expected benefit as an average over a population. It is this personal benefit that the patient will factor into the personal instantaneous benefit-risk weighing. The benefit-risk perceptions and the individual

Table 16.1 Frequency categories for adverse reactions in EU package leaflets (European Commission (EC) 2009) and their numerical descriptions of the range

Verbal description in PI	Numerical description of the lower and upper values in PI	Numerical description of the range with a constant denominator
Very common	≥1/10	1000–10,000 out of 10,000
Common	≥1/100 and <1/10	100–999 out of 10,000
Uncommon	≥1/1,000 and <1/100	10–99 out of 10,000
Rare	≥1/10,000 and <1/1,000	1–9 out of 10,000
Very rare	<1/10,000	<1 out of 10,000
Very common	≥1/10	1000–10,000 out of 10,000

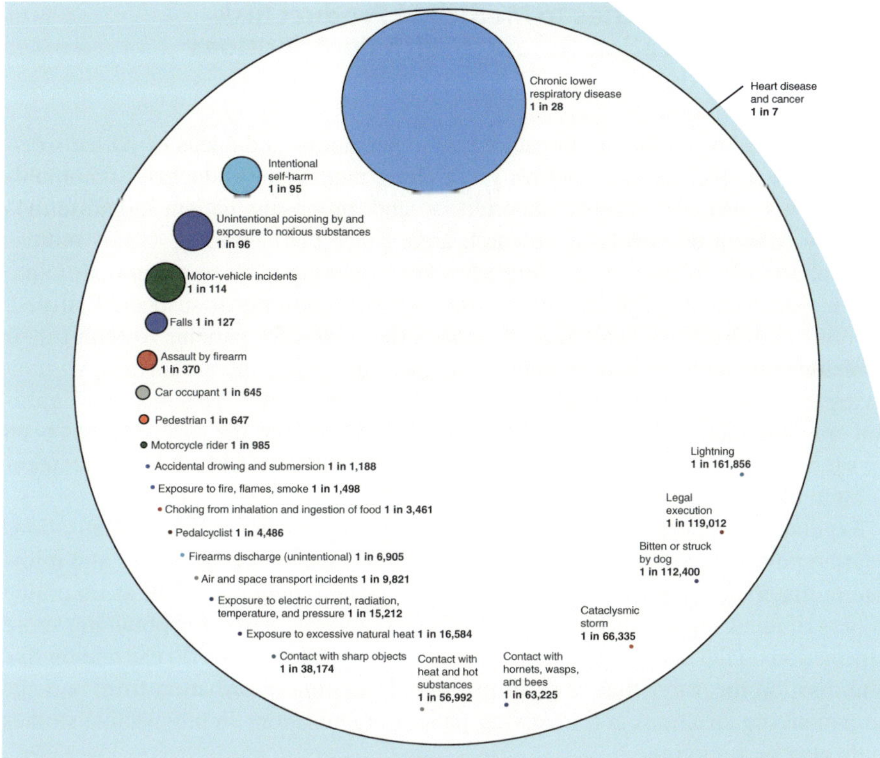

Source: National Safety Council estimates based on from National Center for Health Statistics–Mortality Data for 2014 as compiled from data provided by the 57 vital statistics jurisdictions through the Vital Statistics Cooperative Program. Population and life expectancy data are frome the U.S. Consus Bureau. For mortality figures, estimated one-year and lifetime odds, and external cause classification codes based on the 10th Revision of "The International Classification of Diseases" (ICD) for the causes illustrated, see table on pages 41–42.
[a]Latest official figures.

Fig. 16.2 An example for a risk scale (National Safety Council (NSC) 2017)

decision for a treatment option will depend on the kind of disease. Some diseases affect one main body function and the number of different symptoms is rather limited, while other diseases have heterogeneous clinical manifestations differing from one individual to the next. In the latter case, it is more difficult to select criteria for the expected benefit, in therapeutic decision-making as much as in communication about the therapeutic options.

For example, Friedreich Ataxia (FA) is a neurodegenerative disorder generally characterised by progressive gait and limb ataxia, dysarthria, dysphagia, oculomotor dysfunction, loss of deep tendon reflexes, pyramidal tract signs, scoliosis, and in some patients by cardiomyopathy, diabetes mellitus, visual loss and defective hearing. Treatment of FA is a currently unmet medical need. Attempts have been made to develop a medicine, evaluating the benefit by measuring the change in plasma 8-hydroxy-2'-deoxyguanosine (8OH2'dG). From a patient perspective, however, some clinical outcome assessments could have been used instead, such as in the areas of speech, hand function, bladder control, fatigue and pain, to mention but a few. This example reflects that the needs for evidence and information regarding benefit that is relevant to patients in real life is far more complex than may be seen by those developing and prescribing new medicines.

16.3 New Approaches to Medicinal Product Risk Communication Research with Contributions from Patients

The understanding of factors impacting on expectations and needs of patients discussed in Sect. 16.2 is important for researching medicinal product risk communication. This section presents experiences and proposals patient organisations currently have in this evolving research area. Since the beginning of this millennium, pharmacovigilance as a science has been opening itself to patient participation, in particular through so-called direct patient reporting of suspected adverse reactions (Rolfes 2018). This term describes the option for patients to report their suspicions on side effects they may experience directly to the authorities, without having to see and request a healthcare professional to report it. This means a significant empowerment to patients, as like that they can be sure the suspicion has been reported and will be assessed by the authorities. Patients can add medical documentation to the report and make themselves available for follow-up questions.

Regulatory authorities also seek increasingly input from patient organisations regarding disease experiences, therapeutic preferences, use of medicines and information materials intended for patients and the general public, as well as on policy matters. Patient organisations could also be a potential source for obtaining more information on the benefits and risks of medicines in their real world use and on risk minimisation measures that work in practice. Soliciting information from patients via patient organisations and involving patient organisations in prospective studies could also be an option.

16.3.1 Methods for Collecting Information for Patient-Centred Healthcare

Methods through which data for patient-centred healthcare, such as directly patient-reported outcomes (PROs), quality of life (QoL) parameters and information needs and communication preferences, may be collected from patients include the following:

- randomised trials;
- longitudinal real world studies, which could also be based on patient registries, patient-managed health records and patient diaries in electronic or other formats;
- surveys, which could be based on registration in community or hospital pharmacies, in particular of new users of a medicine;
- focus groups.

Patient organisations can advocate for, participate in or conduct own studies applying these methods, for example, through questionnaires for new or renewing members, meetings at general assemblies or social media platforms.

Methodological advice for applying the methods above can be found in the chapter on the social sciences (see Chap. 8) and the chapter on pharmacoepidemiology (see Chap. 14).

16.3.2 Relevance of Factors Impacting on Patient Needs and Expectations for Researching Communication

While the relevance of health literacy (see Sect. 16.2.1) and numeracy (see Sect. 16.2.2) as a topic of medicinal product risk communication research is fairly obvious, there is more to consider in this respect when designing such research in general. It needs to be recognised that the communication of risk quantification in relation to medicines is challenging due to the limitations and complexity of the data on adverse reactions and their interpretation, as well as to variable risk perceptions. As adverse reactions are rare events, often with some uncertainty whether they were truly caused by the medicine, any quantification is an estimate rather than a true figure. Understanding the meaning of these estimates is already a challenge for specialists in medicines safety, and together with shortcomings in numeracy in the general population, research on the perception, understanding and preferences of different risk communication formats must face that different patients might have limited and diverse understanding of, e.g. survey questions. This should be solved through careful design and testing of the questions, scales and risk comparisons used in the research, and data should be analysed with regard to intrapersonal and intra-audience segment consistency or variability, to interpret the robustness of the research.

Further it needs to be considered for medicinal product risk communication research that benefit perceptions impact on the perception of risks (see Sect. 16.2.3). For example, Alström syndrome (AS) is a multisystem disorder characterised by cone-rod retinal dystrophy in the eye, hearing loss, obesity, insulin resistance and hyperinsulinaemia, type 2 diabetes mellitus, dilated cardiomyopathy and progressive hepatic and renal dysfunction (Orphanet 2014). When determining the value of a new medicine to treat this condition for the patients, mixed methods research can help identify the most patient-relevant outcomes from either or both the patient and the healthcare professional perspectives. When there are many different outcomes, each patient in the study could be asked to select the three symptoms that matter the most to him/her prior to starting the study treatment and these should be monitored as part of the study. These study findings could then be used not only for the evaluation of the medicine and benefit communication in a way that is meaningful to the patient, but also for researching risk perceptions and meaningful contextualisation of risks that need to be communicated.

Methodological advice for studying health literacy and perceptions can be found in the chapter on the cognitive and behavioural sciences (see Chap. 7) and for mixed methods in the chapter on the social sciences (see Chap. 8).

16.3.3 Direct-to-Patient Pharmacovigilance Studies

"Direct-to-patient pharmacovigilance studies" is a not yet commonly used term but is coined here in verbal analogy to another long-established term in the pharmaceutical field, i.e. "direct-to-consumer advertisement" (Ventola 2011). As a method, direct-to-patient pharmacovigilance studies are inspired by longitudinal safety monitoring applying web-based systems (Härmark et al. 2011) and are expected to generate insightful information on how first-time users of a new medicine rate their experiences in terms of benefits and risks. This kind of information could also complete the currently frequency-focussed information on adverse reactions with qualitative characteristics of adverse reactions like time to onset, duration, reversibility and impact on the patient. Patients consider such information relevant for deciding whether to consent and adhering to their medication.

In order to generate an evidence-base that allows for such information to be included in package leaflets, a large and representative data set needs to be collected. Under the term of direct-to-patient pharmacovigilance it is proposed to collect these data directly from patients, who could be asked, in the pharmacy when they obtain their medicine or through membership in a patient organisation, to register in a web-based system and respond to questionnaires which they would receive by e-mail, text or app messages at regular intervals. The data would be analysed, for example, after 1 year of data collection, to identify new suspected adverse reactions or characteristics of known reactions as functions of patient characteristics, dosing and other aspects of medication use. Of course, the data would have to be assessed for causal relationship between the medicine use and the adverse event, for the derived information to be valid. Therefore, direct-to-patient pharmacovigilance studies require a close cooperation between the patients' healthcare professionals, academics with the expertise of data analysis and patient organisations. However, as a proposal currently under discussion by such organisations, this shows the willingness and eagerness of patients to not only passively demand information they consider relevant but also to actively contribute to generating the necessary data. This also illustrates once more that data collection and communication of data, and meaningful safe use advice require integration of pharmacovigilance processes (see Chap. 1).

16.3.3.1 The DIPEx Project in the United Kingdom

As an example, the aim of an initiative at the University of Oxford since 2001, the Personal Experiences of Health and Illness (DIPEx) project, is to conduct and rigorously analyse narrative interviews of people with particular medical conditions, chosen to represent the widest practicable range of experiences. For each condition focused on so far, 40–50 interviews were collected, and the analyses were summarised and made available to patients and healthcare professionals together with extracts from the interviews in written, audio and video format. These summaries can be used to support decision-making in healthcare and enable patients to identify and manage adverse reactions (Herxheimer and Ziebland 2003; Ziebland and Herxheimer 2008).

16.3.4 Studies in Collaboration with Patient Organisations

As said, patient organisations can play a crucial role in facilitating studies collecting data directly from patients or evaluating methods for direct-from-patients data collection and their analysis.

16.3.4.1 The Patient Organisation Collaboration Project by ANSM in France

An example of such a collaborative programme is the annual call for projects targeting patients' organisations started by the French regulatory authority Agence Nationale de Sécurité des Médicaments (ANSM) in 2012. Since then 34 projects have been completed or are in progress, of which twelve are related to pharmacovigilance or communication tools, operating on feasible budgets (Agence Nationale de Sécurité des Médicaments (ANSM) 2017) (see Table 16.2).

16.3.5 Social Media-Based Studies

Since the creation of internet, patients formed online communities to exchange on their experiences with the diseases and treatments. For example, since 1994 the print and online POZ offers daily news for people affected by HIV, in particular on treatments, profiles of personal experiences, investigative features, blogs and an extensive online social network from 150,000 members with constant, day and night, community moderation (POZ 1994). Another internet community called Crix Belly was a major source of reports from patients gaining ten to twenty kilogramme of body weight together with body shape changes such as buffalo neck, fat loss, increased belly while being on HAART. The community derived its name from Crixivan®, the trade name for indinavir, one of the active substances used in HAART. Patient groups contacted the US FDA and the EMA, and it turned out that they—patients themselves rather than healthcare professionals or scientists—were the first who had detected lipodystrophy with these medicines (see Sect. 16.1). This case illustrates the important role of patients can play in observing and contributing data about medicines by means of exchanging and pooling information across patient populations by means of the internet and social media.

More recently, regulators, academic researchers, industry and patient organisations started to explore systematic approaches to analysing public posts on social media. These research projects propose different data mining and analytical approaches to establish and evaluate the role social media-based networks for detecting signals of yet unknown risks with medicines. Examples of such projects are WEB-RADR in the EU (with global partners and leverage) on recognising adverse reactions through web-based technology (WEB-RADR 2019), and in France the Vigi4Med on extracting adverse reaction information from web forums (Audeh et al. 2017) and ADR-PRISM (i.e. the Adverse Drug Reactions from Patient Reports in Social Media) project for providing pharmacovigilance professionals

Table 16.2 Examples of studies with collaboration of patient organisations conducted upon call by the Agence Nationale de Sécurité des Médicaments (ANSM) in France by year (Agence Nationale de Sécurité des Médicaments (ANSM) 2017)

Year	Number of project proposals and examples of selected projects	Funding amount
2012	*39 project proposals received, 9 selected for total costs of*	*261,272 €*
	Patient-reporting of adverse effects related to diethyl-stilbestrol to assess the risk of breast cancer in women exposed in utero and risks of malformation, adverse effects on reproductive organs and cancer in their children	40,000 €
	Patient-reporting of adverse effects related to fingolimod	20,000 €
2013	*38 project proposals received, 8 selected, for total costs of*	*230,500 €*
	Service to support patient-reporting of adverse effects related to medicines used in rare diseases	15,200 €
	Patient-reporting in collaboration with healthcare professionals of adverse effects related to coagulation factor medication, in particular inhibitor development in patients with haemophilia and other rare coagulation disorders	23,600 €
2014	*23 project proposals received, 7 selected for total costs of*	*165,300 €*
	Survey of adolescent patients and patients with cystic fibrosis about the impact of adverse effects on adherence to inhaled medicines	30,000 €
	Translation of package leaflets into sign language	40,000 €
	Creation of a self-evaluation tool for adverse behavioural effects related to anti-Parkinson medicines	20,000 €
	Information to patients for the prevention and the monitoring of adverse effects related to baclofen in alcohol dependency	15,300 €
2015	*17 project proposals received, 6 selected for total costs of*	*149,110 €*
	Establishment of a European paediatric emergency card for children with adrenal insufficiency	7,700 €
	Patient-reporting of adverse effects in bone marrow recipients ("All knowledgeable = All responsible = All vigilant?")	19,000 €
	Analysis of discussions on treatments among patients with kidney disease, dialysis or transplant (Renaloo forum and other social networks)	35,000 €
2016	*16 project proposals received, 4 selected for total costs of*	*80,000 €*
	Reduction of the risk of misuse and early termination of medicines used for post-exposure HIV-prophylaxis	20,000 €

with information from patient discussion forums, which may lead to new hypotheses concerning adverse effects (Bousquet et al. 2017).

While the focus of these projects is more on the detection of signals of adverse reactions and assessing their seriousness, another focus—from a patient perspective—should equally be on gathering data on the impact of adverse reactions on patients' daily life, how to prevent and manage them and on how to most effectively communicate what is known about these risks and practical advice. Within the social media, patients discuss difficulties they have when communicating with their physicians about risks, dose reductions they may desire, interactions with other medicines and the so-called recreational products, the impact of a medicine on their lives and life-styles or challenges they face in obtaining their medicines due to costs, shortages or other reasons. The public content of these discussions could be analysed in order to understand sentiments and information needs of patients, and how they want to be meaningfully presented with the information. Such analyses might also provide the evidence for required training of healthcare professionals and actually support them in building communication capacity in terms of content and skills for fulfilling patient expectations and enabling patients to effectively manage the risks of their medication and hence adhere to treatment.

Research about medicinal product risk communication has to take into account the numerous challenges of risk communication on social networks, from the volatility of the sources (due to, e.g. the evolution of privacy settings or fast ageing technologies), the futility of large volumes of irrelevant data, automatised data mining and the need for human intervention to interpret the data. Furthermore, patients' language, relative lack of precision, abbreviated language or slang renders the understanding of the exchange often difficult. Other methodological challenges lie in image and video analysis and soliciting information from patient organisation members via precise questionnaires, with a view to developing real multi-purpose online platforms. An example is RareConnect, the online community for the Behcet's syndrome (RareConnect 2019).

Methods for conducting social media-based studies are presented in the chapter on social media research (see Chap. 11).

16.4 The Future Role of Patient Organisations for Connecting Pharmacovigilance with Healthcare for Patient Safety

Providing information to patients in healthcare that allows for patient-centred care and shared decisions on the most suitable therapeutic option remains the biggest challenge to fulfil the ultimate pharmacovigilance goal of patient safety and health (Bahri et al. 2015). A dedicated chapter of this book discusses research approaches based on dissemination and implementation science for putting pharmaceutical risk management into the practice of healthcare (see Chap. 13). Patient organisations have already demonstrated that they can conduct surveys among their members that can be useful for deciding on risk minimisation measures and designing communication interventions. For example, surveys on the dissemination of risk information by healthcare professionals to patients constituted important input to the public hearing at the EMA on valproate in 2017 (European Medicines Agency (EMA) 2017). Also, the Council of International Organizations in Medical Sciences (CIOMS) has set up a working group for developing guidance on patient involvement in the development and safe use of medicines (Council for International Organizations of Medical Sciences (CIOMS) 2019). The following section discusses further proposals for how patient organisations could participate more in future communication research that supports connecting pharmacovigilance and healthcare.

Table 16.3 Proposals for regulatory authorities for engaging patients and consumers in pharmacovigilance, derived from (Strengthening Collaboration for Operating Pharmacovigilance in Europe (SCOPE) 2019)

Type of action
Communication campaigns, e.g. on safety issues, the importance of reporting suspected adverse reactions, Adverse Drug Reaction Awareness Week in November of each year
Award of the most informative adverse reaction case report of the year reported directly from a patient
National multi-stakeholder conference on pharmacovigilance
Invitation of patient organisations for specific pharmacovigilance projects
Calls for patients as members of the national pharmacovigilance and risk assessment/ medicines safety committees
Consultation of patients on package leaflets and educational materials
Involvement of patient organisations in the design of new tools for spontaneous reporting of suspected adverse reactions
Contacting patients for detailed review, assessment, follow-up and feedback of spontaneously reported cases of suspected adverse reactions
Verbal and e-mail updates to patient organisations on topical issues
Sharing direct healthcare professional communications (DHCPs) with patient organisations

16.4.1 Interactions Between Patient Organisations and Regulatory Bodies

Patient organisations can provide added value to the work of regulatory bodies. For example, as part of the Joint Action on Strengthening Collaboration for Operating Pharmacovigilance in Europe (SCOPE) a list has been compiled of initiatives authorities in the member states of the EU have taken to engage patients and consumers in pharmacovigilance at national level (Strengthening Collaboration for Operating Pharmacovigilance in Europe (SCOPE) 2019). From these initiatives, proposals can be derived as an inspiration for other countries (see Table 16.3). At EU level, the EMA has set up multiple engagement mechanisms, including management board and scientific committee membership, a working party with patient and consumer organisations, written consultations as well as public and dedicated meetings (European Medicines Agency (EMA) 2019).

16.4.2 A Pharmacovigilance Contact Person at Patient Organisations

A further concrete proposal is that patient organisations appoint their own contact persons for pharmacovigilance, who would be trained by the regulatory body on how pharmacovigilance in the given jurisdiction, including the reporting system for adverse reactions. The person would receive all official safety alerts and direct healthcare professional communications (DHPCs), be kept informed about national and international pharmacovigilance initiatives and overall act as a liaison between the patient organisation and the national pharmacovigilance system for two-way communication and support to putting initiatives as listed above into reality. Tasks would include disseminating information to the members of the patient organisation as well as questions the authority may have regarding the experiences of patients with medicines and their expectations for risk minimisation measures and communication and providing feedback from the members to the authority, and also advising members on information sources and reporting of suspected adverse reactions. The person could also get involved in data analysis, e.g. specifically for communication by analysing frequently asked questions by members and the organisations' social media interactions, and become a facilitator for risk communication research, e.g. regarding the needs and effectiveness of communication. More specifically such research could assess the understanding of proposed key messages from a sample of the audience/test group or support the development of talking points. He/she could possibly also act as contact person vis-à-vis marketing authorisation holders when engaging with patients in pharmacovigilance activities.

16.4.3 Measuring the Impact of Communication on Patient Health

Patient-centred healthcare includes that the individual's health needs and desired outcomes determine the evaluation of healthcare quality (New England Journal of Medicine Catalyst 2017). Patient organisations should therefore engage in measuring the impact of medicinal product risk communication, for example, through:

- determining awareness of changes in package leaflets through surveys among their members or analysing the content of discussion on their online platforms;
- performing a reality check of the implementation of risk minimisation measures in healthcare in terms of delivery, knowledge adoption and changes in safe use behaviours; and
- studying among their members their benefit-risk perception of different medicinal products and therapeutic alternatives.

Working with patients and their organisations is the only approach which can guarantee that patients will truly be at the centre of the action, whatever that action is. Ideally, the decision-making is jointly owned by both researchers or regulators and the public, who work together to achieve a shared understanding. It can be circuitous and unpredictable, but ultimately more worthwhile.

Conclusions

- The AIDS epidemic of the 1980s triggered the rise of patient movements that advocate for the development of new medicines and changes in regulation, and more recently participate in governmental decision-making about medicines.
- Patient organisations work towards patient-centred care, which includes fully informed therapeutic decision-making shared with patients and measuring healthcare quality with regard to the individual's health needs and desired outcomes.

- Patients can and should be proactive in highlighting their information needs and interests and come together in patient organisations that may initiate, contribute to or even conduct research, such as in the area of medicinal product risk communication research.
- Proposals for new research approaches include direct-to-patient pharmacovigilance studies, studies in collaboration with patient organisations and social media-based studies.
- The future role of patient organisations in this respect are proposed to be strengthened through pharmacovigilance contact persons at patient organisations and contributions from measuring the impact of communication on patient health.

References

Agence Nationale de Sécurité des Médicaments (ANSM) (2017) Résultats des appels à projets. ANSM, Saint Denis. Accessible at: https://www.ansm.sante.fr/L-ANSM/Appels-a-projets-Associations/Resultats-des-appels-a-projet/(offset)/0; Last accessed on: 23 Sept 2019

Audeh B, Beigbeder M, Zimmermann A, Jaillon P, Bousquet C (2017) Vigi4Med Scraper: a framework for web forum structured data extraction and semantic representation. PLoS One 12(1):e0169658

Ayer V, Bunn C (2004) Advocacy campaign management. Pact, Phnom Penh

Bacchetti P, Osmond D, Chaisson RE, Dritz S, Rutherford GW, Swig L, Moss AR (1988) Survival patterns of the first 500 patients with AIDS in San Francisco. J Infect Dis 157(5):1044–1047

Bahri P, Dodoo AN, Edwards BD, Edwards IR, Fermont I, Hagemann U, Hartigan-Go K, Hugman B, Mol PG, ISoP CommSIG (2015) The ISoP CommSIG for improving medicinal product risk communication: a new special interest group of the International Society of Pharmacovigilance. Drug Saf 38:621–627

Barbot J (1998) Acting on clinical trials. Experience of organizations for the fight against AIDS [French]. Rev Epidemiol Sante Publique 46:305–315

Batalla J, Gatell JM, Caylà JA, Plasencia A, Jansà JM, Parellada N (1989) Predictors of the survival of AIDS cases in Barcelona, Spain. AIDS 3(6):355–359

Bennett P (1999) Understanding responses to risk: some basic findings. In: Bennett P, Calman K (eds) Risk communication and public health. Oxford University Press, Oxford. (quoting: Fischhoff B, Slovic P, Lichtenstein S, Read S, Coombes B. How safe is safe enough?: a psychometric study of attitudes towards technological risks and benefits. Policy Science. 1978; 9: 127–152.; Gardner GT, Gould LC. Public perceptions of risks and benefits of technology. Risk Analysis. 1989; 9: 225–242.; Slovic P. Informing and educating about risks. Risk Analysis. 1986; 6: 403–415)

Bousquet C, Dahamna B, Guillemin-Lanne S, Darmoni SJ, Faviez C, Huot C, Katsahian S, Leroux V, Pereira S, Richard C, Schück S, Souvignet J, Lillo-Le Louët A, Texier N (2017) The adverse drug reactions from patient reports in social media project: five major challenges to overcome to operationalize analysis and efficiently support pharmacovigilance process. JMIR Res Protoc 6(9):e179

Boyle BA (2000) Adherence and HAART: unique approaches to evaluating and improving adherence discussed. HIV i-base, London. Accessible at: http://i-base.info/htb/4025; Last accessed: 23 Sept 2019

Bozzette SA, Ake CF, Tam HK, Chang SW, Louis TA (2003) Cardiovascular and cerebrovascular events in patients treated for human immunodeficiency virus infection. N Engl J Med 348:702–710

Carr A, Samaras K, Burton S, Law M, Freund J, Chisholm DJ, Cooper DA (1998) A syndrome of peripheral lipodystrophy, hyperlipidaemia and insulin resistance in patients receiving HIV protease inhibitors. AIDS 12:F51–F58

Carr A, Emery S, Law M, Puls R, Lundgren JD, Powderly WG, HIV Lipodystrophy Case Definition Study Group (2003) An objective case definition of lipodystrophy in HIV-infected adults: a case-control study. Lancet 361:726–735

Council for International Organizations of Medical Sciences (CIOMS) (2019) CIOMS Working Group XI – Patient involvement. CIOMS, Geneva. Accessible at: https://cioms.ch/working_groups/working-group-xi-patient-involvement/; Last accessed on: 23 Sept 2019

Data Collection on Adverse Events of Anti-HIV Drugs (DAD) Study Group (2003) Combination antiretroviral therapy and the risk of myocardial infarction. N Engl J Med 349:1993–2003

EMEA/CPMP Working Group with Patients' Organisations (2004) Outcomes of discussions: recommendations and proposals for action. European Medicines Evaluation Agency (EMEA, now European Medicines Agency (EMA), London

Epstein S (1995) The construction of lay expertise: AIDS activism and the forging of credibility in the reform of clinical trials. Sci Technol Human Values 20(4):408–437

European Commission (EC) (2009) Guideline on the readability of the labelling and package leaflet of medicinal products for human use. Rev 1. EC, Brussels

European Medicines Agency (EMA) (2009) Information on benefit-risk of medicines: patients', consumers' and healthcare professionals' expectations. EMA, London

European Medicines Agency (EMA) (2015) EU medicines agencies network strategy to 2020 – theme 3, objective 3: ensure effective communication of and within the network. EMA, London. Accessible at: https://www.ema.europa.eu/en/documents/other/eu-medicines-agencies-network-strategy-2020-working-together-improve-health_en.pdf; Last accessed on: 23 Sept 2019

European Medicines Agency (EMA) (2017) Valproate and related substances – public hearing [webpage]. EMA, London; last updated on: 11 July 2017. Accessible at: https://www.ema.europa.eu/en/medicines/human/referrals/valproate-related-substances-0#public-hearing-section; Last accessed on: 23 Sept 2019

European Medicines Agency (EMA) (2019) Patients and consumers [webpage]. EMA, Amsterdam. Accessible at: https://www.ema.europa.eu/en/partners-networks/patients-consumers; Last accessed on: 23 Sept 2019

European Organisation for Rare Diseases (EURORDIS) (2019) Code of practice between patients' organisations and the healthcare industry. EURORDIS, Paris. Accessible at: https://www.eurordis.org/sites/default/files/thumbnails/0904-PO-Code%20of%20practice.pdf; Last accessed on: 23 Sept 2019

Gigerenzer G, Gaissmaier W, Schwartz LM, Woloshin S (2008) Helping doctors and patients make sense of health statistics. Psychol Sci Public Interest 8:53–96

Härmark L, Puijenbroek E, Grootheest K (2011) Longitudinal monitoring of the safety of drugs by using a web-based system: the case of pregabalin. Pharmacoepidemiol Drug Saf 20: 591–597

Hazard Cards (2019) Hazard Cards: about [webpage]. Accessible at: http://www.hazardcards.com/about/; Last accessed on: 23 Sept 2019

Herxheimer A (2003) Relationships between the pharmaceutical industry and patients' organisations. Br Med J 326(7400):1208–1210

Herxheimer A, Ziebland S (2003) DIPEx: fresh insights for medical practice. J R Soc Med 96:209–210

History.com (2009) "Rock Hudson announces he has AIDS". Accessible at: https://www.history.com/this-day-in-history/rock-hudson-announces-he-has-aids. Last accessed on: 23 Sept 2019

HLS-EU Consortium (2012) Comparative report of the health literacy in eight EU Member States: the European Union Health Literacy Survey (HLS-EU). Accessible at: http://www.health-literacy.eu; Last accessed on: 23 Sept 2019

National Academies of Sciences Engineering, and Medicine (2015) Health literacy: past, present, and future: workshop summary. The National Academies Press, Washington, DC

National Numeracy (NN) (2014–2017) What is numeracy? [webpage]. NN, Lewes. Accessible at: https://www.nationalnumeracy.org.uk/what-numeracy; Last accessed on: 23 Sept 2019

National Safety Council (NSC) (2017) Injury facts®. NSC, Itaska, p 43. (Library of Congress Catalog Card Number: 99-74142; ISBN 978-0-87912-357-4; NSC Press Product No. 02333-0000). Accessible at: http://e57ebfdc25c920958781-6bbae8d59740807b5fdffbff5901a175.r1.cf1.rackcdn.com/files/InjuryFacts-2017.pdf; Last accessed on 23 Sept 2019
New England Journal of Medicine Catalyst. What is patient-centered care?. 1 January 2017
New York Public Library, Manuscripts and Archives Division, New York Public Library Digital Collections 1969–1997 (n.d.) The government has blood on its hands - one AIDS death every half hour. Accessible at: http://digitalcollections.nypl.org/items/510d47e3-3ebe-a3d9-e040-e00a18064a99; Last accessed on: 23 Sept 2019
Nutbeam D (1998) Health promotion glossary. Health Promot Int 13:349–364
Nutbeam D (2008) The evolving concept of health literacy. Soc Sci Med 67:2072–2078
Orphanet (2014) Le syndrome d'Alström [Encyclopédie Orphanet Grand Public]. Orphanet, Paris. Accessible at: https://www.orpha.net/data/patho/Pub/Int/fr/LeSyndromeAlstr-m_FR_fr_PUB_ORPHA64.pdf; Last accessed on 23 Sept 2019
People with AIDS Advisory Committee (1983) The Denver principles. People with AIDS Advisory Committee, Denver. Accessible at: http://www.actupny.org/documents/denver_principles.pdf; Last accessed on 23 Sept 2019
POZ (1994) POZ: About us [webpage]. POZ, New York. Accessible at: https://www.poz.com/page/about-us; Last accessed on: 23 Sept 2019
Price J, Hoy J, Ridley E, Nyulasi I, Paul E, Woolley I (2015) Changes in the prevalence of lipodystrophy, metabolic syndrome and cardiovascular disease risk in HIV-infected men. Sex Health 12:240–248
RareConnect (2019) RareConnect: About us [webpage]. Accessible at http://rareconnect.org/; Last accessed on: 23 Sept 2019
Rolfes L (2018) Patient participation in pharmacovigilance. PhD thesis, Rijksuniversiteit Groningen, Groningen
Rubinelli S, Schultz PJ, Nakamoto K (2009) Health literacy beyond knowledge and behaviour: letting the patient be a patient. Int J Public Health 54:307–311
Selden CR, Zorn M, Ratzan SC, Parker RM (eds) (2000) Health literacy [bibliography]. National Institutes of Health (IoM), US Department of Health and Human Services, Bethesda
Stehr-Green JK, Holman RC, Mahoney MA (1989) Survival analysis of hemophilia-associated AIDS cases in the US. Am J Public Health 79(7):832–835
Strengthening Collaboration for Operating Pharmacovigilance in Europe (SCOPE) (2019) Joint Action. SCOPE: About [webpage]. Accessible at: http://www.scopejointaction.eu/about/; Last accessed on: 23 Sept 2019
US Food and Drug Administration (US FDA) (2018) HIV/AIDS historical time line 1981-1990. White Oak, MA: US FDA; last updated 5 January 2018. Accessible at: https://www.fda.gov/forpatients/illness/hivaids/history/ucm151074.htm; Last accessed on: 23 Sept 2019
Van J (1985) Hudson AIDS case turns spotlight on drug approval process. Chicago Tribune, Chicago. Accessible at http://articles.chicagotribune.com/1985-08-04/news/8502200879_1_new-drugs-fda-aids-therapies; Last accessed on: 16 Dec 2017
Ventola CL (2011) Direct-to-consumer pharmaceutical advertising: therapeutic or toxic? Pharmacy Ther 36:669–684
WEB-RADR (2019) project: Recognising Adverse Drug Reactions working together to improve pharmacovigilance through new technology [webpage]. Accessible at: http://web-radr.eu/; Last accessed on: 23 Sept 2019
Whyte BM, Swanson CE, Cooper DA (1989) Survival of patients with the acquired immunodeficiency syndrome in Australia. Med J Aust 150(7):358–362
Wikipedia (2019) HPA-23. Accessible at: https://en.wikipedia.org/wiki/HPA-23; Last accessed on: 23 Sept 2019
World Health Organization (WHO) Advocacy (2019) Accessible at: http://www.who.int/occupational_health/topics/workplace/en/index2.html. Last accessed on: 1 Dec 2018
Würdemann U (1987) Zulassung von AZT. 2MECS, Berlin; last updated on: 20 March 2019. Accessible at: https://www.2mecs.de/wp/2017/03/30-jahre-azt/; Last accessed on: 23 Sept 2019
Ziebland S, Herxheimer A (2008) How patients' experiences contribute to decision making: illustrations from DIPEx (personal experiences of health and illness). J Nurs Manag 16:433–439

Afterword: The Dimension of Communicating Medicine Risks in Low- and Middle-Income Countries

This book *Communicating about Risks and Safe Use of Medicines: Real Life and Applied Research* offers a framework for research that seeks to understand structures, processes and outcomes of communication. Such research framework deals with the complexities of communication and synergies of research methods from multiple disciplines. The overarching principles for effective communication are applicable everywhere, and the book expresses the desire to support patient safety globally. However, most research to date has happened in Australia, Europe and North America. This constitutes a major gap for medicinal product risk communication research to fill, in particular for countries in Africa, Asia and South America with developing systems. In order to study and improve communication in these regions, researchers have to be aware of the specifically challenging dimension of medicinal product risk communication in these countries, as will be discussed in this afterword.

The objective of communicating risks with medicines, no matter where, is to create understanding and stimulate action for using medicines safely and beneficially. More thinking and an alert mindset should be encouraged, so that signs of harm get noted early and worsening can be prevented. Sometimes there are therapeutic choices to be made based on personal preferences of accepting and tolerating risks.

The most fundamental principle for communication to be effective in reaching its objective is that—as risks, harms and risk tolerance are highly individual—communication should be customised for relevant populations (i.e. specific patients, caretakers, healthcare providers and policymakers), diseases as well as the severity and seriousness of the potential harm. Customisation is supposed to create meaning for those one communicates with and needs to take into account the personal biases, traditions, attitudes and preferences held by these populations, be it a patient, physician, nurse, pharmacist or health worker. The healthcare provider knows more about the science and art of medicine, while the patient knows more about him- or herself, the disease experience and the needs to maintain a good quality of life given the personal circumstances.

© Springer Nature Singapore Pte Ltd. 2020

P. Bahri (ed.), *Communicating about Risks and Safe Use of Medicines*,
https://doi.org/10.1007/978-981-15-3013-5

Considering this customisation, risks of medicines and their communication take a completely different and challenging dimension in low- and middle-income countries with their typical wide variations in socioeconomic status, literacy, communication cultures and access to healthcare providers and medicines. This has implications for the parties responsible for safety of medicines and risk communication.

The first responsibility is with the manufacturer and marketing authorisation holder for a given medicinal product. However, with over 99% of products being developed in countries with advanced economies, marketing authorisation holders in developing economies depend on the officially authorised product information, including the package leaflet, from the marketing authorisation holders in advanced economies. These are at best suited for health systems in countries where legal correctness, lawsuits, insurance and compensation schemes support patient welfare, albeit they may still miss the most meaningful information and care for patients. The package leaflet from advanced economies may not advise on pharmacogenetics and the best use of the product in patients with genetic variations prevalent elsewhere or on interactions with food types taken in other countries, and also not be in the local language, but in English or French only. In any case, a major problem exists in package leaflets not being kept up to date in low- and middle-income countries, even where regulation and national pharmacovigilance programmes exist and the marketing authorisation holder is required to supply and disseminate information about their product by law. Important to note is that—different from many countries with stringent regulatory systems and comprehensive product information requirements for healthcare professionals and patients—in many developing countries package leaflets are considered to inform the healthcare provider and there is no legal requirement for package leaflets to be provided to patients, except for a few like for oral hormonal contraceptives. Thus, the burden of communicating to patients about risks is often entirely on the healthcare provider, who depends on the package leaflet and may not have access to continuing professional development to keep knowledge and skills up to date with scientific and medical progress. Even where policymakers try to support healthcare providers with prescribing, dispensing and communication checklists, they may disregard the wide variation among patients and the need for customisation.

Second, governments are responsible for public health. However, in developing countries, when governmental agencies promote, support or initiate medicinal product-related risk minimisation measures or risk management programmes tailored for the specific country situation by means of standard treatment guidelines, they often do not get reflected in the package leaflets. On the other hand, treatment guidelines in low- and middle-income countries may not be updated, disseminated or used, unlike the prominently successful guidelines from the National Institute for Health and Care Excellence (NICE) in the United Kingdom. For example, in India, health workers in rural tribal areas were found to rely on the package leaflets when using snake venom antiserum, since guidelines from the government had not reached these remote areas. In public health programmes, governmental agencies make attempts to communicate about preventing risks with medicines and risk management strategies. For example, in India a manual on adverse reaction prevention and management for anti-tuberculosis medicines in local language was found to be very useful by health workers, but one made for patients, though considered useful, was not equally well accepted. Famous favourite personalities may increase awareness and acceptance, as they agree to act as health ambassadors and advertise public health messages, such as a famous Indian actor has done for immunisation against tuberculosis with the aim of disease eradication. So far, this "celebrity approach" has rarely been used for medicine risk minimisation. In countries where access to medicines is impaired and drives policymaking, information on medicine-related risks often takes a back seat. Clearly, it needs to be recognised that governments in low- and middle-income countries have to make more efforts to strengthen the customisation and positive impact of official medicinal product risk communication, in order to make access to medicines most effective and build the trust of the population in the benefits of the so-called modern medicines. The reality of fake and substandard products of modern medicines sold in street markets and also in pharmacies in Africa and Asia is a constant threat to trust. At present, the reliance on traditional medicines and the perception that these are completely safe while modern medicines cause adverse effects are so overwhelmingly present that advertisement for modern medicines in developing countries often contains the misinforming catch line "No side effects".

Third, there is the healthcare providers' responsibility to communicate with the patient and carers, both in writing through prescriptions and verbally with instructions about how to take the medicine. However, with overburdened and underresourced health systems in developing countries, this can rarely be achieved properly. In some places, newer technologies such as mobile phone messaging and videos shown in surgery waiting areas are used with good intentions, but these may be lost in the din of competing social messages, entertainments, sales promotions, news and other health risk messages.

In conclusion, communicating risk well is essential for the promotion of the safe, effective and trusted use of medicines. Much more effort is needed from all stakeholders to research and improve the current methods of risk communication. Medicinal product risk communication in low- and middle-income countries has its particular challenges, and how to overcome these poses an important call to researchers. Such research would be part of global mutual learning, as some of these challenges, although to a lesser extent, also exist in countries with advanced economies and stringent regulatory systems. Everywhere in the world, a patient will often rely more on a friendly neighbour and a well-meaning but insufficiently informed community than a package leaflet. Therefore, approaches to communicating risks should not only focus on patients and healthcare providers but on the community and society too. In the same spirit, this book advocates for medicinal product risk communication research to take a communication perspective and study all communication events, whether from official bodies or marketing authorisation holders or within healthcare or social communities, based on the social-ecological model that distinguishes between the individual and social spheres that surround each person. The African proverb "It takes a whole village to bring up a child" could be transposed to "It will take the whole informed community to understand and manage risks of medicines and bring up the patient to recover and society to be healthy".

Delhi, India
October 2019

Nilima A Kshirsagar

Index

© Springer Nature Singapore Pte Ltd. 2020
P. Bahri (ed.), *Communicating about Risks and Safe Use of Medicines*,
https://doi.org/10.1007/978-981-15-3013-5

D

E

U

MIX
Papier aus verantwortungsvollen Quellen
Paper from responsible sources
FSC® C105338

If you have any concerns about our products,
you can contact us on
ProductSafety@springernature.com

In case Publisher is established outside the EU,
the EU authorized representative is:
Springer Nature Customer Service Center GmbH
Europaplatz 3, 69115 Heidelberg, Germany

Printed by Libri Plureos GmbH
in Hamburg, Germany